Bloom & Fawcett's Concise Histology

Second Edition

Don W. Fawcett MD

Hersey Professor of Anatomy, Emeritus
Harvard Medical School

Ronald P. Jensh PhD

Professor of Pathology, Anatomy, and Cell Biology
Jefferson Medical College of Thomas Jefferson University

ARNOLD

A member of the Hodder Headline Group
LONDON • NEW YORK • NEW DELHI

First published in Great Britain in 1997 by Chapman and Hall

This second edition published in 2002 by
Arnold, a member of the Hodder Headline Group,
338 Euston Road, London NW1 3BH

http://www.arnoldpublishers.com

Distributed in the USA by
Oxford University Press Inc.,
198 Madison Avenue, New York, NY10016
Oxford is a registered trademark of Oxford University Press

British Library Cataloguing in Publication Data
A catalogue record for this book is available from the British Library

Library of Congress Cataloging-in-Publication Data
A catalog record for this book is available from the Library of Congress

ISBN 0 340 80677X

1 2 3 4 5 6 7 8 9 10

Commissioning Editor: Georgina Bentliff
Development Editor: Heather Smith
Production Editor: Jasmine Brown
Production Controller: Iain McWilliams
Cover Design: Terry Griffiths

Typeset in 9.5/12 pt Minion by Phoenix Photosetting, Chatham, Kent
Printed and bound in Malta by Gutenberg Press

What do you think about this book? Or any other Arnold title?
Please send your comments to feedback.arnold@hodder.co.uk
http://www.arnoldpublishers.com

Contents

Preface

At his death, in 1928, the distinguished Russian histologist, Alexander Maximov, left behind the unfinished manuscript of a textbook of histology, which was completed by Professor William Bloom. Through seven editions it was the most widely used text on the subject. In 1962, I joined Professor Bloom as co-author of the eighth through the twelfth editions.

With the addition of cell and molecular biology and genetics to the medical curriculum in the 1990s, the courses in histology were greatly shortened. The *Bloom and Fawcett Textbook of Histology* was too detailed for these abbreviated courses, therefore it was considered more suitable as a reference book. To meet the need for a shorter textbook, the *Bloom and Fawcett: Concise Histology* was published in 1997 to provide an adequate understanding of the subject, while giving the students the benefit of many of the instructive illustrations of the larger book. The first edition did not meet the expectations of the author or the contributing editor. The present edition incorporates significant changes in format and in the quality of reproduction of the figures. Chapter One has been expanded to include more of the discoveries in the rapidly advancing field of cell biology. The chapters on the structure and function of the tissues and organs have been up-dated. New colored illustrations have been added, and there have been additions to the questions for self-evaluation at the end of each chapter.

Professor Ronald Jensh has joined me as co-author of the book. I am very grateful to him for his critical appraisal of the text, for the questions at the ends of the chapters, and for many of the colored illustrations. I am also deeply indebted to Professor Jay Angevine for his lucid chapter on the nervous system.

Don W. Fawcett MD

Chapter one

The Cell

The **cell** is the basic structural unit of all living organisms. The human body contains cells of many different kinds that have different specialized functions. This chapter will describe the microscopically visible structural components that are common to most cell types. Cells are enclosed in a **cell membrane**, and are partitioned into two major compartments, the **nucleus** and the **cytoplasm** surrounding the nucleus and making up the greater part of the cell volume. The nucleus contains the **deoxyribonucleic acid** (**DNA**) that encodes the instructions for the synthesis of all structural proteins of the cell, and the enzymes that catalyze the biochemical reactions of its metabolism. In the cytoplasm, where those reactions take place, there are two categories of structures: **organelles** and **inclusions**. The organelles are usually membrane-bounded, and are involved in energy generation, protein synthesis and other vital functions. The inclusions comprise stores of lipid, and inert deposits of waste products of cell metabolism. The organelles and inclusions are suspended in a gel-like matrix called the **cytosol**. The nucleus and some of the organelles are visible, with the light microscope, in living cells and in routine histological preparations. Others require the greater magnification afforded by the electron microscope (Fig. 1.1). In the past 50 years, this powerful optical instrument has revealed structural details in the organelles that have led to a better understanding of their function.

CELL MEMBRANE

The membrane bounding the cell, referred to as the **plasma membrane** (or **plasmalemma**), is a very thin envelope that separates the cytoplasm from the external environment. It is not resolved by the light microscope, but appears in electron micrographs as a pair of parallel dense lines, 2 nm apart, separated by a less dense intermediate layer 3 nm in thickness (Fig. 1.2). It consists of a bimolecular layer of phospholipid molecules, with their hydrophilic heads at the outer and inner surfaces, and their hydrophobic fatty acid chains directed towards the middle of the lipid bilayer (Fig. 1.3). For study with the electron microscope, cells are usually preserved in a solution of osmium tetroxide (the fixative). They are then embedded in plastic, and very thin slices (sections) are cut and stained with lead and uranium salts. The two dense lines in the image of a cell membrane (Fig. 1.2) result from deposition of osmium and lead in the hydrophilic heads of the phospholipid molecules. The paler intermediate zone represents their unstained hydrophobic fatty acid chains. In addition to phospholipids, membranes contain protein and glycoprotein molecules, which may constitute 20–70% of their mass (Fig. 1.3). **Integral proteins** of the membrane extend through the bilayer and their ends are exposed on its outer and inner surfaces. Proteins that are not within the bilayer, but are bound to the

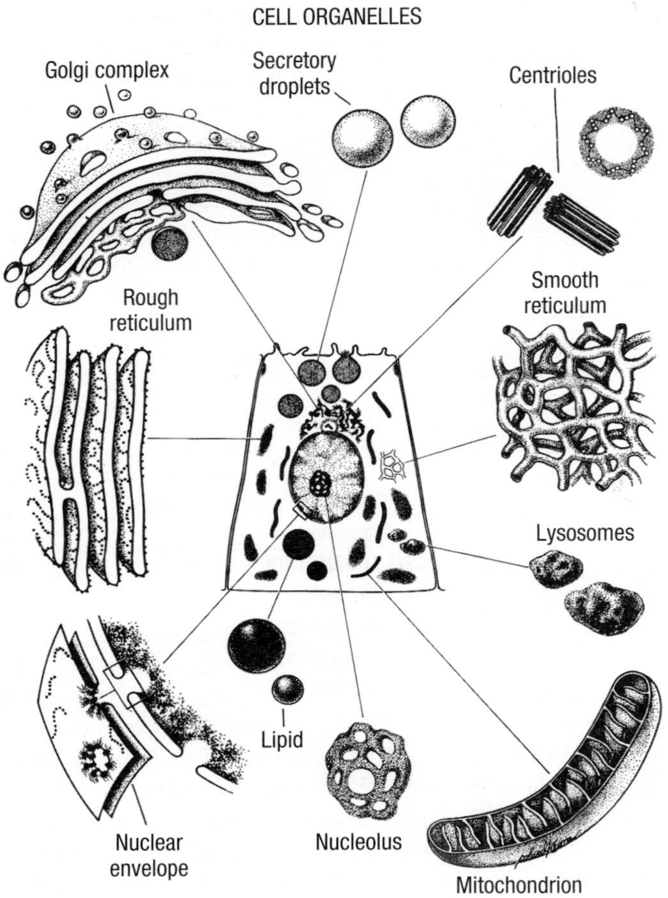

CELL ORGANELLES

Golgi complex

Secretory droplets

Centrioles

Rough reticulum

Smooth reticulum

Lysosomes

Lipid

Nuclear envelope

Nucleolus

Mitochondrion

Figure 1.1 Drawing of the cell organelles, as seen with the light microscope, (center) and their structure revealed by the electron microscope (periphery). (Drawing by Sylvia Keene.)

A relatively constant composition of the cytosol must be maintained. This is possible owing to the selective permeability of the plasma membrane. It is permeable to small uncharged molecules (O_2, CO_2, H_2O), but charged molecules (Na^+, K^+, Cl^-) and larger molecules, such as glucose and amino acids, are unable to diffuse through the phospholipid bilayer of the membrane. The entry of certain molecules depends upon their binding to specific **carrier proteins**, which then change their configuration to translocate their cargo to the other side of the membrane. Certain integral **channel proteins** assemble in the bilayer to form transient pores, through which charged ions can diffuse into, and out of, the cell, down their concentration gradient. Other membrane proteins are **receptors**, which have binding sites for specific hormones, or for other signaling molecules that influence the activity of the cell. Other integral proteins, called **integrins**, have binding sites that anchor the cell to components of the extracellular matrix. Still others, called **cadherins**, are involved in cell-to-cell adhesion. Thus, the plasma membrane must not be regarded as an inert boundary layer, for its proteins are active participants in the vital activities of the cell, and they can be changed to serve different functions. Membranes having the same basic organization as the plasma membrane also bound the organelles in the interior of the cell.

NUCLEUS

The **nucleus** is a large membrane-limited compartment located near the center of the cell. Its size and its strong affinity for basic dyes (basophilia) make it the most conspicuous of the cell organelles (Fig. 1.4). It is usually spherical or ovoid in shape, and it contains the (DNA), the genetic material of the cell that encodes, in the sequence of its nucleotides, the instructions for synthesis of the thousands of proteins of the cell. The nucleus is the command center of the cell and the repository of its archives. It is the site of synthesis of **ribonucleic acids** of several kinds. Three of these, **messenger ribonucleic acids (mRNAs)**, **transfer ribonucleic acids (tRNAs)**, and **ribosomal ribonucleic acids (rRNAs)**, move from the nucleus into the cytoplasm where they participate in the synthesis of the protein constituents of the cell and proteins produced for export from the cell (secretions).

outer or inner end of some of its integral proteins are called **peripheral proteins** (Fig. 1.3). The lipid bilayer has the properties of a two-dimensional fluid, so the integral proteins are free to diffuse within it, if they are not anchored to filaments in the underlying cytoplasm. In some cells, long oligosaccharide chains of integral glycoproteins, project outwards forming a thin carbohydrate outer coat on the surface of the membrane, called the **glycocalyx.**

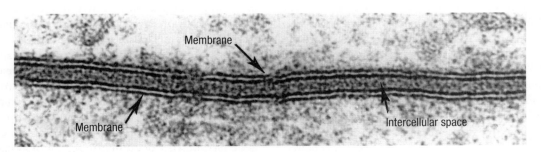

Figure 1.2 Electron micrograph of a segment of the plasma membrane of two cells and the intervening intercellular space. The membranes appear as two dense lines on either side of a line of lower density. The membranes are a bimolecular layer of phospholipid. The dense lines are the result of deposition of osmium in the hydrophilic heads of the phospholipid molecules, and the paler line represents their hydrophobic fatty acid chains.

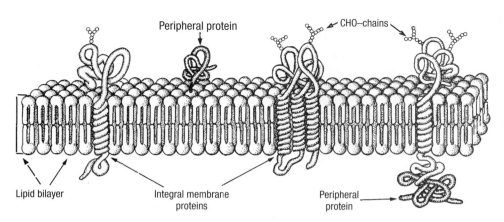

Figure 1.3 Diagram of the organization of a membrane, showing the bimolecular layer of phospholipid molecules, with their heads at the outer and inner surfaces and their tails towards the middle of the bilayer. Integral proteins of the membrane traverse the bilayer one or more times, and may have carbohydrate chains projecting outwards. Peripheral proteins may be bound to the outer or inner end of some integral proteins.

DNA is composed of two chains that spiral around one another in a configuration described as a double helix (Fig. 1.5). Each chain is a polymer of four kinds of nucleotides: **adenine** (**A**), **thymidine** (**T**), **cytidine** (**C**), and **guanine** (**G**), arranged in varying sequences along the length of the molecule. The two chains are held together by hydrogen bonds between each nucleotide on one chain and a complementary nucleotide on the other chain. The pairing is very specific, with A always bound to T, and C to G (Fig. 1.5). Most of the structural elements of cells, the enzymes that catalyze its biochemical reactions, and many of

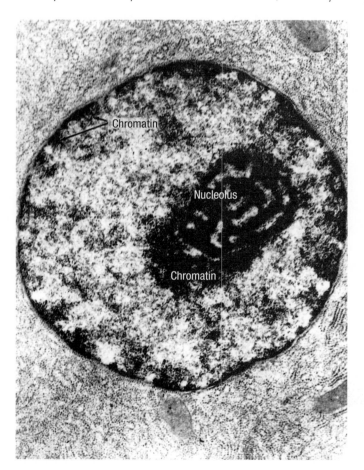

Figure 1.4 Electron micrograph of a typical nucleus. Note the dense clumps of chromatin around the periphery and adjacent to a conspicuous nucleolus in the center.

the secretory products of cells are **proteins**. Proteins are folded polypeptides (polymers of amino acids) and each polypeptide has a unique amino acid sequence. The number of different proteins in cells is estimated to be over 200 000. The instructions for the assembly of each of these are encoded in the sequence of nucleotides in a particular segment of the cell's DNA. Each kind of amino acid is specified by a sequence of three nucleotides, referred to as a **triplet** (or **codon**): for example, AAA specifies the amino acid phenylalanine; CCC glycine; AUG methionine, and so on. Thus, a sequence of 120 nucleotides (40 triplets) would be expressed in the synthesis of a polypeptide chain of 40 amino acids. A **gene** is the sequence of triplets providing the information for the synthesis of a particular protein. For each species of animal, its entire complement of genes is called its **genome**. In preparation for each cell division, the entire genome must be duplicated to insure that both daughter cells will have the same store of information. In this process, called **DNA replication**, the two chains of the helix separate and each serves as a template upon which an enzyme, **DNA polymerase**, assembles a complementary chain of nucleotides (Fig. 1.5). These two chains combine to form a molecule of DNA identical to the original. Occasionally a mistake is made in the replication of one of the genes. Such an abnormal event is called a **mutation**. It may result in the inability to synthesize an essential protein, or it may lead to synthesis of an abnormal protein. Such 'misspellings' in the sequence of nucleotides in a gene are responsible for many of the inherited diseases of humans.

In a remarkable achievement, involving the cooperation of many scientists, analysis of the nucleotide sequence of the entire human genome has recently been completed, and made available to cell and molecular biologists. Its 3 billion pairs of nucleotides have been compared, by Eric Lander, to 78 000 pages of the New York Times filled with combinations of four letters A, T, C, and G. Individual genes are made up of from hundreds to thousands of base pairs. The exact number of genes in the human is still uncertain, but it is estimated to be approximately 33 000. Curiously, only a small fraction of the total number of base pairs are components of functioning genes. The significance of the other, so-called **non-coding segments** of the DNA molecules is unknown. With the entire sequence of the human genome now known, it is often possible to identify the mutated gene that encodes an abnormal protein responsible for a genetic disease, and to specify its location on one of the chromosomes.

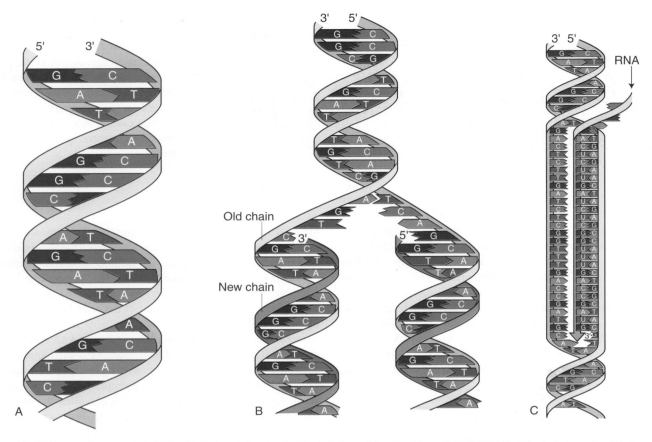

Figure 1.5 (A) Diagram of a segment of a DNA molecule: two chains of nucleotides (adenine, cytidine, thymidine and guanine) held together by hydrogen bonds between complementary nucleotides. (B) During DNA replication, the two chains separate and each serves as a template for polymerization of a complementary chain of nucleotides. (C) In transcription, the two chains dissociate in a segment containing a particular gene, and they serve as templates for polymerization of a molecule of messenger RNA.

For the synthesis of a particular protein, the instructions must be conveyed from a gene in the DNA of the nucleus, to the cytoplasm where protein synthesis takes place. This is accomplished by molecules of ribonucleic acid (RNAs), which are single-stranded polymers of nucleotides. To permit assembly of these RNAs, the two chains of the DNA molecule separate in the segment of the double helix that contains that particular gene, and the nucleotide sequence of the gene then serves as a template for polymerization of a complementary ribonucleic acid, called **messenger RNA (mRNA)** (Fig. 1.5). This transfer of information encoded in DNA to molecules of mRNA is called **transcription**. Two other kinds of RNA, which are synthesized in the nucleus, are transported to the cytoplasm: **transfer RNAs (tRNA)** and **ribosomal RNAs (rRNA)**. Transfer RNAs carry specific amino acids in the cytosol to the site of protein synthesis. Ribosomal RNA is a major component of small granules, called **ribosomes**, that abound in the cytoplasm. These bind to one end of an mRNA molecule and then move along it, assembling a chain of amino acids (a polypeptide) in the order specified by the sequence of nucleotides in the mRNA. This process is called **translation**. Thus, transcription of information encoded in the DNA occurs in the nucleus, and its translation to form a protein takes place in the cytoplasm.

Chromatin

In appropriately stained histological sections, examined under the light microscope, one sees in the nucleus conspicuous clumps of intensely basophilic material, called **chromatin**, located adjacent of the nuclear envelope (Fig. 1.4). Chromatin consists of DNA and associated proteins in a condensed state. The long molecules of a cell's DNA, if placed end-to-end, would be nearly a meter in length. Fitting this length of DNA into a nucleus only a few microns in diameter, requires several orders of coiling, which is the main stratagem involved in the shortening of the DNA. At regular intervals along its length, each DNA molecule is coiled one and a half turns around a cluster of eight molecules of the basic protein, **histone**. Each octomer of histone, and its encircling DNA, constitute a complex called a **nucleosome** (Fig. 1.6). There are about 25 million nucleosomes in the average nucleus, evenly spaced along the DNA molecules like beads on a string, with a single molecule of another histone midway between successive nucleosomes (Fig. 1.6). The coiling of the DNA around the histone octomer of the nucleosomes achieves about a sixfold shortening of the DNA molecules. Further shortening is achieved by helical coiling of these chains of nucleosomes around a central channel to form 30 nm **chromatin fibers** that are the basic structural units of

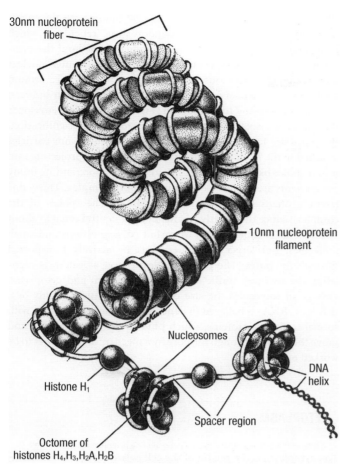

30nm nucleoprotein fiber

10nm nucleoprotein filament

Nucleosomes

Histone H₁

DNA helix

Spacer region

Octomer of histones H₄,H₃,H₂A,H₂B

Figure 1.6 Diagram of a 30 nm chromatin fiber. In the lower part of the figure the fiber is unwound to show the nucleosomes, consisting of DNA wrapped around an octomer of histones. (Redrawn from R. Bradbury *La Recherche* 1978; 9:644 and A. Worcel and Benyai *The Cell* 1978; 12:88.)

the condensed chromatin, observed in the nucleus between cell divisions. The granular appearance of chromatin in electron micrographs is attributed to cross-sections of higher orders of coiling of the 30 nm chromatin fibrils. DNA in this condensed state, commonly called **heterochromatin**, is inactive (i.e. it is not being transcribed). A smaller amount of the DNA is in a less highly coiled state and is referred to as **euchromatin**. It does not stain and is therefore invisible in histological sections, and it is difficult to identify in electron micrographs. The exact structure of euchromatin is not well understood, but it is thought to arise by uncoiling of some of the 30 nm fibers of heterochromatin. In euchromatin, the DNA can dissociate from the histone octomers of the nucleosomes and expose its nucleotide sequences for transcription.

Nucleolus

The **nucleolus** is visible in the living cell as a more-or-less spherical refractile body located eccentrically in the nucleus. In histological sections, it stains deeply with basic dyes and may be surrounded by small clumps of heterochromatin (Fig. 1.4). In electron micro-

graphs, the nucleolus consists of dense strands that branch and rejoin to form a continuous, compact network called the **nucleolonema**. The strands of this network are made up of closely packed, dense granules, comprising the **pars granulosa** of the nucleolus (Fig. 1.7). There are also two or more lighter, non-granular areas within the nucleolus, called **fibrillar centers**. These consist of segments of the DNA of one or more chromosomes that code for rRNA. If fibrillar centers are isolated and dissociated, electron micrographs reveal that they are made up of molecules of DNA, from which numerous chains of newly synthesized rRNA radiate in a configuration that resembles a bottle brush. In the living cell, the molecules of rRNA ultimately detach from the core DNA molecule and round up into granules that become incorporated in the pars granulosa of the nucleolus. There they are further processed, by addition of proteins, to form dense RNA–protein complexes, called **ribosomes**, that are moved into the cytoplasm, where they associate with long molecules of mRNA to participate in the synthesis of new proteins.

Nuclear lamina

Adjacent to the innermost of the two limiting membranes enclosing the nucleus, there is a thin layer, called the **nuclear lamina**. In different cell types, it ranges from 30 to 110 nm in thickness. It is not visible with the light microscope, but is apparent on electron micrographs as a pale layer between the peripheral clumps of heterochromatin and the nuclear membrane. It consists

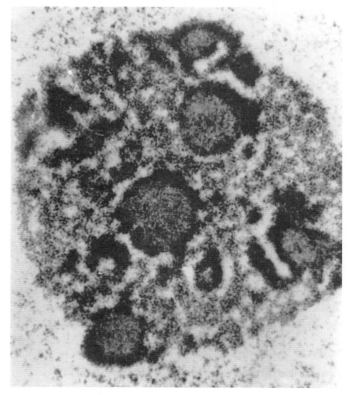

Figure 1.7 Electron micrograph of a nucleolus with a nucleolonema that varies in density along its length. Note also the three paler fibrillar centers.

of a mesh of compacted filaments that are polymers of polypeptides called **lamins**. These are of two kinds, A and B. Filaments of type A lamin are distinguishable from those of type B only by biochemical methods. Both are members of a large class of filaments found in the cytoplasm of various cell types and commonly described as **intermediate filaments**. Type A lamin filaments predominate in the inner half of the nuclear lamina, while the outer half is made up mainly of type B filaments. Associated lamin-binding proteins link the outermost type B filaments to integral proteins of the inner nuclear membrane.

The nuclear lamina makes an important contribution to the structural stability of the interphase nucleus. Its filaments are depolymerized during cell division and reassembled in the daughter cells. Lamins are not confined to the nuclear lamina. They are also found in the interior of the nucleus where they are believed to form structural elements of unknown configuration that may influence the disposition of chromosomes at the earliest stages of cell division.

Nuclear envelope

The nucleus is bounded by a **nuclear envelope** consisting of two parallel membranes separated by a 20–30 nm space called the **perinuclear cisterna** (Fig. 1.8). At a few sites around the perimeter of

the nucleus, the outer membrane is continuous with the membrane of another organelle, the endoplasmic reticulum, which consists of a network of tubules ramifying throughout the cytoplasm. At many sites around its periphery, the outer nuclear membrane is continuous with the inner membrane, around **nuclear pores** that serve as avenues of communication between the nucleoplasm and the cytoplasm (Fig. 1.8). In nuclear envelopes that have been isolated, stained, and viewed at high magnification, the pores are found to be lined by two rings of 15 nm particles attached to the inner and outer lips of the pore and projecting into it in a spoke-like pattern (Fig. 1.8, inset). The pore and its lining components are now called the **nuclear pore complex**. Thirty different proteins have been identified in it. The spokes of the complex reduce the effective diameter of its central canal to about 10 nm. This is large enough to permit passage of ions and small molecules, but larger molecules must be actively transported through the pores. The pore complexes serve as gateways regulating the two-way traffic between nucleoplasm and cytoplasm. Passage of molecules the size of proteins or nucleic acids (e.g. tRNA or rRNA) is believed to depend upon their association with special transport proteins, which bind to the pore complex and move their cargo through the pore by a mechanism that is yet to be worked out in detail.

CYTOPLASM

The cytoplasm is the region of the cell between the plasma membrane and the nuclear envelope. It contains cell organelles and inclusions suspended in a semi-fluid cytosol. Each of the membrane-bounded organelles (mitochondria, endoplasmic reticulum, Golgi complex, lysosomes and peroxisomes) is specialized to carry out a specific function in cell metabolism (e.g. energy generation, protein synthesis, product processing and packaging, or waste disposal). The inclusions, which include lipid droplets, pigment granules, and accumulations of non-degradable waste products, do not have a limiting membrane and are not active participants in cell metabolism.

Mitochondria

Mitochondria are organelles that generate the chemical energy necessary for most of the biochemical reactions that take place in the cytoplasm. They are present in nearly all cell types, but are most numerous in those that have unusually high energy requirements (such as muscle and neurons). In living cells, viewed with the phase contrast microscope, they are slender sausage-shaped structures 4–9 μm in length and 0.4–0.8 μm in diameter. They exhibit some variation in shape in different cell types. They are quite flexible and can be seen to bend and straighten as they move about in the cytosol of living cells. In transmission electron micrographs, each mitochondrion is found to have two membranes: a smooth outer membrane and an inner membrane that is plicated into thin folds of varying length, called the **cristae**

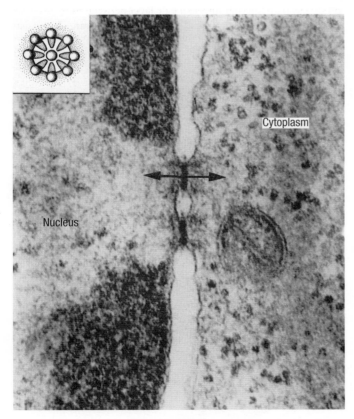

Cytoplasm

Nucleus

Figure 1.8 Electron micrograph of two of the many nuclear pores that cross the perinuclear cisterna, permitting molecules to move from the nucleoplasm to the cytoplasm. The dense line across the pore is caused by rings of dense spokes that project inwards from the limiting membrane of the pore (see inset).

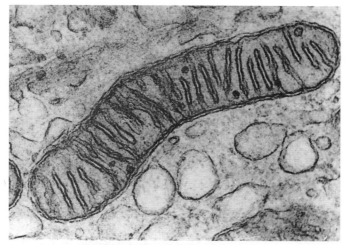

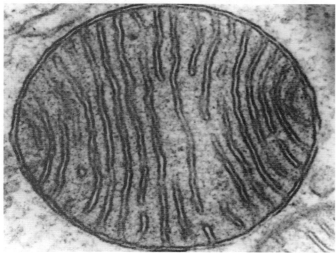

Figure 1.9 Micrographs of mitochondria showing their two limiting membranes and the cristae that project into their interior. Mitochondria are usually rod-like but they may be spherical in some cell types.

mitochondriales, which project into the interior of the organelle (Fig. 1.9). The cristae are a device for increasing the surface area of the enzyme-rich inner membrane of the mitochondrion. The mitochondria of cell types that have high energy needs have a larger number of cristae than those of cells that are less active. The two mitochondrial membranes are similar in appearance, but differ greatly in their chemical properties. The outer membrane contains proteins, called **porins**, which form channels to allow free diffusion of small molecules. The inner membrane is less permeable, but has a very high content of enzymes. Its protein content is higher than that of any other membrane of the cell. Associated with its inner surface are minute protein granules, which are the principal sites of generation of **adenosine-5-triphosphate (ATP)**, a very important molecule that serves as a store of the free energy needed for many of the chemical reactions of cell metabolism. The narrow space between the outer and inner membrane, and extending into the cristae, is called the **intermembrane space**. It has no visible content. The interior of the mitochondrion, is occupied by a **mitochondrial matrix**, which contains a few dense **matrix granules** (calcium phosphate),

and the **mitochondrial DNA**, which is a single, circular double-helix about 5.5 μm in diameter. Mitochondrial DNA very closely resembles the DNA of bacteria, and it is believed that mitochondria evolved, about 1.5 billion years ago, from symbiotic bacteria that subsequently relinquished the coding and synthesis of many of their proteins to the nucleus and cytoplasm of their host cell. Mitochondria do retain some tRNAs and rRNAs of their own, but they are dependent upon those in the surrounding cytosol for synthesis of many of their protein components. Like their ancestral bacteria, mitochondria reproduce by binary division. Mutations of the mitochondrial genome may occur during its replication, prior to mitochondrial division, and these are responsible for certain heritable diseases of humans. Such diseases are transmitted only through the mother, because the mitochondria of the fertilizing spermatozoon do not enter, or do not survive in, the zygote (the fertilized ovum).

In the disease, **Leber's heritable optic neuropathy**, a mutation in the mitochondrial DNA results in reduced capacity to carry out oxidative phosphorylation and generate ATP. Nerve tissue is highly dependent upon oxidative metabolism, and persons inheriting this disease often become blind between 15 and 30 years of age as a result of degeneration of the optic nerve.

Endoplasmic reticulum

The largest of the cytoplasmic organelles, the **endoplasmic reticulum (ER)**, is usually not visible in histological sections viewed with the light microscope. However, if thin intact cells, grown in tissue cultures, are stained with a lipophilic fluorescent dye, a lace-like network of delicate branching and anastomosing strands can be seen extending throughout the cytoplasm. In the preparation of tissues for electron microscopy, the continuity of the reticulum is disrupted and only short segments of it are visible in the ultrathin sections. These appear as branching membrane-bounded tubules. At some places along their length, the tubules are widened into flat

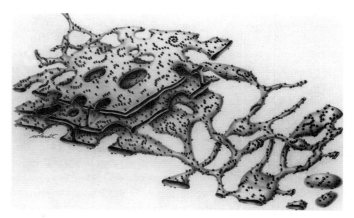

Figure 1.10 The rough endoplasmic reticulum consists of branching and anastomosing tubules and flat saccules, called cisternae. The cisternae are often arranged parallel to one another. The small granules on the surface, called ribosomes, may be aligned in rows, arcs, or circles referred to as polyribosomes.

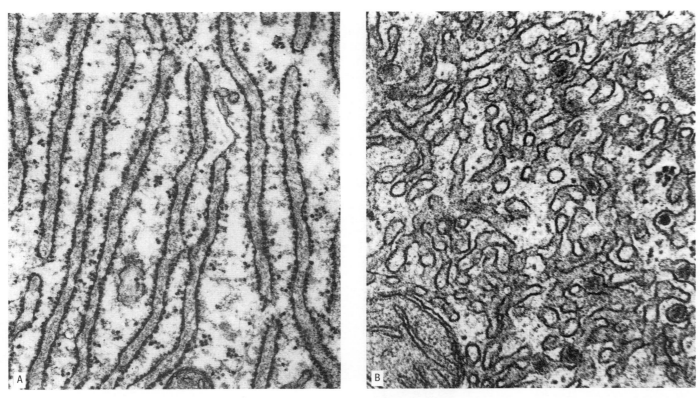

Figure 1.11 (A) Electron micrograph of parallel cisternae of the rough endoplasmic reticulum. (B) Smooth endoplasmic reticulum is a network of tubules devoid of adherent ribosomes.

saccules, called **cisternae**, which have a tendency to become arranged in parallel arrays (Fig. 1.10).

Two forms of the ER are distinguished: **rough endoplasmic reticulum (rER)**, so named because its surface is studded with small granules, called ribosomes (Fig.1.11A); and **smooth endoplasmic reticulum (sER)**, which consists of tubules without adherent ribosomes. The sER forms networks with smaller meshes than those of the rER (Fig.1.11B). The two forms of ER are continuous with one another, and can be considered regional variations of the same organelle, performing different functions. At high magnification, the ribosomes on the rER are seen to be composed of two distinct subunits, each of which has its own characteristic proteins and RNAs. Ribosomes occur free in the cytosol, as well as on the rER and they may number as many as 10 million in rapidly growing cells, or in cells specialized for production of a protein-rich secretion. In surface views of the rER, single ribosomes are rarely observed. Instead ten or more are evenly spaced on a long molecule of mRNA, like beads on a string, forming complexes called **polyribosomes** (Fig.1.12A).

Proteins of various kinds are the most abundant, and probably the most important, constituents of cells. Some are synthesized on polyribosomes free in the cytosol. Others, destined to become membrane proteins, or a secretory product, are synthesized on the polyribosomes of the rER. In this process, long molecules of mRNA, transcribed from the DNA of the nucleus, are moved into the cytoplasm. Each mRNA molecule has an **initiation site** at one end, to which a free ribosome binds. The

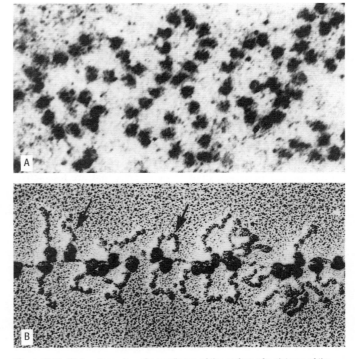

Figure 1.12 (A) A surface view of a small area of the surface of a cisterna of the rough endoplasmic reticulum showing four polyribosomes. (B) Scanning electron micrograph of an isolated polyribosome showing (at arrows) nascent polypeptide chains radiating from each ribosome. (Micrograph B courtesy of E. Kiseleva.)

ribosome, with the mRNA molecule in a groove between its sub-units, then binds to a receptor in the membrane of the ER. It then moves along the mRNA molecule, reading each codon (nucleotide triplet, CGG, UUC, etc.), and adding the specified amino acid to a nascent polypeptide chain (Fig.1.13). As soon as the first ribosome moves on, a second ribosome binds to the vacated initiation site. This is followed by a third, and fourth, and so on until as many as 20 ribosomes may be moving along the same mRNA molecule, each assembling the same polypep-tide. Each amino acid is brought to the ribosomes by a molecule of tRNA, bearing an anticodon that identifies the codon on the mRNA that is being read. The amino acid, bound to the other end of the tRNA molecule, is then added, by the ribosome, to the polypeptide chain being assembled. Approximately the first dozen amino acids assembled will not be part of the definitive protein, but constitute a **signal sequence** that appears to guide the lengthening polypeptide chain into a pore in the underlying membrane, through which it will extend into the lumen of the ER (Fig.1.13). The signal sequence is subsequently cleaved off by an enzyme (signal peptidase) located on the inner surface of the ER membrane. As each ribosome approaches the distal end of the mRNA molecule, it encounters a **stop codon**. Addition of amino acids ceases, the subunits of the ribosome separate and leave the membrane, and the completed polypeptide chain is released into the lumen of the ER. There it undergoes folding and disulfide bonding to achieve its native configuration. The newly formed protein molecules remain only transiently in the lumen of the ER, and are then transported in small vesicles to the Golgi complex, for further processing.

The sER has various functions unrelated to protein synthesis. Its membrane contains enzymes that are involved in the synthesis of cholesterol and steroid hormones. It is, therefore, exceptionally abundant in the interstitial cells of the testis (secreting testos-terone), and in cells of the adrenal cortex (secreting corticosteroids). In the liver, the sER has an important role in detoxification of drugs and alcohol, and also participates in the synthesis of glycogen. In muscle, a special form of sER, sarcoplas-mic reticulum, is the site of storage of calcium that is released to trigger contraction.

Golgi complex

The **Golgi apparatus**, or **Golgi complex**, named after its discov-erer, the 19th century Italian histologist, Camilio Golgi, is the organelle in which newly synthesized proteins, received from the rER, are further processed, sorted and packaged for transport to their final destinations in the cell. To be visible with the light microscope, it must be impregnated with silver or osmium (Fig.1.14). During the past 50 years, it has been studied mainly using the electron microscope. A Golgi complex is present in nearly all cell types, but it varies greatly in size. It is largest in secretory cell types. It consists of a stack of parallel, membrane-bounded, flat saccules and associated small vesicles. The saccules, commonly referred to as the **Golgi cisternae**, are usually slightly curved and thicker at their margins (Fig.1.15). They range in number from four to eight. Vesicles transporting newly synthe-sized protein from the rER fuse with the cisterna on the convex *cis-*

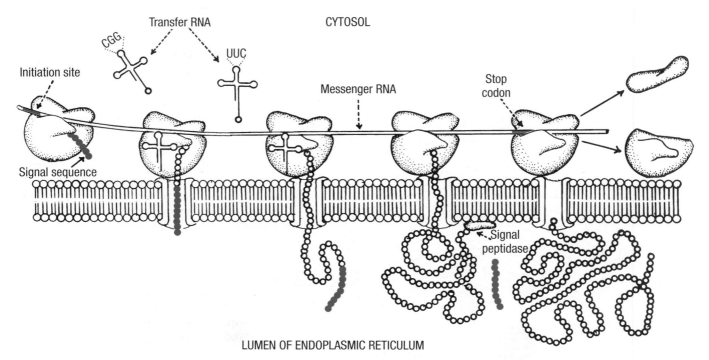

Figure 1.13 Diagram of a translation unit (polyribosome) consisting of several ribosomes moving along a molecule of mRNA, reading each codon and adding the specified amino acid to a polypeptide. The lengthening polypeptide chain passes through a pore in the underlying membrane into the lumen of the endoplasmic reticulum. Also shown are molecules of tRNA that bring to the ribosome the amino acid designated by the codon then being read. When the ribosomes reach a stop codon, their subunits separate and leave the rough endoplasmic reticulum.

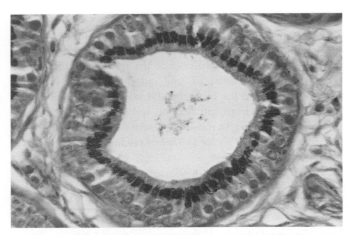

Figure 1.14 Photomicrograph showing epithelial cells, in which the Golgi complex has been impregnated with a metal. The Golgi complex is always in a supranuclear location in polarized epithelial cells.

face of the Golgi, and the processed protein exists in vesicles derived from the cisterna at the concave *trans* face of the organelle. There is a distinct polarity within the organelle. Histochemical staining reactions reveal that the enzymes present in the membrane of the first two to three cisternae, called the **cis-compartment** of the Golgi, differ from those of the remaining cisternae, which constitute its **trans-compartment** (Fig. 1.15). The cisterna on the exit face of the Golgi is fenestrated and therefore is often referred to as the **trans-Golgi network**.

In the final stage of protein synthesis by the rER, oligosaccharide chains are added to the protein, and, in the Golgi complex, the N-linked oligosaccharides of the resulting glycoproteins are

extensively modified in an ordered sequence of reactions involving removal of certain sugar residues, and addition of others in its cis-compartment, followed by addition of N-acetylglucosamines, galactose and sialic acid residues, in the trans-Golgi compartment. Intermediate products in this process are moved through the stack of Golgi cisternae by small vesicles that bud off one cisterna and fuse with the next until the modified protein reaches the terminal cisterna. This may seem to be a slow process, but tracer experiments have shown that vesicles having a total surface area approaching that of a cisterna are moved from one cisterna to the next every few minutes.

Some of the proteins that the Golgi complex receives from the rER are destined to be secreted, others will become components of other organelles (e.g. the lysosome). Proteins of these different kinds are processed differently in the Golgi and reach the trans-Golgi network bearing distinctive N-linked oligosaccharide chains. Once there, they are sorted, and aggregations of molecules of the same kind are enclosed in vesicles for transport to their respective destinations. The membranes of the different kinds of transport vesicles formed at the terminal cisterna of the Golgi have surface coats of different composition that serve as 'addresses' insuring that each will fuse with the appropriate target membrane. The most thoroughly studied of these are the so-called **coated vesicles**, which are targeted to the lysosomes. These are enclosed in a basket-like lattice of the protein **clathrin**. When such vesicles arrive at their destination, the clathrin coat is disassembled, permitting fusion of the transport vesicle with the lysosome. Other Golgi-associated vesicles that have other missions, are all very similar in appearance, but have different coat proteins, which are now being investigated. Two coat proteins (COP-I and COP-II) have recently been identified. It is believed that vesicles with a COP-I

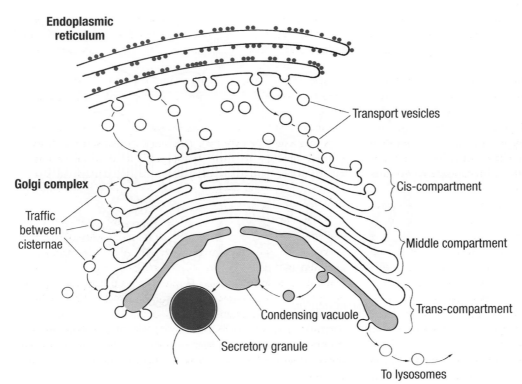

Figure 1.15 Diagram of the Golgi complex. In secretory cells, small vesicles transport newly synthesized proteins from the rough endoplasmic reticulum to the uppermost cisterna of the Golgi. The protein is then transported between successive cisternae in small vesicles. During its passage through the organelle, carbohydrate chains are added, and in the terminal cisterna it is concentrated and packaged into vesicles for transport to other organelles. In glandular cells, the vesicles fuse to form secretory granules, which release their content at the apical surface of the cell.

coat transport proteins from the rER to the Golgi complex. It is still unclear whether COP-II vesicles transport proteins between Golgi cisternae, or recycle membrane from the Golgi complex back to the rER.

In glandular cells, small vesicles containing their secretory product are budded off the trans-Golgi network and coalesce to form larger membrane-bounded **secretory granules**, which accumulate in the apical cytoplasm in considerable numbers. When the cell is stimulated by a nerve, the limiting membrane of the secretory granules fuses with the plasma membrane and their content is discharged into a system of ducts, or, in certain secretory cells of the connective tissue, into the extracellular fluid. This mode of secretion, described as the **regulated secretory pathway**, is largely confined to glandular cells, which are specialized for the secretion of large amounts of a specific product. However, in nearly all cell types, smaller amounts of various products are synthesized and continuously transported, in small vesicles, from the trans-Golgi network to the plasma membrane, where they are released without awaiting an external signal. This is called the **constitutive secretory pathway**.

Lysosomes

Lysosomes are membrane-bounded organelles 0.3–0.8 μm in diameter. They vary in shape, and in the appearance of their interior, with some being dense throughout, while in others there is an intermingling of light and dark areas (Fig. 1.16). Lysosome numbers in different cell types range from a few to over a hundred. They contain more than 30 hydrolytic enzymes that have acid pH optima, and they function as the 'digestive system' of the cell, decomposing substances taken into the cell, and disposing of excess, or damaged, cell organelles. Unlike mitochondria, lysosomes are not self-duplicating. They are assembled by fusion of vesicles from the Golgi complex, with vacuoles originating from the plasma membrane.

Large molecules that cannot diffuse, or be actively transported, across the cell membrane are taken up by **endocytosis**, a process in which small depressions in the plasma membrane deepen, constrict at their neck and separate from the membrane as vesicles, free in the cytoplasm. Such vesicles, containing fluid and macromolecules taken up from the extracellular environment, coalesce to form larger vacuoles, called **early endosomes** (Fig. 1.17). These serve as sorting compartments in which ligands are separated from their receptors, and the exogenous macromolecules that were taken up by endocytosis are transported in vesicles to lysosomes for degradation. The receptors and other membrane proteins are recycled to the plasma membrane in vesicles that bud off from the endosome. As an early endosome moves deeper into the cytoplasm, and matures into a **late endosome**, it receives, from the trans-Golgi network, vesicles containing newly synthesized hydrolytic enzymes. The enzymes are inactive at the pH in the interior of these vesicles. However, the membrane of the late endosome contains integral protein complexes that act as proton pumps, lowering the pH in its interior to pH 5.5 or lower. This low pH activates the

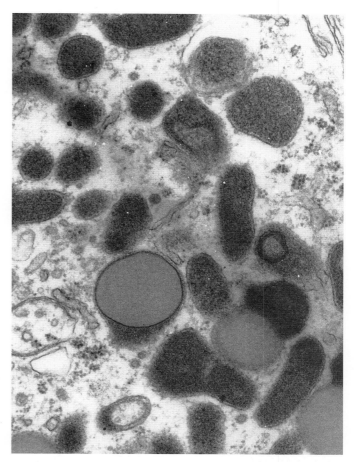

Figure 1.16 Electron micrograph of an area of cytoplasm containing a number of lysosomes varying in shape and density.

enzymes, and the exogenous macromolecules taken up by endocytosis are broken down to small molecules that can be utilized in cell metabolism. By continuing to accumulate enzymes of many kinds, late endosomes are believed to mature into lysosomes. This explanation of the origin of lysosomes is offered with the caveat that probably only some of the late endosomes mature into lysosomes, for endocytosis is continuous, and maturing late endosomes are not observed in cells in the numbers that would be expected. This suggests that some endosomes do not proceed to form lysosomes, but may be eliminated before maturation via a progressive loss of volume to vesicles targeted to existing lysosomes, and others recycling membrane proteins to the plasma membrane.

A few cell types are able to take large particulates (including bacteria or erythrocytes) into their cytoplasm, enclosed in a single, very large vacuole. Lysosomes then fuse with this vacuole, discharging into it hydrolytic enzymes that completely digest its contents. Lysosomes are also involved in a similar process, called autophagy, that disposes of excess or damaged cell organelles. A membrane is first assembled around the organelle selected for destruction (e.g. a mitochondrion), isolating it from the surrounding cytoplasm in a large vacuole. Lysosomes then fuse with the vacuole, and the organelle is digested by their hydrolytic enzymes.

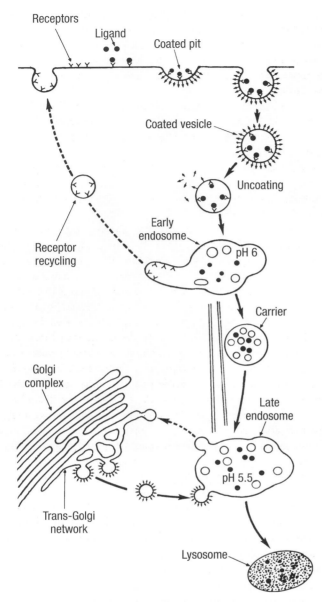

Figure 1.17 Diagram of the endocytic pathway. (1) Aggregation of receptors and their ligands in the membrane of coated pits. (2) Formation of coated vesicles. (3) Fusion of vesicles to form endosomes. (4) Transport of enzymes from Golgi to the endosome. (5) Lowering of pH in the interior of the late endosome activating the enzymes. (6) Transformation of late endosome to a lysosome.

There are a number of so-called **lysosomal storage diseases** that result from a mutation in the gene for one of the many different lysosomal enzymes. The most common of these is **Gaucher's disease**, in which there is a mutation of the gene for the enzyme that breaks down glycolipids. In these patients, undigested glycolipids accumulate to such an extent that they interfere with cell function. The organs principally involved are the spleen and liver, which become greatly enlarged. In **Pompe's disease** the enzyme acid maltase is deficient, or entirely absent, resulting in a massive accumulation of its substrate, glycogen, in the cells of liver, muscle and other organs. There are 15, or more, other diseases in which a single lysosomal enzyme is missing. The various substances that accumulate in cells include, glycolipids, glycopeptides, and sphingomyelin. In addition to the resulting physiological deficiencies, there is often severe mental retardation.

Peroxisomes

Peroxisomes bear some resemblance to lysosomes, but they are more consistently spherical and their content is less dense. In some species, they contain a crystalline inclusion, called the **nucleoid** (Fig. 1.18). Peroxisomes are present in small numbers in most cell types and they participate in a number of important biochemical pathways. They are especially abundant in liver cells, where they are involved in detoxification of alcohol, drugs, and other potentially harmful substances which are carried to the liver in the blood. Peroxisomes contain over 40 different enzymes, including D-amino acid oxidase, hydroxyacid oxidase, and catalase. Their oxidative reactions break down amino acids, uric acid, and fatty acids. The oxidation of fatty acids by peroxisomes is an important source of metabolic energy. Hydrogen peroxide (H_2O_2) is produced as a by-product of some of their oxidative reactions, but the enzyme catalase rapidly breaks H_2O_2 down to water and oxygen, preventing its potentially harmful effects upon the cell.

The protein constituents of peroxisomes are not synthesized on the rER, and are not processed in the Golgi complex. Instead, they are synthesized on free polyribosomes within the cytosol. The post-translational targeting of these proteins to peroxisomes is

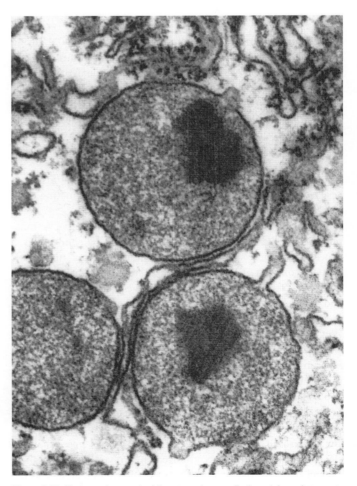

Figure 1.18 Electron micrograph of three peroxisomes. Each contains a dense inclusion called the nucleoid, which is a crystal of urate oxidase. (Micrograph courtesy of D. Friend.)

dependent upon a signal sequence on each protein that is recognized by a receptor in the peroxisome membrane. When peroxisomes reach a certain size, they divide by a mechanism that is still poorly understood.

Centrosome and centrioles

The **centrosome** consists of two **centrioles** in the center of a sphere of material of low density, described as the **pericentriolar matrix** (Fig. 1.19). Unlike other organelles, the centrosome is not enclosed by a membrane and its outer boundary is indistinct. On routine electron micrographs, no ordered substructure is visible in the pericentriolar matrix, but special methods have revealed within it a delicate lattice consisting of two proteins, **pericentrin** and **γ-tubulin**. Small rings of tubulin, of the same diameter as a microtubule, have also been observed near the periphery of the pericentriolar matrix. The two centrioles in the center of the centrosome are hollow cylinders 0.5 μm in length and 0.2 μm in diameter. Their wall has a complex structure consisting of nine evenly spaced triplet microtubules (Fig. 1.19). When viewed in cross-section, each triplet is seen to be positioned at an angle of 40° to its respective tangent, resulting in a pattern reminiscent of

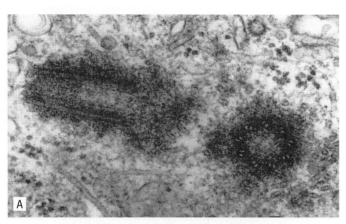

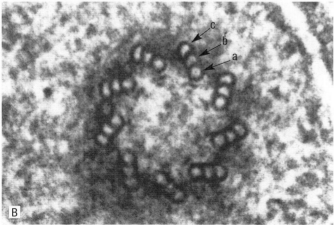

Figure 1.19 (A) Centrioles are short cylindrical structures located in the center of the centrosome, and oriented with their long axes perpendicular. (B) The wall of the centriole is made up of nine triplet microtubules in which the subunits are designated a, b, and c.

the blades of a turbine. The three subunits of each triplet are designated **microtubules a, b**, and **c**, with microtubule a nearest to the central cavity of the cylinder. Only microtubule a has a complete circular profile, for microtubule b shares a portion of the wall of microtubule a, and microtubule c shares a portion of the wall of microtubule b.

The function of the centrosome, in the non-dividing cell, is to nucleate the polymerization of long, single **microtubules** that radiate throughout the cytoplasm. These contribute to the maintenance of cell shape, and also serve as tracks along which transport vesicles and organelles are moved from place to place by motor proteins. Polymerization of the microtubules is initiated on γ-tubulin rings associated with the pericentrin-γ-tubulin lattice of the pericentriolar matrix.

In preparation for cell division, the centrioles replicate. A new centriole is assembled, in end-to-side relationship to each of the pre-existing centrioles. The two members of the original pair then separate, and each, together with its newly formed daughter centriole and a portion of the surrounding matrix, moves to opposite poles of the cell. There the centrosomes nucleate the polymerization of the microtubules of the **mitotic spindle** (see Cell division).

The structure of the wall of centrioles is duplicated in the so-called **basal bodies** of cilia, motile cell processes that project from the apical surface of certain types of epithelial cells. In the differentiation of such cells, hundreds of basal bodies are assembled and aligned in rows beneath the plasma membrane. Each basal body then nucleates polymerization of nine doublet microtubules and two single microtubules, that form the core structure of a cilium. Similarly, in the development of a spermatozoon, one member of the juxtanuclear pair of centrioles initiates polymerization of nine doublet microtubules in a long flagellum that executes undulant (or helical) movements to propel the spermatozoon, and aid in its penetration of the layer of cells that surrounds the ovum. Thus, both centrioles and basal bodies have the ability to nucleate polymerization of the doublet microtubules of motile cell processes.

CYTOPLASMIC INCLUSIONS

The several kinds of **organelles** described above are common to nearly all cells. Each has a distinctive structure and an indispensable function in cell metabolism. In addition to these, there are other structures, less essential to cell viability, that are collectively classified as **cytoplasmic inclusions**. These are not found in all cell types and within the same type; they may be present in some cells and not in others.

Glycogen

Glycogen is a polymer of the simple sugar **glucose**, which is the major product of photosynthesis in plants. In animals, glucose is absorbed in the digestion of fruits and vegetables, and it circulates in the blood after meals. It is metabolized by cells to enable them to synthesis ATP, which provides the energy for most of the biochemical reactions taking place in the cell. Even a brief deficiency of blood glucose can severely impair brain function. After a meal, when the level of blood glucose is high, it is taken up and stored by some cells in the form of its polymer, glycogen. In histological sections stained with a dye that binds to carbohydrates (Best's carmine), cells that contain a significant amount of glycogen stain a deep pink. In electron micrographs, glycogen is identifiable as dense particles 20–30 nm in diameter. These are widely distributed in the cytoplasm and may occur singly, or in aggregations of larger size (Fig. 1.20). Glycogen is found in abundance in the cytoplasm of liver cells, and in lesser amounts in muscle and many other cell types. Between meals, when the concentration of blood glucose declines, glycogen is hydrolyzed to yield glucose that is utilized by the cell or returned to the blood.

Lipid

Some cells also store triglycerides in their cytoplasm in the form of spherical **lipid droplets**. These are extracted in the preparation of histological sections, leaving behind only round, clear areas in the cytoplasm in their place. Lipid droplets are well preserved by the fixatives used for electron microscopy, and are identifiable, in micrographs, as perfectly round, jet-black structures of varying diameter (Fig. 1.21). Lipid droplets are not surrounded by a membrane, and they are not found in all cell types. Their sporadic occurrence evidently depends upon the nutritional state of the animal, and upon the varying energy needs of the different kinds of cells. One type of cell, the **fat cell**, or **adipocyte**, is specialized for storage of triglycerides, and contains a single, very large droplet of lipid that occupies 90% of the cell volume. Multiple small lipid droplets containing cholesterol esters, as well as triglycerides, are commonly seen in cells specialized for synthesis of steroid hormones.

Lipofuchsin pigment

Some cells contain irregularly shaped masses of a material that is yellow in the living cell, and black after fixation in osmium. These are called **lipofuchsin pigment**, or **residual bodies**. They are most common in cells that have a relatively long lifespan, such as neurons. Residual bodies are believed to be accumulations of indigestible residues of lysosomal activity. In electron micrographs,

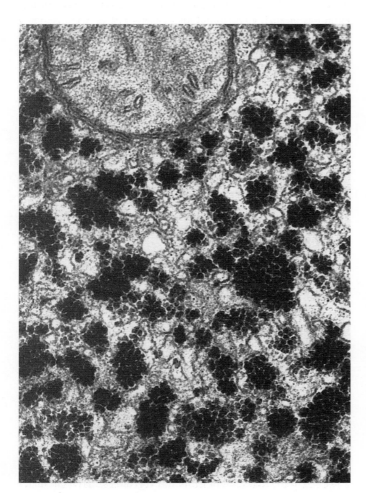

Figure 1.20 Electron micrograph of a small area of liver cell cytoplasm after a meal. It contains aggregations of small granules of glycogen.

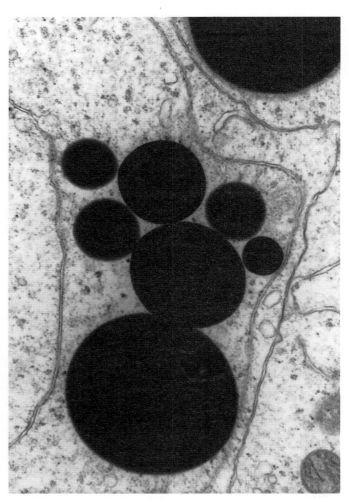

Figure 1.21 Lipid droplets in the cytoplasm of a cell fixed in osmium tetroxide, which preserves and stains the lipid black. Lipid is extracted in the preparation of tissues for light microscopy.

they may be of the same density throughout, or may have a mottled appearance, suggesting that they are aggregates of materials of differing density. While stores of glycogen and lipid are transient, lipofuchsin deposits are permanent and increase in size with age. They have no metabolic value, but the cell seems to have no way of eliminating them.

CYTOSKELETON

The cytoplasm of cells contains three categories of filaments: **microfilaments** (actin filaments), **intermediate filaments**, and **microtubules**. These collectively constitute the **cytoskeleton**, which determines cell shape and many of the physical properties of the cytoplasm. It is not the static, rigid, structural framework that the term 'cytoskeleton' might imply. It is very dynamic, with its filamentous components continually depolymerizing, and repolymerizing in different arrangements to alter the shape of the cell, to move its membranous organelles, or to move the cell as a whole.

Microfilaments (actin filaments)

The microfilaments, which are polymers of the protein **actin**, may account for up to 5% of the protein content of the cell (Fig. 1.22). Actin occurs in the cytoplasm as single globular molecules (**G-actin**), and in the form of filaments (**F-actin**) generated by polymerization of G-actin monomers. As a result of the eccentric position of binding sites on the globular monomer, it polymerizes to form two helically entwined actin chains, that constitute an **actin microfilament**. During F-actin assembly, monomers are added more rapidly at one end (the plus end) than at the other (the minus end), giving the filaments a polarity. Actin filaments are 7 nm in thickness and of varying length. **Actin-binding proteins** link them together in different arrangements for differing functions (internal support, cell attachment, or cell motility). Short actin filaments are especially abundant in a zone immediately beneath the plasma membrane, where they are interwoven to form a dense meshwork (Fig. 1.23) that gives this peripheral region of the cytoplasm, referred to as the **cell cortex**, the properties of a firm gel. Within this meshwork, the actin filaments are cross-linked at their sites of intersection by molecules of the actin-binding protein, **filamin**, and the outermost filaments are bound to integral proteins of the plasma membrane by another actin-binding protein, **ankyrin**. Changes of cell shape and movements of the cell, as a whole, are dependent upon interaction of actin filaments of this cortical meshwork with a motor protein **myosin** (Fig. 1.24). There are many isoforms of myosin, involved in different functions, including changes of cell shape, movement of its organelles, cell locomotion, and cell division. Which myosin isoform is involved in each kind of movement of cells in general is still a subject of research. However, the mode of actin–myosin

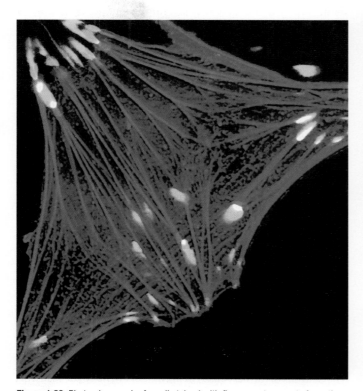

Figure 1.22 Photomicrograph of a cell stained with fluorescent reagents for actin and integrins. Bundles of actin filaments (red) cross the cell and end in focal adhesions (yellow and green), which consist of clusters of integrin molecules within the plasma membrane. (Reproduced from G. Gundersen *Science* 1999; 286:1173.)

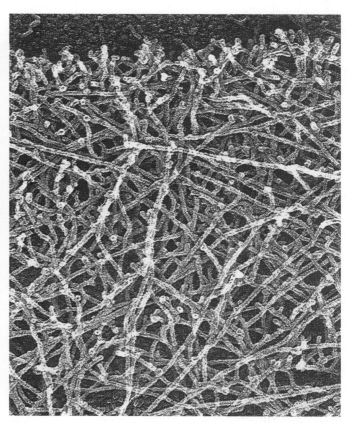

Figure 1.23 A high magnification electron micrograph of the dense network of interwoven actin filaments in the cell cortex. (Micrograph courtesy of T. Svitkina and G. Borisy.)

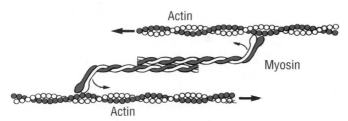

Actin

Myosin

Actin

Figure 1.24 The ability of the cells to extend cell processes or change their shape is attributed to interaction of actin filaments with a motor protein, myosin. Shown here are two filaments of F-actin that have myosin-binding sites. ATP-activated bending of the heads of the myosin molecules is believed to slide the actin filaments in opposite directions, resulting in contraction. (Drawing by Sylvia Keene.)

interaction in the shortening of muscle cells is now well understood. Long molecules of myosin form bundles (thick filaments) that are oriented parallel to thin filaments of actin. The heads of the multiple myosin molecules, of the thick filaments, bind to the neighboring actin filaments. Release of products of ATP hydrolysis then causes a change in configuration of the bound heads of the myosin molecules, which results in a sliding of the actin filaments with respect to the thick myosin filaments. In non-muscle cells, the interaction of actin and myosin may have some features in common with that in muscle, but their short actin filaments are less well organized, and the associated myosin molecules do not form bundles and therefore exert less motive force. Changes in shape of non-muscle cells are thought to be attributable, in large measure, to three-dimensional forces generated by rapid polymerization and depolymerization of the actin filaments in the cell cortex, but in some movements myosin plays an ancillary role.

Actin microfilaments may be organized by another actin-binding protein into very long thin bundles, referred to as **stress fibers**. These extend across the interior of the cell in various directions. At their ends some bind to the plasma membrane at specialized structures, called **focal adhesions**, which attach the cell to adjacent cells, or to its substrate. Although microfilaments are usually studied with the electron microscope, the long stress fibers can also be seen with the light microscope in cells stained with a fluorescent antibody to actin (Fig. 1.22). Other bundles of actin filaments are anchored to transmembrane proteins of the plasma membrane, called **integrins**, which bind at their outer end to components of the extracellular matrix.

In certain highly specialized cells, actin filaments are deployed in unusual arrangements adapted to the unique function of those cells; for example, erythrocytes, the cells of the blood which are specialized for transport of O_2, and CO_2 have an odd shape, best described as a biconcave disc. This cell shape is maintained by a thin layer of actin filaments immediately beneath the plasma membrane. In this layer, unusually short actin filaments are linked together by the actin-binding protein, **spectrin**, to form a network which is bound to integral proteins of the plasma membrane by the protein, **ankyrin**. The thin, resilient network, so formed, permits deformation of the erythrocytes as they pass through narrow capillary blood vessels, and restores their normal shape when they pass on to larger vessels.

In muscle cells, which are specialized for contraction, a protein called **dystrophin** links short actin filaments beneath the plasma

membrane, to form a network that is bound to specific proteins in the plasma membrane. These transmembrane proteins are also bound to fibrous proteins of the extracellular matrix. This cortical cytoskeleton, anchored to extracellular components, is believed to prevent damage to the cell membrane by the forceful contractions of the muscle cell.

Muscular dystrophy is a disabling inherited disease caused by a mutation in the gene coding for the actin-binding protein **dystrophin**. The gene is one of the largest in the human genome, and, depending upon the extent of its mutation, its product may be abnormal or entirely lacking. The disease has an onset in childhood, with progressive degeneration of muscle cells resulting in weakness, and inability to walk. Ultimately, degeneration of diaphragmatic and intercostal muscles leads to respiratory failure.

Intermediate filaments

Intermediate filaments were so named because they have a diameter (10 nm) that is intermediate between that of microfilaments (7 nm) and of microtubules (25 nm) (Fig. 1.25). Intermediate filaments are not a single entity, but a class of filaments of similar appearance and diameter, but composed of proteins of widely differing molecular weight. Seven or more different kinds can be distinguished microscopically by using specific immunocytochemical staining methods.

The intermediate filaments in fibroblasts of connective tissue are polymers of the 58 kDa protein, **vimentin**. They may be randomly oriented in a loose network throughout the cytoplasm, or they may aggregate into bundles that traverse the entire cytoplasm and bind, at their ends, to the cell membrane at sites of its attachment to the neighboring cells. In muscle cells, intermediate filaments are composed of the 53 kDa protein, **desmin**. These filaments transmit the tension developed by interaction of actin and myosin, and insure a uniform distribution of force throughout the cell. In cells of the epidermis of the skin, the intermediate filaments consist of **keratins**, a large and diverse family of proteins of differing molecular weights. Keratin filaments usually form a network around the nucleus from which bundles of similar filaments radiate towards the cell surface, where they terminate in membrane specializations for cell-to-cell attachment, called **desmosomes**. In the uppermost cells of the skin, keratin filaments occupy a large fraction of the total volume of the cytoplasm, and make these cells exceptionally resistant to mechanical injury.

Epidermolysis bullosa is a disease in which a mutation of one of the genes for **keratin** prevents assembly of intermediate filaments of this type in cells of the epidermis. In patients with this disorder, the cells of the epidermis are very fragile, and the slightest blow to the skin results in lysis of cells and formation of large bullae (blisters) at the site.

The neurons of the nervous system contain intermediate filaments of yet another kind, commonly referred to as **neurofilaments**. These are of great importance in providing internal support for the axon, a very long cell process that may be as much as a meter in length in cells of the spinal cord.

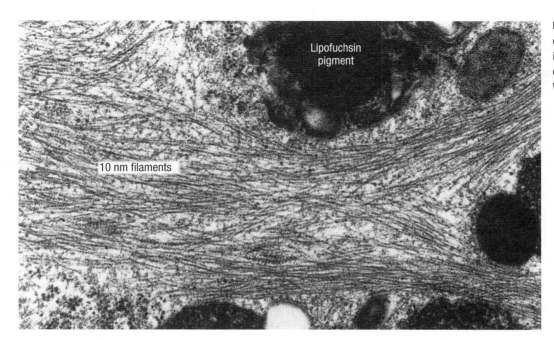

Figure 1.25 Electron micrograph of cytoplasm containing many 10 nm intermediate filaments of the cytoskeleton (Micrograph courtesy of W. Vogl.)

Microtubules

Microtubules differ from the filamentous components of the cytoskeleton, both in structure and function. They are straight tubules 25 nm in diameter with a wall 9 nm thick around a 15 nm lumen (Fig. 1.26). They may be many microns in length. Microtubules are polymers of the protein, **tubulin**, which is present in the cytosol as a heterodimer of two 55 kDa polypeptides, α-**tubulin** and β-**tubulin**. These heterodimers polymerize to form 13 linear protofilaments that are bonded laterally to make up the wall of the microtubule. Microtubule formation is usually initiated at the centrosome, on rings of another form of tubulin, γ-**tubulin**, which are 25 nm in diameter and serve as templates, nucleating polymerization of the heterodimers of α- and β-tubulin. The lengthening microtubules radiate outwards from the centrosome towards the cell surface. They may later dissociate from the centrosome and assume other orientations. Some microtubules of the cytoskeleton are relatively stable, while others undergo cycles of assembly and disassembly. During assembly, dimers are added preferentially to one end, designated the plus-end of the microtubule.

In addition to their cytoskeletal functions, the microtubules also serve as tracks, along which transport vesicles and organelles are moved from one region of the cytoplasm to another. Their movement is effected by two motor proteins, **kinesin** and **dynein**, which move them in opposite directions along microtubules. Kinesin is a 350 kDa protein that has two diverging globular heads and a long α-helical segment (tail), which has a cargo-binding domain at its end. Each globular head has binding sites for tubulin and ATP. The tail of the molecule has a binding site for a protein in the membrane of the vesicle or organelle that is being translocated. During transport, one of the diverging heads

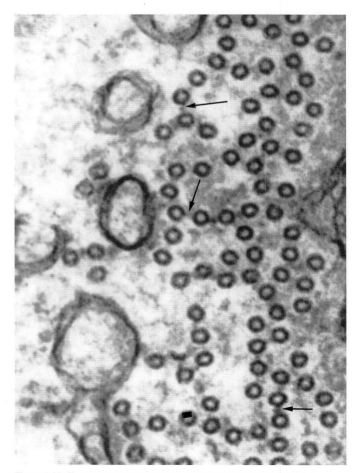

Figure 1.26 Electron micrograph showing cross-sections of microtubules. A microtubule-associated protein can be seen (at arrows) cross-linking some of the microtubules.

of the kinesin molecule binds to a tubulin dimer in the wall of a microtubule (Fig. 1.27). A conformational change in the molecule, coupled to the release of ADP and P_i, then swings the unbound head 180° around the bound head to bind to the next tubulin dimer of that protofilament. The first head is then released and swings around the bound head to bind to the next tubulin dimer, and so on. By repetition of these steps, the kinesin molecule 'walks' along the microtubule, moving its cargo towards the plus-end of the microtubule, at a rate of about 0.3 µm per second. Because the minus-ends of the microtubules tend to be at, or near, the centrosome, kinesin commonly moves vesicles towards the cell periphery. Kinesin-based transport of small vesicles is especially important in neurons, which synthesize neurotransmitters and package them into small vesicles that are then moved along microtubules in the very long axon, to reach a nerve ending that may be thousands of microns away from the cell body. Microtubules and the motor protein kinesin are also involved in movement of the secretory granules of glandular cells from the Golgi complex to the apical cytoplasm, for storage and ultimate release.

The other major microtubule-associated motor protein, **dynein**, is a large molecular complex of about 2000 kDa. Like kinesin, it has two globular heads that bind to tubulin and hydrolyze ATP, and tails that bind to a protein in the membrane of the structure being transported. Dynein's mode of progression along a microtubule is very similar to that of kinesin, but in the opposite direction (towards the minus-end) It can move a wide range of cargoes, including small vesicles and larger organelles, such as mitochondria and chromosomes. Dynein also generates the movements of cilia and flagella by driving the sliding of the microtubules, in their interior, relative to one another.

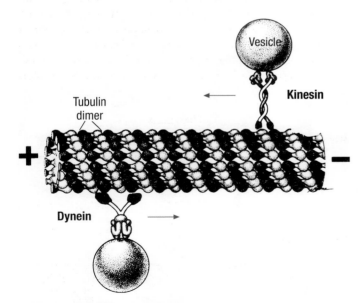

Figure 1.27 Microtubules serve as tracks along which vesicles are moved by motor proteins, kinesin and dynein. The tail of these proteins binds to a vesicle and the two heads of the molecule bind alternately to successive tubulin dimers of a protofilament in the wall of a microtubule. Kinesin thus 'walks' towards the plus-end of the microtubule. Dynein moves cargo similarly, but towards the minus-end of the microtubule. (Drawing by Sylvia Keene.)

CILIA AND FLAGELLA

Continuous sheets of closely adherent cells (epithelia) that line portions of the respiratory and reproductive tracts have, on their free surface, motile cell processes called **cilia** (Fig. 1.28A). These slender processes, about 10 µm long and 0.25 µm in diameter, are constantly in motion, all bending to-and-fro in parallel, and in synchrony. Their coordinated activity moves fluid, or an overlying layer of mucus, over the surface of the epithelium in a consistent direction. The movements of each cilium are generated by a core complex, called the **axoneme**, made up of nine **doublet microtubules** uniformly spaced around a central pair of single microtubules (Fig. 1.28B). In the doublets, the wall of one member (the a-microtubule) has the usual 13 protofilaments, while the wall of the other member (the b-microtubule) has only 10 protofilaments, and shares three protofilaments of the wall of the a-tubule. Spaced at 24 nm intervals along the length of the a-tubule, are pairs of short projections that extend in a clockwise direction, towards the b-tubule of the adjacent doublet. These are made up of the motor protein dynein and are commonly referred to as the **dynein arms**. The a-tubules of the nine doublets are connected to a thin sheath around the central pair of microtubules by

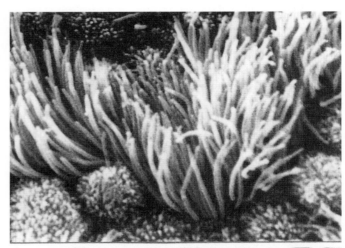

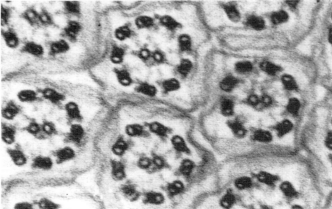

Figure 1.28 (A, top) Scanning micrograph of cells with cilia projecting from their apical surface. (B, bottom) A higher magnification transmission micrograph of several cilia in cross-section.

nine radial **spokes**. The doublets are linked to each other by tenuous strands of a protein called **nexin**. In the cytoplasm at the base of each cilium, there is a short cylindrical **basal body**, which has a wall composed of nine **triplet microtubules** identical to those seen in the wall of the centrioles (described earlier in the chapter). Each doublet of the axoneme is continuous with two subunits of a triplet microtubule in the wall of the basal body. In the development of the anoneme, the basal body nucleates the assembly of its doublet microtubules.

Many species of protozoa are moved through their aqueous environment by the action of cilia on their surface. Other species are propelled by a single **flagellum**, several times the length of a cilium, which has an undulant (or helical) motion, with waves of bending moving along its length from base to tip. The internal structure of a flagellum, viewed in cross-section, appears to be identical to that of a cilium. The only mammalian cell that possesses a flagellum is the spermatozoon. In some species, this may be over 200 μm in length. The initial portion of its axoneme is enveloped by a sheath of closely spaced mitochondria that synthesize ATP to provide the large amount of energy required for propagation of waves of bending along the length of the flagellum. The underlying mechanism of motility in both cilia and flagella is the sliding of doublet microtubules of the axoneme, relative to neighboring doublets, by the action of their dynein arms. To account for the alternation in direction of bending of cilia, it is suggested that the dynein arms of doublets on one side of the axoneme are active during the forward power stroke, and the dynein arms of doublets on the other side of the axoneme are active in its return stroke.

> Verification of the essential role of dynein in the motility of cilia and flagella is found in humans with the rare inherited disease **Kartagener's syndrome**, in which the dynein arms of the doublet microtubules of the axoneme are absent. Persons with this disorder have serious pulmonary problems because the cilia on the epithelium lining the trachea are immotile, and fail to clear the upper respiratory tract of mucus by moving it up the tract to the pharynx, where it is normally swallowed. Males with Kartagener's syndrome are sterile because the spermatozoa are not motile. In females, the chance of successful reproduction is diminished by immotile cilia in the oviducts. In rare instances, movements of the fimbriae of the oviduct, generated by smooth muscle cells, compensates for impaired ovum transport by their cilia.

ENDOCYTOSIS

Endocytosis is the taking of extracellular materials into the cell in invaginations of the cell membrane that pinch off to form vesicles, which move into the cytoplasm. Three modes of endocytosis are distinguished: (1) **pinocytosis** (drinking by cells), in which extracellular fluid and its solutes are continuously taken up in multiple small vesicles; (2) **receptor-mediated endocytosis**, the selective uptake of substances that bind to specific receptors in patches of membrane that invaginate to form vesicles; and (3) **phagocytosis** (eating by cells), in which a sizable particle is taken up in a single large vacuole. Pinocytosis and receptor-mediated endocytosis are observed in nearly all cell types. Phagocytosis is confined to a few

motile cell types, such as macrophages and neutrophil leukocytes that patrol the tissues of the body, ingesting and digesting cellular debris and any invading bacteria that they may encounter.

Pinocytosis

Pinocytosis is a non-selective form of endocytosis in which small and large molecules in solution are taken up in the concentration prevailing in the extracellular fluid. A shallow depression is first formed, which deepens into a small flask-shaped invagination of the plasma membrane. Initially, this is open at its neck to the extracellular space, but subsequent narrowing and closure of the neck detaches it from the membrane as a small vesicle, free in the cytoplasm (Figs 1.29A, 1.30A). These small vesicles are 60–80 nm in diameter. The molecular events responsible for the membrane invagination, and for membrane fusion at their necks, are still unclear.

Receptor-mediated endocytosis

Receptor-mediated endocytosis is a mechanism for the selective concentration and uptake of specific protein molecules from the extracellular fluid. It depends upon the presence of receptors for that protein in the plasma membrane, which move within the fluid, lipid bilayer to gather in shallow depressions of the cell surface, called coated pits. These are so-named because their cytoplasmic surface is coated by a 180 kDa protein, called **clathrin**. Molecules of clathrin, which have three arms, with a binding site at the end of each, polymerize to form a cage-like lattice, which is bound to the underside of the membrane of the pit. In scanning electron micrographs, this network presents a pattern of of pentagons and octagons that resembles the framework of a geodesic dome (Figs 1.29B, 1.30B). Polymerization of clathrin progresses as the pit deepens, and another cytosolic protein **dynamin** forms a ring around its neck. Contraction of the ring of dynamin constricts the neck and releases a coated vesicle into the cytoplasm. The coated vesicles, containing the receptors

Pinocytosis

Non-specific uptake

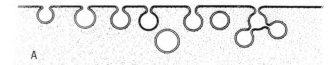

A

Selective uptake

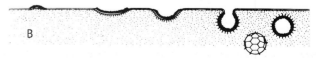

B

Figure 1.29 (A) In fluid-phase pinocytosis, minute invaginations of the cell surface detach and move into the cytoplasm as smooth-surfaced vesicles. This process is non-selective. (B) In receptor-mediated endocytosis, specific receptors and their ligands cluster, and this portion of the membrane invaginates to form a vesicle that is enclosed in a lattice of clathrin. This type of endocytosis is selective.

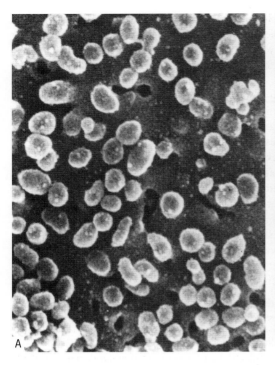

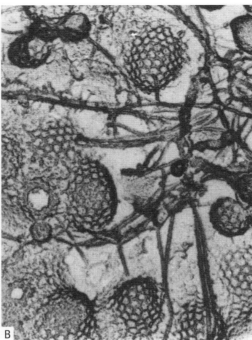

Figure 1.30 (A) Scanning micrograph of the cytoplasmic surface of the plasmalemma of a cell engaged in pinocytosis. Notice the large number of membrane invaginations that will pinch off to form vesicles. (B) A comparable image of receptor-mediated endocytosis, showing several forming vesicles covered by a lattice of clathrin. (Micrographs courtesy of (A) T. Inoue and H. Osatako, and (B) N. Hirokawa and J. Heuser.)

and their ligands, rapidly lose their clathrin coat and fuse with endosomes, which are vesicular compartments that process materials taken up by endocytosis. Endosomes maintain an acid pH in their interior that dissociates the ligands from their receptors, and the latter are returned to the plasma membrane in vesicles that bud off the endosome (Fig. 1.17). The molecules taken up in coated vesicles are sorted in the endosome for transport to other destinations in the cell. Receptors for 30 or more different proteins have been identified in coated pits. Among them is a receptor for low-density lipoprotein (**LDL**), an important class of serum proteins that contains cholesterol. Cells take up blood-borne LDL by receptor-mediated endocytosis, and it is broken down by lysosomal enzymes to release cholesterol for use in the biosynthesis of membranes, steroid hormones, bile salts or vitamin D.

In the disease **familial hypercholesterolemia**, cells have defective LDL receptors and fail to take up LDL from the blood. Continuing formation and absorption of LDL by the intestines, combined with increased cholesterol synthesis by the liver, results in very high levels of cholesterol in the blood. This leads to its deposition in the walls of arteries (arteriosclerosis). Patients with blood cholesterol levels above 200 mg per 100 ml of blood are at great risk of heart attack, because plaques of cholesterol crystals in the lining of the coronary arteries present a rough surface that promotes the formation of a blood clot, which may occlude the vessel and deprive an area of heart muscle of oxygen.

Phagocytosis

Phagocytosis is the internalization of particles, such as bacteria, for destruction within the cell. This activity is largely confined to motile cell types (macrophages, neutrophils, and dendritic cells) that are involved in the body's defense against invading microorganisms. Contact of one of these cells with a bacterium triggers

actin assembly and myosin-generated motor activity in its cortex, which results in formation of two broad surface projections, called **pseudopodia**, on either side of the point of contact (Fig. 1.31). The

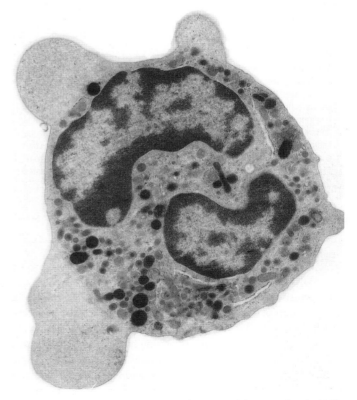

Figure 1.31 A neutrophilic leukocyte beginning to extend three pseudopods. At this early stage, they are simply thickened regions of the cell cortex formed by polymerization and cross-linking of new actin filaments. At a later stage of their elongation, cytosol extends into their interior.

pseudopodia are advanced over the surface of the bacterium until it is completely surrounded. Their tips then fuse, enclosing the bacterium in a large vacuole, or **phagosome**, bounded by membrane derived from the plasma membrane. Lysosomes subsequently fuse with the membrane of the phagosome, discharging hydrolytic enzymes into it to digest its contents.

The phagocytic activity of macrophages is not directed against invading bacteria alone. They also phagocytize any dead, or damaged cells, that they encounter; for example, the 5.5 l of blood in the human circulation contain about 5 million red blood cells (erythrocytes) per cubic millimeter. A small percentage of this great number are nearing the end of their normal 120 day lifespan. These senescent erythrocytes are filtered out of the blood in the spleen, where they are taken up and digested by the large population of macrophages residing in that organ. Macrophages also take up any inorganic particulates that they may encounter in the tissues. Any of these that are resistant to digestion by lysosomal enzymes are sequestered in the cytoplasm as components of residual bodies (lipochrome pigment). Macrophages in the lungs of smokers have many residual bodies, containing indigestible, small particulates inhaled in tobacco smoke.

CELL LOCOMOTION

During embryonic development, active movement of cells is necessary to establish the primary germ layers (endoderm, mesoderm, and ectoderm), and later for assembly of cells into organs (organogenesis), and for shaping of the body as a whole (morphogenesis). In the adult, the great majority of cell types are relatively immobile, but they may become active during normal wound-healing, or in the spread (metastasis) of cells that have undergone malignant transformation (cancer).

The crawling movement of a mammalian cell, such as the fibroblast of connective tissue, depends upon its ability to extend forward a type of cell process, called a **lamellipodium**. This is a broad, thin fold of the plasma membrane and the underlying cell cortex. Its extension is brought about by the regulated assembly and cross-linking of actin filaments of the cell cortex. The leading edge of the lamellipodium binds to the cell substrate at focal adhesions on its underside. Contraction of the cell body by interaction of the actin and myosin in its cortex then detaches, and quickly draws the trailing end of the cell into the cell body. The lamellipodium then extends and anchors its leading edge farther forward on the substrate, and contraction of the cell cortex again retracts the trailing end of the cell. The cell is moved forward a short distance with each repetition of this sequence of events. Other thin, tapering processes, called **filopodia**, may attach transiently to neighboring structures, but these do not appear to play a significant role in advancing the cell.

While the great majority of cells in the adult are relatively quiescent, there is a population of blood cells, called **leukocytes** (neutrophils, monocytes, and eosinophils) that leave the circulation and continually migrate through the tissues on a search-and-destroy mission against any bacteria, or parasites, that may have invaded the body. These cells extend forward a process,

called a **pseudopodium**, which is thicker than a lamellipodium and more-or-less cylindrical, with a blunt end. This is anchored to the substrate and the cell body then contracts and cytosol flows into the pseudopodium, expanding it and encorporating it into the cell body, and a new pseudopodium is then extended and anchored. Thus, the cell is moved forward by the length of the pseudopodium, and this sequence of events is repeated. This mode of progression is described as 'amoeboid', because of its resemblance to the movements of the protozoon, *Amoeba proteus*. Forward progress by amoeboid motility is more rapid than the movement of fibroblasts. Pseudopodia involved in this kind of cell locomotion are similar in appearance to those that are extended around large particles to draw them into the cytoplasm during phagocytosis.

CELL DIVISION

Chromosomes

Chromosomes are structural units of the genetic material of the cell, each consisting of a linear double-stranded DNA molecule and associated proteins. Chromosomes are not identifiable in the nucleus of the non-dividing cell, but in preparation for cell division, the chromatin of the nucleus decondenses and its molecules of DNA are reorganized into chromosomes, sausage-shaped structures of varying length that are visible under a light microscope. In electron micrographs, they are found to consist of loops of a 30 nm fiber, which radiate from an axial **chromosome scaffold** of non-histone protein (Fig. 1.32B). The nucleus of all somatic cells, of a given species, contains a constant number of **chromosomes**. The number and length of the chromosomes are distinctive for each species and are referred to as its **karyotype**. In the human karyotype, the chromosome number is 46, of which 23 were received from the mother, and 23 from the father. For each of the chromosomes received from the mother (maternal chromosomes), there is a matching chromosome of the same length among the paternal chromosomes (except in the male, where in one pair, called the **sex chromosomes**, one is shorter than its mate). The pairs of matching maternal and paternal chromosomes are referred to as **homologous chromosomes**.

Chromosomes have long been studied in 'squash preparations' made by crushing dividing cells between two microscope slides, then staining them. This crude procedure spreads the chromosomes apart so that their number and size can be observed (Fig. 1.32A). In such preparations, the staining accentuates a cross-banded pattern along the length of the chromosomes. Homologous chromosomes are identified in such preparations, by their having the same length and the same pattern of cross-banding. The 23 pairs of human chromosomes have been assigned numbers, and distinctive bands along their length are designated by letters. Genes newly discovered by molecular biologists can often be localized to a particular band on one of the numbered chromosomes. The 22 pairs of chromosomes containing most of the genome are called the **autosomes**. The remaining pair, the sex

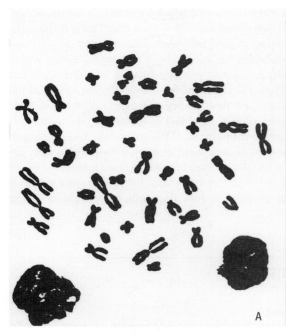 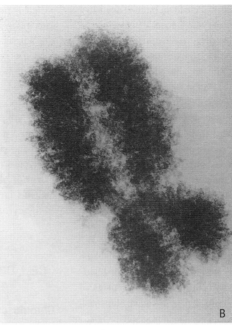

Figure 1.32 (A) Photomicrograph of a squash preparation of the chromosomes of a dividing cell. 22 pairs of autosomes and the X and Y sex chromosomes are identified. (B) Micrograph of an unsectioned metaphase chromosome showing the two chromatids, the primary constriction, and loops of DNA radiating from an axial scaffold of non-histone protein in each chromatid. ((A) courtesy of H. Lisco; (B) courtesy of H. Ris.)

chromosomes, contain only a small fraction of the genome, but determine the gender of the individual. These are not assigned numbers, but are identified by the letters **X** and **Y**. Cells of a female have two sex chromosomes of equal length, and the pair is designated **XX**. Cells of the male contain two sex chromosomes that differ in length. The longer of the two has been assigned the letter X, the shorter, the letter Y, and the pair is designated XY. Thus, the chromosome complement of the human female is 44XX, and that of the male 44XY.

At the ends of the DNA molecule of chromosomes there are multiple repeats of a short sequence of nucleotides, constituting a non-coding segment called the **telomere**, which caps and protects the ends of the chromosomes. In DNA replication prior to cell division, new DNA molecules are assembled by the enzyme DNA-polymerase, on the template provided by the pre-existing DNA. However, replication of the telomeres requires a separate enzyme, **telomerase**, which carries its own template. In tissue cultures of human fibroblasts, it has been observed that the telomeres become shorter with each successive cell division, and after a certain number of divisions, the cells are no longer able to divide. It has been inferred from this that the limited proliferative lifespan of cells is attributable to depletion of the telomeres in cells lacking telomerase activity. Premature conclusions have been drawn from this observation with regard to the relation of telomere shortening to aging and limitation of human lifespan. This interpretation has recently been challenged by the finding that Schwann cells isolated from peripheral nerves are able to proliferate *in vitro* indefinitely, with no morphological evidence of senescence.

The cell cycle

Some cells of the adult spend long periods of time in a steady state, in which segments of DNA are constantly being transcribed into sets of mRNAs specifying proteins needed to carry out the normal functions of the cell. Concurrently, proteins are being degraded at the same rate, by large protein complexes called **proteasomes**. The synthesis of new proteins and the degradation of old proteins are so regulated that the cell neither grows nor changes its function; for example, nerve cells and muscle cells may remain indefinitely in this balanced state, referred to as G_0. Other cell types undergo a regular sequence of biochemical and morphological changes, which lead to their division into two daughter cells. The **cell cycle** is the ordered sequence of events that a cell undergoes from its origin to its division. The length of the cycle in different cell types varies. In cells of the early embryo it may be less than 24h. In the adult, some cells of the intestine also have a very short cycle, dividing often to replace the large numbers of senescent cells that are lost into its lumen. The cycle of the parenchymal cells of the liver may be months in length. In the cycle of cells, in general, two major segments are distinguished, **interphase**, and **mitosis**. Interphase is the period between the origination of the cell and its division, and it occupies 95% of the cycle. Mitosis, its division into two daughter cells, occupies only a few hours.

Interphase

It is customary to consider the biochemical and structural events of interphase in four stages, designated G_1, **S**, G_2 and **mitosis**. Throughout the relatively long G_1 phase, the cell carries out its normal functions with little change in its appearance, other than some increase in size. It is in this phase of the cycle that certain cell types may cease cycling and enter the G_0 phase, described above. In cycling cell types, the centrosome is replicated, near the end of the G_1 phase, with the two resulting centrosomes remaining in a juxtanuclear location (Fig.1.33A). The cell then proceeds into **S** phase, during which there is some further increase in size. During the latter part of this phase, its chromatin decondenses and the DNA molecules are uncoiled by an enzyme called **helicase**. Each of the resulting, linear nucleotide chains then serves as a template for its replication by the enzyme **DNA-polymerase**. This replication of the DNA, in S phase, insures that the two daughter cells of the division will each possess the normal two copies of the entire genome. These events are followed by a very brief G_2 phase of the cycle, during which there is further increase in cell volume, and synthesis of enzymes and other proteins, including **cyclins**, which will control its progression through the successive stages of cell division (mitosis). Tubulin and accessory proteins also accumulate in the cytoplasm in this phase of the cycle in anticipation of the formation of the mitotic spindle (see Mitosis).

Mitosis

The fourth phase of the cycle, **mitosis**, is divided into five stages: **prophase**, **prometaphase**, **metaphase**, **anaphase**, and **telophase**. Early in prophase, the nucleus takes on an altered appearance, with slender strands of uncoiled DNA tracing a meandering pattern throughout the karyoplasm. Owing to the DNA replication that occurred in **S** phase of the cycle, each of the original chromosomes is now represented by two strands of DNA, which later condense into a pair of rod-shaped structures, called **chromatids** (Fig.1.33B). The chromatids of each pair are bound together at a narrow segment midway along their length, called the **centromere**. While these changes are in progress, the nucleolus disappears and the nuclear envelope disintegrates (Fig.1.33B). Late in prophase, the two centrosomes begin to migrate to opposite poles of the cell, where they initiate polymerization of tubulin to form the **mitotic spindle**, an array of many microtubules, of which some radiate towards the membrane at the ends of the cell, while others extend from the centrosomes towards the chromosomes that are randomly dispersed in the cytoplasm after disintegration of the nuclear envelope (Fig.1.33C). The cell then enters **prometaphase**, a transitional stage during which microtubules emanating from opposite poles of the spindle attach, at their plus-ends, to **kinetochores**, multilayered protein structures on either side of the **centromeres** of each pair of chromatids. Because the kinetochores are oriented on opposite sides of the centromere region of each pair of chromatids, they bind the plus-ends of microtubules emanating from opposite poles of the spindle. In **metaphase**, the pairs of chromatids all become aligned across the middle of the cell in the same transverse plane, called the **equatorial plate** (Figs 1.33D, 1.34). In **anaphase**, the sister chromatids are separated from one another by the action of a specific protease on their centromeres, and they move towards

Figure 1.33 Drawing of mitosis. (A) Late interphase cell in which the centrosome has divided. (B) Prophase. Nuclear membrane breaking up; chromatids of two pairs of homologous chromosomes condensing. (C) Prometaphase. Centrosomes at opposite poles; spindle developing; chromatids condensed. (D) Metaphase. Spindle formation completed, and pairs of chromatids aligned on the equatorial plate. (E) Anaphase. Single chromatids moving to the poles. (F) Telophase. Two nuclei being reconstituted; cleavage furrow deepening in cytokinesis. (G) The two diploid cells produced.

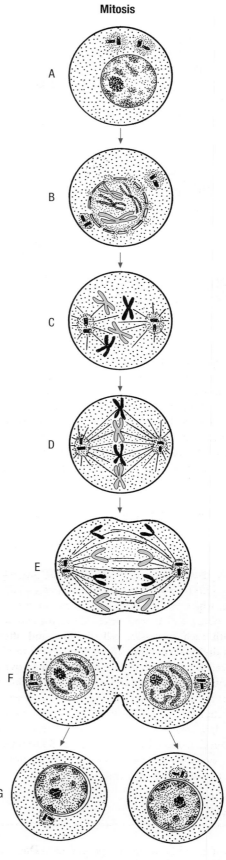

Mitosis

Two diploid cells

opposite poles of the spindle as the chromosomes of the two daughter cells (Fig.1.33E). **Telophase** of mitosis begins when the movement of chromosomes towards the poles ceases. The microtubules of the spindle depolymerize, and a nuclear envelope is assembled around each of the two groups of chromosomes. These undergo decondensation, and their DNA and associated histones coil and condense into heterochromatin. With the appearance of a nucleolus, the assembly of two interphase nuclei is complete. While these nuclear changes were in progress, a local polymerization of additional actin filaments, had resulted in a ring-like thickening of the cell cortex around the middle of the elongated cell. Actin–myosin interaction in this ring during telophase, forms a circumferential furrow (Fig.1.33F), which deepens and, ultimately, cleaves the elongated cell into two spherical daughter cells. The division of the cell into two by contraction of the encircling thickening of the cell cortex is called **cytokinesis**.

Just how the scattered pairs of chromatids of prometaphase are moved to the equatorial plate, and how they are moved to the poles in anaphase, has long puzzled cytologists. Clarification of the mechanisms of these movements has come with the recent identification of four of the motor proteins involved: **C-terminal kinesin**, **bipolar kinesin**, **chromokinesin**, and **dynein**. The movement of chromatids to the equatorial plate is believed to be brought about by one member of the large family of kinesins, called **chromokinesin**, which has a binding site for DNA at the tail end of the molecule that binds to one member of a pair of chromatids. The two heads of the motor domain, at the other end of the molecule, bind alternately to successive tubulin dimers in the wall of a microtubule and thus move the chromatids towards its plus-end, which is located at the site of the future equatorial plate (Fig.1.35).

The mitotic spindle is made up of three groups of microtubules: (1) **astral microtubules**, which radiate from each centrosome towards the plasma membrane at the ends of the dividing cell; (2) **kinetocore microtubules**, which extend inwards and attach to kinetochores of the pairs of chromatids; and (3) **interpolar microtubules**, which cross the equatorial plate, passing between the pairs of chromatids and extending some distance beyond the plate (Fig.1.35). Thus, the interpolar microtubules from opposite ends of the spindle overlap in a region on either side of the equatorial plate. Because the plus-ends of these overlapping parallel microtubules are pointed towards opposite poles, they are described as antipolar microtubules. In anaphase, antipolar microtubules are moved with respect to one another to elongate the spindle and move the pairs of chromatids apart. The motive force for this movement is provided by two co-operating, plus-end directed, motor proteins: **C-terminal kinesin**, and **bipolar kinesin**. Molecules of C-terminal kinesin bind, at their tail end, to an interpolar microtubule, and their two heads move from tubulin dimer to tubulin dimer along a protofilament in the wall of a neighboring interpolar microtubule of opposite polarity, moving the two microtubules in opposite directions. Bipolar kinesin is a symmetrical molecule with motor domains at both ends that bind to neighboring antipolar microtubules. The motor domains at both ends of the bipolar kinesin molecule are active. Therefore, it is more efficient than C-terminal kinesin in moving adjacent interpolar microtubules in opposite directions. By sliding antiparallel microtubules past one another, these plus-end motor proteins, move the spindle poles (and the attached chromatids) apart, and contribute to further elongation of the dividing cell. Some additional separation of the spindle poles is believed to be achieved by the minus-end-directed motor protein **dynein**, bound to actin filaments of the cell cortex and pulling astral microtubules towards the ends of the dividing cell. Whether shortening of the kinetochore microtubules, by depolymerization at their minus-end, is also involved in movement of the chromatids to the poles is still debated.

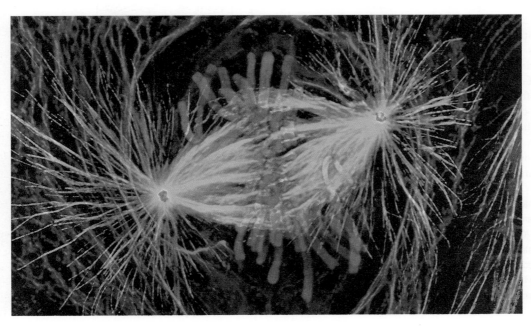

Figure 1.34 Photomicrograph of a dividing cell in metaphase, stained with immunofluorescent reagents: chromosomes, blue; spindle microtubules, green; centrosomes, magenta; and intermediate filaments, red. (Reproduced courtesy of MacMillan Magazines and A. Khodjakov from *Nature Rev, Mol Cell Biol* 2000; 1:246.)

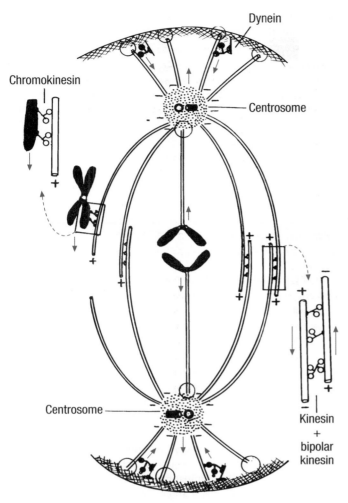

Dynein

Chromokinesin

Centrosome

Centrosome

Kinesin
+
bipolar
kinesin

Figure 1.35 Diagram of the spindle microtubules, and at upper left, the motor protein, chromokinesin, that moves the chromosoms to the equatorial plate. At the lower right, the motor proteins, kinesin and bipolar kinesin, that move the chromosomes apart.

Meiosis

In mitosis of a somatic cell, prior replication of the DNA in the S phase of the cycle, insures that both daughter cells of a mitotic division will receive 46 chromosomes. However, in the genesis of the gametes (ova and spermatozoa), the chromosome number must be reduced by half to prevent a doubling of the chromosome number at fertilization. This is accomplished by **meiosis**, a kind of cell division that occurs only in the production of the ova and spermatozoa. It consists of two successive divisions, **meiosis**-I and **meiosis**-II, which result in four daughter cells, each containing 23 chromosomes. The gametes are described as **haploid**, while the somatic cells, containing 46 chromosomes, are **diploid**.

In meiosis I, as in mitosis, replication of DNA has already occurred before onset of division, and each of the homologous chromosomes is represented by a pair of chromatids (Fig. 1.36B). In meiotic prophase, the two centrosomes migrate towards

opposite poles of the cell, the nuclear envelope disintegrates, and assembly of a spindle is begun (Fig. 1.36). In a later event, called **synapsis**, the pairs of conjoined chromatids derived from homologous chromosomes, come together on the equatorial plate to form groups of four chromatids, called **tetrads** (Fig. 1.36C). Within the tetrad, one member of each pair of chromatids is bound along its entire length to a member of the other pair, by a zipper-like protein structure called the **synaptonemal complex**. The other two chromatids of the tetrad are only attached to their partner at their centrosome. In anaphase of meiosis-I, the synaptonemal complex breaks down and pairs of chromatids move to opposite poles of the spindle (Fig. 1.36C). In telophase, cytokinesis divides the original cell into two diploid daughter cells, terminating the first phase of meiosis, **meiosis**-I (Fig. 1.36E). Before the chromosomes in the daughter cells have completed their decondensation, a second division, **meiosis**-II, is initiated in both daughter cells *without prior replication of DNA*. Therefore, at metaphase-II, pairs of chromosomes (instead of tetrads), become aligned on the equatorial plate (Fig. 1.36F), and in anaphase-II, the two chromosomes of each pair separate and move to opposite poles of the spindle. In telophase of meiosis-II, cytokinesis of the daughter cells of meiosis-I divides each of them into two cells that have only half the number of chromosomes present in the cell that entered meiosis-I (Fig. 1.36G). In summary, mitosis produces two **diploid** cells (46 chromosomes), while meiosis results in four **haploid** cells (23 chromosomes). The diploid number is restored in the fertilization of the ovum by a spermatozoon.

The movements of chromosomes in meiosis described above do not account for the diversity of physical features and personality traits observed among children of the same marriage. Before meiosis one member of each homologous pair of chromosomes came from the mother, and the other from the father. DNA replication before meiosis-I resulted in pairs of maternal chromatids and pairs of paternal chromatids that assembled to form tetrads. The orientation of those tetrads on the equatorial plate is random and microtubules from the poles of the spindle will attach to kinetochores of whichever chromatid happens to be oriented toward that pole. Thus, daughter cells of that division will have some paternal chromosomes and some maternal chromosomes, but their numbers may differ. Therefore, the gametes (spermatozoa or ova) developing from those cells will have different mixtures of the parental genomes.

There is another important source of genetic diversity resulting from meiosis. In the tetrads, one member of each pair of chromatids is attached, along its entire length, to a member of the other pair by the **synaptonemal complex**, but the other two chromatids of the tetrad are bound to their mate only at the centromere. The flexible free portions of these chromatids may bend across one another, and at such sites of crossing-over (**chiasmata**), they may fuse with one another, exchanging segments containing a number of genes. This random interchange of genome segments, occurring in some of the 23 tetrads results in widely differing proportions of maternal and paternal genes in the **recombinant chromosomes** of the daughter cells, and in the gametes that develop from them. Thus, it is not surprising that one child may have its mother's hair color and disposition, but

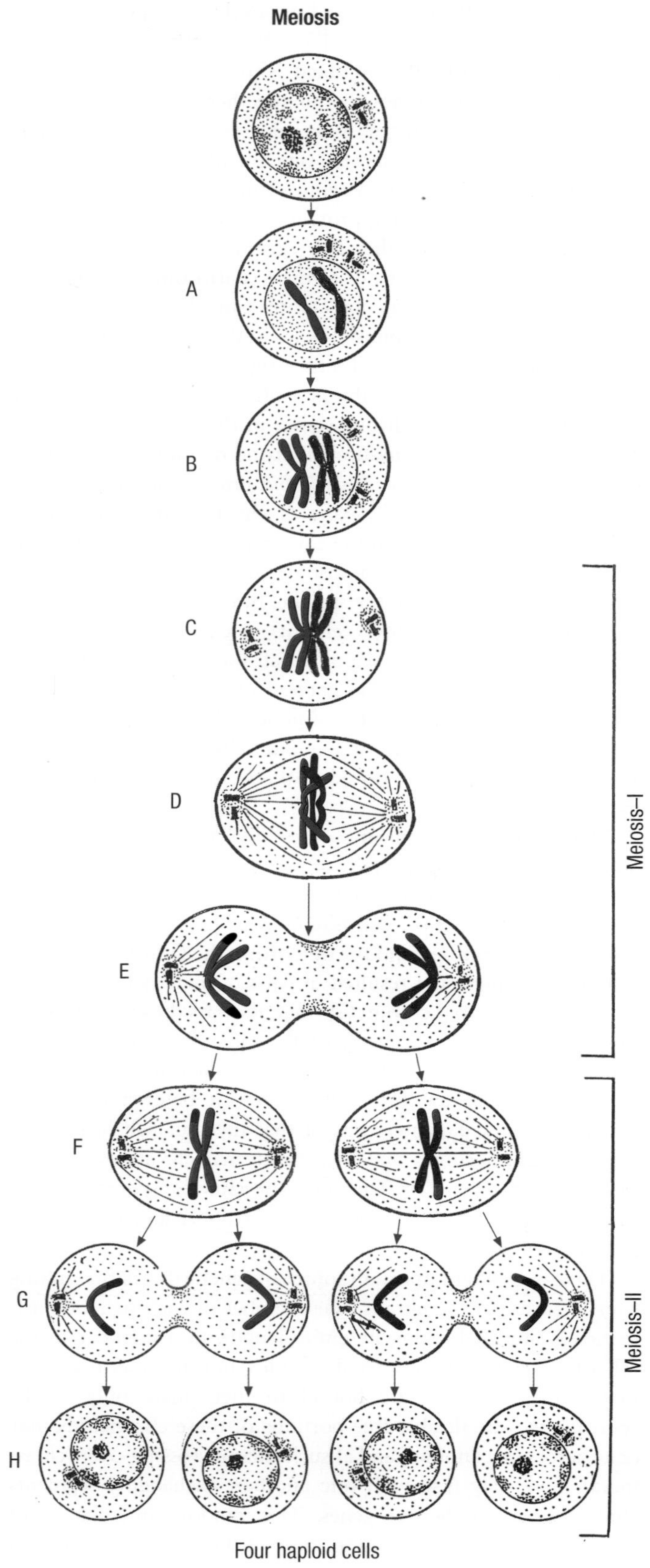

Meiosis

A

B

C

D

E

F

G

H

Meiosis-I

Meiosis-II

Four haploid cells

facial features resembling those of the father. Another child may have the mother's features but the father's disposition, etc.

Several developmental disorders of humans are attributable to errors during meiosis, with one or more of the chromosomes being distributed unequally to the daughter cells of meiosis-I. Individuals with **Down's syndrome** have three copies of chromosome 21, resulting in mongoloid features, short fingers, short stature, and mental retardation. In **Klinefelter's syndrome** there is an extra X chromosome (XXY) resulting in infertility, and mild mental retardation. Women with **Turner's syndrome**, have only a single X chromosome (XO) and their ovaries fail to develop.

CELL DEATH

Two different kinds of cell death are distinguished: **apoptosis** and **necrosis**. In the early stages of embryonic development, and in the subsequent remodeling of its tissues and organs, elimination of certain cells is an essential part of normal development. In postnatal life, the different cell types have lifespans ranging from a few days to 80 years, or more, and cell death is essential to eliminate senescent cells that are no longer able to carry out their normal functions. In both of these circumstances, death occurs by a process called **apoptosis** or **programmed cell death**. This is an active, energy-dependent, gene-directed process, a kind of cell suicide. An early biochemical event in the process is the activation of a specific endonuclease that cleaves the DNA between nucleosomes. The resulting short segments of DNA condense into conspicuous basophilic clumps in the nucleoplasm. The nucleus then breaks up into several fragments. Numerous small blebs appear on the surface of the cell body, and it soon breaks up into a number of small membrane-bounded globules. The fate of these is uncertain, for the involvement of macrophages that would be expected to destroy them is not evident.

Cell **necrosis**, on the other hand, is not a programmed process. It may result from anoxia, mechanical injury, invasion of the cell by viruses, exposure to toxins or to irradiation. The successive stages in this form of death are swelling, disintegration of the organelles, and lysis of the cell, followed by phagocytosis and digestion of the debris by macrophages.

Figure 1.36 Diagram of meiosis. (A) For simplification, only a single pair of homologous chromosomes is shown. (B) Pairs of chromatids resulting from DNA replication prior to onset of division. (C) Conjugation of chromatid pairs to form a tetrad. (D) Chromatids on the equatorial plate. (E) Separation of chromatid pairs, movement towards poles, and beginning of cytokinesis. (F) Daughter cells do not reconstitute a nucleus, but enter meiosis-II with chromatid pairs realigned on the equatorial plate. (G) Separation of the chromatids and completion of cytokinesis, resulting in four haploid daughter cells.

Questions

1 The motor protein kinesin moves vesicles along microtubules towards
   a the minus-end
   b the plus-end
   c either end
   d in neither direction
   e the centrosome

2 One of the functions of the Golgi complex is to
   a synthesize protein
   b nucleate polymerization of microtubules
   c synthesize lysosomal enzymes
   d process and package secretory products
   e synthesize carbohydrates

3 In cell motility actin generally interacts with
   a kinesin
   b dynein
   c myosin
   d fibronectin
   e laminin

4 During mitosis chromosomes are aligned in the middle of the spindle during
   a prophase
   b telophase
   c anaphase
   d metaphase
   e interphase

5 The microtubules of the mitotic spindle attach to
   a telomeres of chromosomes
   b kinetochores
   c synaptonemal complex
   d intermediate filaments
   e Golgi

6 In receptor-mediated endocytosis the membrane vesicles are initially enclosed in
   a calmodulin
   b clathrin
   c syndesmin
   d dystrophin
   e actin

7 The human female karyotype is
   a 24 XY
   b 48 XX
   c 44 XY
   d 44 XX
   e 23 XX

8 An enzyme involved in transcription is
   a DNA polymerase
   b ribonuclease
   c RNA polymerase
   d hyaluronidase
   e peptidase

9 Connexons are characteristic features of
   a the trans-Golgi network
   b the rough endoplasmic reticulum
   c the smooth endoplasmic reticulum
   d gap junctions
   e lysosomes

10 Synthesis of steroids and drug detoxification are functions of
   a rough endoplasmic reticulum
   b Golgi complex
   c smooth endoplasmic reticulum
   d mitochondria
   e perinuclear cisterna

11 What organelle belongs to the cytoskeleton of the cell?

12 Indigestible waste products of metabolism are stored as what?

13 Glucose derived from food is stored in what form?

14 What is the microtubule cytoskeleton of a cilium called?

15 What is the non-selective uptake of fluid in small membrane vesicles called?

16 What is the site of assembly of ribosomal subunits?

17 What is a group of ribosomes associated with a molecule of mRNA called?

18 What does the Golgi apparatus produce?

19 What motor protein is responsible for the bending movement of cilia?

20 Groups of three nucleotides that encode a particular amino acid are called what?

Epithelium

An **epithelium** is a continuous sheet of closely adherent cells covering a naturally occurring surface in the body. It may consist of a single layer of cells, or may have multiple layers. An epithelium forms a boundary layer that controls the movement of substances between the external environment and the interior of the body, or between its internal compartments. The epithelia of different organs may be made up of cells specialized for absorption, secretion, or ion transport. In all epithelia, the lowermost cells rest upon a thin, continuous supporting layer, the **basal lamina**, which comprises a very fine meshwork of filaments in an amorphous matrix.

CLASSIFICATION OF EPITHELIA

To lend precision to their description of organs, histologists have defined several types of epithelium, based upon the number of cell layers, the shape of the cells, and the presence or absence of specializations of the free surface. The student should be familiar with the defining characteristics of the several kinds of epithelium. An epithelium consisting of a single layer of cells is a **simple epithelium**; if there are multiple layers, it is a **stratified epithelium**. The modifiers *squamous*, *cuboidal* or *columnar* are added to indicate the shape of the cells. Thus, a single layer of flat cells is a **simple squamous epithelium**; a single layer of tall prismatic cells is a **simple columnar epithelium** (Fig. 2.1). If these cells have slender motile processes on their free surface, it is a **ciliated columnar epithelium**.

Simple epithelium

A simple **squamous** epithelium is made up of closely adherent cells that have a polygonal outline in surface view, and thus resemble a tiled floor. In sections perpendicular to the plane of the epithelium, the cells have a flat rectangular outline, or are fusiform (i.e. tapering towards either end) (Fig. 2.2A). Epithelium of this kind lines the thoracic, abdominal, and pericardial cavities of the body. In a simple **cuboidal** epithelium, the cells are polygonal in surface view, and, in section, have a rectangular or square outline (Fig. 2.2B). Such an epithelium lines the ducts of many glands and some of the tubules of the kidney. In simple **columnar** epithelium, the cells have a tall, narrow, rectangular profile, and their nuclei are all aligned at the same level (Fig. 2.2C). Occasional mucus-secreting **goblet cells** may be found among the non-secretory cells of the epithelium. In other simple columnar epithelia, all cells are secretory and their apical cytoplasm is filled with secretory granules (Fig. 2.2D).

Traditionally, histologists referred to an epithelium and its underlying connective tissue as either a **serous membrane**, or a **mucous membrane**. A simple squamous epithelium, and its supporting connective tissue, lining a body cavity was called a serous membrane. One that lined tubular organs that ultimately opened externally (e.g. the gastrointestinal tract) was called a mucous membrane. Regrettably, this terminology may still be encountered. However, reference to an epithelium and its underlying connective tissue as a 'membrane' is discouraged in order to avoid confusion with true membranes (lipid bilayers) that enclose the cell or its organelles. The preferred term for the simple squamous epithelium lining a body cavity is **mesothelium**,

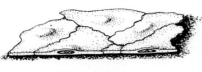

A   Simple squamous

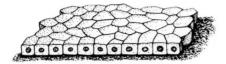

B   Simple cuboidal

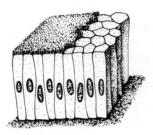

C   Simple columnar

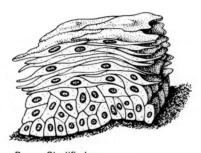

D   Stratified squamous

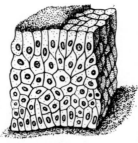

E   Stratified columnar

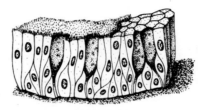

F   Pseudostratified columnar

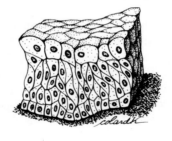

G   Transitional

Figure 2.1 Drawings illustrating the shape and arrangement of cells in the principal types of epithelium.

and for that lining blood vessels, **endothelium**. Neither of these terms includes the underlying connective tissue.

Stratified epithelium

In **stratified squamous epithelium** there are multiple layers, and the cell shape changes from the basal to the uppermost layer of the epithelium. Those at the base have a rounded or beveled upper side; the cells above this layer are irregularly polyhedral, but become increasingly flattened in successive layers and are flat (squamous) cells in the uppermost layer (Figs 2.1D, 2.2F). This type of epithelium constitutes the epidermis of the skin, and is found in the lining of the oral cavity, the esophagus, and the vagina. Cell division is limited to the cells of the lowermost layer, and the new cells formed move slowly upwards and are ultimately sloughed off at the surface of the epithelium. In the epidermis of skin on the palms of the hands and the soles of the feet, the cells synthesize increasing amounts of the fibrous protein **keratin** as they move upwards in the epithelium. This accumulates

to such an extent that the uppermost cells become dry, lifeless scales, which are continually shed from the surface (Fig. 2.2H). Such an epithelium is described as a **keratinized stratified squamous epithelium**.

In **stratified columnar epithelium**, the basal cells are cuboidal, or low columnar, and the cells of the upper row are tall columnar. The nuclei are aligned in two distinct rows. If the epithelium has more than two layers of cells, those intervening between the basal and upper layers vary in size and shape and there is no alignment of their nuclei (Figs 2.1E, 2.2B). This type of epithelium is uncommon, occurring only in the conjunctiva of the eye, the cavernous urethra, and in the large excretory ducts of some glands.

Pseudostratified epithelium

In **pseudostratified columnar epithelium**, all cells rest on the basal lamina, but some are columnar in form and extend upwards to the free surface, while others located between them have a tapering upper end, which extends only part way to the surface. The nuclei

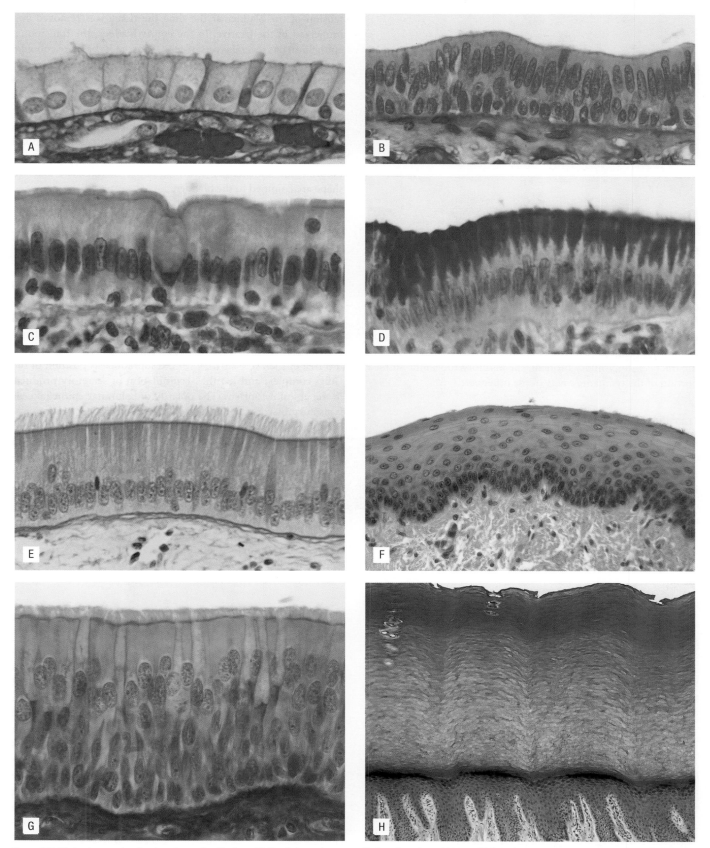

Figure 2.2 Photomicrographs of various types of epithelium. (A) Simple low columnar epithelium from duct of kidney. (B) Stratified columnar epithelium from duct of salivary gland. (C) Simple columnar epithelium of intestine. (D) Columnar epithelium of mucus-secreting cells. (E) Simple ciliated columnar epithelium. (F) Stratified squamous epithelium from esophagus. (G) Ciliated pseudostratified epithelium from trachea. (H) Keratinized stratified squamous epithelium from epidermis of the sole of the foot.

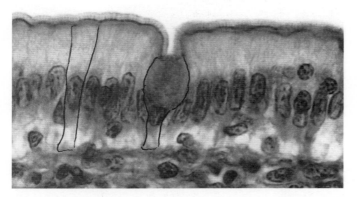

Figure 2.3 Columnar epithelium of intestine containing one goblet cell. Profiles of columnar cell and goblet cell outlined to show their shape.

of these two kinds of cells are aligned at different levels, creating a false impression of stratification (Figs 2.1F, 2.2G). This kind of epithelium is found in the male urethra and the duct of the parotid gland. **Ciliated pseudostratified epithelium** occurs in a portion of the trachea, the primary bronchi, the auditory tube, and lining a portion of the tympanic cavity of the inner ear.

Transitional epithelium

Transitional epithelium lines the urinary bladder, an organ that undergoes major changes in volume during its filling and emptying. A special kind of epithelium has evolved to permit these changes without interruption of its continuity. The appearance of this epithelium varies greatly, depending upon the degree of dis-

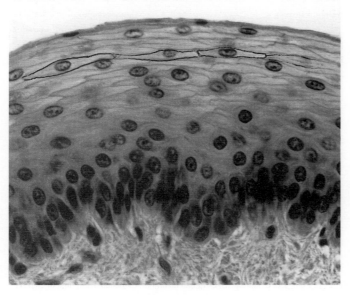

Figure 2.4 Stratified squamous epithelium. Three cells near the surface are outlined to show their shape and horizontal orientation.

tension of the bladder at the time the tissue was removed and immersed in the fixative. In the empty bladder, the transitional epithelium has several layers of cells. Those at its base are cuboidal and are overlain by two, or more, rows of polyhedral cells. The uppermost cells are much larger than the others and have a rounded free surface (Fig. 2.1G). The shape and number of layers of cells change during bladder filling. In the full bladder, there are only two layers of cells, a basal layer of cuboidal cells overlaid by a layer of large squamous cells. Transitional epithelium is found throughout the urinary tract, from the calyces of the kidneys to the urethra, but the changes described above in thickness and cell shape are confined to the bladder.

EPITHELIAL POLARITY

A cell is said to be **polarized**, if its functions are preferentially directed towards one end. Epithelial cells are polarized to carry out functions such as secretion of a product, or transepithelial movement of ions and small molecules. Morphological evidence of cell polarity is found in: (1) apical specializations that amplify the area of their free surface; (2) the supranuclear position of the Golgi complex; and (3) the accumulation of secretory products in the apical cytoplasm. The polarity of columnar epithelial cells is also expressed in the segregation of certain of their biochemical activities in functionally distinct portions of the plasma membrane, namely an **apical domain** and a **basolateral domain** (Fig. 2.5). The apical domain is especially rich in glycolipids, cholesterol, H^+/K^+-ATPase, and anion channels. The lateral portion of the basolateral domain contains proteins involved in attachment to neighboring cells, and in cell-to-cell communication. The basal portion of the basolateral domain also contains binding sites for constituents of the basal lamina, and receptors for hormones and other signaling molecules that regulate the function of the cell.

CELL COHESION

Maintenance of the cohesion and arrangement of cells in an epithelium is dependent upon a family of glycoproteins in the cell membranes, collectively called **cell adhesion molecules (CAM)**. One category of these, called **cadherins**, are responsible for the mutual recognition and cohesion of similar cells. In electron micrographs of columnar epithelial cells, their lateral surfaces appear to be separated by a very narrow intercellular space throughout most of their length. However, long carbohydrate chains of cadherin molecules in the membranes of neighboring cells extend into this space and bind to one another. In addition to cell cohesion dependent upon cadherin molecules, there are conspicuous local specializations of the opposing membranes that are collectively called **junctional complexes** (Fig. 2.6). These are of four kinds: the **zonula occludens**, **zonula adherens**, **desmosome**, and **gap junction**.

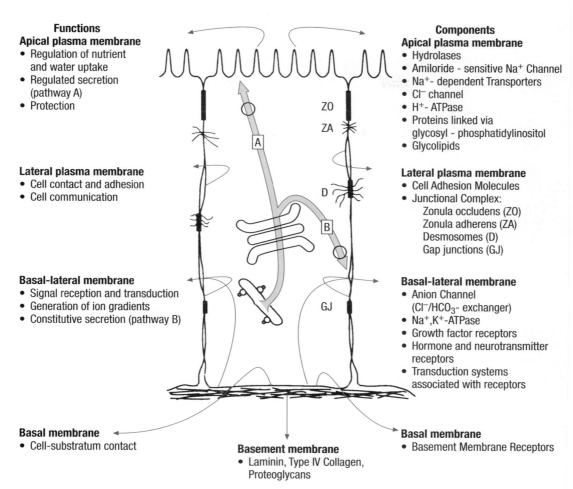

Functions
Apical plasma membrane
- Regulation of nutrient and water uptake
- Regulated secretion (pathway A)
- Protection

Lateral plasma membrane
- Cell contact and adhesion
- Cell communication

Basal-lateral membrane
- Signal reception and transduction
- Generation of ion gradients
- Constitutive secretion (pathway B)

Basal membrane
- Cell-substratum contact

Basement membrane
- Laminin, Type IV Collagen, Proteoglycans

Components
Apical plasma membrane
- Hydrolases
- Amiloride - sensitive Na$^+$ Channel
- Na$^+$- dependent Transporters
- Cl$^-$ channel
- H$^+$- ATPase
- Proteins linked via glycosyl - phosphatidylinositol
- Glycolipids

Lateral plasma membrane
- Cell Adhesion Molecules
- Junctional Complex:
   Zonula occludens (ZO)
   Zonula adherens (ZA)
   Desmosomes (D)
   Gap junctions (GJ)

Basal-lateral membrane
- Anion Channel (Cl$^-$/HCO$_3$- exchanger)
- Na$^+$,K$^+$-ATPase
- Growth factor receptors
- Hormone and neurotransmitter receptors
- Transduction systems associated with receptors

Basal membrane
- Basement Membrane Receptors

Figure 2.5 Diagram of the polarity of a columnar epithelial cell as expressed in functionally and biochemically distinct apical, lateral, and basal domains of the plasmalemma. (Reproduced from Rodriguez-Boulan and Nelson *Science* 1989; 245:718.)

Zonula occludens

The **zonula occludens** (or **tight junction**) is a belt-like membrane specialization that encircles the columnar cells just below the free surface of the epithelium. There, the intercellular space is narrowed and at several points the opposing membranes appear to fuse. Additional details of the structure of this region can be obtained from freeze-fracture preparations, in which the lipid bilayer of the membrane is cleaved, displaying either its inner half-membrane, called the P-face, or its outer half-membrane, the E-face. Electron micrographs of such preparations reveal, in the zonula occludens, a network of ridges or strands on the P-face of the membrane (Fig. 2.7). These strands, composed of a protein called **occludin**, correspond to the sites of apparent fusion of opposing membranes that are seen in electron micrographs of thin sections. Just how the networks in adjacent membranes are joined to one another is not yet certain. However, it is clear that the apices of all columnar cells of an epithelium are firmly bound together at the zonula occludens, and that the intercellular space is occluded by this junctional complex.

A columnar epithelium, such as that lining the gastrointestinal tract, constitutes a selectively permeable barrier between the lumen and the underlying blood vessels. It permits passage of some ions and small molecules and excludes others. There are two possible pathways across an epithelium: (1) the **transcellular pathway**, which involves the active uptake of substances at the free surface by pinocytosis, followed by transport of the vesicles across the cell and release of their content at the cell base; or (2) the **paracellular pathway**, in which molecules passively diffuse through the intercellular spaces of the epithelium. The zonula occludens is a means of closing the paracellular pathway and enabling the cells to exercise selectivity as to what passes across the epithelium. The zonula occludens also serves as a barrier between the apical and basolateral domains of the plasma membrane, preventing movement of integral proteins from one to the other.

Zonula adherens

Another junctional specialization, the **zonula adherens**, encircles the apical portion of the cells below the zonula occludens (Fig. 2.6). Here, the opposing cell membranes are 15–20 nm apart,

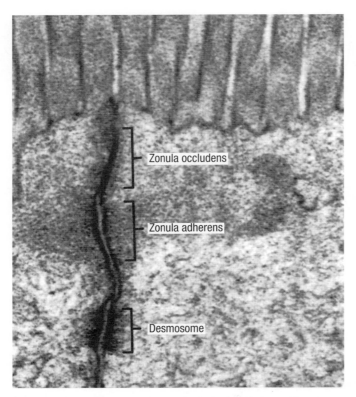

Figure 2.6 An electron micrograph of junctional complexes between adjacent epithelial cells. The zonula occludens, zonula adherens, and desmosome (macula adherens) are shown.

intramembranous components that distinguish this zone from other regions of the membrane. The most conspicuous feature of the zonula adherens, in electron micrographs, is the greater density of the cytoplasm adjacent to the junctional membranes. At high magnifications this is found to be caused by a dense mat of interwoven fine filaments. Some of these appear to continue inwards and mingle with those of the **terminal web**, a meshwork of cross-linked actin filaments that crosses the apex of the cell below the brush border. Histochemical staining methods have revealed the presence of myosin, α-actinin, and vinculin in the zonula adherens. These are believed to be involved in cross-linking its filaments and binding them to the membrane. The function of the zonula adherens is less apparent than that of the zonula occludens. It is certainly a site of cell-to-cell adherence, and it may have a role in stabilizing the epithelium by connecting the terminal webs of adjoining cells.

Desmosomes (macula adherens)

Other sites of cell cohesion are small, round, junctional specializations on the sides of adjoining epithelial cells, called **desmosomes** (Fig. 2.8). Their most conspicuous component, as seen on electron micrographs, is a dense plaque on the cytoplasmic sides of the opposing membranes, which are about 20 nm apart. A thin, dense line parallel to the membranes, and midway between them, can sometimes be seen. Very thin filaments, called **transmembrane linkers**, extend across the intercellular space and apparently bind the membranes and their associated dense plaques together. Bundles of intermediate filaments in the cytoplasm of adjoining cells terminate in the dense plaques of the desmosome. Thus, in addition to being sites of cell-to-cell attachment, the desmosomes

but very fine transverse striations between them are detectable at high magnification, and a specific cell adhesion molecule has been identified in the interspace. Freeze-fracture preparations reveal no

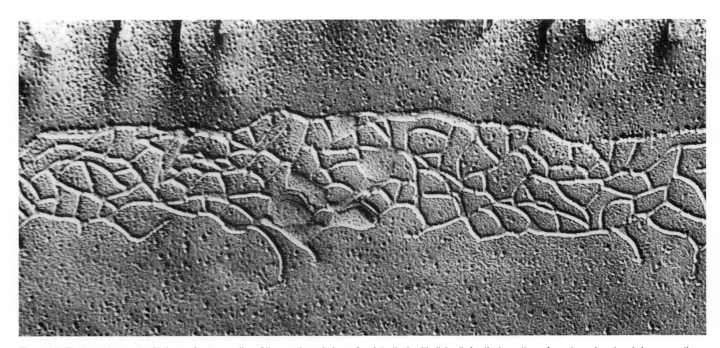

Figure 2.7 Electron micrograph of a freeze-fracture replica of the zonula occludens of an intestinal epithelial cell. A reticular pattern of anastomosing strands is seen on the P-face of the cleaved membrane, just below the brush border of the cell. (Micrograph courtesy of J.P. Revel.)

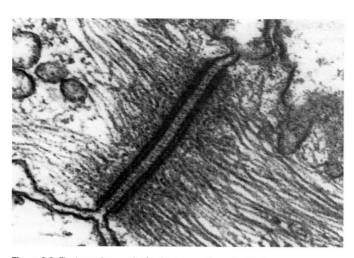

Figure 2.8 Electron micrograph of a desmosome from stratified squamous epithelium. Notice the intermediate filaments of the cytoskeleton terminating in the dense plaque of the desmosome. (Micrograph courtesy of D. Kelly.)

contribute to the stability of the epithelium as a whole by linking the cytoskeletons of adjoining cells.

In the stratified squamous epithelium of the skin, **hemidesmosomes** are regularly spaced along the cell membrane where it is in contact with the basal lamina. Hemidesmosomes are not found in simple squamous epithelium, simple columnar epithelium, or pseudostratified epithelium. The hemidesmosomes of the stratified squamous epithelium of the epidermis apparently enable this epithelium to withstand the blows and shearing stresses to

which the skin is exposed, without becoming separated from the basal lamina.

CELL COMMUNICATION

Gap junction (nexus)

The **gap junction**, or **nexus**, is a junctional complex that is primarily concerned with cell-to-cell communication. At this junction, the intercellular space is narrowed to about 3 nm and there is no increased density of the neighboring cytoplasm. Freeze-fracture preparations reveal a round area of closely packed particles called **connexons**, in the membrane of both cells (Fig. 2.9). Each of these consists of six protein particles, about 7 nm in diameter around a central pore 1.5–2.0 nm in diameter. Connexons of the opposing membranes project into the intercellular space, where they are linked end to end. Their central pores thus form a continuous channel, connecting the cytoplasm of the two cells. Ions, amino acids, cyclic AMP, and other molecules less than 2 nm in diameter would be able to pass freely through these channels. These connections are believed to permit coordination of the activities of cells throughout the epithelium. Gap junctions are not confined to epithelia. They are abundant in smooth and striated muscle, where they provide low resistance pathways through which excitation passes rapidly between cellular units, insuring their simultaneous contraction.

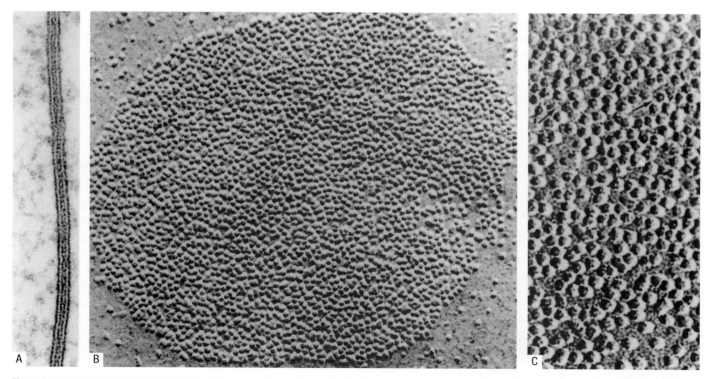

Figure 2.9 (A) Micrograph of a gap junction as it appears in section. No intercellular gap is seen between the two membranes. (B) Freeze-fracture replica of the P-face of a gap junction, showing the large number of particles within the membrane. (C) At higher magnification a small pore can be resolved in each particle, through which ions and small molecules can pass from cell to cell.

BASAL LAMINA

An extracellular layer found beneath all epithelia was formerly called the **basement membrane**. The term **basal lamina** is now preferred. It has two ill-defined layers 45–50 nm in thickness, with little visible substructure in either. The rather transparent layer adjacent to the epithelium, called the **lamina lucida**, is composed of molecules of a large proteoglycan, **laminin**, and an atypical **collagen** (type IV). The collagens, which are major structural components of the extracellular matrix throughout the body, polymerize to form filaments that assemble, in parallel, to form cross-striated fibers. The unusual type of collagen found in the inner layer of the basal lamina does not form filaments, but simply binds together laminin and other minor constituents of the lamina lucida. The outer layer of the basal lamina, called the **lamina densa**, is a meshwork of fine filaments of another uncommon type of collagen (type VII). Slender **anchoring fibers** of this collagen extend downwards from the basal lamina, looping around type I collagen fibers in the underlying extracellular matrix (Fig. 2.10). The anchoring fibers are especially numerous beneath the stratified squamous epithelium of the skin, but few anchoring fibers are found beneath the basal lamina of other epithelia that are less subject to shearing forces.

SURFACE SPECIALIZATIONS

The cells of the body are not simply building blocks of predetermined form, assembled according to some architectural design. They are dynamic living units capable of adapting their shape and internal structure for different functions. The solitary cells that migrate through the tissues must constantly change their shape in order to move over their substrate. The cells of differentiated epithelia are relatively immobile, but during their development they undergo shape changes that lead to a final form that is most favorable for their specific function. There are basic respiratory and nutritional requirements that are better served by some shapes than

by others. The vital exchange of O_2 and CO_2 between the cells and their extracellular environment takes place across the cell membrane. The efficiency of this exchange depends in large measure upon the surface area of plasma membrane in relation to cell volume. A cell with a large surface area can sustain a more active metabolism than one with less surface area. In this context, the shapes of cells have functional significance. Cells of the same volume, but differing in shape, also differ in surface area (Fig. 2.11). An ovoid cell has a greater surface area than a spherical cell, a columnar cell has more than a cuboidal cell, a squamous cell more than a columnar cell of the same volume. In epithelium viewed from above, the closely adherent cells have a pentagonal or hexagonal outline imposed by mutual deformation. Their lateral membranes, which are specialized for cohesion and cell-to-cell communication, are not directly exposed to the external environment. Therefore any modification of cell shape to amplify surface area for greater efficiency, takes place at the apical or basal surfaces.

Brush border

Under high magnification with the light microscope, some columnar epithelia have a refractile apical border, which exhibits fine vertical striations. On electron micrographs, this so-called **brush border** is found to be made up of closely spaced, slender, cell processes 1–2 μm long, and 80–90 nm in diameter, called **microvilli**. Very fine branching filaments extending from their tips may form a furry coat over the border, called the **glycocalyx** (Fig. 2.12). Its delicate filaments are terminal oligosaccharides of integral proteins of the membrane covering the tips of the microvilli. Each microvillus contains an axial bundle of 20–30 actin filaments, which are attached to the membrane at its tip, and extend downwards into the cytoplasm, where they mingle with the filaments of the terminal web. The filaments of this core bundle are bound together by slender transverse bridges, consisting of a polypeptide called **villin**. At regular intervals along its length, the core bundle of filaments is linked to the membrane by another protein, as yet unnamed.

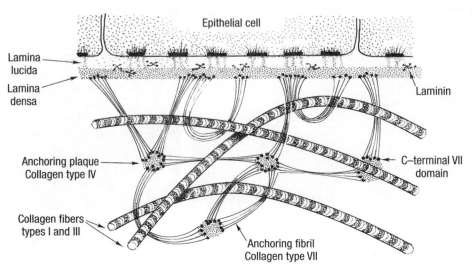

Lamina lucida

Lamina densa

Epithelial cell

Laminin

Anchoring plaque
Collagen type IV

C–terminal VII domain

Collagen fibers types I and III

Anchoring fibril
Collagen type VII

Figure 2.10 Drawing of the anchoring fiber network beneath a stratified squamous epithelium. The anchoring fibrils are believed to be aggregates of type VII procollagen molecules. They originate in the basal lamina and inset into anchoring plaques of type IV collagen. (Redrawn from D.R. Keene et al. *J Cell Biol* 1987; 104:611.)

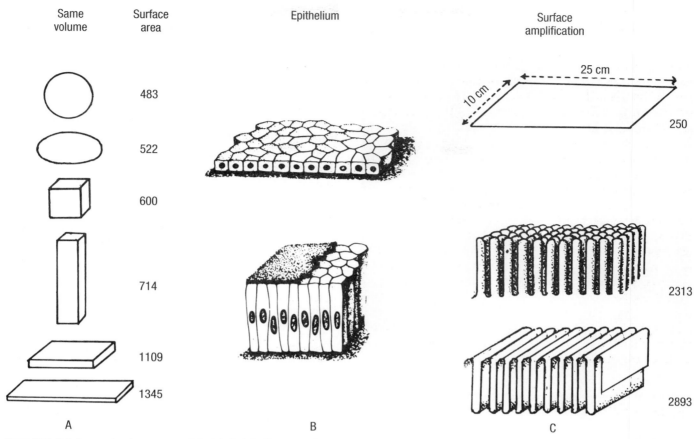

Same volume	Surface area	Epithelium	Surface amplification

Figure 2.11 Cell shape and surface area are of physiological significance. (A) Six figures of the same volume and their respective surface areas. (B) In columnar epithelia, only the apical and basal surfaces are directly exposed to the extracellular environment. (C) Surface area of a planar surface compared to an area of the same dimensions, bearing slender cylindrical projections, or narrow folds.

A brush border occurs on epithelia specialized for absorption; for example, on cells of the epithelium lining the intestine: the apical domain of their membrane is rich in enzymes that complete the digestion of carbohydrates, which began in the lumen. The microvilli of the brush border result in a 20- to 30-fold increase in the surface area of membrane exposed to the lumen of the intestine, and thus greatly increase the efficiency of the epithelium in absorption of nutrients. It is estimated that the total surface area of the intestinal epithelium is about 200 m², an area comparable to the floor space of an average house.

In epithelia specialized for rapid absorption of water and electrolytes, and their transport to the underlying capillaries (e.g. in the tubules of the kidney), the brush border is supplemented by **basal infoldings** of the plasmalemma, which further amplify its surface area. Mitochondria are lodged between the basal infoldings to provide the energy for active transport across the membrane.

Cilia

The **cilia**, described in Chapter 1, are motile cell processes 7–10 μm in length and 0.3 μm in diameter, which are present in great numbers on the free surface of certain epithelia. They execute to-and-fro oscillations at a rate of 10–17 times per second. Cilia may be present on all cells of an epithelium, or may occur only on small clusters of cells among many others that bear only short microvilli (Fig. 2.13). They are arranged in rows, and all beat in the same direction. Direct observation of their movement is unrewarding, but by using high speed cinematography, each cilium can be seen to stiffen on the rapid forward stroke and then bend and move back more slowly in the recovery stroke. Cilia on some protozoa have an **isochronal rhythm**, in which all beat synchronously, but on mammalian epithelia they have a **metachronal rhythm**, in which the cilia in successive rows start their beat in sequence. The cilia of each row are therefore slightly more advanced in their cycle than the cilia in the row behind. This results in waves of movement that can be seen sweeping over the epithelium, like the waves that run before the wind in a field of grain. The effect of this coordinated activity is to move a blanket of mucus and particulate matter along a tubular organ; for example, if pollen grains are placed on the layer of mucus on the epithelium of the trachea, at its bifurcation, the grains traverse the length of the trachea and reach the pharynx in about 6 min.

EPITHELIAL RENEWAL

Epithelial cells have a limited lifespan, and some are continually lost by exfoliation, or by programmed cell death, and are replaced

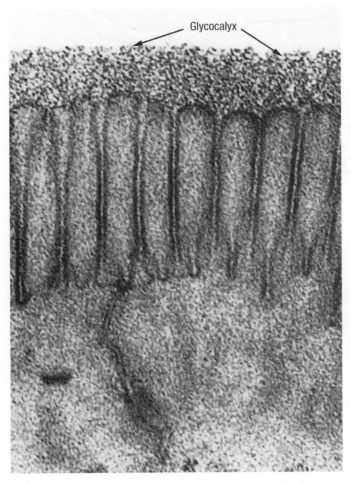

Figure 2.12 Electron micrograph of a few microvilli of the brush border of an intestinal epithelial cell, showing the glycocalyx.

by mitotic division of other cells. In some simple epithelia, all cells retain the ability to divide. In the development of a stratified epithelium, assembly of the cells into layers is followed by their

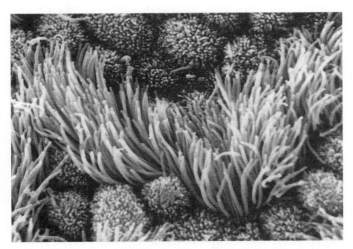

Figure 2.13 Scanning electron micrograph of the lumenal surface of a human oviduct showing the apical ends of ciliated and non-ciliated cells. The latter have short microvilli. (Reproduced from P. Gaddum-Rosse, R. Blandau and R. Tiersch, *Am J Anat* 1973; 138:269.)

differentiation (the acquisition of the biochemical machinery appropriate to their function). In this process, the majority of the cells lose their ability to divide. However, a few cells at the base of the epithelium remain undifferentiated and serve as **stem cells**. As needed, these undergo asymmetrical division yielding one daughter stem cell that remains on the basal lamina, and one daughter cell that differentiates as it moves up to replace a lost cell. In the repair of a gap in an epithelium caused by injury, the cells at the margins of the defect migrate over the denuded basal lamina to restore a single continuous layer of cells. Stem cells at the margins then proliferate and their daughter cells restore the epithelium to its original thickness.

Thin sheets of undifferentiated cells from the basal layer of the stratified squamous epithelium of human skin can now be grown *in vitro*, and these are commercially available to surgeons to hasten the healing process in badly burned patients in whom large areas of skin have been destroyed.

Stem cells are normally committed exclusively to production of cells of the kind making up the epithelium in which they reside, and are said to be **monopotential**. However, recent studies have shown that some stem cells can be transferred elsewhere and will give rise to differentiated cells of the host tissue. This suggests that some stem cells of adults are **pluripotential**. There is now great interest in transplanting stem cells from bone marrow or muscle to the brain to see whether they will replace the neurons lost in Alzheimer's disease, multiple sclerosis, and other degenerative diseases of the nervous system.

ABSORPTIVE EPITHELIA

The function of some organs requires an **absorptive epithelium** composed of cells specialized for uptake of ions and small molecules from the lumen, and their movement across the epithelium to the extracellular fluid beneath the basal lamina. Reference has already been made to the lining of the intestine as an example of such an epithelium. Glucose and amino acids in the intestinal lumen bind to **carrier proteins** in the membrane of the microvilli. These proteins then change their configuration to move these small molecules to the cytoplasmic side of the membrane. The entry of ions depends upon **channel proteins** that form small pores through which the ions are actively transported against their concentration gradient. The ions or molecules entering at the free surface then diffuse across the cell to the basolateral domain of the cell membrane, where they bind to integral carrier or channel proteins that move them out of the cell. Absorptive epithelia commonly have both a brush border and multiple infoldings of the basal cell membrane to increase their surface area.

SECRETORY EPITHELIA

The cells of **secretory epithelia** are specialized for the synthesis of a specific product and its release onto an external or internal surface. The cells typically contain an extensive rough endoplasmic reticulum (rER), which is the site of synthesis of the protein, or glycoprotein, cell product. This is transported, in small vesicles, from the rER to the Golgi complex and, after further processing in this organelle, it is concentrated and packaged into membrane-bounded **secretory granules** (Fig. 2.14). These accumulate in the apical cytoplasm until a signal is received to release their content by fusion of their membrane with the apical domain of the plasmalemma. Organs composed mainly of secretory epithelium are called **glands**.

Exocrine glands

Glands that deliver their secretion onto the surface of an external or internal surface of the body are called **exocrine glands**. Solitary secretory cells may be found widely distributed among the absorptive cells of an epithelium such as that lining the small intestine. These are called **goblet cells** because they have a narrow basal region and a greatly expanded apical region, containing stored secretory product. Goblet cells can be considered unicellular glands. Multicellular glands range in size from simple tubular invaginations of a surface epithelium (e.g. the sweat glands) to large organs (e.g. the pancreas). The secretory units of glands may be **tubules** lined by secretory epthelial cells, or they may be made up of pyramidal secretory cells arranged around a small lumen to form a spherical **acinus** (Fig. 2.15). The acini are usually located at the ends of a branching system of small **ducts** that converge upon a single larger duct which opens into the intestinal lumen (in the pancreas), or into the oral cavity (in the salivary glands). The

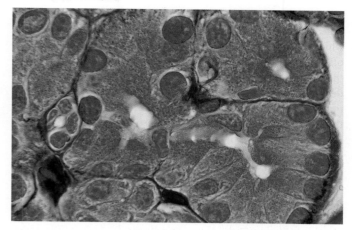

Figure 2.15 Photomicrograph of three acini, consisting of pyramidal glandular cells around a small lumen.

epithelium lining the ducts is not secretory but it may concentrate the secretory product of the glandular cells during its passage through the duct system.

Glands are classified according to the arrangement of their ducts and secretory units. Those that have a single unbranched duct are termed **simple glands**; those with a highly branched duct system are **compound glands**. Modifiers are added to indicate whether the secretory portion is straight, coiled, or branched: **simple tubular**, **simple coiled tubular**, or **simple branched tubular**. If the secretory units of the gland are acini, they are named according to the configuration of their duct system: **simple acinar**, or **branched acinar**. Not uncommonly, the secretory units at the ends of a branching system of ducts are short tubules that have acini along their sides and at their ends. Such glands are described as **compound tubuloacinar glands** (Fig. 2.16).

Different types of glands may be classified more simply according to the physical properties of their secretory product. Glands

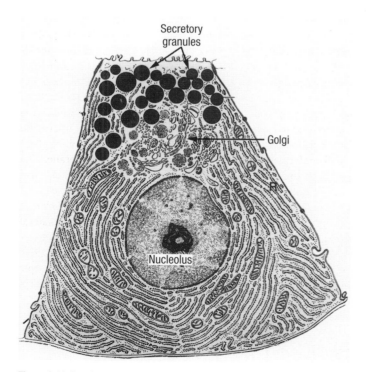

Figure 2.14 Drawing of a typical glandular cell. Note the extensive rough endoplasmic reticulum, a supranuclear Golgi complex and dense secretory granules in the apical cytoplasm.

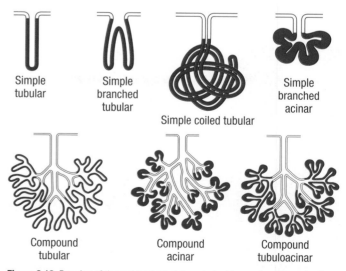

Figure 2.16 Drawing of the architecture of the principal types of exocrine glands. The portion consisting of secretory cells is shown in black. The glands in the lower row are depicted at lower magnification than those above. (Redrawn after L.C. Junquiera, J. Carniero, and R.O. Kelly, *Basic Histology*, 7th edn. Appleton and Lange.)

that produce a viscous surface layer of mucopolysaccharide are called **mucous glands**. Others that produce a watery secretion, which is often rich in enzymes, are described as **serous glands**. Still others are **mixed glands**, in which a mucous product is made by the acini, and a watery secretion is added by cells in **serous demilunes**, which are crescentic cap-like structures over one side of each acinus. Finally, different glands may be characterized by the way in which they release their product. If their product is released by fusion of the membrane of secretory granules with the cell membrane, it is called a **merocrine gland**. The great majority of glands fall into this category. If whole cells are exfoliated and the secretion consists of residues of those cells as well as the product they have synthesized, it is called a **holocrine gland**. The only example of holocrine secretion, in the human, is in the sebaceous glands of the skin. If the secretory cells pinch off their apical portion containing the secretory product, it is an **apocrine gland**. The only example of apocrine secretion, in the human, is in the mammary gland, where a portion of the cell membrane and a film of cytoplasm surrounding a very large lipid droplet, are pinched off from the cell body. The protein constituents of the milk are contributed by other cells exhibiting merocrine secretion.

Endocrine glands

Endocrine glands do not deliver their secretion through a system of ducts; their product is a protein, or steroid **hormone** that is released into the surrounding extracellular fluid and diffuses into the blood, which carries it to distant target organs that have specific receptors for that hormone. The cells of most endocrine glands do not form sheets, tubules or acini, but are simply compact aggregations of cells permeated by a dense network of capillary blood vessels.

Endocrine glands may be separate organs (e.g. thyroid and adrenal glands), or they may consist of small islands of endocrine cells scattered through the parenchyma of an exocrine gland (e.g. the islets of Langerhans of the pancreas, and the Leydig cells of the testis). In some endocrine cells, their product is released at the same rate that it is synthesized, and they do not accumulate secretory granules in the cytoplasm. Other endocrine cells do contain a few small secretory granules. The major endocrine glands are the hypophysis, thyroid, adrenals, ovaries, and testes. Their microscopic structure will be considered in Chapter 19.

Questions

1 One of the principal biochemical constituents of the basal lamina is
   a collagen type I
   b collagen type II
   c collagen type III
   d collagen type IV
   e collagen type V

2 The cell junction specialized for cell–cell communication is called a
   a zonula adherens
   b zonula occludens
   c gap junction
   d macula adherens
   e hemidesmosome

3 Which phrase best defines a serous membrane?
   a contains mesothelium with underlying connective tissue
   b contains glands but no connective tissue
   c contains goblet cells and connective tissue
   d generally has a brush-bordered epithelium with a basement membrane
   e lines all organs of the body

4 Organs subject to large changes in volume are likely to have
   a stratified columnar epithelium
   b stratified squamous epithelium
   c pseudostratified columnar epithelium
   d transitional epithelium
   e simple cuboidal epithelium

5 Which cell type lines blood vessels?
   a simple cuboidal epithelium
   b mesothelium
   c pseudostratified columnar epithelium
   d stratified squamous epithelium
   e endothelium

6 Stratified squamous epithelia subject to abrasion are rich in
   a vimentin
   b ankrin
   c keratin
   d desmin
   e filamin

7 Secretion, in which an apical portion of the cell becomes the secretory product, is called
   a merocrine
   b holocrine
   c apocrine
   d endocrine
   e exocrine

8 What lines the natural free surfaces of tissue that is in contact with the exterior?
   a mucosa
   b serous membrane
   c endothelium
   d serosa
   e mesothelium

9 The epithelial cell modification most suitable for vastly increasing the absorptive surface of that cell is the
   a cilium
   b microvillus
   c stereocilium
   d goblet cell
   e desmosome

10 Which phrase best defines cilia?
   a are found in the esophagus
   b are non-motile
   c are significantly smaller than microvilli
   d significantly increase the absorptive surface of cells
   e are adapted to move luminal material

11 What type of epithelium lines the esophagus?

12 What cell type may be observed in both mesothelium and endothelium?

13 What tissue lines the peritoneal cavity?

14 What is the term for the band-like impermeable junctional specialization that surrounds the columnar cell near its apex?

15 What type of epithelium lines the bronchi of the lungs?

16 What is the name of the epithelial membrane specialization involving two attachment plaques on adjacent cells?

17 What type of epithelium lines the trachea?

18 What type of epithelium lines the urinary bladder?

19 What is the term for the cytoskeleton of the cilium?

20 Connexons are components of what type of junction?

Chapter three

Blood

Blood is made up of several kinds of cells suspended in a fluid matrix, the **blood plasma**. Its cells are divided into three major categories: **erythrocytes** (red blood cells), **leukocytes** (white blood cells), and **platelets**. Unlike the cells of epithelia, the blood cells are unattached and make no enduring contact with one another. Blood circulates in the blood vessels to maintain logistical support and communication between all other tissues of the body. It distributes oxygen from the lungs and nutrients from the gastrointestinal tract. It carries carbon dioxide from the tissue back to the lungs for exhalation, and nitrogenous wastes from the tissues to the kidneys for excretion. It also plays an essential role in integrating the functions of the organs, by carrying hormones from their site of production to their distant target tissues.

A knowledge of the normal form and number of the several kinds of blood cells is important to physicians, for no tissue is examined more often for diagnostic purposes. Examination of stained blood-smears not only yields information about diseases that primarily affect the blood, it also provides indirect evidence of viral, bacterial, or parasitic infections, and thus enables the physician to follow the course of the infection and evaluate the effectiveness of treatment.

ERYTHROCYTES

Erythrocytes are minute anucleate corpuscles that impart a red color to the blood because they contain the oxygen-carrying pigment, **hemoglobin**. They number from 5.1×10^6 to $5.8 \times 10^6/mm^3$ in the male, and from 4.3×10^6 to $5.2 \times 10^6/mm^3$ in the female. In total, they present a surface area of $3800\,m^2$ (about the size of a football field) for gas exchange. The function of the erythrocytes is transport of oxygen (O_2) and carbon dioxide (CO_2). As blood passes through the capillaries of the lung, oxygen binds to the hemoglobin of the erythrocytes, converting it to **oxyhemoglobin**, which gives arterial blood its bright pink color. An erythrocyte contains about 250 million molecules of hemoglobin, each binding four molecules of oxygen, so each erythrocyte is able to transport about a billion molecules of oxygen. As they pass through the peripheral capillaries, O_2 is released and diffuses into the tissues. Concurrently, CO_2 diffuses from the tissues into the blood, combining with hemoglobin to form the **carbaminohemoglobin**, which imparts a bluish color to the venous blood. In the lungs, the CO_2 dissociates from the hemoglobin, diffuses into the air spaces and is eliminated in exhalation.

Erythrocytes develop in the bone marrow from nucleated precursor cells, but before they enter the blood, the nucleus and organelles are extruded and they are reduced to membrane-limited corpuscles. Hemoglobin accounts for 30% of their weight. Their shape is best described as a biconcave disc 7.6–$7.8\,\mu m$ in diameter. Their thickness is $1.9\,\mu m$ near their periphery and somewhat less at their center (Fig. 3.1). This shape is well adapted to their function of gas exchange for it presents a surface area 20–30% greater than that of a sphere of the same volume.

In blood-smears, the great majority of the erythrocytes stain pink, but a small number that have only recently entered the blood from the bone marrow have a bluish or greenish tint as a result of the basophilic staining of residual ribosomes in their cytoplasm. Such erythrocytes are commonly called **reticulocytes**, because, when stained with Brilliant Cresl Violet, their ribosomes are precipitated by the dye into a delicate basophilic network in an otherwise acidophilic cytoplasm. Within 24 h of entering the

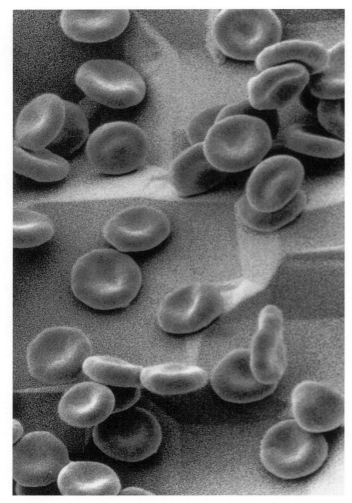

Figure 3.1 A scanning electron micrograph of erythrocytes, showing their biconcave discoid shape (color added). (Micrograph courtesy of David Scharf, copyright Peter Arnold, Inc.)

by **actin**. Actin in erythrocytes does not form filaments as it does in the cytoskeleton of other cells. Instead, it forms very short polymers, only 7 nm in length. These bind to **tropomyosin**, forming nodal structures that join the ends of the spectrin filaments together to form a network beneath the erythrocyte membrane. Near the middle of each spectrin filament there is a binding site for a phosphoprotein called **ankyrin**, which links the network to integral proteins of the cell membrane. This simple cytoskeleton helps to maintain the shape of the erythrocytes while, at the same time, giving them the resilience necessary to resist the frequent deformations to which they are subjected in thousands of passages through small vessels of the vascular system.

Departures from the normal size and shape of erythrocytes are found in certain kinds of anemia. Those in which all erythrocytes have a diameter greater than 9μm are described as **macrocytic anemias**, and those in which they are smaller than 6μm are **microcytic anemias**. The term **anisocytosis** is used to describe a finding of large numbers of erythrocytes of varying size.

The membrane of human erythrocytes contains certain integral glycoproteins that are antigens (substances causing a severe immune response if transfused into another person). Two of these are designated **antigen A** and **antigen B**, and are the basis of the **ABO blood-group typing system**. The erythrocytes of some individuals have antigen A on their membrane, others have antigen B, others have both, and still others have neither. Thus, there are four major blood groups **A**, **B**, **AB**, and **O**. For reasons that are not entirely clear, all individuals have, in their blood plasma, antibodies against the antigens that do not occur on their own erythrocytes. Therefore, before giving a transfusion it is necessary to determine which antigens occur on the erythrocytes of the donor, and which antibodies are present in the plasma of the recipient. Failure to carry out this cross-matching may result in a massive intravascular agglutination and lysis of erythrocytes in the recipient of the transfusion.

blood, they lose their basophilia. In the adult human, the number of reticulocytes averages about 8% of the total erythrocyte population. The **reticulocyte count** is used clinically as a rough measure of the rate of new erythrocyte production. In patients with anemia, an elevated reticulocyte count is an encouraging sign of response to treatment.

> **Anemia** is the term applied to a significant reduction in the total number of erythrocytes, or in their content of hemoglobin, resulting in reduced oxygen-carrying capacity of the blood. A deficient dietary intake of the iron needed to synthesize hemoglobin may result in **iron-deficiency anemia**. Deficiencies of vitamin B$_{12}$ or folic acid may lead to **megaloblastic anemia**, in which there is a retarded production of erythrocytes and those produced are of greater than normal size.

Examination of thin sections of erythrocytes under the electron microscope reveals the structural elements that maintain their unusual biconcave shape. Immediately beneath the membrane there is a so-called **membrane skeleton**, a network made up of filaments of **spectrin** 200 nm in length, bound together at their ends

BLOOD PLATELETS

Blood platelets are very small, colorless corpuscles 2–3 μm in diameter. They are ovoid in surface view and fusiform in longitudinal section (Fig. 3.2). They are present in the blood of all mammals, and in the human they number from 200 000 to 400 000/m³ of blood. In stained blood smears, they exhibit two concentric zones: a thin, pale peripheral zone, the **hyalomere**, and a darker central region, the **granulomere**. The latter contains small granules. Blood platelets are essential for the clotting of the blood to limit bleeding after injury. Their numbers are regulated by a hormone, **thrombopoietin**.

Inactive platelets

Electron micrographs of equatorial sections of a platelet reveal a circumferential band of 10–15 microtubules in the hyalomere immediately beneath the membrane. In cross-sections, these appear as a cluster of small circular profiles at either end of the platelet (Fig. 3.2).

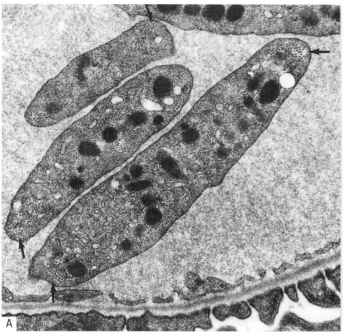
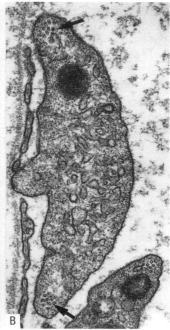

Figure 3.2 (A) Electron micrograph of platelets. The arrows indicate cross-sections of a bundle of circumferential microtubules that maintain the flat shape of the platelets. (B) Cross-sections of microtubules are more clearly visible in this platelet adjacent to the wall of a fenestrated capillary. ((A) Courtesy of D. Bainton. (B) Courtesy of Daniel Friend.)

The hyalomere contains no other visible elements, but the presence of actin and myosin can be demonstrated by histochemical methods. The actin is normally present in monomeric form, but when platelets are activated in the clotting process, it polymerizes into filaments that are necessary for contraction of platelets in clot formation. In electron micrographs, small aggregations of glycogen may be found in the granulomere. There are also small membrane-limited canaliculi that traverse the hyalomere to open at several sites on the surface of the platelet. These are believed to serve as pathways for discharge of secretory products of activated platelets. The most conspicuous components of the granulomere are small granules. These are called **alpha granules** and they correspond to the azurophilic granules that are seen in platelets under the light microscope. They contain several substances that have important functions in blood clotting: (1) **platelet factor IV**, which counteracts the anticoagulant effect of heparin; (2) **von Willebrand's factor**, a glycoprotein that promotes the adhesion of platelets to sites of injury in the wall of blood vessels; (3) **platelet-derived growth factor**, which initiates the process of repairing the damaged blood vessel; (4) **thrombospondin**, a glycoprotein responsible for platelet aggregation and adhesion in the clotting process. The platelets of some species also contain **beta granules**, which store serotonin and other molecules that are potent promoters of platelet aggregation.

Activated platelets

Platelets in the circulating blood continually patrol the vascular system to detect any damage to the lining of the blood vessels. The magnitude of their mission is evident from the estimate that each minute approximately 10^{11} platelets pass over 1000 m of capillary surface, lined by 7×10^{11} endothelial cells. They normally show no tendency to adhere to one another or to the vessel wall, but if any break in the endothelial lining is detected, they adhere to it, and to

one another, to initiate formation of a blood clot. Platelets also adhere to collagen fibers of connective tissue exposed at the site of injury, via specific receptors in their membrane. Adhesion activates the platelets, causing them to release a glycoprotein that is a potent inducer of platelet aggregation, resulting in adhesion of many more platelets to those already bound to the site of injury. These events lead to formation of a **platelet thrombus**, a semisolid mass of platelets that partially occludes the lumen of the blood vessel (Fig. 3.3).

Concurrent with platelet aggregation, other complex reactions of the clotting process are set in motion. A complex called **prothrombin activator** and other substances released by injured cells initiate a series of reactions in the blood plasma that convert **prothrombin** to **thrombin**. This, in turn, catalyzes conversion of a

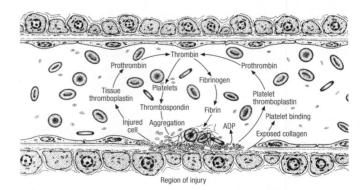

Figure 3.3 Schematic representation of early events in formation of a blood clot in an injured blood vessel. Platelets adhere to the site and release ADP and adhesive glycoproteins, which results in platelet aggregation. Thromboplastin from the damaged cells of the vessel wall converts prothrombin to thrombin, which catalyzes polymerization of fibrin from plasma fibrinogen. Fibrin filaments enmesh platelets and erythrocytes to form a gelatinous clot.

constituent of plasma called **fibrinogen** to **fibrin**, which polymerizes to form a network of fibrils among the aggregated platelets (Fig. 3.4). This binds the platelets together in a gelatinous **blood clot** (or **thrombus**) that prevents further outflow of blood from the injured blood vessels.

Pathological changes in the endothelium lining a coronary artery of the heart may cause platelet adhesion and formation of a clot that occludes its lumen, resulting in a 'heart attack.' A number of inherited diseases result from platelet abnormalities, or from a deficiency of one of the plasma proteins that are involved in blood clotting.

> **Hemophilia** is an inherited defect in factor VIII, one of the clotting factors. Daughters of hemophiliacs are carriers, and the sons of such carriers have a 50% chance of inheriting the disease. These patients bleed into muscles, joints and body cavities for days after an injury. Surgery and even dental extraction must be carried out with extreme care to prevent excessive bleeding.

LEUKOCYTES

Leukocytes (white blood cells) include several cell types involved in the defense of the body against invasion by bacteria, viruses, parasites, and foreign proteins. They are classified as, **granular leukocytes (granulocytes)**, or **agranular leukocytes**, depending upon the presence or absence of specific granules visible in their cytoplasm in stained blood-smears. There are three types of granular leukocytes, **neutrophils**, **eosinophils**, and **basophils**, and two types of agranular leukocytes, **monocytes** and **lymphocytes** (Fig.3.5). Leukocytes spend a relatively small fraction of their lifespan in the circulation. Neutrophils and eosinophils spend no more than 2 days in the blood, and lymphocytes less than 1 day, before migrating across the wall of capillaries into the surrounding tissues. They are spherical and inactive in the blood, but exhibit varying degrees of ameboid motility as they wander over the solid substrate afforded by the collagen fibers of the connective tissues.

The number of leukocytes in the circulation ranges from 5000 to 9000/mm³ of blood. This number varies somewhat with the age of the individual, and even with the time of day. The much larger number in the tissues and organs cannot be quantified. Minor variations in the numbers of leukocytes are of little clinical significance, but if there is an infection anywhere in the body, the blood leukocyte count may rise to 20 000–40 000/mm³. The relative numbers of the several kinds of leukocytes, the so-called **differential leukocyte count**, are normally fairly constant: neutrophils 55–60%; eosinophils 1–3%; basophils 0.0–0.7%; lymphocytes 25–30%; monocytes 3–7%. Different diseases affect the number of certain types more than others, and therefore the differential leukocyte count may be helpful in making a diagnosis.

GRANULAR LEUKOCYTES

Neutrophilic leukocytes

Polymorphonuclear leukocytes (**neutrophils**), are the most abundant of the granular leukocytes. They number 3000–6000/mm³ and 20 × 10⁶ or more in the entire circulation. They are 7 μm in diameter in blood-smears and are easily recognized by their unusual nucleus, which has two to four lobules connected by narrow constrictions (Figs 3.5A, 3.6). Neutrophils, that have only recently entered the circulation from the bone marrow, have a simple elongated nucleus with no constrictions. These are referred to as **band forms**. An increase in the number of band forms in a differential leukocyte count suggests that the number of neutrophils is increasing in response to an infection. In the neutrophils of the human female, the chromatin representing the X chromosome, may form an additional minute lobule that is often referred to as the 'drumstick' because of its characteristic shape. Thus, it is possible to determine the sex of an individual by examining a large number of neutrophils for the presence, or absence, of this nuclear appendage.

A small Golgi complex is found between the lobules of the nucleus and there are a few mitochondria. Small clusters of glycogen granules are not uncommon. The cytoplasm of neutrophils is stippled with numerous small granules of two kinds: the **specific granules**, which have little affinity for dyes, and the **azurophilic granules**, which are slightly larger and stain more deeply.

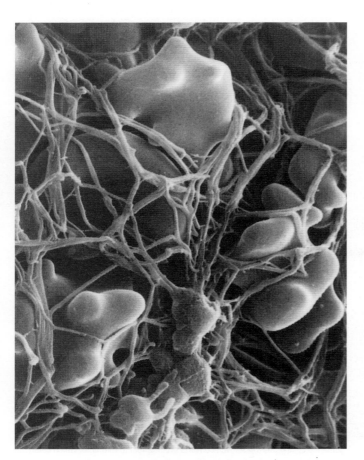

Figure 3.4 Scanning micrograph of a forming blood clot showing crenated erythrocytes and platelets in a meshwork of fibrin.

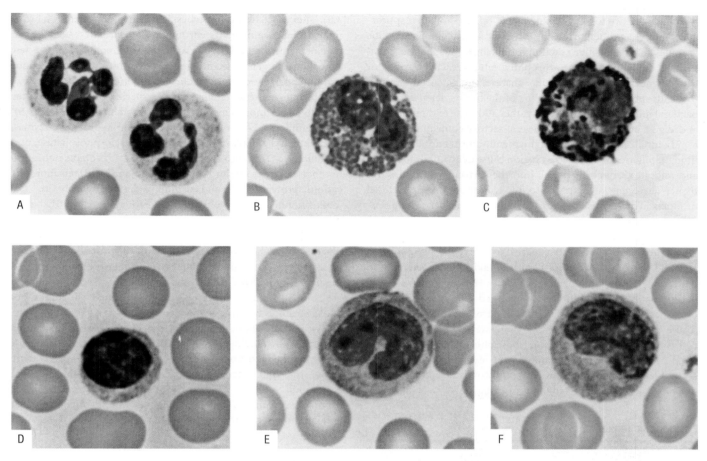

Figure 3.5 Photomicrographs of the leukocytes as they appear in blood-smears. (A) Neutrophilic leukocyte. (B) Eosinophilic leukocyte. (C) Basophilic leukocyte. (D) Lymphocyte. (E,F) Monocytes.

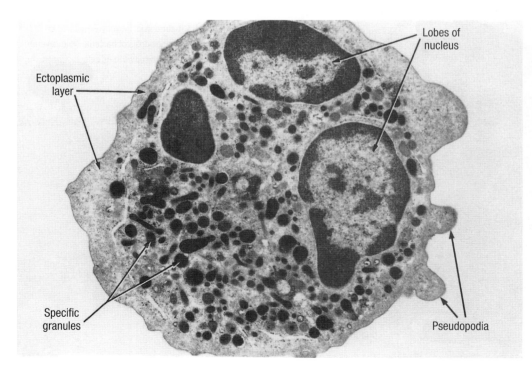

Figure 3.6 Electron micrograph of a polymorphonuclear leukocyte (neutrophil). Thin sections create the erroneous impression that this cell is multinucleate. The three lobes shown here are continuous with one another in other planes of section.

Although the two kinds of granules are rather similar in appearance, they react differently to histochemical reagents. The specific granules show a positive reaction for alkaline phosphatase, collagenase, and lysozyme. The azurophil granules react positively for the enzymes peroxidase, acid phosphatase, and glucuronidase.

Neutrophils are in the front line of the body's defenses against bacterial infections. They rapidly gather at the site and phagocytize and digest bacteria (Fig. 3.7). Several factors contribute to their rapid mobilization. Changes in the membrane of endothelial cells lining capillaries in the infected region cause neutrophils to adhere and migrate through their wall into the surrounding connective tissue. There they are exposed to low concentrations of bacterial products. Their cytoskeleton is reorganized and becomes polarized for migration towards the source of those products. Migration up the concentration gradient of a chemoattractant is called **chemotaxis**. When they reach the source they stop migrating and become avidly phagocytic, taking in bacteria and destroying them with lysosomal enzymes (Fig. 3.7). Mobilization of circulating neutrophils is augmented by their release of cytokines, which are carried in the blood from the site of infection to the bone marrow, where they stimulate release of additional neutrophils into the blood to join those already at the site of bacterial invasion. The **inflammatory exudate** ('pus') that accumulates at such a site consists mainly of dead and dying neutrophils that have completed their mission.

Eosinophilic leukocytes

Eosinophilic leukocytes (**eosinophils**) are 9 μm in diameter in suspension and about 12 μm in diameter in blood-smears. They are easily distinguished from neutrophils by their larger specific granules, which stain pink with Wright's blood stain (Figs 3.5B,

3.8). Their nucleus has two lobes, which are connected by a broad intermediate segment. Its chromatin pattern is less coarse than that of neutrophils. There is a small Golgi complex and a few mitochondria. The specific granules are the most conspicuous component of the cytoplasm. On electron micrographs, these vary in appearance in different mammalian species. In the human, they contain one or more dense crystals in a less dense matrix (Fig. 3.8). The granules of eosinophils contain several hydrolytic enzymes, including aryl sulfatase, β-glucuronidase, acid phosphatase, and ribonuclease. They also contain three cationic proteins not found in other cell types, **major basophilic protein (MBP)**, **eosinophilic cationic protein (ECP)**, and **eosinophil-derived neurotoxin**.

Eosinophils circulate in the blood for only 6 to 10 h before migrating into the connective tissues of the body, where they spend the remainder of their 8 to 10-day lifespan. They do not phagocytize and destroy bacteria. One of their functions is to take up and break down antigen–antibody complexes that are formed in allergic conditions, such as asthma and hay fever. Eosinophils are especially numerous beneath the epithelium of the respiratory and gastrointestinal tracts where entry of foreign proteins is most likely to occur. They are attracted to sites of release of **histamine**. The enzymes in their granules are capable of degrading histamine, and other mediators of allergic reactions. Eosinophils play a more active role in certain parasitic infections of humans. The eosinophil cationic proteins MBP and ECP are toxic to *Schistosoma mansoni*, and *Trypanosoma cruzi*, two parasites that are common in the tropics.

Basophilic leukocytes

Basophilic leukocytes, (**basophils**) are the least numerous of the granulocytes, accounting for only 0.5% of the total leukocyte

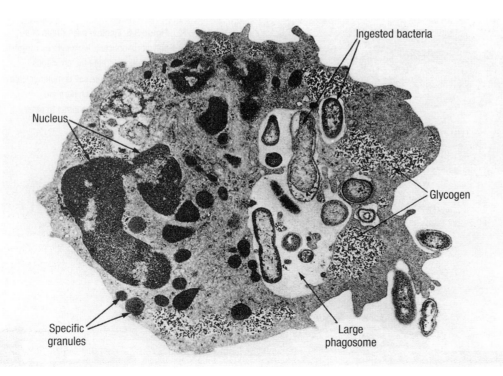

Figure 3.7 Electron micrograph of a neutrophilic leukocyte engaged in phagocytosis of bacteria. Note several large vacuoles in its cytoplasm.

Ingested bacteria

Nucleus

Glycogen

Specific granules

Large phagosome

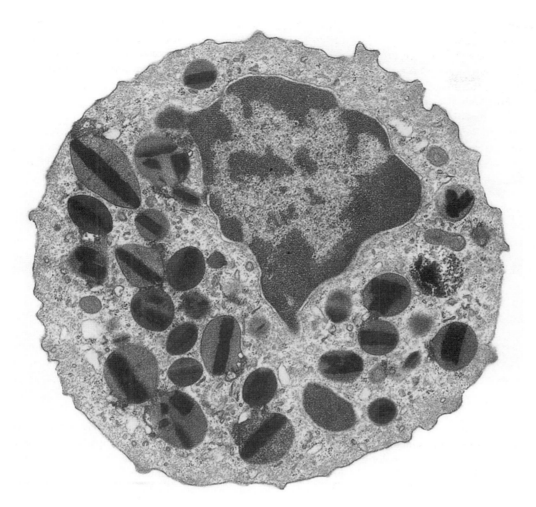

Figure 3.8 Electron micrograph of a human eosinophilic leukocyte. Notice the large specific granules, containing dense rhomboidal crystals. The crystals are not found in eosinophils of other mammalian species.

count. They are about the same size as neutrophils, but are easily distinguished by their very large specific granules (Figs 3.5C, 3.9). The nucleus is curved, but not distinctly lobulated. In electron micrographs, basophils have a small Golgi complex, a few mitochondria, and endoplasmic reticulum. The latter is somewhat more prominent in these cells than in other leukocytes. Particles of glycogen are often present in the cytoplasm. The specific granules are round or ovoid and up to 0.5 μm in diameter. They contain **heparin** and **histamine**, but no lysosomal hydrolases.

The basophils of the blood and the mast cells of connective tissue share certain properties. Both have large metachromatic granules containing histamine and heparin, but mast cells are larger and have many more granules. Basophils are short-lived and mast cells long-lived. Mast cells are relatively sessile, whereas basophils are motile, as shown by their assembly at sites of inflammation. Both release histamine and heparin and they evidently have similar functions. Whether they arise from the same, or different stem cells, is not yet settled. They both contribute to the discomforts associated with severe allergic reactions. They bind to one class of antibodies (immunoglobulin-E) and respond by releasing histamine and heparin. Histamine causes dilatation of small blood vessels, which then leak fluid constituents of the blood plasma into the tissues, resulting in local swelling (edema). The symptoms of these histamine-generated events include runny nose, watery eyes, and, in asthmatic patients, constriction of the airways of the lung, which makes breathing difficult. The role of heparin in hypersensitivity responses is less clear. It is an anticoagulant, slowing the clotting of blood, but it may have other less well known effects.

AGRANULAR LEUKOCYTES

The **agranular leukocytes** include monocytes and lymphocytes, in which granules are not a prominent feature of the cytoplasm. The alternative term in common use, **mononuclear leukocytes**, is etymologically misleading, for 'mono'-nuclear, implies that the other leukocytes have more than one nucleus. Actually, all leukocytes have a single nucleus, but that of the granular leukocytes may have two or more lobes.

Monocytes

Monocytes account for 3–8% of the circulating leukocytes. They are spherical cells 10–12 μm in diameter in suspension, but may

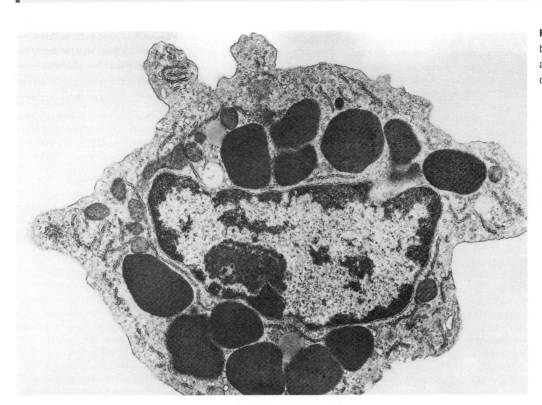

Figure 3.9 Electron micrograph of a basophilic leukocyte. The dense granules are considerably larger than those of other kinds of granular leukocyte.

be up to 17 μm in diameter in blood-smears. The nucleus is kidney-shaped or bilobed. Its chromatin is less deeply stained than that of other leukocytes. The cytoplasm stains a pale blue color, and, under the light microscope, appears to be devoid of granules (Figs 3.5E,F, 3.10).

On electron micrographs, the monocyte has a few short microvilli or lamelliform processes. The cytoplasm contains a small Golgi complex, a few mitochondria, occasional cisternal profiles of endoplasmic reticulum, and numerous free ribosomes. Scattered glycogen particles may also be present. There are also a

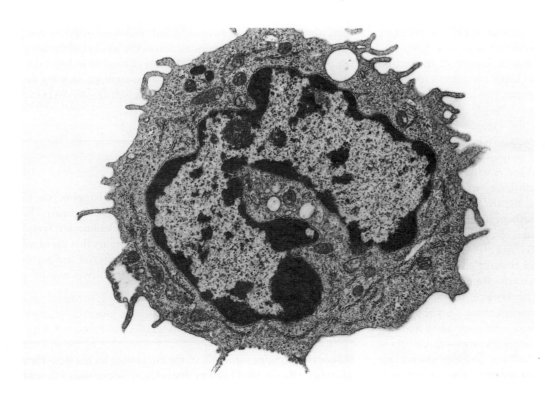

Figure 3.10 Electron micrograph of a monocyte. It has a deeply indented nucleus, and a few mitochondria and cisternae of endoplasmic reticulum in a cytoplasm rich in ribosomes. It contains no specific granules.

few dense granules that correspond to the azurophilic granules of other leukocytes.

Monocytes originate in the bone marrow and circulate in the blood for 1–4 days before entering the connective tissues of the body. There they differentiate into **tissue macrophages**, voracious phagocytic cells that take on the housekeeping function of ingesting senescent cells and any foreign matter they encounter, including invading bacteria. Macrophages also play an indispensable role in immune responses by processing foreign proteins (antigens) and presenting them to lymphocytes to initiate the production of protective antibodies.

Lymphocytes

Lymphocytes are the second most numerous class of leukocytes, comprising 20–30% of the circulating white blood cells. In blood-smears they are small, round cells 7–12 μm in diameter, with a deeply staining, slightly indented nucleus, surrounded by a thin rim of clear blue cytoplasm (Figs 3.5D, 3.11). They contain no specific granules but there may be very few small azurophilic granules. One or two mitochondria are present, but a Golgi complex is seldom observed. An endoplasmic reticulum is lacking, but free ribosomes are numerous.

The great majority of lymphocytes are at the lower end of their size range and are referred to as **small lymphocytes**. Others, with a somewhat wider rim of cytoplasm, are called **large lymphocytes**. The functional implications of these size differences are not clear, and these traditional descriptive terms based upon size are no longer widely used. Advances in our understanding of the immunological functions of lymphocytes, have made it more useful to distinguish two major categories, **B-lymphocytes** and **T-lymphocytes**. These differ in their development, lifespan, and functions. They are not morphologically distinguishable, but they have distinctive surface molecules, which make it possible to identify them by immunocytochemical methods.

The lymphocytes are the principal agents of the body's immunological defenses against invasion by bacteria and viruses. How they accomplish this will be the subject of a separate chapter on the Immune System (Chapter 10). It suffices here to state that B-lymphocytes produce specific **antibodies** against invading microorganisms. There are two major categories of T-lymphocytes: **helper T-lymphocytes**, which release signaling molecules to attract and activate B-lymphocytes, and **cytotoxic T-lymphocytes** which secrete toxic substances that kill virus-infected cells, or cells transplanted from another individual and recognized as foreign. In addition to their respective roles in immune responses, B- and T-lymphocytes secrete a dozen or more signaling molecules (**lymphokines** or cytokines) that influence each other's behavior, and have important roles in coordinating and regulating the body's immune defenses.

Lymphocytes are present in vast numbers in the parenchyma of the spleen and lymph nodes, accessory organs of the immune system. The great majority of these are B-lymphocytes, which have arisen from precursors in the bone marrow and have been carried to these organs in the blood. After a stay of varying duration in these organs, they are returned to the blood either directly or via the lymph. B-lymphocytes have a normal lifespan of many months. During this time, they recirculate through the blood, lymph nodes, spleen, and lymph many times in quest of any invading microorganisms. T-lymphocytes have a very different life history. The stem cells destined to give rise to T-lymphocytes originate in the bone marrow, but soon after birth, they enter the blood and settle in the thymus, where they proliferate. As their progeny move through the cortex of the thymus and into the medulla, they differentiate, acquiring the surface markers and receptors characteristic of T-lymphocytes. Upon entering the blood from the thymus, they join the continuously recirculating population of lymphocytes. They make up 70% or more of the lymphocytes of the blood, and have a lifespan, in humans, that may extend over several years.

HEMOPOIESIS

The generation of new blood cells is called **hemopoiesis**. Because the several kinds of blood cells have a very short lifespan, they must be continually replaced by new cells. The number of cells generated in this process is astonishing. In the adult human, approximately 10^{10} erythrocytes, and 4×10^8 leukocytes are formed each day. The principal site of hemopoiesis, in the adult, is the **bone marrow**, which occupies the medullary cavities of the long bones and the spongiosa of the vertebrae, ribs and sternum.

In early embryonic life, when the skeleton is still entirely cartilaginous, no marrow cavities exist, and the earliest formation of blood cells occurs in small islands of precursor cells in the yolk sac and body stalk of the embryo. This is called the **mesoblastic phase** of hemopoiesis. At about 6 weeks of gestation, erythrocyte formation begins in the primordium of the liver, initiating the **hepatic phase** of hemopoiesis. Later in pregnancy, when cartilage is being replaced by bone, blood cell formation declines in the liver, and

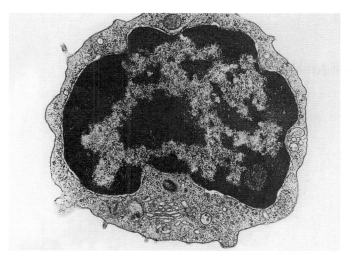

Figure 3.11 Electron micrograph of a lymphocyte. It has a heterochromatic nucleus, surrounded by a thin layer of cytoplasm. A small Golgi complex, a centriole and a single mitochondrion are also visible in this section.

begins in the newly formed medullary cavities of the developing bones, initiating the **myeloid phase** of hemopoiesis which continues throughout postnatal life.

BONE MARROW

Bone marrow occurs in two forms, distinguishable with the naked eye: **red marrow**, which is active in hemopoiesis, and **yellow marrow**, which is inactive and consists mainly of adipose cells that give it its yellow color. At birth, red marrow is found throughout the skeleton, but after the age of 6 years it is gradually replaced by yellow marrow in many of the bones. By age 10 years, red marrow persists only in the vertebrae, ribs, pelvis, and in the proximal ends of the humerus and femur.

Active red marrow is a soft, highly cellular tissue consisting of stem cells and precursors of the blood cells, supported by a loose stroma of reticular cells and reticular fibers (Fig. 3.12). Its organization can best be described in relation to its blood supply. The nutrient artery and accompanying vein of a long bone course longitudinally in the center of the medullary cavity (marrow cavity). Radial branches of the artery carry blood towards the wall of the bone, giving rise to large numbers of smaller vessels that are confluent with capacious venous sinuses. The majority of the exchanges between the blood and the marrow take place through the very thin walls of these vessels. The blood flows from the sinuses inwards to the central vein. Hemopoietic cells proliferate and differentiate in the interstices of the stroma between the sinusoidal vessels. The principal non-hemopoietic cells of the marrow are **macrophages** and **reticular cells**. The tips of long cell processes of the reticular cells adhere to form a loose cellular network. The spaces within this supporting network are occupied by closely packed differentiating blood cells. The reticular cells, and possibly the macrophages, release cytokines called **colony stimulating factors**, that promote proliferation and differentiation of the blood cell precursors.

Development of the several kinds of blood cells depends upon the existence of **pluripotential hemopoietic stem cells (PHSCs)** in the bone marrow. Stem cells found in other organs divide to produce progeny committed to differentiate into only the effector cell type of that particular organ. The stem cells of the marrow (Fig. 3.13) are described as 'pluripotential' because they give rise to all of the different cell types of the blood. They make up a very small fraction of the total cell population, probably no more than 1 in 10000 of the nucleated cells of the marrow. At any one time, a great many of them are dormant, but they are able to resume proliferation in response to a need for blood cells of any type. Stem cells that are cycling may undergo either **self-renewing divisions**, to maintain the pool of stem cells, or **differentiating divisions**, that give rise to four kinds of precursor cells (Fig. 3.14). These all have a euchromatic nucleus and a highly basophilic cytoplasm and are so similar in appearance that they cannot be distinguished in histological sections of bone marrow. The clones of cells derived from these precursors differentiate into all of the cell types of the peripheral blood (Fig. 3.14).

Our knowledge of the existence of four types of precursor cells and of the cell types arising from each is based upon ingenious animal experiments that could not be carried out in humans. These studies took advantage of the fact that the spleen provides an environment sufficiently similar to that of the bone marrow to permit hemopoiesis. A suspension of cells isolated from the bone marrow was injected into the blood stream of a syngyneic animal

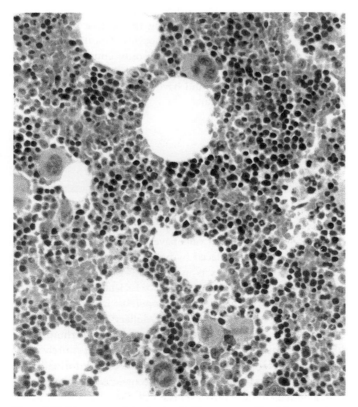

Figure 3.12 A low-power photomicrograph of bone marrow. The pink areas are erythrocytes in the sinuses. Blue areas are nuclei of precursors of the various blood cell types. The large, clear areas are adipose cells from which the lipid has been extracted.

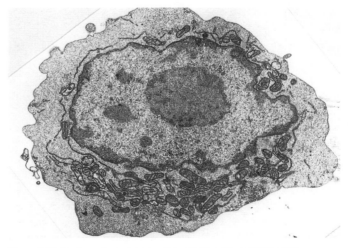

Figure 3.13 Electron micrograph of a stem cell. Its nucleus contains little chromatin and a very large nucleolus. The cytoplasm contains many mitochondria and a few cisternae of endoplasmic reticulum.

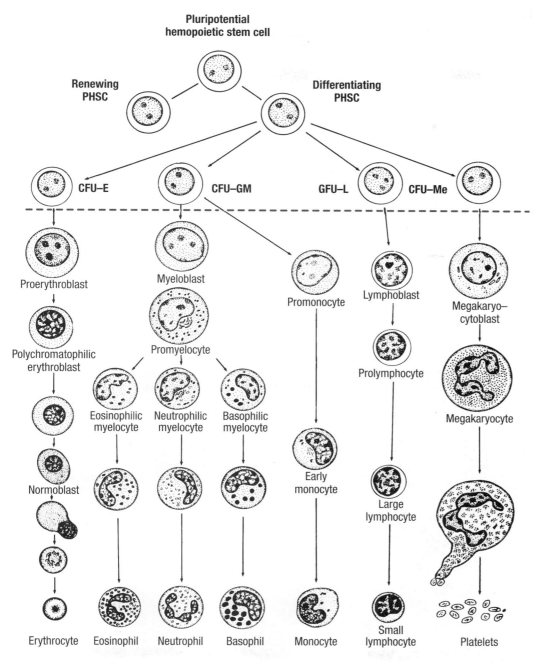

Pluripotential hemopoietic stem cell

Renewing PHSC

Differentiating PHSC

CFU–E

CFU–GM

GFU–L

CFU–Me

Proerythroblast

Myeloblast

Promonocyte

Lymphoblast

Megakaryo–cytoblast

Polychromatophilic erythroblast

Promyelocyte

Prolymphocyte

Eosinophilic myelocyte

Neutrophilic myelocyte

Basophilic myelocyte

Megakaryocyte

Normoblast

Early monocyte

Large lymphocyte

Erythrocyte

Eosinophil

Neutrophil

Basophil

Monocyte

Small lymphocyte

Platelets

Figure 3.14 Diagram of the stages of hemopoiesis. Save for the pluripotential hemopoietic stem cell (PHSC), the cells above the dotted line are not easily distinguishable with the light or electron microscope. Those below the line can be identified in sections or smears of bone marrow. CFU-E, colony-forming unit erythrocyte; CFU-GM, colony-forming unit granulocyte-monocyte; CFU-L, colony-forming unit lymphocyte; CFU-Me, colony-forming unit megakaryocyte.

that had previously been exposed to sufficient X-irradiation to prevent proliferation of its own bone marrow or spleen cells. Some of the injected cells lodged individually at different sites in the spleen, where they proliferated and differentiated. After several days, colonies each derived from a single precursor cell of the donor animal were clearly visible in the spleen of the irradiated recipient. The cell types in each colony were then examined microscopically. If only developmental stages of erythrocytes were found in a colony, the precursor cell was designated a **colony-forming unit erythrocyte (CFU-E)**. If another colony contained only developmental stages of granulocytes and monocytes, the single cell of origin was designated a **colony-forming unit granulocyte-monocyte (CFU-GM)**. If only cells of the lymphocyte

lineage were found, their cell of origin was called a **colony-forming unit lymphocyte (CFU-L)**, and finally, if a colony contained only the developmental stages of megakaryocytes, the cell of origin was called a **colony-forming unit megakaryocyte (CFU-Me)**. These experimental findings are the basis for the labeling of the four different precursor cell types illustrated in Fig. 3.14, and for the application of the same terms (CFU-E, CFU-GM, CFU-L, and CFU-Me) for the corresponding hemopoietic precursor cell types of the human bone marrow. Although these cells are visually indistinguishable, they subsequently pass through a series of developmental stages that are microscopically identifiable (Fig. 3.15). The characteristics of the intermediate states of each lineage will now be briefly described.

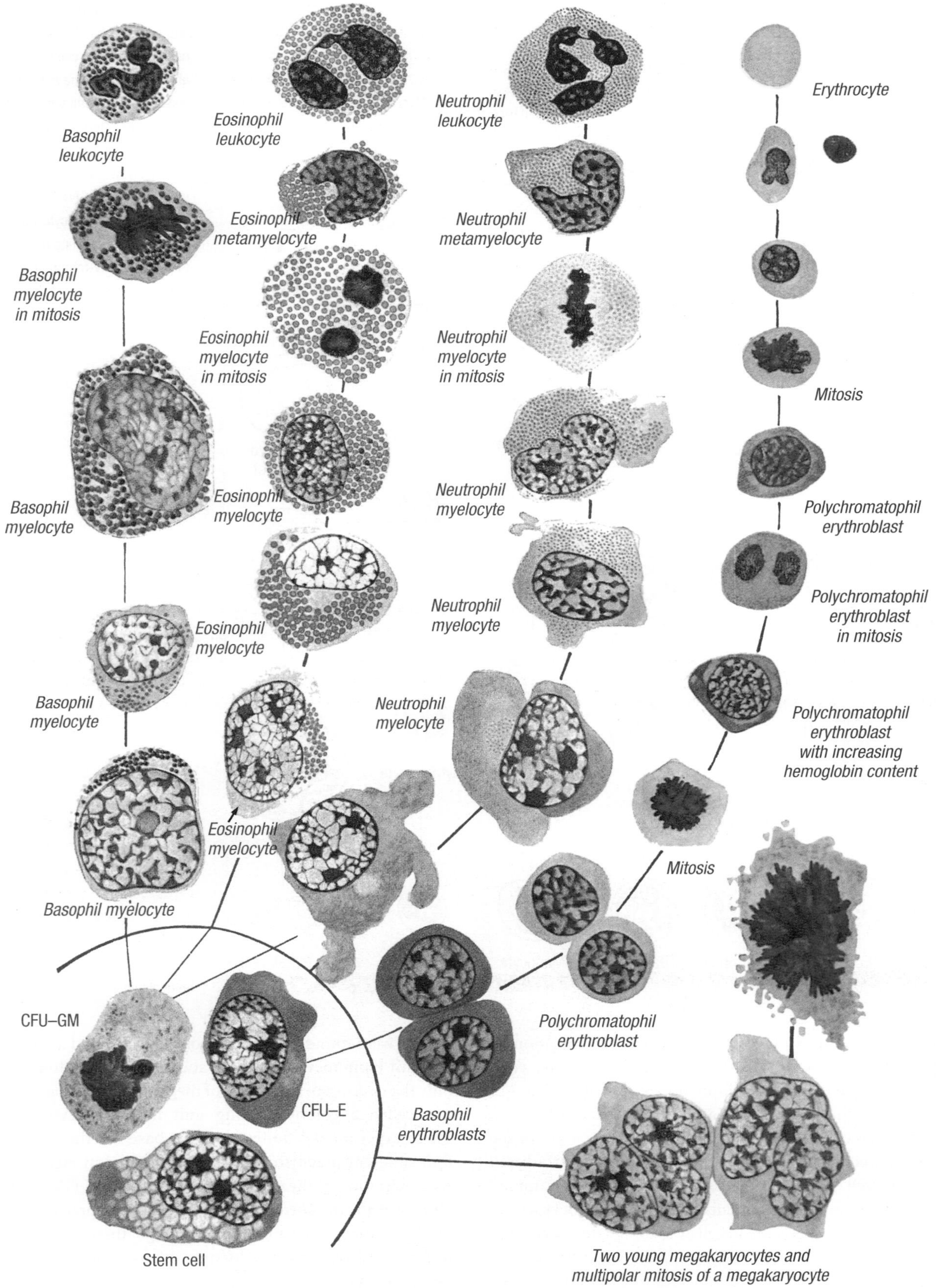

Figure 3.15 Drawing of the successive stages in the development of erythrocytes, neutrophils, eosinophils, and basophils, as seen with the May–Gruenwald–Giemsa stain. Development of lymphocytes and monocytes is not shown. CFU-GM, colony-forming unit granulocyte-monocyte; CFU-E, colony-forming unit erythrocyte.

Erythrocytopoiesis

The CFU-E differentiates into a **proerythroblast**, the earliest recognizable stage of the erythrocyte lineage. It is a spherical cell up to 16 μm in diameter, with a rim of moderately basophilic cytoplasm around a large nucleus containing two or three nucleoli. It undergoes several mitotic divisions that yield somewhat smaller progeny, called **basophilic erythroblasts**, which have a more heterochromatic nucleus and an intensely basophilic cytoplasm. On electron micrographs, their cytoplasm contains abundant polyribosomes, and moderate numbers of smaller and less dense particles of hemoglobin (Fig. 3.16). The next stage, called the **polychromatophilic erythroblast**, is so named because the color of its cytoplasm, in stained smears, is no longer blue but ranges from blue-gray to olive green. This color change results from a further increase in the number of acidophilic hemoglobin particles in the cytoplasm (Fig. 3.17, right column). These cells are smaller than their precursors and their deeply stained heterochromatic nucleus lacks a nucleolus. As their development progresses to the next stage, the **orthochromatic erythroblast** (or **normoblast**), there is a further increase in hemoglobin and a relative decrease in the number of polyribosomes, resulting in a more eosinophilic cytoplasm. Chromatin condensation has progressed and the nucleus is smaller. Towards the end of this stage, the nucleus is extruded (Figs 3.16, 3.18), and the remainder of the cell then assumes a biconcave shape to become an immature **erythrocyte**. At this stage the erythrocytes enter the lumen of the sinusoids and complete their maturation in the circulation. The immature erythrocyte is eosinophilic but has a slight blue tint because of the small numbers of basophilic ribosomes remaining in its cytoplasm. As stated earlier in the chapter,

these newly formed erythrocytes are called **reticulocytes**. Their number, in appropriately stained blood-smears, is used by doctors as a convenient measure of the rate of erythropoiesis. The polyribosomes soon break down and the reticulocytes are then **mature erythrocytes**. The developmental events from proerythroblast to mature erythrocyte take about 7 days.

Any significant reduction in the number, or hemoglobin content, of erythrocytes, resulting in diminished oxygen-carrying capacity, is called **anemia**. Vitamin B is required for normal erythrocytopoiesis. In the disorder **pernicious anemia**, certain cells in the gastric mucosa fail to secrete a protein that is necessary for absorption of this vitamin. **Iron-deficiency anemia** results from a diet lacking sufficient iron. **Sickle-cell anemia** is an inherited disease in which the hemoglobin molecules are abnormal. When exposed to low oxygen tensions the hemoglobin crystallizes within the erythrocyte, resulting in their deformation to the shape of a sickle blade. The symptoms of all severe anemias are much the same: pallor, shortness of breath, increased heart rate, and low exercise tolerance. Treatment varies depending upon the underlying cause of the anemia.

Granulocytopoiesis

Further differentiation of the progenitor cell, CFU-GM, leads through several intermediate stages, to either granulocytes (neutrophils, eosinophils, basophils), or to monocytes (Fig. 3.14). The first stage of the granulocyte lineage is the **myeloblast**, a cell 16 μm in diameter, that has a large nucleus with finely dispersed chromatin and three or more nucleoli. Its cytoplasm is basophilic and contains no specific granules. Myeloblasts undergo several

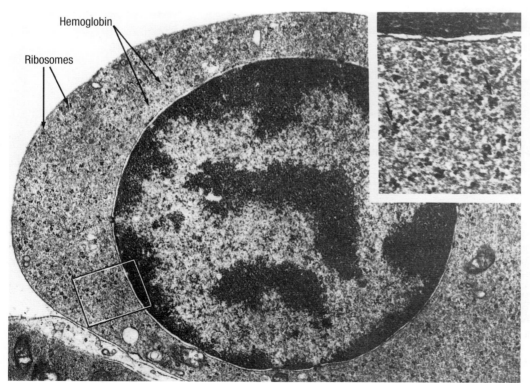

Figure 3.16 Electron micrograph of a late polychromatophilic erythroblast, showing its coarse clumps of heterochromatin in the nucleus, and a cytoplasm filled with clusters of ribosomes and smaller particles of hemoglobin. At higher magnification (inset) the ribosomes (at arrows) can be distinguished from the paler granules of hemoglobin.

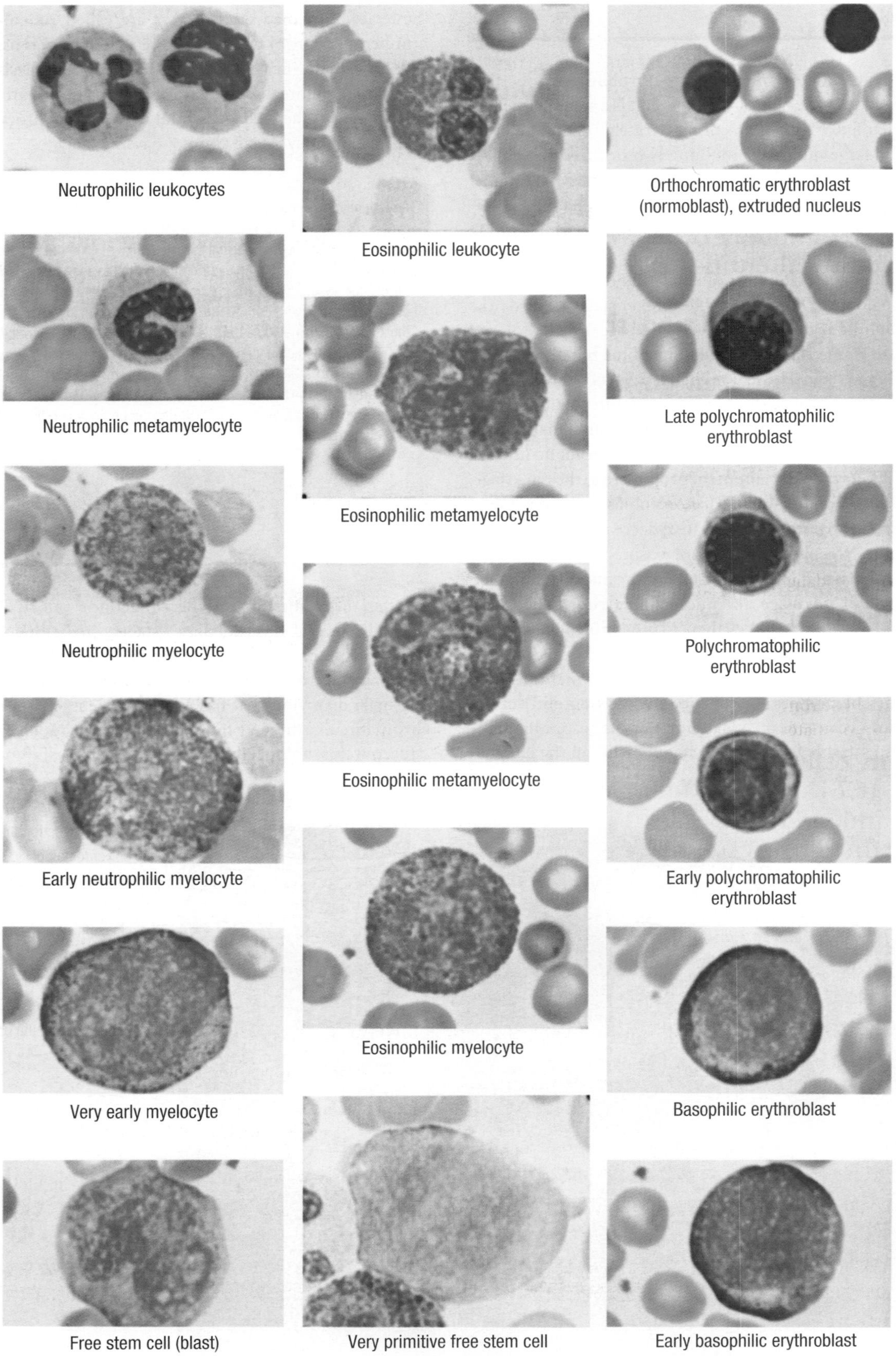

Neutrophilic leukocytes

Eosinophilic leukocyte

Orthochromatic erythroblast (normoblast), extruded nucleus

Neutrophilic metamyelocyte

Eosinophilic metamyelocyte

Late polychromatophilic erythroblast

Neutrophilic myelocyte

Eosinophilic metamyelocyte

Polychromatophilic erythroblast

Early neutrophilic myelocyte

Eosinophilic myelocyte

Early polychromatophilic erythroblast

Very early myelocyte

Basophilic erythroblast

Free stem cell (blast)

Very primitive free stem cell

Early basophilic erythroblast

Figure 3.17 Stages in the differentiation of neutrophils, eosinophils, and erythrocytes, as seen in bone marrow smears stained with Wright's blood stain. Neutrophils (left column), eosinophils (middle column) and erythrocytes (right column). Early stages are at the bottom of the figure and mature stages at the top.

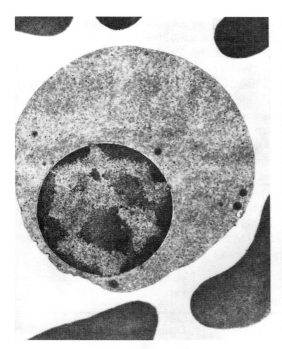
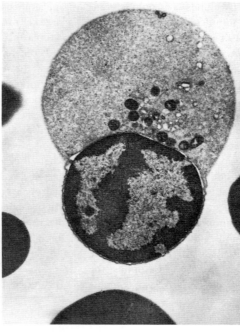

Figure 3.18 Electron micrographs of orthochromatic erythroblasts. The cell on the right is in the process of extruding its nucleus to become an erythrocyte.

divisions, producing daughter cells called **promyelocytes**. These attain a diameter of 20 μm. The nucleus is similar to that of the myeloblast, but the cytoplasm is more basophilic. In electron micrographs, rough endoplasmic reticulum (rER) is abundant, a Golgi complex is present, and there are numerous azurophilic granules (Fig. 3.19). Promyelocytes undergo divisions, and the daughter cells differentiate into **myelocytes**. These cells are smaller

and have a nucleus that stains more intensely than that of the promyelocyte. The cytoplasm is less basophilic and contains many azurophilic granules. There are three kinds of myelocytes destined to develop into the three kinds of granulocytes, but these are difficult to distinguish. The separate paths of differentiation can only be identified with certainty in the next, **metamyelocyte**, stage. The **neutrophilic metamyelocyte** has a deeply indented nucleus and

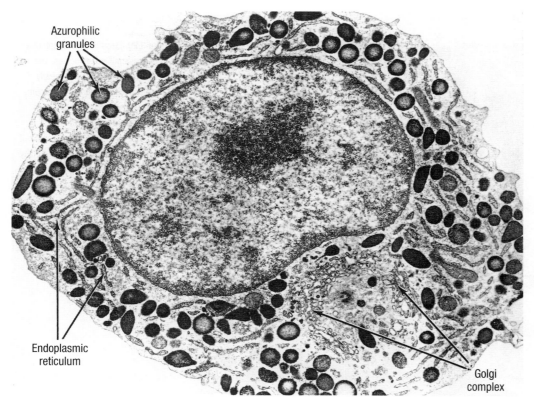

Azurophilic granules

Endoplasmic reticulum

Golgi complex

Figure 3.19 Electron micrograph of a promyelocyte, the largest precursor stage of the neutrophil. The preparation was stained for the enzyme peroxidase, and the azurophilic granules give a positive reaction. The specific granules have not yet developed. (Reproduced from D. Bainton et al. *J Exp Med* 1971; 134:907.)

the cytoplasm contains granules of two kinds, **azurophilic granules** that stain deeply, and **specific granules** that are only faintly stained. In subsequent development of neutrophilic metamyelocytes into neutrophils, the granules increase in number, the nucleus becomes long and narrow and is often displaced to one side of the cell. In the mature neutrophil, the long nucleus is narrowed at several places along its length, resulting in distinct nuclear lobules connected by very slender segments.

Eosinophilic metamyelocytes can be distinguished from neutrophilic metamyelocytes by the larger size and eosinophilic staining of their cytoplasmic granules in marrow smears examined with the light microscope (Fig. 3.17, middle column). On electron micrographs, they are readily identifiable by the larger size and greater density of their granules (Fig. 3.20). The nucleus is indented, but even in the mature eosinophil, it never attains the degree of lobulation seen in neutrophils. **Basophilic metamyelocytes** are rarely observed because of their small numbers, and the difficulty of preserving their granules. In mature **basophils**, the nucleus is deeply indented or bilobed and the cytoplasm contains large, intensely basophilic granules.

The development time from stem cells to mature granulocytes is about 18 days. A great number of neutrophils are retained in the bone marrow as a ready reserve. It may contain as many as 10 times the normal daily production, and these can be rapidly mobilized in case of a bacterial infection anywhere in the body.

Monocytopoiesis

Monocytes develop from CFU-GM progenitor cells, with the next stage being the **monoblast**, a large basophilic cell very similar in appearance to a myeloblast. It differentiates into a **promonocyte**, a large cell (16–18μm) with a euchromatic nucleus and a basophilic cytoplasm devoid of granules. Promonocytes divide repeatedly and some of the daughter cells differentiate into **monocytes** that enter the circulation as rapidly as they are formed. Other promonocytes divide more slowly and constitute a reserve of monocyte precursors in the marrow. Their maturation can be accelerated in response to a need for more monocytes and macrophages in the tissues. Monocytes normally circulate in the blood for no more than 36h before they migrate into the tissues, where they increase in size, acquire granular endoplasmic reticulum and a conspicuous Golgi complex, and begin to synthesize hydrolytic enzymes that are incorporated in numerous lysosomes. These changes transform the monocyte into an actively phagocytic **macrophage** equipped to ingest and destroy bacteria, or any other foreign matter encountered.

Thrombocytopoiesis

The blood of lower vertebrates contains nucleated cells, called **thrombocytes**, that promote blood clotting to limit the loss of blood after an injury. The functional equivalent of the thrombocytes in mammals are the anucleate blood platelets. These are generated by detachment of small, membrane-bounded fragments from the cytoplasm of very large cells of the bone marrow, called **megakaryocytes**, that are found adjacent to the sinusoids of the bone marrow. Megakaryocytes originate from a unipotential precursor, CFU-Me, that differentiates into a **megakaryocytoblast**, a cell up to 50μm in diameter with a lobulated nucleus containing many nucleoli. The cytoplasm is basophilic and initially devoid of granules.

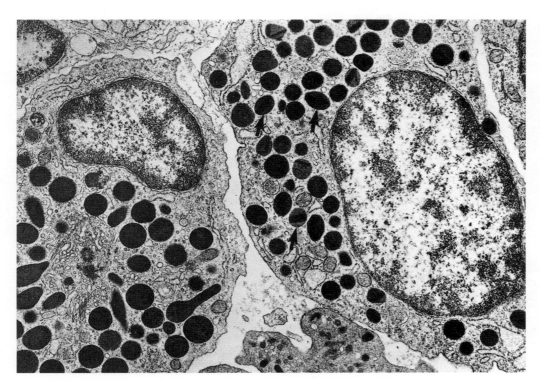

Figure 3.20 Electron micrograph of a pair of eosinophilic myelocytes. The formation of granules is now nearly complete, and endoplasmic reticulum, which was abundant in the previous stage, is now greatly diminished. Crystals are forming in the granules but are difficult to see, owing to the density of the granule matrix.

In the initial differentiation of this cell, the DNA undergoes multiple replications without division of the cytoplasm (endomitosis). This results in a giant polyploid cell. It is the largest cell type of the marrow and may attain a diameter of $100\mu m$ (Fig.3.21). The chromatin of its very large, multilobular nucleus may contain the DNA of as many as 14 sets of chromosomes. The basophilic cytoplasm contains great numbers of small azurophilic granules that are arranged in clusters, separated by aisles of granule-free cytoplasm. Electron micrographs reveal pairs of membranes in the cytoplasm that are oriented in intersecting planes, partitioning it into units $1-3\mu m$ in diameter, each containing a cluster of granules. These so-called **platelet demarcation channels** (Figs 3.21, 3.22), are located in the aisles between clusters of granules, outlining areas that will form individual platelets upon subsequent fragmentation of the cytoplasm. The megakaryocytes extend long processes into the lumen of a neighboring sinus. These may consist of as many as 1000 platelet subunits. Fragmentation of these processes along the platelet demarcation channels releases individual **platelets** into the bloodstream. A single megakaryocyte may be able to release as many as 8000 platelets before it degenerates and is replaced.

Any deficiency in the number of circulating blood platelets is called **thrombocytopenia**. It may be caused by inadequate production, or accelerated destruction of platelets. In the chronic autoimmune disease called **thrombocytopenic purpura**, platelet production is normal but antibodies bind to a protein on their surface and interfere with their aggregation to form a blood clot. These patients have prolonged bleeding after minor lacerations, and there are often numerous black-and-blue spots on their body resulting from unintended contact with hard objects. The condition is more common in women than men and results in prolonged menstrual flow.

Lymphocytopoiesis

Stem cells of the bone marrow give rise to a precursor, CFU-L, whose daughter cells become **lymphoblasts**. After several divisions, their smaller progeny develop into **prolymphocytes**. These have nuclei with deeply staining condensed chromatin sur-

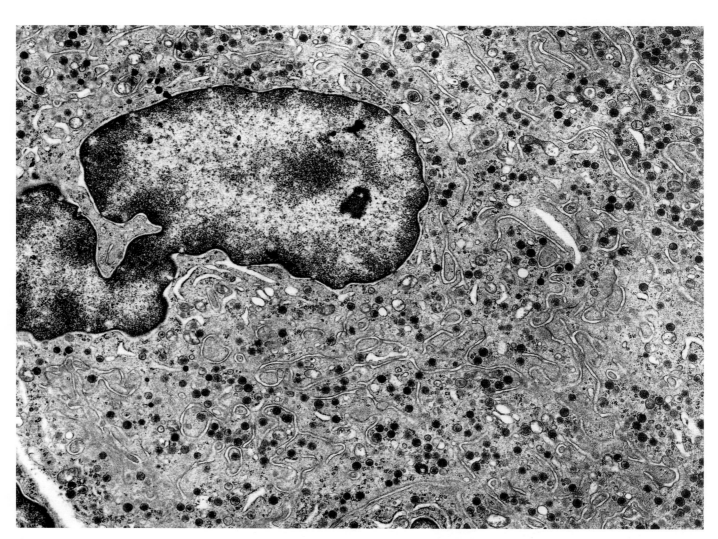

Figure 3.21 Electron micrograph of a portion of a megakaryocyte. It is a huge polyploid cell with a nucleus having several lobes. The small granules seen throughout the cytoplasm will be the azurophilic granules of future platelets, which will be formed by fragmentation of the megakaryocyte cytoplasm.

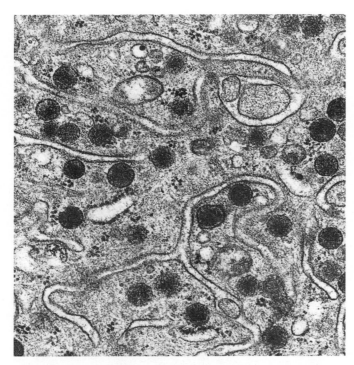

Figure 3.22 An area of megakaryocyte cytoplasm at higher magnification, showing the platelet demarcation channels outlining future platelets.

rounded by a small amount of basophilic cytoplasm containing very few organelles. Some of the prolymphocytes remain in the bone marrow and divide throughout life, producing **lymphocytes** that are released into the blood bearing surface markers identifying them as B-lymphocytes. Other prolymphocytes enter the blood and are carried to the spleen and lymph nodes where they complete their differentiation into B-lymphocytes.

In embryonic and early postnatal life, lymphoblasts are also carried in the blood, from the bone marrow to the cortex of the thymus, where they proliferate and differentiate into lymphocytes. As these move through the cortex and into the medulla of the thymus, they generate surface markers characteristic of **T-lymphocytes** and are then released into the blood. Thus, mature B-lymphocytes are produced in the bone marrow, spleen, and lymph nodes, and T-lymphocytes are generated in the thymus. We will return to this subject again in the chapter on the Immune System (Chapter 10).

Malignant transformation of the hemopoietic precursors of the leukocytes results in the dreaded forms of cancer called **leukemias**. In **myelogenous leukemia**, the cells are derived from the granulocytopoietic line, and in **lymphatic leukemia**, the cells are malignant lymphocyte precursors. In myelogenous leukemia, rapid proliferation and accumulation of the malignant cells in the bone marrow displaces normal hemopoietic cells, resulting in anemia, and increased susceptability to infection. In lymphatic leukemia, the cells proliferate in the spleen and lymph nodes, resulting in their enlargement and impaired function. The leukemias may occur in an acute form leading to death in a few months, or in a chronic form that has a much slower course.

HISTOPHYSIOLOGY OF BONE MARROW

Red bone marrow is unique among the tissues of the body in the diversity of the cell types it produces. In normal health, the normal numbers of each type in the blood are maintained within quite narrow limits, but in emergencies, such as blood loss or infection, the marrow is able to respond rapidly with increased production of the appropriate cell type. This requires a rather complex system of controls that we are only recently beginning to understand.

Erythrocytes have the life-sustaining function of transporting oxygen from the lungs to all other tissues, and maintenance of adequate numbers in the circulation is essential. The rate of their production is regulated, in large part, by a glycoprotein hormone, **erythropoietin**, which is produced by certain cells in the kidneys. These cells are very sensitive to hypoxia (low oxygen concentration in the blood), which may result from diseases of the lungs that interfere with oxygen uptake, or from anemia (deficiency of red blood cells). The kidney cells respond to hypoxia by releasing erythropoietin which is carried in the blood to the marrow where it binds to committed erythrocyte precursors, stimulating their proliferation and differentiation. The amount of erythropoietin produced varies with the degree of hypoxia.

Progenitor cells and blast cell precursors of other blood cell types are unable to proliferate and differentiate without continuing stimulation. That stimulation depends upon contact with stromal cells, binding of signaling molecules they release, and upon cytokines called **colony-stimulating factors** (CSFs). Five distinct CSFs have been identified and each is named by a prefix indicating the blood cell type or types they control: **granulocyte-monocyte-CSF** (GM-CSF), **granulocyte-CSF** (G-CSF), **monocyte-CSF** (M-CSF) and one with a broader range of target cells, **multi-CSF** (or **leukotriene-3**) produced by activated T-lymphocytes. All are glycoproteins of varying molecular weight and there are specific receptors for each on the appropriate progenitor cells of the marrow. CSFs not only stimulate proliferation of precursors, they enhance the functional activity of the mature cells formed, and they are effective in very low concentration. It has been possible to increase the neutrophil count in the peripheral blood of mice from 1000/ml to 100000/ml by giving daily injections of G-CSF. CSFs are synthesized by stromal cells, macrophages, and possibly by endothelial cells of the marrow. At sites of infection, bacterial toxins immediately activate genes for synthesis of CSFs in monocytes and macrophages, and in T-lymphocytes that have bound antigen. The resulting increase in the level of CSFs in the blood stimulates increased production of those cell types responsible for defense of the organism against bacteria. Certain CSFs (e.g. GM-CSF) are also chemotactic, attracting neutrophils, monocytes, macrophages and eosinophils to the site of bacterial invasion and enhancing their functional activities.

Questions

1 A differential count of the white blood cells in a smear of normal human peripheral blood would reveal that
 a basophils predominate (>50%)
 b eosinophils are quite rare (2–5%)
 c monocytes are quite abundant (>30%)
 d neutrophils predominate (>50%)
 e lymphocytes are quite rare (<10%)

2 Which of these statements best describes white blood cells?
 a their primary function is within blood vessels
 b they leave blood vessels to perform most of their functions
 c they function equally well, no matter what their location
 d they remain inside blood vessels
 e they all possess a round nucleus

3 The macrophage found in connective tissues of the body
 a is derived from monocytes in the circulation
 b arises from a macrophage-forming clonal unit
 c is phagocytic in suspension and when attached to a substrate
 d has a bilobed nucleus
 e never has cytoplasmic granules

4 Which of these statements best describes basophils?
 a they leave the circulation to become mast cells of the connective tissue
 b they are highly phagocytic
 c they are a rich source of aryl sulfatase
 d they contain histamine and heparin
 e they possess a round nucleus

5 Which of the following blood granulocytes contains very large metachromatic granules?
 a basophil
 b mast cell
 c monocyte
 d neutrophil
 e lymphocyte

6 Circulating antibodies are produced by
 a neutrophils
 b eosinophils
 c plasma cells
 d mast cells
 e monocytes

7 Megakaryocytes of the bone marrow
 a are the source of platelets found in the circulation
 b undergo cytokinesis without benefit of karyokinesis
 c are haploid
 d are diploid
 e are about the same size as neutrophils

8 In the early stages of an inflammatory response, which of the following cell types will predominate?
 a macrophages
 b monocytes
 c basophils
 d neutrophils
 e plasma cells

9 Cytokines such as interleukin-1 are responsible for
 a maturation of erythroblasts
 b differentiation of monocytes to macrophages
 c activation of platelets
 d production of erythropoietin
 e release of neutrophils from bone marrow

10 Which statement best describes granulopoiesis?
 a it gives rise to monocytes as well as granulocytes
 b it results in mature red blood cells
 c it produces blood platelets
 d when stimulated, it produces enormous numbers of proerythroblasts
 e it is not influenced by cytokines

11 What blood cell would be in abundance during an active parasitic infection?

12 What is the most common nucleated cell in the circulation?

13 What is the largest hemopoietic cell in human bone marrow?

14 What is the component of peripheral blood provided by megakaryocytes?

15 What is the smallest white blood cell found in peripheral blood?

16 What cell in the bone marrow is the earliest recognizable stage of the red blood cell line?

17 What cell is the first identifiable precursor of the neutrophil line?

18 What cell type has a pyknotic nucleus that will be subsequently expelled?

19 What hematopoietic cell is polyploid?

20 What cell derives directly from the myeloblast?

Chapter four

Connective Tissue

Connective tissue supports and binds together other structural elements throughout the body. It forms the capsules of organs, and the thin septa between the epithelial subunits. It is the tissue through which arteries and nerves enter, and veins and lymphatics leave, the organs. Its aqueous phase is the medium through which nutrients and waste products of metabolism diffuse to and from the parenchymal cells of the organs. **Connective tissue** is made up of cells and fibers embedded in a gel-like extracellular matrix, commonly called the ground substance. The relative abundance of cells, fibers and ground substance in the connective tissue varies from region to region depending upon the architecture of the tissues and the stresses to which they are exposed. To express these differences, several kinds of connective tissue are distinguished: **loose connective tissue, reticular connective tissue, dense irregular connective tissue**, and **dense regular connective tissue**. The defining characteristics of each will be presented after the components that they have in common have been defined.

GROUND SUBSTANCE

The **ground substance** occupies all of the space between the cells and fibers of connective tissue. It is a colorless, translucent substance with the consistency of a highly hydrated gel. It is poorly preserved in routine histological preparations, but residues of it can be detected because it stains with histochemical methods for detection of carbohydrates. Its major components are **glycosaminoglycans**, large molecules that are linear polymers of disaccharide subunits. The major glycosaminoglycans of connective tissue are **chondroitin sulfate, keratan sulfate, heparin sulfate**, and **hyaluronic acid**. These are usually covalently bound to a core protein to form still larger molecules called **proteoglycans**. In these molecules, the glycosaminoglycans radiate from the core protein like the bristles on a bottle brush (Fig. 4.1).

Hyaluronic acid is exceptional among the glycosaminoglycans in not being bound to a core protein. It is a very large polymer of some 5000 disaccharides in a chain that, if straightened, would be

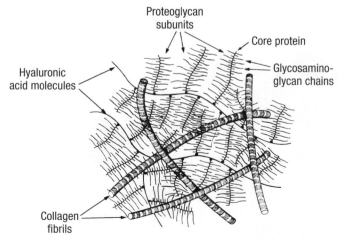

Figure 4.1 Drawing of the components of the ground substance. The matrix between collagen fibers is made up of long entwined proteoglycan molecules that have hundreds of polysaccharide side-chains.

nearly 2.5 μm in length. One of its important properties is its high viscosity in aqueous solution, which is largely responsible for the gel-like consistency of the ground substance. The hyaluronic acid and proteoglycans are no barrier to diffusion of metabolites through the aqueous phase of the ground substance, but they are probably a significant barrier to the spread of any bacteria that may enter the body. Indirect evidence for this is the finding that, in the course of evolution, some very invasive species of bacteria have acquired the ability to synthesize the enzyme hyaluronidase, which depolymerizes the hyaluronic acid of the connective tissue and facilitates their spread.

In addition to the long, entwined proteoglycan molecules that occupy most of the space between the fibers of connective tissue, there are lesser amounts of three **adhesion proteins**, which bind cells to the fibers of the connective tissue. One of these, **fibronectin**, is a large glycoprotein (440 kDa) that is made up of two long polypeptide chains. Regularly spaced along their length are binding sites for cells, for collagen fibers, and for proteoglycans. Thus, fibronectin is able to interconnect all three components of connective tissue. Many cell types are dependent upon fibronectin for their attachment. The plasma membrane of others contains integral proteins, called **integrins**, that are able to bind directly to collagen fibers. Another very large glycoprotein,

laminin, has binding sites for cell membranes, collagen fibers, and heparin sulfate proteoglycan. It copolymerizes with type IV collagen and entactin to form the **basal lamina**, to which the cells of epithelia adhere. Although cell attachment is the primary function of the adhesion proteins, there is also evidence that they indirectly influence the state of differentiation of the cells and the organization of their cytoskeleton.

EXTRACELLULAR FIBERS

Collagen fibers

Collagen fibers are the most abundant fibrous component of connective tissue. In histological sections, they appear pink with the hematoxylin-eosin stain, blue with Mallory's trichrome stain, and green with Masson's stain. In unstained spreads of connective tissue, they are randomly oriented, thin, colorless strands, ranging from 0.5 to 10.0 μm in diameter (Fig. 4.2A). In electron micrographs they are seen to be made up of smaller **unit fibrils**, 50–90 nm in diameter (Fig. 4.3). In preparations

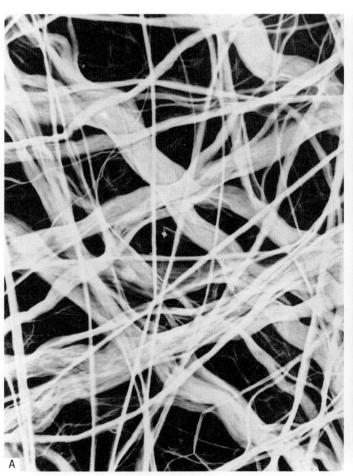
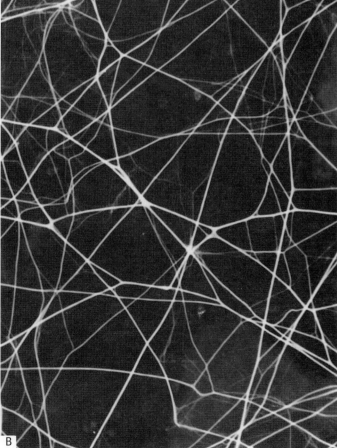

Figure 4.2 Photomicrograph of the extracellular fibers in a thin spread of mesentery. (A) Collagen fibers. (B) Elastic fibers. The preparation was stained with a silver method and printed as a negative to simulate more closely their appearance *in vivo*.

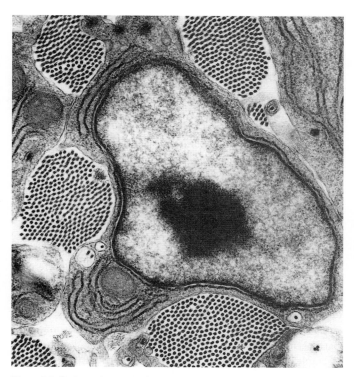

Figure 4.3 Electron micrograph of a developing tendon, showing bundles of unit fibrils of collagen fibers around a fibroblast. (Reproduced from D. Birk and R. Trelstad *J Cell Biol* 1986; 103:231.)

stained with lead, collagen fibers appear cross-striated, with denser transverse bands spaced at 64 nm intervals along their length. This cross-banding is also evident in metal-shadowed preparations of isolated unit fibrils (Fig. 4.4). The unit fibrils are polymers of **tropocollagen** molecules 280 nm in length and 1.4 nm in diameter. Each tropocollagen molecule consists of three polypeptide chains (alpha chains) entwined in triple helical configuration. In the assembly of these molecules into unit fibrils, there is a short gap between the ends of successive molecules (Fig. 4.5). At intervals of 64 nm along the length of the unit fibril a number of these gaps are in register across its width. Penetration of stain into these gaps results in uniformly spaced dark bands across the fibril. The intervening light bands are

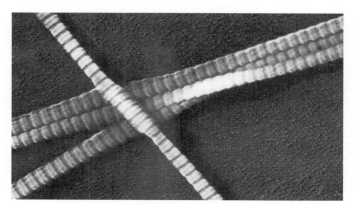

Figure 4.4 Electron micrograph of collagen fibrils isolated from human skin and shadowed with lead to show their 64 nm periodicity.

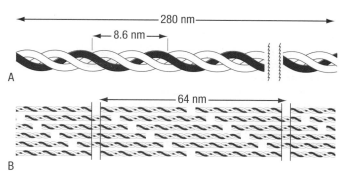

Figure 4.5 (A) Each molecule of type I collagen is composed of two alpha-1 polypeptide chains and one alpha-2 chain entwined in a double helix. (B) Drawing of several rows of the molecules in a collagen fibril. The molecules are aligned with a gap between their ends, and molecules of adjacent rows overlap in a step-wise manner. At 64 nm intervals the intermolecular gaps are aligned across the fibril. Penetration of contrast medium into these is responsible for the cross-striations at these sites. (Reproduced from L.C. Junquiera and J. Carniero *Basic Histology*, 3rd edn, Lange Medical Publications, 1980.)

regions in which overlap of tropocollagen molecules prevents penetration of the stain.

Collagen is not a single entity, it is a family of proteins that share the same molecular configuration, but are composed of polypeptide chains that differ slightly in amino acid sequence. Eleven or more collagens have been identified and designated by Roman numerals. Common to all are two amino acids, hydroxyproline and hydroxylysine, which are virtually unique to collagen. The amount of collagen in any tissue can be quantified by analysis for either of these amino acids. Type I, type II, and type III collagen are the most common. They form fibrils of slightly different diameter. Although the different types of collagen cannot be easily distinguished in sections stained with hematoxylin and eosin, they can be identified by using labeled type-specific antibodies.

Type I collagen is ubiquitous, forming fibers and fiber bundles of varying size in the connective tissue of the skin, in bone and tendon, and in the capsules of organs. **Type II collagen** forms very thin fibers in the abundant ground substance of cartilage, the nucleus pulposus of the intervertebral discs, and the vitreous body of the eye. **Type III collagen** forms slender fibers arranged in loose networks. Collagen types I to III, which form fibers, are often referred to as the **interstitial collagens**. **Type IV collagen** does not form fibers, but copolymerizes with laminin and entactin to form the basal lamina of epithelia. Collagen **types V to X** are quite restricted in their distribution, and, in a first course of histology, may be considered less deserving of student attention than types I to IV.

The collagens are not the product of a single cell type. Most of the type I collagen is synthesized by **fibroblasts**, which are the dominant cell type of the connective tissues, but it is also produced by the osteoblasts of bone and several other cell types. Type II collagen is a product of the chondrocytes of cartilage. Type III collagen is synthesized by fibroblasts, smooth muscle cells, liver cells, and many other cell types. Type IV collagen is synthesized by epithelia cells.

There are several inherited diseases attributable to aberrant regulation of fibroblast proliferation and collagen synthesis. Either too much, or too little, collagen may have undesirable consequence. In **Ehler–Danlos syndrome** insufficient collagen results in lax ligaments and hyperextensible knee joints that make walking difficult. The skin is thin, and a fold of it, grasped between the thumb and forefinger, can be stretched 2 in (5 cm), or more, away from the underlying structures. In **scleroderma**, collagen fibers are formed in great excess. The skin is thick and taut and may interfere with flexion of the fingers, and limit movement of other joints. Thickening of the wall of the esophagus may make swallowing difficult, and increased perivascular connective tissue may interfere with blood flow.

Reticular fibers

Reticular fibers are thin fibers that form networks throughout the parenchyma of many organs. They are composed of fibrils of type III collagen and associated glycoproteins. Their fibrils are only 25–45 nm in diameter compared to those of the coarser collagen fibers, which range from 50 to 90 nm in diameter. They are not seen in routine hematoxylin and eosin preparations, but can be blackened by impregnation with silver salts (Fig. 4.6). Because of this staining property they are also described as **argyrophilic**

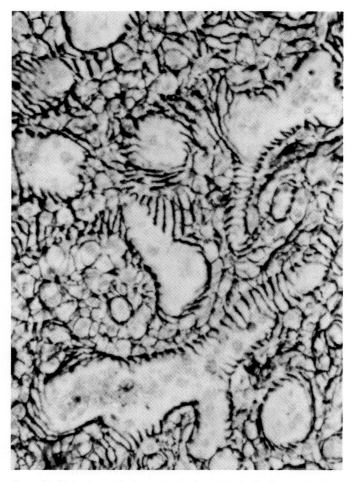

Figure 4.6 Photomicrograph of a section of spleen stained with silver to show the abundant argyrophilic reticular fibers.

fibers. They are most abundant in hemopoietic and lymphoid tissues, and in hollow organs, such as the bladder, intestines, and uterus, which are subject to large changes in volume.

Elastic fibers

Connective tissue also contains **elastic fibers**. These are not easily identifiable in routine preparations, but they can be selectively stained with resorcin-fuchsin. If a thin spread of mesentery is so stained, a network of slender branching fibrils is revealed (Fig. 4.2B). These fibers are composed of an amorphous, rubber-like glycoprotein, **elastin**, in the core of a bundle of microfibrils. The polymers of elastin are cross-linked by covalent bonds between two uncommon amino acids, desmosine and isodesmosine. These fibers have rubber-like properties, stretching under tension and snapping back when the tension is relieved. They can be stretched to 1.5 times their length and will immediately return to their original length when released. Elastin is synthesized by the fibroblasts of connective tissue and by smooth muscle cells of large arteries, and is assembled extracellularly. In the walls of arteries, some of the elastin synthesized does not form networks of fibrils, but instead is assembled into fenestrated sheets, called **elastic laminae**, that are arranged concentrically in the wall of the blood vessel. The wall of the aorta (the large artery that conducts blood away from the heart), is distended by the outflow of blood from each contraction of the heart. The elastic recoil of its wall is essential to maintain continuous flow from intermittent contractions of the heart.

Elastic fibers are especially abundant in the connective tissue of organs that must yield to externally or internally applied force. The lungs, for example, are expanded with each inspiration and must have sufficient elasticity to return to their original volume upon expiration. An abundance of elastic fibers in the alveolar septa of the lungs makes this possible.

CELLS OF CONNECTIVE TISSUE

The cells of connective tissue will be considered in two categories: **fixed cells** and **free cells**. The fixed cells include the **fibroblasts** and **adipose cells** (fat cells). In normal connective tissue, they constitute a stable population of relatively immobile cells. The fibroblasts produce and maintain the extracellular components of connective tissue. The adipose cells store lipids after meals and later release them into the blood to serve as an energy source during periods of fasting.

The so-called free cells are an ever-changing population of motile cells that emigrate from the blood and wander through the connective tissue on various missions. They include **neutrophils, eosinophils, monocytes**, and **lymphocytes**. Some of these are short-lived and are continually replaced from the pool of leukocytes in the circulation. Lymphocytes may return to the blood or lymph, and are transported to connective tissue elsewhere in the body. Soon after their migration from the blood into the connective tissue, monocytes differentiate into **macrophages**. These highly mobile phagocytic cells ingest any invading bacteria encountered. They also interact with lymphocytes in the generation of protective antibodies against the invaders. Some lymphocytes that have been activated in response to a bacteria, differentiate into **plasma cells** that reside for some time in the connective tissue, and continue to produce antibodies for long-term immunological defense against that species of bacteria.

FIXED CELLS OF CONNECTIVE TISSUE

Fibroblasts

Fibroblasts are the principal cell type of connective tissue. Their shape varies in different locations, but where they are stretched out along collagen fibers they are usually fusiform, tapering towards both ends (Figs 4.7, 4.8). In other locations they may take on a flat, stellate form with several slender radiating processes. On electron micrographs, their elongated nucleus contains one or two nucleoli and small clumps of heterochromatin adjacent to the nuclear envelope. Long, slender mitochondria are found in the perinuclear cytoplasm, but may extend a short distance into the tapering cell processes. The endoplasmic reticulum is sparse in inactive cells, but is more extensive in fibroblasts actively engaged in collagen synthesis. There is a small Golgi complex. A few microtubules may be seen radiating from a juxtanuclear centrosome into the cell processes.

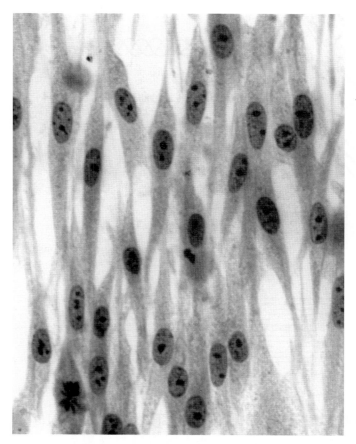

Figure 4.7 Photomicrograph of fibroblasts in tissue culture. They retain, *in vitro*, the same elongated form that they have *in vivo*, where their shape is often obscured by surrounding collagen fibers.

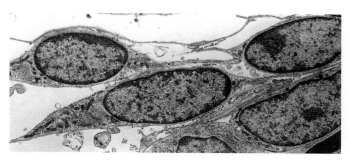

Figure 4.8 Electron micrograph of fibroblasts, illustrating their tapering ends, elongate nucleus, and relatively few organelles.

The principal functions of fibroblasts are the synthesis of collagen, elastin, and the proteoglycans of the ground substance of connective tissue. In the synthesis of collagen, amino acids taken into the cytoplasm are assembled by polyribosomes of the rER, into polypeptides, with the amino acid sequences encoded in two different mRNAs. The two resulting polypeptides, designated α-**chains** and β-**chains**, accumulate in the lumen of the endoplasmic reticulum, where their signal sequences are clipped off by a peptidase, and one α-chain and two β-chains entwine in a triple helical configuration to form molecules of **procollagen**. These are transported to the Golgi complex for glycosylation and packaging for exocytosis. After release into the extracellular space, short registration peptides on either end of the chains are cleaved off by another peptidase, converting the procollagen molecules to **tropocollagen molecules** and these polymerize to form unit fibrils of collagen. These, in turn, are assembled into collagen fibers. These events in collagen synthesis are portrayed in Figure 4.9.

Collagen fibers are a principal source of strength for bone. In the disease **osteogenesis imperfecta**, a mutation in one of the genes for Type I collagen results in synthesis of structurally abnormal α-chain or β-chains. This prevents their assembly in triple helical configuration to form tropocollagen. Patients with this disease have extremely fragile bones that fracture very easily. The most severe cases may be in people born with fractures sustained in the birth process. In milder cases, fractures may occur in childhood but become less common after puberty and the individual can live a nearly normal life. Deficiency of collagen fibers in the dermis results in thin, mobile skin. The sclera of the eyes is thinner than normal and often has a bluish tint. There is no specific therapy for the disease.

Many of the fibroblasts bound to collagen fibers of connective tissue remain sessile for long periods, but in the event of an injury that destroys tissue, they are capable of migrating to the site at a rate of about 1 μm/min to participate in repair of the damage. Dividing fibroblasts are rarely seen in normal tissue, but they proliferate in response to tissue damage and become active in synthesis of the fibrous and amorphous components of connective tissue needed for repair of the injury.

Adipose cells (fat cells)

Both fibroblasts and adipose cells arise from **mesenchymal cells** of the embryo. Some of these pluripotential cells differentiate

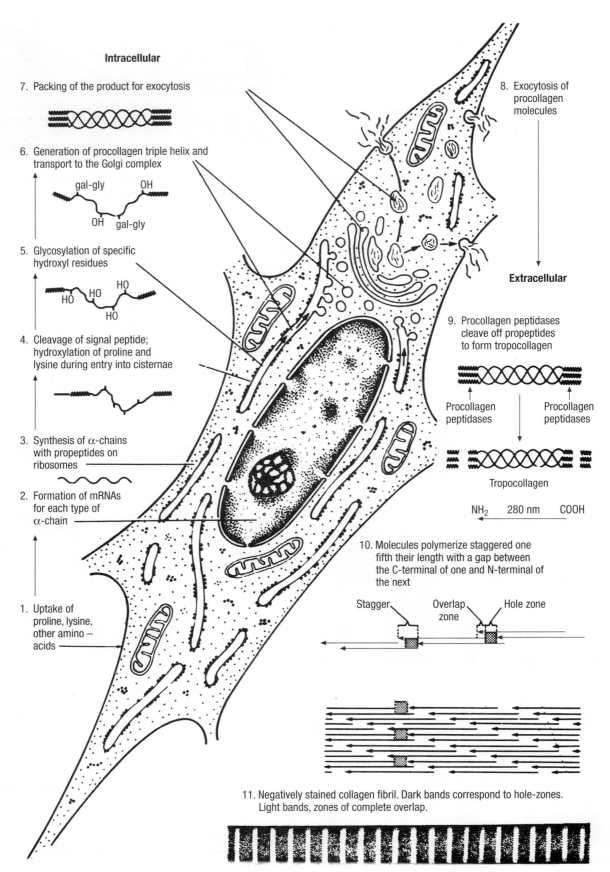

Intracellular

7. Packing of the product for exocytosis

6. Generation of procollagen triple helix and transport to the Golgi complex

gal-gly   OH

OH   gal-gly

5. Glycosylation of specific hydroxyl residues

HO   HO

HO   HO

HO

4. Cleavage of signal peptide; hydroxylation of proline and lysine during entry into cisternae

3. Synthesis of α-chains with propeptides on ribosomes

2. Formation of mRNAs for each type of α-chain

1. Uptake of proline, lysine, other amino – acids

8. Exocytosis of procollagen molecules

Extracellular

9. Procollagen peptidases cleave off propeptides to form tropocollagen

Procollagen peptidases

Procollagen peptidases

Tropocollagen

NH_2 280 nm   COOH

10. Molecules polymerize staggered one fifth their length with a gap between the C-terminal of one and N-terminal of the next

Stagger   Overlap zone   Hole zone

11. Negatively stained collagen fibril. Dark bands correspond to hole-zones. Light bands, zones of complete overlap.

Figure 4.9 Drawing presenting the biochemical events and organelle participation in the synthesis of collagen by a fibroblast. On the left the intracellular steps and on the right the extracellular events in assembly of collagen fibrils are defined. (Reproduced from L.C. Junquiera and J. Carniero *Basic Histology*, 3rd edn, Lange Medical Publications, 1980.)

into **lipoblasts**, which are scattered throughout the connective tissue. When dietary intake exceeds metabolic needs, some of these differentiate into **adipose cells**. These cells take up and store triglycerides (neutral fats) in a very large droplet, which displaces the nucleus and flattens it against the plasma membrane. Adipose cells may be found singly, or in small groups in connective tissue anywhere in the body, but in certain regions they accumulate in great number, replacing the other components of connective tissue to constitute **adipose tissue** (fat). Its organization and physiology are sufficiently distinct from ordinary connective tissue to be considered separately later in this chapter.

FREE CELLS OF CONNECTIVE TISSUE

Macrophages

Macrophages are motile phagocytic cells found in connective tissues throughout the body. In their unstimulated state, they may be fusiform or stellate in shape and adherent to the collagen fibers. They are distinguishable from fibroblasts by their slightly smaller, and more deeply stained nucleus, and by a cytoplasm that contains a number of granules of varying size that are identifiable on electron micrographs as lysosomes. When stimulated, they become actively motile cells of varying shape, which have a remarkable capacity for phagocytosis. They participate in the maintenance of the connective tissue by clearing it of dead cells, cellular debris, bacteria, and any other foreign particulate material. At sites of infection, they gather in large numbers and voraciously ingest and destroy the bacteria.

The mechanisms involved in their ingestion of bacteria have been thoroughly studied. Upon entering the tissues of the body, bacteria become coated with **immunoglobulins** (antibodies) and **complement** (a group of serum proteins that enhance inflammatory responses). This surface coating renders the bacteria more vulnerable to phagocytosis by macrophages, which have surface receptors for these serum proteins. Ingestion of a bacterium by a macrophage begins with a zipper-like progressive binding of receptors in its membrane to the proteins on the surface of the bacterium. This proceeds until pseudopodia of the macrophage completely surround the bacterium. Upon membrane fusion at the leading edges of the pseudopodia, the bacterium is enclosed in a vacuole, or **phagosome**, within the cytoplasm. Lysosomes then fuse with the phagosome, discharging into it **lysozyme**, an enzyme that digests the bacterial wall. Several other lysosomal hydrolases complete the digestive process.

Macrophages also mobilize other cell types to participate in the body's defense against infection. They synthesize and release a number of **cytokines** (short range signaling molecules) that diffuse from the site of infection, into the capillaries to stimulate leukocytes to migrate into the connective tissue. One of the cytokines, **interleukin-1**, is a chemoattractant that induces neutrophils to migrate up its concentration gradient to join the macrophages in phagocytosis of bacteria. It is also chemotactic for

lymphocytes, which gather around the macrophages and are stimulated to proliferate and produce specific antibodies against that species of bacteria. Macrophages have an essential role in the immune response by presenting foreign proteins (antigens) to lymphocytes in a more immunogenic form.

Macrophages belong to a heterogeneous group of phagocytic cell types that was formerly designated the **reticuloendothelial system**. Cells belonging to this system were originally identified by injecting the vital dye Trypan Blue into experimental animals. Cells that were found to take up the dye were considered to share the phagocytic properties of macrophages. On the basis of these experiments, various free cells resembling macrophages were assigned to this system, as well as the endothelial cells lining sinusoids in certain organs. The term reticuloendothelial system is still in use and is strongly defended by its proponents. However, more recently the Trypan Blue technique has been abandoned in favor of isotopically labeled monoclonal antibodies against specific surface markers. This has made it possible to identify legitimate members of this system with greater accuracy, and the newer term **mononuclear phagocyte system** is now widely accepted. This now includes all highly phagocytic cell types of whatever shape or location, but it excludes the controversial sinusoidal endothelia, which evidently took up the dye in small amounts by pinocytosis instead of phagocytosis. The members of the mononuclear phagocyte system as currently interpreted are: **monocytes** and **macrophages** of connective tissue; **alveolar phagocytes** of the lung; **Kupffer cells** of the liver; **osteoclasts** of bone; and **dendritic cells** of the skin and lymph nodes.

Neutrophils

Neutrophils are few in normal connective tissue, but they gather in great numbers at sites of infection. The mechanisms involved in their mobilization have recently been clarified. Cytokines released by macrophages at the site induce endothelial cells of capillaries to synthesize, and incorporate in their membrane, molecules of a protein called **endothelial adhesion molecule-1** (selectin). The surface of the neutrophils contains receptors for this protein and they adhere to the endothelium of capillaries at the site of infection. The neutrophils then migrate through the wall of the capillaries, and up the concentration gradient of bacterial products and cytokines released by macrophages. These mechanisms insure rapid mobilization of neutrophils to join the macrophages in phagocytosis of bacteria. The 'pus' that accumulates at sites of infection consists mainly of dead and dying neutrophils that have completed their mission.

Eosinophils

Eosinophils are present in small numbers in normal connective tissue, but they are greatly increased in allergic conditions, and around nematode worms and other parasites. In normal individuals, eosinophils are most abundant in the connective tissue beneath the epithelia that are most likely to be exposed to foreign protein (e.g. those of the alimentary and respiratory tracts). They do not phagocytize bacteria, but are involved in damage control in allergic reactions, disposing of antigen–antibody complexes. They also release the enzymes **aryl sulfatase** and **histaminase**, which break down histamine and heparin, the chemical mediators of allergic reactions. In parasitic diseases, eosinophils also secrete cationic proteins that form pores in the membrane of the parasite, and they release superoxide ions and hydrogen peroxide that damage parasite membranes by lipid peroxidation.

Lymphocytes

Lymphocytes are present in considerable numbers in normal connective tissue, where they are involved in protective immunosurveillance. At sites of invasion by bacteria, they gather in large numbers and contact macrophages already assembled at the site. Lymphocytes are not phagocytic and are unable to respond directly to bacteria. These must first be phagocytized by macrophages, which insert into their membrane a peptide product of bacterial digestion. When a foreign protein (an antigen) is presented to B-lymphocytes in this form, they respond with the production of specific immunoglobulins (antibodies). The different types of lymphocytes, and their respective functions in the immune response, will be discussed in greater detail in Chapter 10, Immune System.

Plasma cells

Plasma cells are spherical, or ovoid cells much larger than lymphocytes. Their eccentrically located nucleus often has a radial pattern of coarse clumps of heterochromatin. The cytoplasm is intensely basophilic. On electron micrographs, the cytoplasm is found to be filled with closely spaced cisternae of rER (Fig. 4.10). Plasma cells develop by further differentiation of lymphocytes that have encountered an antigen and produced specific antibodies against it. As plasma cells they continue to produce the same antibody in large amounts for weeks after the initial immune response. Plasma cells produce antibody (immunoglobulin-E, IgE) of slightly different structure than that produced by their lymphocyte precursors (immunoglobulin-G, IgG). No secretory granules are formed; their product is released continuously by exocytosis of small vesicles formed in the Golgi and transported to the cell surface. Plasma cells probably live no more than 3 or 4 weeks. They are replaced by terminal differentiation of other B-lymphocytes that have reacted to an antigen.

Mast cells

Mast cells are widely dispersed in connective tissue and are the largest of its cells, measuring 20–30 μm in diameter. They are easily identified by the intensely basophilic granules that fill the cytoplasm, often obscuring the nucleus (Fig. 4.11). Mast cells contain short profiles of rER, a small Golgi complex, and a few mitochondria. The granules contain **heparin**, a glycosaminoglycan. When stained with Toluidine Blue, the granules are metachromatic (i.e. they take on a color different from that of the stain applied), a property common to glycosaminoglycans. Other components of the granules include **histamine**, and the enzymes **tryptase** and **chymase**. On electron micrographs of human connective tissue, the granules of some mast cells contain a cylindrical scroll-like inclusion. In cross-section, this appears to be made up of concentric laminae about the thickness of a lipid bilayer. In other mast cells, the granules have a dense outer matrix surrounding a pale central area,

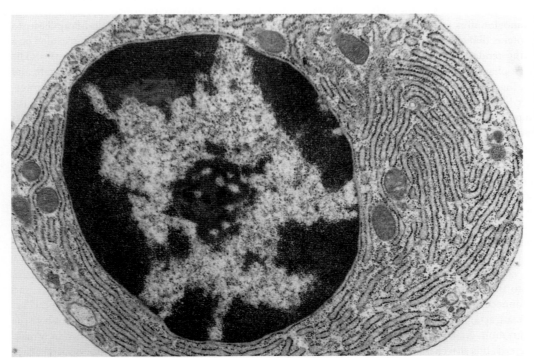

Figure 4.10 Electron micrograph of a plasma cell, illustrating the coarse pattern of heterochromatin in its nucleus, and the extensive rough endoplasmic reticulum in its cytoplasm. Plasma cells synthesize large amounts of immunoglobulin, but it is not stored in secretory granules.

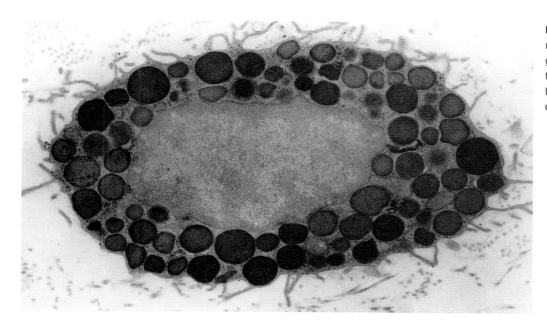

Figure 4.11 Electron micrograph of a mast cell. It contains many secretory granules. When stimulated by an antigen to which the organism has previously been exposed, there is a massive release of the histamine content of the granules.

which contains parallel linear densities. The significance of these variations in granule ultrastructure is unknown.

Mast cells are sensitive sentinels for the immune system, detecting foreign proteins in the tissues and rapidly releasing potent mediators of an inflammatory reaction, followed by a slower release of cytokines that recruit other participating cell types. Molecules of immunoglobulins (antibodies) produced by plasma cells bind to the surface of mast cells. These cells are then prepared to respond immediately, by massive release of their granules, whenever the corresponding antigen re-enters the body. Allergic individuals produce antibodies to pollens and a host of other foreign proteins. Upon re-exposure to one of these, it binds to IgE molecules on the surface of mast cells and cross-links them, triggering their release of **histamine** and other products. The response may be local or general. In hay fever, for example, histamine released by mast cells in the connective tissue of the nasal mucosa causes increased permeability of the capillaries and consequent swelling of the mucosa, accompanied by sneezing, stuffy nose and nasal discharge. In asthma, the response is mainly in the lungs, where histamine plays a less important role than the cytokines that are released. These cause contraction of smooth muscle in the wall of the bronchi, and narrowing of the airway, making breathing difficult.

Mast cell granules also contain β-glucuronidase and aryl sulfatase, enzymes that play no part in inflammatory or immune responses, but degrade glycosaminoglycans of the extracellular matrix. This has led to the suggestion that mast cells have a continual low level of secretory activity, which may contribute to the turnover of the ground substance of connective tissue. This remains to be verified.

TYPES OF CONNECTIVE TISSUE

Local differences in the organization and relative abundance of cells, fibers, and ground substance in connective tissue are indicated by use of different descriptive terms. The term **loose connective tissue** (areolar tissue) is applied to areas in which the collagen fibers are relatively small, moderately abundant and loosely interwoven. The term **dense connective tissue** is applied to areas in which the fibers are coarse and very abundant. Modifiers are added to this term to indicate the arrangement of the fibers. Where they are closely interwoven in seemingly random orientation, the tissue is described as **dense irregular connective tissue**. Where they are closely packed in parallel bundles the tissue is referred to as **dense regular connective tissue**.

Loose connective tissue

Loose connective tissue is a loose network of randomly oriented fibers in an abundant ground substance. It is the most widespread of the connective tissues, occurring in sites where relatively little resistance to stress is required. It supports the epithelial parenchyma of many organs and is the tissue through which their blood vessels and nerves are distributed. It occupies the spaces around and between muscles, and surrounds blood vessels. It is found beneath the dermis of the skin, and immediately beneath other epithelia. It forms thin layers beneath the mesothelium lining the thoracic and peritoneal cavities, and in the mesenteries that suspend the organs from the posterior wall of the abdominal cavity. Its most numerous cells are fibroblasts, but macrophages and other motile cells of connective tissue are present in small numbers.

Reticular connective tissue

Reticular connective tissue is a form of loose connective tissue in which a network (reticulum) of argyrophilic fibers is the dominant fibrous component. The cells tend to be stellate, with their slender radiating processes deployed along the intersecting fibers of the reticulum. They are probably simply fibroblasts of atypical shape. They synthesize type III collagen and relatively little ground substance. Reticular connective tissue surrounds the functional units of epithelial organs, and forms the stroma of the bone marrow, spleen, lymph nodes, and thymus. In the lymphoid organs, the spaces within the network are occupied by large numbers of lymphocytes, and in the marrow, by closely packed precursors of the blood cells.

Mucous connective tissue

Mucous connective tissue is an uncommon form of loose connective tissue, containing a very large amount of ground substance, which is rich in hyaluronic acid. Collagen fibers make up a very small fraction of its volume. Its widely spaced cellular elements are stellate fibroblasts. This kind of connective tissue is rare in adults, but is common in the embryo. It is the principal component of the umbilical cord, where it was formerly called **Wharton's jelly**.

Dense connective tissue

Dense irregular connective tissue differs from loose connective tissue in the preponderance of fibrous elements and the paucity of cells. Collagen fibers make up most of its volume. The fiber bundles are relatively coarse and interwoven in a compact meshwork with little space occupied by cells and ground substance. A network of elastic fibers intermingles with the collagen fiber bundles. Long fusiform fibroblasts are present between the bundles of collagen fibers, but usually only their nuclei are visible in histological sections. Macrophages are present in small numbers, but they are distinguishable from fibroblasts only after supravital staining. Other free cells are very few. Dense irregular connective tissue is found in the dermis of the skin, in the capsule of the liver, and other organs, in the tunica albuginea of the testes, in the dura mater enclosing the brain, and in the sheaths of large nerves.

In **dense regular connective tissue** the bundles of collagen fibers are oriented parallel to one another and closely packed, with little intervening ground substance. The fibroblasts are aligned between fiber bundles with most of their cytoplasm in thin, fin-like processes that extend between, and partially surround, neighboring fiber bundles. Usually, only their elongated nuclei are visible in histological sections. The compact fiber bundles are all oriented in the direction best suited to resist the stresses to which the tissue is subjected. The most common examples of this kind of connective tissue are the tendons that transmit the tension produced by muscles. The primary bundles of type I collagen fibers in tendons are assembled into larger secondary bundles that are surrounded by a very thin layer of loose connective tissue containing capillaries and small nerves. At the periphery of the tendon, a layer of dense irregular connective tissue forms the tendon sheath. The parallel arrangement of collagen fibers in a tendon forms a structure that is flexible, but offers great resistance to a pulling force.

Certain broad, flat muscles of the body do not have cylindrical tendons, but are attached to their insertions by sheets of dense regular connective tissue called **aponeuroses**. These consist of multiple layers of coherent bundles of collagen fibers. Within any one layer, the fiber bundles are parallel, but their direction changes in successive layers. Separation of the layers is prevented by some fibers that cross over between layers.

HISTOPHYSIOLOGY OF CONNECTIVE TISSUE

As the name implies, connective tissue binds other components of the body together. Loose connective tissue is the avenue through which blood vessels pass to reach other tissues. Oxygen and nutrients diffuse through the aqueous phase of its ground substance. This fluid and the small amount of free tissue fluid, are continually renewed. Hydrostatic pressure at the arterial ends of the capillaries causes water, electrolytes, and small molecules to pass through the walls of these vessels. Some of this fluid re-enters the blood at the venous end of the capillaries where the pressure is lower, and some of it is returned to the blood via the lymph vessels. Fluid normally enters and leaves the ground substance at the same rate. However, damage to the capillaries, or obstruction of lymphatics, may result in accumulation of excess fluid in the ground substance (edema).

During the growth period, there is considerable turnover of the collagen fibers of connective tissue, but in the adult these are relatively stable. The degradation of collagen is carried out by specific collagenases produced by fibroblasts and certain other cell types.

ADIPOSE TISSUE

Adipose tissue is included in this chapter because histologists have traditionally considered it to be loose connective tissue in which some of the fibroblasts have stored excess lipid and become transformed into adipose cells. In recent years, this interpretation has fallen into disfavor as evidence has accumulated that adipose tissue not only stores lipid as a reserve of energy-rich material, but also produces hormones that influence the carbohydrate and lipid metabolism of other tissues, and act upon the brain to control appetite. Many now consider adipose tissue sufficiently distinct from connective tissue, in its organization and function, to be considered a separate tissue type.

The classical interpretation that fibroblasts anywhere in the body can store lipid and become adipose cells, fails to account for their preferential distribution. The characteristic differences in the body form of males and females is, in large measure, a result of different sites of predilection for subcutaneous fat disposition. In the male, the principal sites are over the nape of the neck, in the lumbosacral region, and on the buttocks. In the female, fat is most abundant in the breasts, buttocks, over the trochanter of the femurs, and the anterior and lateral aspects of the thighs. With advancing age, the male tends to accumulate subcutaneous fat over the anterior abdominal wall. To account for these differences, many histologists now consider it likely that fat cells arise from mesenchymal cells of the embryo that differentiate into **lipoblasts** (adipose cell precursors), which have a pattern of distribution, in the adult, that is distinct from that of the ubiquitous fibroblasts. Verification of this interpretation is difficult because mesenchymal cells, lipoblasts and fibroblasts are very similar in appearance in histological sections.

There are two forms of adipose tissue that differ in color, vascularity, metabolic activity and distribution. One is called **white adipose tissue** and the other **brown adipose tissue**. The cells of white adipose tissue store lipid in a single very large droplet, and are described as **unilocular** fat cells. Those of brown adipose tissue contain multiple small droplets of lipid and are called **multilocular** fat cells.

WHITE ADIPOSE TISSUE

White adipose tissue varies in color from white to pale yellow, depending upon the dietary content of a group of pigments called

carotenoids. As described earlier, single fat cells in loose connective tissue are spherical, but where they are closely packed together in adipose tissue, they take on a polyhedral shape as a result of mutual deformation. Some 80% of the cell volume is occupied by a single large drop of stored lipid that displaces the nucleus to one side of the cell and flattens it against the plasmalemma. The cytoplasm is reduced to a thin rim around the lipid drop. During their development, fat cells may contain several smaller lipid droplets, but these coalesce into a single drop as the cell matures.

Unfixed adipose tissue, stained with the lipid-soluble dye Sudan Black, appears as a mosaic of large lipid drops that are polygonal in outline and of nearly uniform size (Fig. 4.12A). In the preparation of histological sections, the lipid is extracted, leaving behind only their thin rim of cytoplasm, containing the greatly flattened nucleus. In well-preserved specimens, the polygonal shape of the mutually deforming cells is retained and the tissue appears as a network with large polygonal meshes (Fig. 4.12B). However, during dehydration of a specimen prior to embedding, the thin rims of cytoplasm often collapse to varying degrees, giving the cells an irregular outline that does not accurately represent their form *in vivo*. Fat cells are 50–150 μm in diameter, three or four times the diameter of the capillaries supplying the tissue.

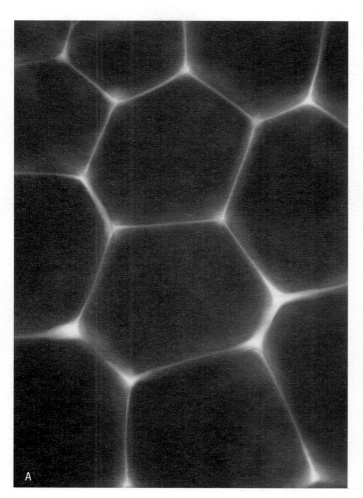
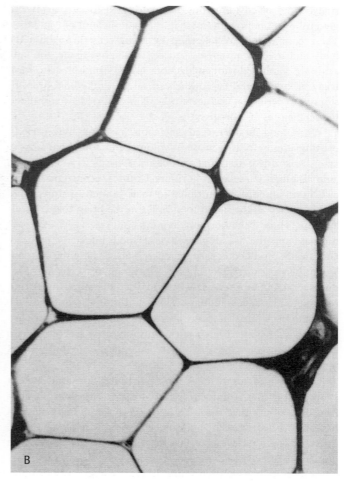

Figure 4.12 (A) A thin spread of unilocular adipose tissue stained with Sudan Black without previous exposure to lipid solvents. The lipid has been retained and is stained by the fat-soluble dye, while the surrounding rim of cytoplasm is unstained. (B) Unilocular adipose tissue prepared by the routine method involving dehydration before staining. The lipid drop has been extracted and only the thin rim of cytoplasm remains.

Each cell is surrounded by a loose network of reticular fibers, and the tissue as a whole is partitioned by thin connective tissue septa into lobules that are discernible with the naked eye. This lobulation is most obvious in subcutaneous tissue such as that over the buttocks, where the adipose tissue has a cushioning or shock-absorbing function.

On electron micrographs, a small Golgi complex, a few long mitochondria, and occasional fenestrated cisternae of rER can be found in the thicker region of cytoplasm near the nucleus. The lipid drop is not enclosed by a membrane, but may be surrounded by a layer of 10 nm intermediate filaments of vimentin. The thin layer of cytoplasm contains many small pinocytotic vesicles. There may also be small lipid droplets that have not yet fused with the main lipid drop. These are usually not seen in sections examined with the light microscope.

Histophysiology of white adipose tissue

Lipids in the diet are absorbed as triglycerides and monoglycerides and are combined with cholesterol, phospholipid, and protein in the intestinal cells to form water-soluble particles called **chylomicrons**, which enter the blood. In the circulation, the triglycerides of chylomicrons are hydrolyzed to fatty acids and glycerol by a lipoprotein lipase in the endothelium of capillaries. These compounds are taken up by tissue cells throughout the body and used as an energy source. In adipose tissue, the fatty acids are combined with endogenous glycerol phosphate to form triglycerides (neutral fats), which are added to the lipid drop for storage. In periods of fasting, fatty acids are released into the blood to fuel the cells of other tissues.

When food intake exceeds metabolic need for long periods, existing adipose cells increase in volume, and additional adipose cells are formed, resulting in obesity. Obesity is very rare in animals other than man. A hormone **leptin** is secreted by adipose cells in an amount proportional to their content of stored lipid and is carried in the blood to a center in the brain that controls appetite. Thus, if the hormone reports lipid reserves in excess of normal, appetite is suppressed and food intake is reduced. Genetically modified experimental animals, lacking the gene for leptin, become extremely obese. Human adipose cells also produce leptin, but for reasons that are not yet understood, it does not restrain food intake in humans. This is unfortunate, for half of the people in the United States are overweight, and one-third are clinically obese. Obesity is associated with increased risk of diabetes and cardiovascular disease, and is a public health problem of increasing magnitude.

Leptin is proving to be a multifunctional hormone. Recent studies show that it influences carbohydrate and lipid metabolism of cells in other tissues; stimulates the immune system of undernourished animals; and affects the growth of capillaries. There is, as yet, no evidence that these functions are impaired in humans.

Adipose cells have been found to secrete a second hormone, **resistin**. Obese individuals are at increased risk of developing type II diabetes, in which insulin is produced but fails to have its normal effect on the processing of glucose for use by muscles and other tissues. Administration of excess resistin to experimental animals causes a similar insulin resistance. This recent discovery sheds new light upon the relation of obesity to type II diabetes, and suggests approaches to development of drugs to treat or prevent this common disease.

The common assumption that lipid stores in adipose tissue are only drawn upon in periods of fasting has proven to be erroneous. Isotopic studies have clearly established that the lipid is constantly being turned over, even if the animal is eating and in caloric balance. In laboratory rodents, the half-life of depot lipid is about 8 days, which means that almost 10% of the fatty acids in adipose tissue is replaced each day. Continuous renewal also occurs in humans, but the exact rate of turnover has not been determined.

Lipid is a poor conductor of heat, and human babies have a continuous layer of subcutaneous fat, called the **panniculosus adiposus**, that helps maintain body temperature. This insulating function of adipose tissue is well developed in adult aquatic mammals (whales, seals, walrus), which have a very thick layer of subcutaneous adipose tissue (blubber) to minimize loss of heat to the arctic seawater.

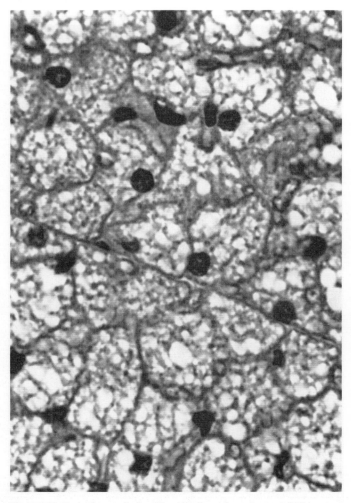

Figure 4.13 Photomicrograph of multilocular adipose tissue (brown fat). The polygonal cells contain many small droplets of lipid instead of a single large drop. The lipid was extracted in preparation of the tissue for sectioning.

BROWN ADIPOSE TISSUE

The **brown adipose tissue** ranges in color from tan to reddish brown. Its color results, in part, from its rich vascularity and, in part, from cytochromes in its exceptionally abundant mitochondria. The cells are polygonal in section and considerably smaller than those of white adipose tissue. Their cytoplasm is relatively abundant and contains multiple lipid droplets of varying size (Fig.4.13). The spherical nucleus is eccentric in position, but is not displaced to the periphery of the cell, as in white fat. In electron micrographs, large spherical mitochondria occupy a large part of the cytoplasm between lipid droplets (Fig.4.14). They have numerous cristae that often traverse the entire width of the organelle. Rough endoplasmic reticulum is virtually absent, but there are occasional tubular profiles of smooth endoplasmic reticulum. Free ribosomes and variable amounts of glycogen are also present.

Brown fat has a lobular organization, and the pattern of distribution of its blood vessels is reminiscent of that of a gland. In animals subjected to prolonged fasting, their brown fat gradually loses lipid, becoming more deeply colored and reverting to a glandlike mass of epithelioid cells that bear no resemblance to the fibroblasts of connective tissue.

The blood supply of brown adipose tissue is very rich and fibrous components of connective tissue are few. Its cells are, therefore, in more intimate relation to one another and to the capillaries than in white fat. Silver stains and electron micrographs reveal numerous small unmyelinated nerves in brown adipose tissue. Their axons are frequently found in close apposition to the surface of the cells. This contrasts with the nerves in white adipose tissue, which appear to innervate only the blood vessels.

Brown adipose tissue is found in all mammalian species that have been investigated, but it is best developed in those species that have a period of winter dormancy (hibernation). In the common laboratory rodents, it occurs in two symmetrical interscapular fat bodies and in lobules between the muscles of the shoulder girdle. In humans, it is found in the posterior triangle of the neck, and in the interscapular region. It also occurs on the posterior wall of the abdominal cavity on either side of the vertebral bodies, and around the kidneys.

The embryological origin of brown fat is debated, but it is now believed that mesenchymal cells give rise to **lipoblasts** of two kinds, one developing into unilocular adipose cells (white fat) and the other into multilocular adipose cells (brown fat) (Fig.4.15). In rodents, brown fat retains its multilocular character in adults. Brown fat cells in humans are multilocular at birth and

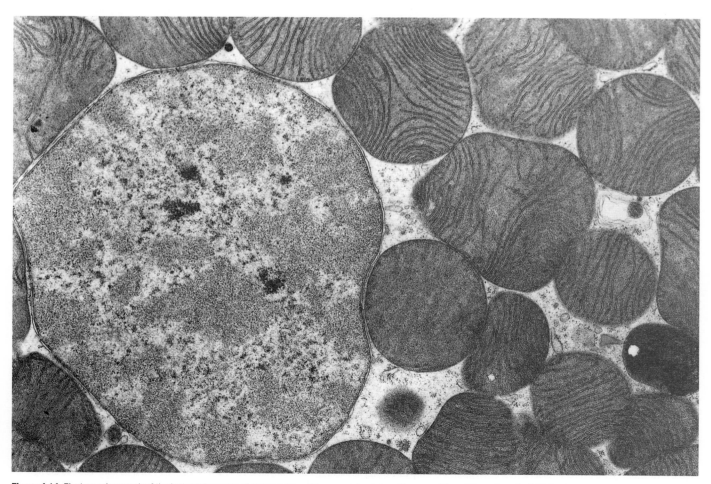

Figure 4.14 Electron micrograph of the juxtanuclear area of a brown fat cell from an animal recently aroused from hibernation. No lipid droplets remain. Note the very large spherical mitochondria characteristic of this tissue.

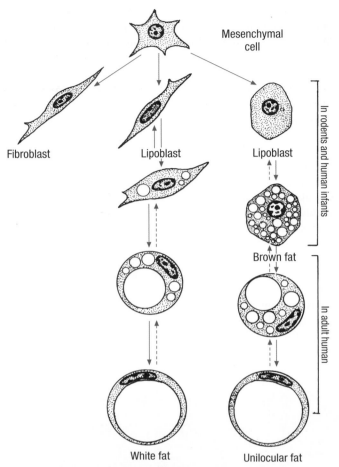

throughout early childhood, but the droplets later tend to coalesce, and in the adult, the cells may closely resemble those of white adipose tissue. Although in well nourished adults, these may be difficult to distinguish microscopically from white adipose cells, there is compelling evidence that two physiologically distinct types of adipose tissue persist. In prolonged fasting, or in emaciated elderly individuals suffering from a chronic wasting disease, multilocular fat again becomes apparent in the same regions in which it is found in the newborn. Further support for two types of fat is derived from the observation that there are two distinct types of **lipomas** (tumors of fat).

Histophysiology of brown adipose tissue

Brown adipose tissue serves as an energy reserve but has little, or no, insulating function. One of its major functions is heat generation. Its very numerous mitochondria give it an unusual capacity for generating heat by oxidation of fatty acids. The rate of substrate oxidation by brown fat cells, *in vitro*, is as much as 20 times that of white fat cells. Each milliliter of oxygen consumed in the process contributes about five calories of body heat. Brown fat cells are activated in a cold environment and may treble their heat production.

Adult animals in a cold environment produce heat as a by-product of the muscular activity involved in shivering. Newborn and very young animals are unable to shiver and rely on their brown adipose tissue for non-shivering thermogenesis. Upon exposure to cold, sensory receptors in the skin send nerve impulses to the temperature-regulating center in the brain, which relays impulses along sympathetic nerves to the brown adipose tissue. Some of these nerves act upon the blood vessels to increase blood flow, others terminating on brown adipose cells, release norepinephrine, which activates the enzyme that splits triglycerides to fatty acids and glycerol, thereby triggering a heat-producing cycle of fatty acid oxidation and triglyceride regeneration, which converts chemical-bond

Figure 4.15 In the development of adipose tissue, mesenchymal cells give rise to fibroblasts and two kinds of lipoblasts. One of these differentiates into unilocular adipose tissue (white fat), and the other into multilocular adipose tissue (brown fat). In the adult human the droplets of the latter coalesce and it comes to resemble white adipose tissue but remains physiologically distinct.

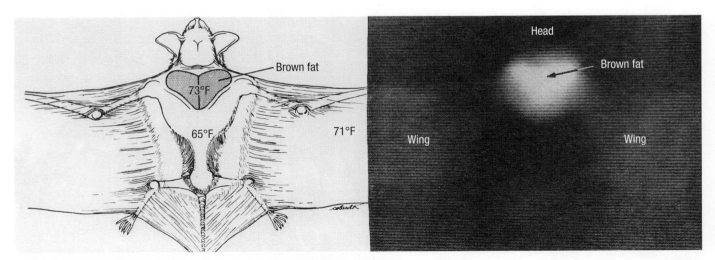

Figure 4.16 Drawing of a bat during arousal from hibernation. The temperature over its interscapular brown fat is 73°F, compared to 65°F over its lower back. At the right is a thermogram, made by scanning the animal for infra-red radiation. It reveals a 'hot spot' over the interscapular brown fat which serves as a chemical furnace, producing heat that is carried in the blood to warm the rest of the animal.

energy to heat energy. This is made possible by a unique uncoupling protein, **thermogenin**, in the inner membrane of the mitochondria of brown fat cells that permits the energy generated in the above reactions to be dissipated as heat instead of being used in the synthesis of ATP, which is its fate under other circumstances. The heat warms the blood flowing through the brown adipose tissue and this heat is carried in the circulation to other parts of the body.

Brown adipose tissue is especially abundant in animal species that hibernate. Its heat production is believed to be essential for their rapid warming during arousal from the torpid state (Fig. 4.16). In the adult human, a physiological role for brown fat in temperature regulation is less well established, but in the newborn and in young infants, it is believed to be essential for maintenance of normal body temperature.

Questions

1   Which of the following is released by mast cells?
  a   interleukin-1
  b   IgE
  c   histamine
  d   lymphokines
  e   erythropoietin

2   Macrophages are derived from
  a   fibroblasts
  b   osteocytes
  c   plasma cells
  d   monocytes
  e   adipocytes

3   Dense regular connective tissue is present in which of the following?
  a   organ capsules
  b   basement membranes
  c   ligaments
  d   cartilage
  e   skin

4   Which of the following are not permanent residents of connective tissue?
  a   fibroblast
  b   mast cell
  c   mesenchymal cell
  d   plasma cell
  e   adipocyte (fat cell)

5   The cells (adipocytes) of white adipose tissue are characterized by which of the following?
  a   well-defined darkly stained cytoplasm
  b   no basal lamina
  c   a single large fat droplet
  d   abundant mitochondria
  e   a round nucleus

6   Which of the following cells does not belong to the mononuclear phagocytic system?
  a   histiocyte
  b   osteoclast
  c   Kupffer cell
  d   alveolar macrophage
  e   mast cell

7   Which statement best describes the fibroblast?
  a   it is involved in the synthesis, maintenance, and turnover of the extra-cellular matrix

  b   it assembles collagen into fibrils intracellularly and then secretes the fully formed fibril into the extracellular matrix
  c   it is found only in loose connective tissue and dense regular connective tissue
  d   it does not synthesize hyaluronic acid or proteoglycans in most tissues
  e   it is derived from a bone marrow precursor that migrates out of the blood into connective tissues

8   Which of the following statements about brown adipose tissue is correct?
  a   it is also termed unilocular adipose tissue
  b   individual cells exhibit a 'signet ring' appearance
  c   it is present during intrauterine life
  d   it is present postnatally
  e   it contains few mitochondria

9   Which of the following is not considered a transient cell of connective tissue?
  a   eosinophil
  b   neutrophil
  c   plasma cell
  d   fibroblast
  e   none of the above

10 Which of the following arises from activated B-lymphocytes?
  a   T-lymphocytes
  b   macrophages
  c   pericytes
  d   mast cells
  e   plasma cells

11 What type of collagen predominates in hyaline cartilage?

12 What connective tissue fibers are argyrophilic?

13 What type of fiber contains 6–12% hexosamine, allowing it to be positive in a periodic acid-Schiff reaction?

14 A 'signet ring' appearance is characteristic of what connective tissue cell?

15 Monocytes can develop into what type of connective tissue cell?

16 What cell is responsible for the synthesis, maintenance, and turnover of extra-cellular matrix?

17 What is the precursor of collagen?

18 What cell is the largest of the connective tissue cells?

19 Name the cell type that can release histamine near small blood vessels

20 What connective tissue fiber has the ability to recoil after being stretched?

Chapter five

Cartilage

Cartilage is a specialized type of connective tissue in which cells called **chondrocytes** are distributed some distance apart in an exceptionally firm gel-like ground substance (Fig. 5.1). Unlike other connective tissues, it is not penetrated by blood vessels. Its cells are isolated in small cavities in the ground substance, called **lacunae**, and are nourished by diffusion of small molecules

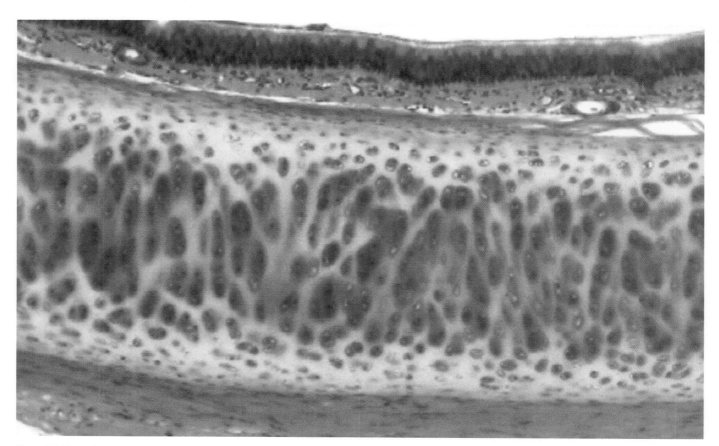

Figure 5.1 Photomicrograph of hyaline cartilage of the trachea. The tracheal epithelium is visible at the top of the figure. The eosinophilic layers on either side of the cartilage are the perichondrium. Beneath this, small chondrocytes are uniformly distributed in a pale staining matrix. Deeper in the cartilage are groups of larger chondrocytes surrounded by deeply basophilic territorial matrix.

through the aqueous phase of the matrix from capillaries in the connective tissue around the cartilage. The unique viscoelastic properties of its ground substance give cartilage great firmness and it is able to retain this property during rapid growth. This makes cartilage an ideal skeletal material for the developing embryo. Most of the skeleton is initially formed of cartilage, and this is gradually replaced by bone later in development. The amount of cartilage is progressively reduced in postnatal life, but it continues to play an important role in the growth in length of the long bones of the extremities, throughout childhood. By the time adult stature has been attained, all cartilage has been replaced by bone except on the joint surfaces of the limb bones, the ventral ends of the ribs, the intervertebral discs of the spine, and in the nose, larynx, and trachea.

Three types of cartilage are distinguished on the basis of the relative abundance of collagen and elastin in their extracellular matrix: **hyaline cartilage**, **elastic cartilage**, and **fibrocartilage**. Of these, hyaline cartilage is the most widespread. Elastic cartilage, and fibrocartilage can be regarded as variants, with properties adapted to special local needs.

HYALINE CARTILAGE

Histogenesis

At sites of cartilage formation in the embryo, mesenchymal cells withdraw their cell processes and gather together to form a dense aggregation of round cells that will constitute a **center of**

chondrification (Fig. 5.2B). Other mesenchymal cells form the **perichondrium**, a layer of fusiform cells and collagen fibers that envelopes the center of chondrification. The cells of the perichondrium continue to divide and add more cells to the periphery of the expanding center of chondrification. In its interior, the cells begin to secrete hyaline matrix around themselves. The continuing deposition of matrix between the cells (now called **chondrocytes**) moves them apart (Fig. 5.2C) and they become isolated in small cavities in the hyaline matrix, called **lacunae**. The growth in size of developing cartilage thus depends upon: (1) **appositional growth**, addition of cells at its periphery; and (2) **interstitial growth**, accumulation of an increasing amount of hyaline matrix between cells. In the embryo, the lacunae are single and are uniformly distributed in the matrix. However, for some time after birth, the chondrocytes retain the ability to divide, and after division, only a small amount of matrix is deposited between the daughter cells. Thus, in adult cartilage, the lacunae occur in pairs or groups of four to six (Fig. 5.3). The cells of each group are said to be **isogenous**, because they represent the progeny of a single chondrocyte. Cell division ceases in childhood after formation of the isogenous groups, and in the cartilage that persists into adulthood, the chondrocytes remain quiescent.

Chondrocytes

In histological sections of adult cartilage, the lacunae near the perichondrium are elliptical, with their long axis parallel to the surface. Those in isogenous groupings, deeper in the matrix, are hemispherical or roughly triangular. *In vivo*, the chondrocytes

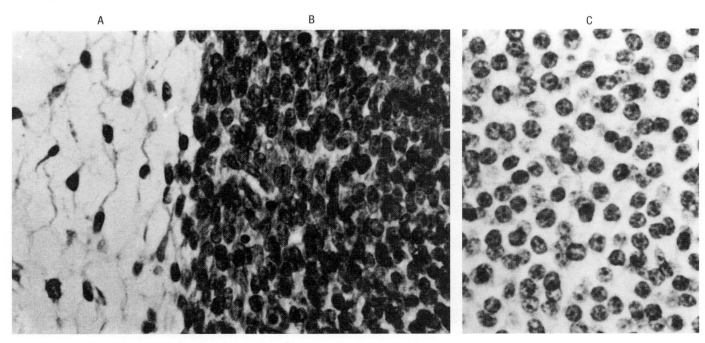

Figure 5.2 Early stages of development of cartilage in the embryo. (A) An area of mesenchymal cells. (B) An adjacent area in which the mesenchymal cells have withdrawn their processes and have become closely aggregated to form a center of chondrification. (C) A later stage in which the cells have been moved apart by deposition of intercellular hyaline matrix.

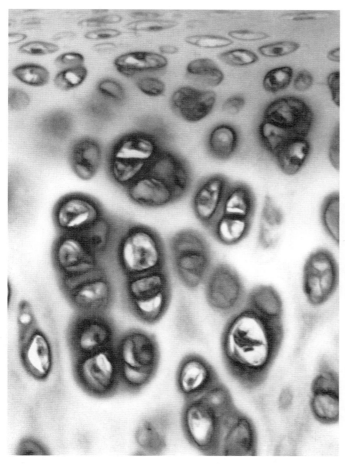

Figure 5.3 Postnatal hyaline cartilage. Notice that the cells immediately beneath the perichondrium (top), which have recently been added in appositional growth, are single and elongated. Those below are larger and occur in isogenous groups formed in interstitial growth of the cartilage. These are surrounded by matrix that stains more deeply with basic dyes.

conform to the shape of their lacuna, but during preparation of histological sections they often shrink and retract from the wall of the lacuna and may appear stellate. The matrix immediately surrounding each cluster of isogenous cells stains more intensely with basic dyes than the matrix elsewhere, and is termed the **territorial matrix**. Between cell groups it is less basophilic and is called the **interterritorial matrix** (Fig. 5.3). In preparation of cartilage for electron microscopy, there is less cell shrinkage and chondrocytes fill their lacunae. The nucleus is well preserved, and a Golgi complex, a few mitochondria, and cisternae of rough endoplasmic reticulum (rER) can be seen in the cytoplasm (Fig. 5.4). The endoplasmic reticulum is more extensive, and the mitochondria more numerous, in chondrocytes that are still actively engaged in synthesis of matrix components.

Chondrocytes secrete and maintain the surrounding matrix. They are also able to depolymerize the fibrous and amorphous constituents of the surrounding matrix to enlarge their lacunae. This ability is shown most dramatically during the early stages of **endochondral ossification**, the replacement of cartilage by bone. The chondrocytes hypertrophy at the expense of the surrounding matrix, enlarging their lacunae and reducing the interterritorial

matrix to thin plates or spicules, which become the sites of deposition of calcium phosphate. The chondrocytes then degenerate and their lacunae coalesce and are invaded by blood vessels from the perichondrium, accompanied by cells that differentiate into bone-forming cells, **osteoblasts**.

Near the ends of the cartilage models of the long bones (e.g. femur or tibia), the chondrocytes become rearranged into longitudinal columns parallel to the long axis of the cartilage model, to form cartilaginous **epiphyseal plates** between the epiphysis and the shaft at either end of the developing long bone (Fig. 5.5). Growth in length of the bone depends on continuing chondrocyte proliferation at the distal end of the epiphyseal plate, followed by their maturation, hypertrophy, and ultimate degeneration at the other side of the plate, where they are replaced by bone-forming osteoblasts. This will be explained in more detail in Chapter 6, Bone.

The joint surfaces of the long bones are covered by a layer of **articular cartilage**, 2-7 mm in thickness, that is bathed by lubricating **synovial fluid**. The cartilage provides a very smooth surface that allows an almost frictionless movement of the joint. The chondrocytes near its surface are small, elongated and flattened parallel to the articular surface. Cells deeper in the cartilage are larger and more rounded. The collagen fibers, at different levels within the articular cartilage, are arranged to best resist the great stresses to which they are subjected in weight bearing. The chondrocytes of cartilage are exceptionally long-lived, but articular cartilage does become thinner and less cellular with advancing age, as cells degenerate without being replaced.

Cartilage matrix

Like the extracellular matrix of connective tissue, the matrix of hyaline cartilage consists of collagen fibers in an amorphous matrix, rich in proteoglycans. Collagen makes up 40% of its dry weight, but this is not apparent in histological sections, for the collagen fibers and the matrix have approximately the same refractive index.

The arrangement of the collagen fibers can be studied with polarization optics in sections from which the proteoglycans have been extracted. Type II collagen predominates and occurs in cross-striated fibers, 15–45 nm in diameter, that do not assemble into large bundles. Fibers at the smaller end of this range form a loose, three-dimensional network throughout the matrix. The larger fibers are deployed in a pattern suggesting that their orientation is adapted to resist the strains to which that particular cartilage is normally subjected. Collagen types IX, X, and XI have been identified in cartilage, in small amounts, and these may serve to cross-link and stabilize the network of type II collagen fibers. Proteoglycans are present in higher concentration than in any other connective tissue, and they form a much firmer gel. They consist of a core protein 200–300 nm in length, from which many glycosaminoglycan molecules radiate in a bottle-brush configuration. The principal glycosaminoglycans of cartilage are **chondroitin sulfate** and **keratan sulfate**.

The proteoglycans of cartilage are among the largest molecules

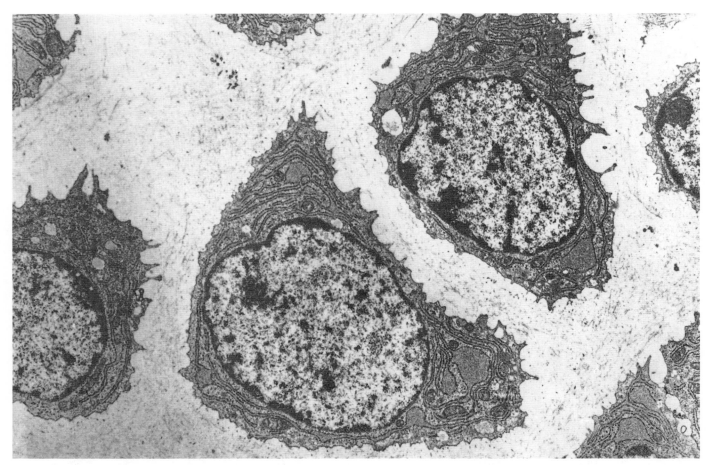

Figure 5.4 Electron micrograph of chondrocytes and the intervening matrix. Note the shape and irregular surface of the cells, and their extensive rough endoplasmic reticulum. (Reproduced from R. Seegmiller, C. Ferguson, and H. Sheldon *J Ultrastr Res* 1972; 38:288.)

produced by cells, having molecular weights ranging up to 3.5×10^6 Da. Proteoglycan molecules of the matrix are bound at their globular head to a long molecule of **hyaluronic acid** and are spaced along its length at intervals of 30 nm, forming a large **proteoglycan aggregate**. A single molecule of hyaluronic acid may have as many as 100 proteoglycan molecules linked to it. These aggregates interact with specific sites on the cross-banded collagen fibers. On electron micrographs prepared by high-pressure freezing, freeze-substitution, and low-temperature embedding, it is possible to see what appear to be the core proteins of the proteoglycans, and around these, a network of thin filaments that are believed to be their glycosaminoglycan side-chains. Chondrocytes also synthesize **chondronectin**, a large molecule involved in the adherence of the chondrocytes to the collagen fibers of the surrounding matrix.

> The **chondrodystrophies** are a group of diseases characterized by disturbance of cartilage growth and its subsequent replacement by bone. One member of this group, **achondroplasia**, is an inherited disorder in which there is reduced proliferation of chondrocytes in the epiphyseal plate of the long bones, resulting in a form of dwarfism in which the trunk is of normal length but the extremities are very short.

ELASTIC CARTILAGE

Elastic cartilage is found in the external ear, in the wall of the external auditory and eustachian canals, and in certain small cartilages of the larynx. It differs from hyaline cartilage in its greater opacity, yellowish color, and its greater flexibility. Its chondrocytes are indistinguishable from those of hyaline cartilage and are housed in lacunae that are scattered singly or in pairs. The matrix is somewhat less abundant than that of hyaline cartilage, and a significant fraction of its substance consists of branching fibers of **elastin**. In histological sections stained for elastin, the fibers deep in the cartilage may be so closely packed that the amorphous portion of the matrix is not apparent (Fig. 5.6). Nearer to the periphery of the cartilage, the network of elastic fibers is looser and its fibers can be seen to continue into the perichondrium.

As in hyaline cartilage, the viscoelastic properties of elastic cartilage are largely dependent on the proteoglycans of its matrix. If the enzyme papain is injected intravenously into a rabbit, its ears soon collapse as the enzyme degrades the proteoglycans of their elastic cartilage. The chondrocytes quickly respond by secretion of proteoglycans and other matrix components, and the ears are restored to their erect position in 48 h.

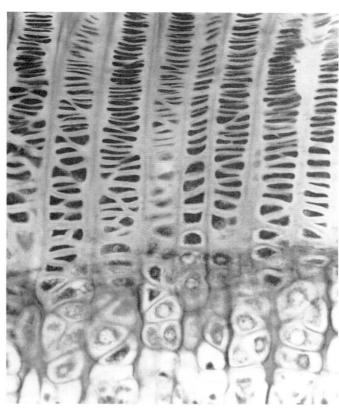

Figure 5.5 Photomicrograph of cartilage of the epiphyseal plate of a long bone. The chondrocytes are arranged in parallel columns. Growth in length of the bone depends upon division of the cells at the top of the columns, their maturation in the mid-zone and their apoptosis and replacement by osteocytes at the bottom of the columns.

Figure 5.6 Photomicrograph of elastic cartilage from the epiglottis of a child. Darkly stained bundles of elastic fibers can be seen in the matrix between groups of chondrocytes.

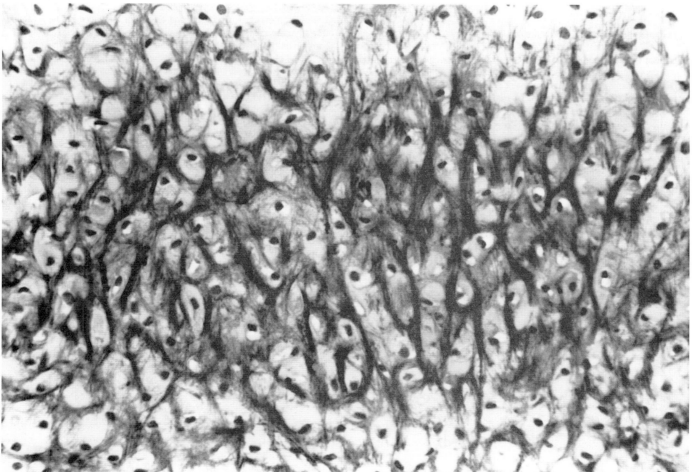

FIBROCARTILAGE

Fibrocartilage is found in the vertebral column, the pubic symphysis, and at sites of insertion of ligaments and tendons into bone. It resembles dense regular connective tissue, and the two are often continuous without any clear line of demarcation. Chondrocytes, surrounded by a small amount of matrix, are aligned in rows between coarse parallel bundles of type I collagen fibers. A thin basophilic territorial matrix can be identified around the lacunae, but the interterritorial matrix is largely replaced by the bundles of collagen. The tissue as a whole is acidophilic. A well-defined perichondrium is usually lacking.

Fibrocartilage with a somewhat different organization is found in the **intervertebral disks** between successive vertebrae. In the center of the disk, there is a soft viscous **nucleus pulposus**. This consists of a small population of cells in a semi-fluid matrix rich in hyaluronic acid and type II collagen fibers. This is surrounded by a thick ring of fibrocartilage, called the **annulus fibrosus**, which is made up of multiple concentric lamellae of collagen fibers. Some of these terminate in a thin layer of hyaline cartilage on the surface of the vertebrae above and below the disk. A few chondrocytes can be found between the lamellae of the annulus. The orientation of the collagen fibers in successive lamellae changes, giving the fibrocartilage the ability to resist any forces that would tend to displace the vertebrae with respect to one another.

Herniated intervertebral disk is a spinal injury common in contact sports. Forceful asymmetrical compression of an intervertebral disk ruptures the annulus fibrosus. The nucleus pulposus herniates into the spinal canal and presses upon nerve roots, causing pain and neurological disturbances in the region supplied by those nerves. Treatment is by surgery to remove the tissue projecting into the spinal canal. In some cases, removal of the disk and fusion of the vertebrae above and below may be necessary.

HISTOPHYSIOLOGY OF CARTILAGE

In adult life, the firm extracellular matrix of the articular cartilages enables them to withstand great compressive forces, and their smooth surface permits frictionless joint movement. In children, growth in stature depends on the rapid interstitial growth of epiphyseal cartilage and its replacement by bone. Such growth is indirectly controlled by the hypophyseal hormone **somatotrophin** (growth hormone). This hormone regulates production by the liver of another hormone, **somatomedin-C**, which stimulates the proliferation of the chondrocytes in the epiphyseal plates of the long bones.

Cartilage is an avascular tissue, and cartilages are limited in size by the distance that small molecules can diffuse through the matrix to nourish the chondrocytes. The matrix is also a barrier to the entry of lymphocytes, and immunoglobulins (antibodies) cannot diffuse into the matrix. This property is of clinical importance for cosmetic and reconstructive surgery, for cartilage can be transplanted from one individual to another without fear of rejection by the immune system.

Rheumatoid arthritis is a very common disease of unknown cause, characterized by a chronic inflammatory reaction in the synovial lining of the joints. The joint capsule and its lining are thickened and infiltrated by mononuclear cells, especially monocytes, macrophages, T-lymphocytes and helper T-lymphocytes. The chronic inflammatory reaction causes persistent pain, breakdown of articular cartilage, and erosion of the underlying bone. Anti-inflammatory drugs provide little improvement, and treatment is usually limited to pain relief. **Osteoarthritis** is a common disease of the elderly. The articular cartilage of joints in the fingers, knees and hips thins and breaks. The bone beneath the cartilage is affected. There is a conspicuous widening of the interphalangeal joints of the hands, and bony spurs may develop around the knee joints. Painful hip joints may ultimately make walking impossible. Treatment is limited to anti-inflammatory and analgesic drugs.

Questions

1 Isogenous groups are best described as
   a direct derivatives of blood monocytes
   b multinucleated cells
   c the progeny of a single chondrocyte
   d precursors to osteoclasts
   e consisting of between 30 and 40 cells

2 Concerning the territorial matrix, which one of the following statements is correct?
   a it surrounds fibroblasts
   b it surrounds chondroclasts
   c it surrounds fibrocytes
   d it surrounds chondrocytes
   e it surrounds chondroblasts

3 Interstitial growth of hyaline cartilage does not involve
   a formation of isogenous cells
   b mitoses
   c growth of perichondrium
   d formation of daughter cells
   e formation of territorial matrix

4 Fibrocartilage contains predominantly which type of collagen?
   a type I
   b type II
   c type III
   d type IV
   e type V

5 In the adult human, perichondrium fibers consist of which one, if any, of the following
   a collagen type I
   b collagen type II
   c collagen type III
   d collagen type IV
   e collagen type VII

6 The matrix of hyaline cartilage does not contain
   a type II collagen
   b blood capillaries
   c chondroitin sulfate
   d keratan sulfate
   e hyaluronic acid

7 Chondrocytes are nourished by
   a the rich vascularity of its matrix
   b intrachondral canals
   c capillaries opening directly into the lacunae
   d diffusion of metabolites via the matrix
   e Volkmann's canals

8 Chondrocytes of hyaline cartilage are located in spaces called
   a lamellae
   b cisternae
   c interterritorial matrix
   d blastemae
   e lacunae

9 Which statement is correct regarding cartilage?
   a it contains an abundance of calcium
   b it is characterized by the presence of Haversian canals
   c it may contain elastic fibers
   d it has little or no influence in the growth of long bones
   e it contains chondroblasts embedded within the matrix

10 Elastic cartilage is not found in
   a external ear
   b larynx
   c epiglottis
   d tracheal rings
   e eustachian (auditory) tube

11 What type of collagen is contained in the perichondrium?

12 Ground substance of cartilage is composed of chondroitin sulfate and what other substance?

13 What is the predominant type of collagen in hyaline cartilage?

14 What is the name of the cell found within the cartilage?

15 What is the process by which chondrocytes are nourished?

16 What is the name for the connective tissue lining of cartilage?

17 What type of cartilage is observed in the pinna of the ear?

18 What hormone, produced in the liver, stimulates chondrocytes in the epiphyseal plates of long bones?

19 What type of cartilage can be seen in the tracheal rings?

20 What is the name of a group of chondrocytes derived from a single chondrocyte?

Chapter six

Bone

Bone is a connective tissue in which the cells and fibers are embedded in a matrix (ground substance), that contains crystals of a complex calcium salt, **hydroxyapatite** ($Ca_{10} [PO_4]_6 [OH]_2$). The calcification of its matrix makes bone a hard unyielding substance, ideally suited for its supportive and protective role in the skeleton. Bones provide attachment and levers for muscles involved in locomotion; they protect the vital organs of the cranial and thoracic cavities; and they constitute a mobilizable store of calcium that can be drawn upon in the regulation of the concentration of this ion in the blood and body fluids.

A layer of dense, uncalcified connective tissue, the **periosteum**, covers the outer surface of bones, and a similar, but thinner layer, the **endosteum**, lines their interior. In addition to fibroblasts, both of these layers contain **osteoprogenitor cells**, inactive precursors of the cells that form bone. The cells of bone include the **osteoblasts**, which secrete the collagen, proteoglycans, and hydroxyapatite of bone matrix; **osteocytes**, which reside in lacunae within the ground substance; and **osteoclasts**, which remove bone in the continual resorption and remodeling of bone that occurs throughout life.

MACROSCOPIC STRUCTURE

Understanding of the histology of bone will be facilitated by a preliminary description of the macroscopic structure of a typical long bone, such as the tibia. In longitudinal section, the shaft or **diaphysis**, consists of dense bone, the **substantia compacta**, surrounding a voluminous central **medullary cavity** (marrow cavity). Towards the ends of the diaphysis, the compact bone becomes thinner and the medullary cavity contains a three-dimensional network of branch-

ing bone spicules (trabeculae) that constitutes the **substantia spongiosa**, also described as **cancellous bone** (Fig. 6.1). The central cavity of the shaft is occupied by the **bone marrow**, and this extends a short distance into the labyrinthine system of spaces among the trabeculae of cancellous bone. At the ends of a long bone, where it forms a joint with another bone, the thin layer of compact bone is covered by a layer of hyaline cartilage, referred to as the **articular cartilage**.

In the growing long bones of children, a short segment of bone at either end, called the **epiphysis**, is separated from the diaphysis by a thin zone of hyaline cartilage called the **epiphyseal plate** (Fig. 6.2). This is the principal site of growth in length of the bone.

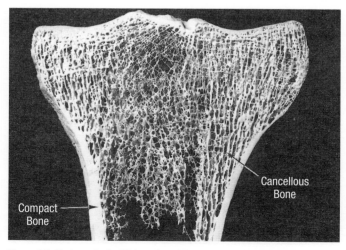

Figure 6.1 Photograph of a thick section of the upper end of the tibia, from an adult, illustrating the cortical compact bone of the shaft, and the lattice of trabeculae of cancellous bone in the interior.

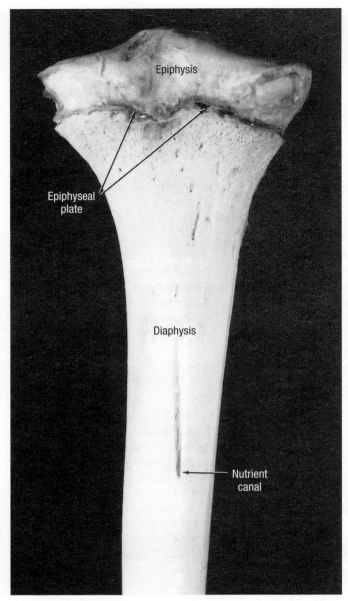

Figure 6.2 Photograph of the upper portion of the tibia, from a child, showing the epiphysis, the cartilaginous epiphyseal plate and the diaphysis.

When adult stature is attained, this layer of cartilage is eliminated and bone of the epiphyses and the diaphysis becomes continuous. In the flat bones of the skull, compact bone forms outer and inner layers, generally referred to as the **outer table** and **inner table** of the bone. The intervening space, corresponding to the medullary cavity of a long bone, is called the **diploe**.

MICROSCOPIC STRUCTURE

Osteoprogenitor cells

The dense connective tissue forming the **periosteum**, on the outer surface of a bone, and the **endosteum**, on its inner surface,

contains fusiform **osteoprogenitor cells**, which are not easily distinguishable from the fibroblasts. Their elongated nucleus is pale staining and the cytoplasm is acidophilic, or very faintly basophilic. These cells are the inactive precursors of the **osteoblasts**, the bone forming (osteogenic) cells of growing bone.

Osteoblasts

During deposition of new bone matrix, **osteoblasts** are cuboidal, or low columnar cells aligned on bone surfaces (Fig.6.3). They do not form a typical epithelium. They are spaced a short distance apart, but maintain contact with neighboring osteoblasts via short lateral processes. The nucleus is near the rounded upper end of the cell and the underlying cytoplasm is basophilic and contains abundant rough endoplasmic reticulum (rER) and free ribosomes. Osteoblasts synthesize the type I collagen, glycoproteins, and proteoglycans of the ground substance, and several minor protein components (**osteocalcin**, **osteonectin**, **osteopontin**, and **osteoprotegerin**). The osteoblast membrane contains receptors for various hormones, vitamins, and cytokines that control the activity of the cell. When they become inactive, osteoblasts are flattened against the underlying bone and their basophilia and content of endoplasmic reticulum are reduced. Osteoblasts appear to be polarized towards the surface that is in contact with the underlying bone, but their release of matrix components is not confined to that surface. On a growing bony surface, some of the osteoblasts become enveloped by their own secretions, and are imprisoned in lucunae within the newly synthesized bone matrix and are transformed into **osteocytes**.

Osteocytes

The **osteocytes** residing in lacunae within the calcified matrix are the principal cells of adult bone (Fig.6.4). A number of slender, tapering cell processes radiate from the cell body. The elongated nucleus is more heterochromatic than the nucleus of the

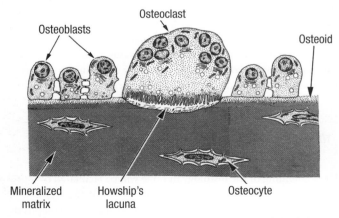

Figure 6.3 A drawing of the three principal cell types of bone and their relation to a trabeculum of mineralized bone matrix. Note the contact between processes of neighboring osteoblasts, and the Howship's lacuna beneath the ruffled border of the multinucleate osteoclast.

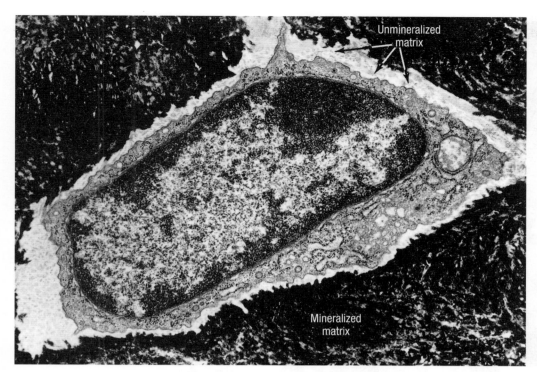

Figure 6.4 Electron micrograph of an osteocyte surrounded by mineralized bone matrix. The cell fills its lacuna. The clear area around the cell is unmineralized matrix. The mineralized matrix appears black owing to the electron scattering of the apatite crystals. (Micrograph courtesy of Marie Holtrop.)

osteoblast, and the cytoplasm contains a smaller Golgi complex and less endoplasmic reticulum. Although osteocytes do not have the appearance of synthetically active cells, there is evidence that they play an active role in maintenance of the surrounding matrix.

The shape of each **lacuna** conforms to that of the osteocyte within it, and the slender cell processes occupy **canaliculi** that radiate from the lacuna. The ends of the processes of neighboring cells meet within the canaliculi and have gap junctions at their site of contact. Thus, unlike the cells of cartilage, osteocytes are not completely isolated in the matrix, but are in communication with one another via gap junctions that permit the passage of ions and small molecules from cell to cell. Diffusion of nutrients from the blood vessels to the osteocytes through the surrounding calcified bone matrix is very limited, however, there is a thin film of fluid between the osteocytes and the surrounding matrix, which may permit diffusion of small molecules to the lacunae via the continuous system of canaliculi.

The canaliculi are not visible in routine histological preparations, but if a section of dry bone is ground down to a thin translucent sheet and then examined with the microscope, the air-filled lacunae and their radiating canaliculi are clearly visible (Fig.6.5). Much of our knowledge of the complex organization of this tissue has been learned from such ground sections of dry bone.

Osteoclasts

Throughout adult life, bone undergoes a continuous process of internal remodeling and renewal that involves removal of calcified bone matrix, and its replacement by newly deposited bone. In this process, the agents of bone removal are the **osteoclasts**. These are very large cells up to 15 µm in diameter and containing from 4 to 40 nuclei. The cytoplasm contains multiple Golgi complexes, multiple centrosomes, numerous mitochondria, and a large number of lysosomes. Beneath each osteoclast there is a shallow depression on the surface of bone that has traditionally been called a **Howship's lacuna**. This concavity is created by enzymatic digestion of the underlying bone matrix by lysosomal enzymes released by the osteoclast.

Osteoclasts exhibit an obvious polarity. The nuclei are congregated beneath the smooth-contoured, round, upper surface of the cell, and its lower border has a striated appearance when viewed with the light microscope. On electron micrographs, this appearance is found to be caused by deep folds of the plasmalemma that delimit a large number of clavate (club-shaped) or foliate (leaf-like) cell processes. These are quite unlike the static microvilli of an epithelial brush-border. Cinematographic observations of living osteoclasts reveal frequent changes in shape of the processes as they are extended and retracted. This active surface specialization is referred to as a **ruffled border**, to distinguish it from the more orderly brush border of epithelia. Around the periphery of the ruffled border, the plasmalemma of the osteoclast is very firmly attached to the underlying bone, in what is termed the **sealing zone** (Fig.6.6). This circumferential attachment bounds a closed compartment between the ruffled border and the surface of the bone. Osteoclasts secrete H$^+$ ions into the underlying compartment, acidifying its content to dissolve the bone mineral. In addition, collagenase and other hydrolytic enzymes are released into the compartment by abundant lysosomes in the basal cytoplasm, and these digest the organic

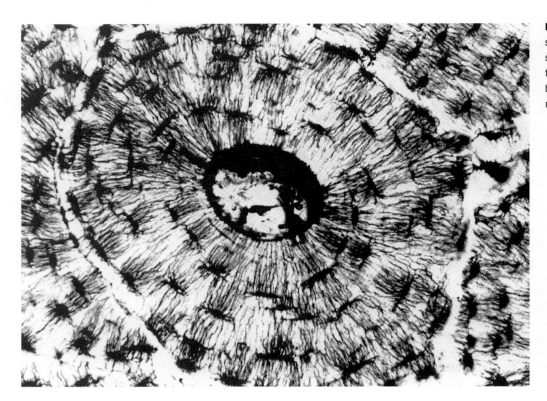

Figure 6.5 Photomicrograph of a ground section of bone, showing a Haversian system in cross section. The lucunae and their slender radiating canaliculi appear black, and the surrounding mineralized matrix is white.

components of the bone matrix. This is one of the very few examples of extracellular release of lysosomal enzymes. Small crystals of calcium salts and incompletely digested collagen fibers can be identified in the subosteoclastic compartment. The ultimate products of digestion are taken up at the ruffled border in small vesicles. These move across the cell and fuse with the membrane on the apical surface, releasing their contents into the extracellular fluid, and thence into the blood in neighboring capillary blood vessels.

For a long time it was thought that the multinucleate osteoclasts arose by coalescence of blood-borne monocytes generated in the bone marrow. There is now some evidence that they arise from precursors that resemble monocytes, but differ from them in containing a distinctive tartrate-resistant acid phosphatase.

Bone matrix

The organic portion of bone matrix is made up of proteoglycans and type I collagen fibers, with collagen accounting for more than 50% of its volume. The ground substance of bone has many similarities to that of cartilage, but its proteoglycans tend to have shorter core proteins and fewer side-chains. Chondroitin sulfate and keratan sulfate are major components of its glycosaminoglycans. Other matrix proteins, unique to bone, are **osteopontin** and **osteocalcin**. These bind tightly to crystals of the mineral hydroxyapatite and have amino acid sequences that are thought to be involved in binding osteoblasts to the underlying bone matrix. In the first bone deposited (primary bone), the collagen fibers are interwoven in random orientation, but in the lamellar bone, deposited later (secondary bone), they have a highly ordered arrangement, with the fibers within each lamella parallel to one another.

The inorganic matter of bone matrix consists of **hydroxyapatite**, a mineral nearly identical to geological deposits of calcium phosphate. Although some of the bone mineral may be amorphous, the great bulk of it is in the form of rod-like hydroxyapatite crystals 40nm in length and 1.5–3.0nm in thickness. These are regularly spaced at intervals of 60–70nm along the length of the collagen fibers. Bone matrix also contains a significant

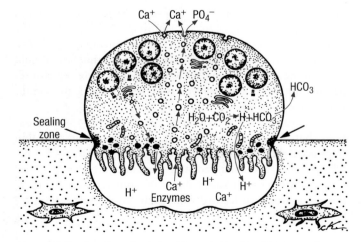

Figure 6.6 Drawing of an osteoclast and the underlying Howship's lacuna. From water and carbon dioxide, the cell produces hydrogen ions and bicarbonate. The hydrogen ions acidify the underlying compartment to dissolve bone mineral. Lysosomes release enzymes into the compartment to digest the organic matrix of bone.

concentration of citrate and carbonate ions. A layer of water, termed the **hydration shell**, surrounds each hydroxyapatite crystal and is believed to facilitate the exchange of ions between the crystals and the extracellular fluid outside of the bone.

ORGANIZATION OF LAMELLAR BONE

The compact bone of adults is made up of cylindrical subunits called **Haversian systems**, or **osteons**, each composed of 5–15 lamellae of calcified matrix arranged around a **central canal** that contains a capillary blood vessel (Figs 6.7, 6.8A). Osteons branch with the bifurcation of the blood vessel in their central canal. The collagen fibers within each lamella are parallel to one another and have a helical course along the length of the osteon. The pitch of the helix in the successive lamellae is such that, at any given point along the osteon, the fibers in adjacent lamellae are nearly at right angles to one another. Thus, when the osteons are viewed in cross-section, with the polarizing microscope, bright birefringent lamellae alternate with dark isotropic lamellae (Fig. 6.8B). The central canals of the osteons are connected to each other and to

the marrow cavity via occasional oblique channels that pass through the lamellae. These are called **Volkmann's canals** (Fig. 6.7). They are distinguishable from central canals by their transverse course, and by the fact that they are not encircled by concentric lamellae.

Angular areas between the osteons are occupied by parallel lamellae of varying length, called the **interstitial lamellae**. These are remnants of pre-existing osteons that were largely eroded away by osteoclasts in the continual remodeling of bone. The outer boundary of each Haversian system, or osteon, is distinctly outlined by a thin refractile layer called a **cement line**. This is a rather inappropriate term, for no 'cementing' substance has been identified. This boundary appears to be simply a layer of mineralized bone matrix that is deficient in collagen fibers and, therefore, has different refractile properties. In cross-sections, compact bone appears as a mosaic of circular and angular units outlined by thin, dense lines (Fig. 6.8A).

Immediately beneath the periosteum, on the shaft of a bone, there are a number of lamellae that extend, without interruption, around the entire circumference of the shaft. These are called the **outer circumferential lamellae** (Fig. 6.7). Comparable lamellae beneath the endosteum are designated the **inner circumferential**

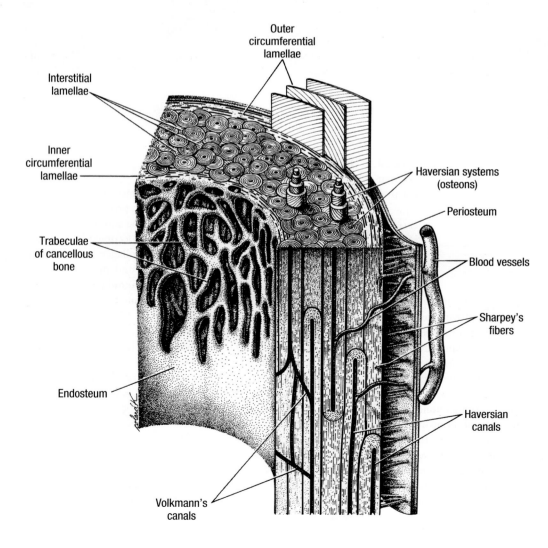

Figure 6.7 Drawing of a sector of the shaft of a long bone, showing the arrangement of lamellae in the osteons, the interstitial lamellae, and the outer and inner circumferential lamellae. (Redrawn from A. Benninghof, *Lehrbuch der Anatomie des Menschen*, Urban and Schwartzenberg, Berlin, 1935.)

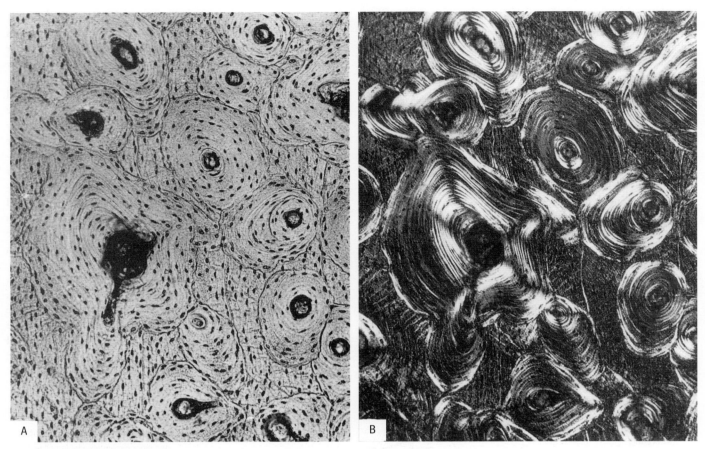

Figure 6.8 (A) Photomicrograph of a ground section of bone from a human tibia. (B) The same section photographed through the polarizing microscope. Alternating light and dark concentric lamellae in the Haversian systems result from differing orientation of the collagen fibers in successive lamellae. (Micrographs courtesy of R. Amprino.)

lamellae. The periosteum is fixed to the outer circumferential lamellae by bundles of collagen fibers, called **Sharpey's fibers**, that penetrate these lamellae and extend a short distance deeper into the bone.

HISTOGENESIS OF BONE

Bone always develops by replacement of a pre-existing connective tissue. In the embryo, two different modes of osteogenesis are observed. Where bone is formed by replacing primitive connective tissue (mesenchyme), the process is called **intramembranous ossification**. Where bone formation takes place in pre-existing cartilage, it is called **endochondral ossification**. The flat bones of the skull develop by intramembranous ossification, while the long bones of the appendicular skeleton develop by endochondral ossification. In both processes the deposition of bone matrix is essentially the same, but in endochondral ossification the bulk of the cartilage matrix must be removed before bone deposition begins. In both processes, bone is first laid down as a network of trabeculae, called the **primary spongiosa**, and this is subsequently transformed into compact bone by filling in the interspaces between trabeculae.

Intramembranous ossification

In this mode of ossification, the embryonic mesenchyme first condenses into a richly vascularized layer of primitive connective tissue. Its stellate cells are in contact with one another via long cell processes, and the intercellular spaces are occupied by a ground substance containing randomly oriented collagen fibers. Certain of the mesenchymal cells then aggregate and differentiate into osteogenic cells that deposit bone matrix around themselves. This process results in thin trabeculae of eosinophilic bone matrix (Fig. 6.9). These tend to form equidistant between neighboring blood vessels, and, because the blood vessels form a network, the trabeculae in the **primary spongiosa** also have a branching and anastomosing pattern (Fig. 6.10A). Other mesenchymal cells enlarge and become intensely basophilic **osteoblasts**, which gather on the surface of the primary trabeculae. They secrete additional matrix, which results in the trabeculae becoming larger and thicker. As more and more osteoblasts become incarcerated in lacunae within the matrix as **osteocytes**, they are replaced at the surface of the trabeculae by new osteoblasts, formed by further differentiatiion of osteoprogenitor cells present in the perivascular connective tissue. The area of primitive connective tissue where in these events are taking place is called a **primary center of ossification**. In portions of the resulting primary spongiosa that are

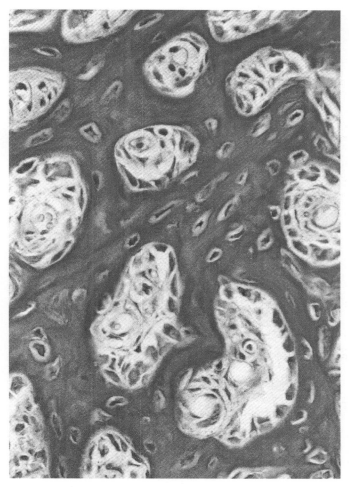

Figure 6.9 Photomicrograph of intramembranous ossification. Notice the osteocytes within the branching trabeculae and the osteoblasts on their surface.

destined to become compact bone, progressive thickening of the trabeculae encroaches upon the perivascular spaces until they are reduced to narrow spaces surrounding the blood vessels. These will become the central canals of Haversian systems when the primary woven bone is replaced by lamellar bone during the continuous remodeling of bone (Fig. 6.10A,B). Bones so formed are described as **membrane bones** to distinguish them from bone that develops in pre-existing cartilage.

Endochondral ossification

Long bones of the skeleton (e.g. humerus and femur) develop by **endochondral ossification**, replacement of cartilage with bone. In the early embryo, cartilages are formed that have a shape roughly similar to that of the long bones of the mature skeleton. These are commonly referred to as the **cartilage models** of the future bones. The first indication of beginning endochondral ossification is an enlargement (hypertrophy) of the chondrocytes at the middle of the shaft of the cartilage model. As their lacunae continue to enlarge, the matrix between lacunae is gradually reduced to irregularly shaped spicules or trabeculae of cartilage matrix. The

hypertrophied chondrocytes then die and small aggregations of calcium phosphate crystals form within the residues of cartilage matrix. This process of hypertrophy and degeneration of chondrocytes spreads from the original center towards both ends of the model.

While these changes are occurring in the interior of the cartilage, osteoprogenitor cells in the perichondrium differentiate into osteoblasts that deposit a thin **periosteal collar** of bone around the middle of the shaft of the cartilage model (Fig. 6.11B,C). At the same time, capillaries and associated osteoprogenitor cells invade the spaces left behind by the degeneration of hypertrophied chondrocytes. The vessels branch and grow towards either end of the cartilage model (Fig. 6.11D–F), forming loops that extend into the blind ends of cavities in the calcified cartilage. The osteoprogenitor cells, accompanying the invading blood vessels, differentiate into osteoblasts that congregate on the surface of the remaining irregular spicules of calcified cartilage, and begin to deposit bone matrix on them. The resulting trabeculae have a mottled appearance in histological sections as a result of the difference in staining properties of the core of cartilage and the coating of bone matrix (see Figs 6.12B, 6.13).

This stage of development is usually reached by the third month of fetal life. The developing long bones then have expanded ends (**epiphyses**) of hyaline cartilage and a shaft (**diaphysis**) consisting of an hour-glass-shaped region of endochondral ossification, surrounded by a collar of bone of periosteal origin (Fig. 6.11F). The term **primary center of ossification** embraces all of the events described above and is intended to distinguish the diaphyseal center of ossification, which develops first, from **secondary centers of ossification**, which appear later in the epiphyses (Fig. 6.11F,G).

Growth in length of long bones

While cartilage continues to be replaced by bone in the expanding diaphyseal center of ossification, the epiphyseal centers of ossification are also expanding. The cartilage between the epiphysis and diaphysis is gradually reduced to a relatively thin layer, called the **epiphyseal plate** (Fig. 6.11H,I). Its proliferating chondrocytes become arranged in longitudinal columns separated by columns of cartilage matrix (Figs 6.12A, 6.13). As ossification progresses, the chondrocytes in these longitudinal columns undergo changes similar to the early events in the primary center of ossification. Four zones become recognizable along their length. At their epiphyseal ends, there is a **zone of proliferation**, where frequent mitosis of the chondrocytes insures continuing elongation of the developing bone. Below this is a **zone of maturation**, in which the cells undergo significant enlargement, which reaches its peak in a **zone of hypertrophy**, where the cells are very large and highly vacuolated. The matrix between columns in this zone is undergoing calcification, and this region is also referred to as the **zone of provisional calcification**. Finally, at the diaphyseal end of the columns is the **zone of degeneration**, where the hypertrophied chondrocytes are dying and the open ends of their vacated lucunae are being invaded by capillary loops and associated osteoprogenitor cells from the

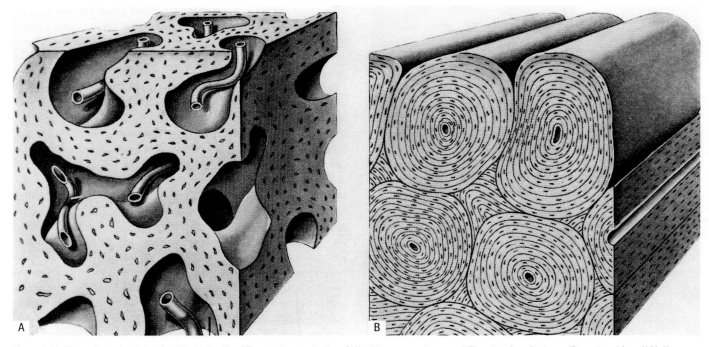

Figure 6.10 Three-dimensional drawings illustrating the difference in organization of (A) primary woven bone, and (B) mature lamellar bone. (Reproduced from N.M. Hancox, *Biology of Bone.* Cambridge University Press, Cambridge, 1972.)

marrow cavity. The osteoprogenitor cells differentiate into osteoblasts that deposit bone matrix on the spicules of calcified cartilage that remain between the cell columns (Fig.6.12).

A center of ossification appears in the proximal epiphysis somewhat later than that in the distal epiphysis (Fig.6.11H), but ossification centers are present in both epiphyses soon after birth. During their progressive expansion, all cartilage is replaced by bone except for the **epiphyseal plate**, and a thin layer at the ends of the bone that persists as its **articular cartilages**. All subsequent growth in length of the long bones during childhood is attributable to proliferation of chondrocytes in the zone of proliferation in the epiphyseal plates and their replacement by bone. At the end of the growing period, proliferation of the cartilage cells slows and finally ceases. Continuing replacement of cartilage by bone results in obliteration of the epiphyseal plate (Fig.6.11I,J). This **closure of the epiphyses** occurs at the age of about 18years. Thereafter, no further growth is possible.

Growth in diameter of long bones

While growth in length of the long bones is occurring at the epiphyseal plate, growth in the diameter of the diaphysis is occurring by circumferential deposition of membrane bone beneath the periosteum. The thickening of the shaft by deposition of bone on its outer surface is accompanied by mobilization of osteoclasts on its inner surface. These resorb bone there and thus enlarge the marrow cavity. Deposition of bone on the outside, and resorption of bone on the inside of the shaft, continue until the diameter of the adult bone is attained. Early in this process, all of the

spicules of endochondral bone formed in the primary center of ossification are removed by osteoclasts during the enlargement of the marrow cavity and, thereafter, the entire shaft consists of membrane bone deposited by the periosteum. The respective rates of deposition of bone on the outside, and osteoclastic erosion of bone on the inside of the shaft, are such that the thickness of the wall soon reaches its definitive thickness, and thereafter remains nearly constant.

Surface modeling of bones

Throughout their growth, long bones retain approximately the same external form. Obviously, this would not be true if new bone were deposited at a uniform rate at all points beneath the periosteum. Instead, approximately the definitive shape of the bone is maintained throughout its growth by a continual modeling or sculpturing of its surface that involves subperiosteal bone deposition in some areas, and bone resorption in other areas. If a bone-seeking radioisotope is given to a growing rat, and autoradiographs are then made of longitudinal sections of its tibia, the sites of new bone formation are disclosed by the distribution of silver grains in the overlying photographic emulsion. In the conical regions towards the ends of the bone, the grains are aligned immediately beneath the endosteum, whereas in the cylindrical mid-portion of the shaft, they are found beneath the periosteum. Study of parallel histological sections reveals numerous osteoclasts beneath the periosteum of the conical region, and beneath the endosteum in the cylindrical shaft.

Thus, it is clear that in surface modeling of this bone, the periosteum plays opposite roles in the two regions of the bone:

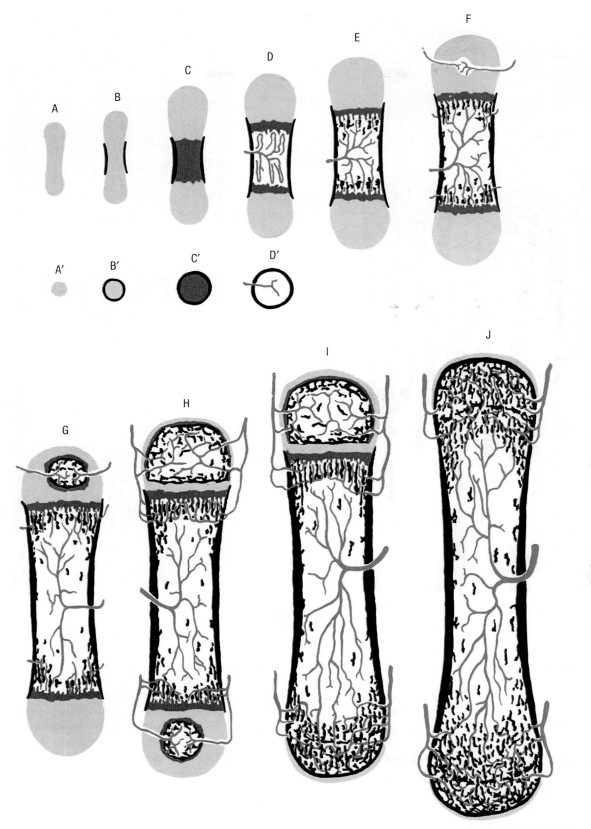

Figure 6.11 Diagram of successive stages in the development of a typical long bone. Pale blue, cartilage; purple, calcified cartilage; black, bone; red, arteries. (A) Cartilage model. (B) Periosteal bone collar. (C) Cartilage begins to calcify. (D) Blood vessels enter calcified matrix and divide it into two zones of ossification (E). (F) Blood vessels enter upper epiphyseal cartilage and establish secondary ossification center. (G) Ossification center forms in lower epiphysis. (H) Lower epiphyseal plate disappears. (I) Closure of upper epiphyseal plate. (J) Growth in length ceases and marrow cavity becomes continuous throughout the length of the bone.

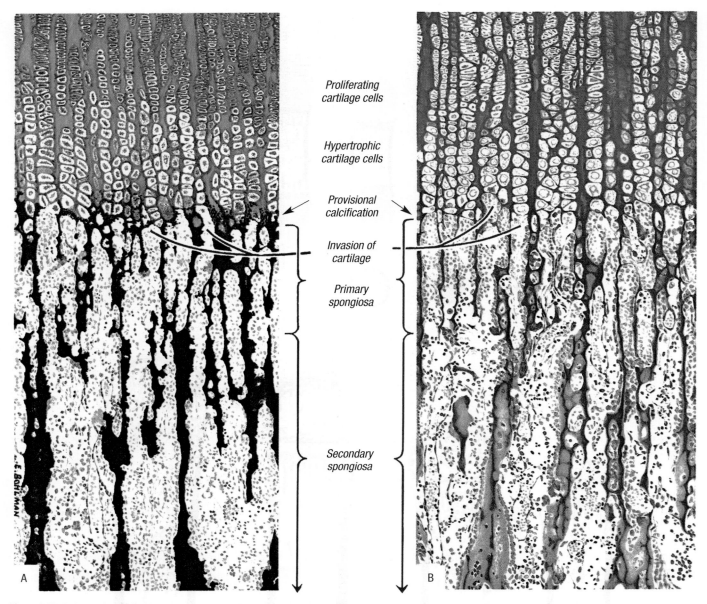

Figure 6.12 Endochondral ossification in longitudinal section through zone of epiphyseal growth. Notice the alignment of chondrocytes in columns in the epiphyseal cartilage, above. (A) Calcified bone matrix stained black. (B) Persisting cores of cartilage matrix in trabeculae stain blue or purple, while bone matrix stains pink.

subperiosteal bone deposition is occurring in the cylindrical portion of the shaft, while subperiosteal bone resorption is taking place in the conical region towards the ends. Thus, the diverging walls of the conical region are being straightened and are contributing, at their lower end, to a lengthening of the cylindrical portion of the shaft. How the local variations in function of the endosteum and periosteum are controlled in space and time in order continually to mold the shape of the bone, is a fascinating unsolved problem in morphogenesis.

Internal reorganization of bone

In the conversion of primary spongiosa to compact bone, progressive thickening of the trabeculae largely obliterates the perivascular spaces. In this process, bone with randomly oriented collagen fibers is deposited by osteoblasts in ill-defined concentric layers, but true Haversian systems, with precisely oriented collagen, are first formed during secondary bone formation.

In this process, **absorption cavities** appear in primary compact bone as a result of osteoclast activity. Long, cylindrical cavities are formed and these are then invaded by blood vessels, and accompanying osteoprogenitor cells from the bone marrow. When bone resorption ceases, the osteoclasts lining the cavities are replaced by osteoblasts that deposit concentric lamellae of bone on the inner aspect of the absorption cavity. These lamellae have the ordered arrangement of collagen fibers characteristic of Haversian systems of adult bone. From the age of 1 year onwards, only lamellar bone is deposited in the shafts of long bones and this secondary bone ultimately replaces all of the primary bone.

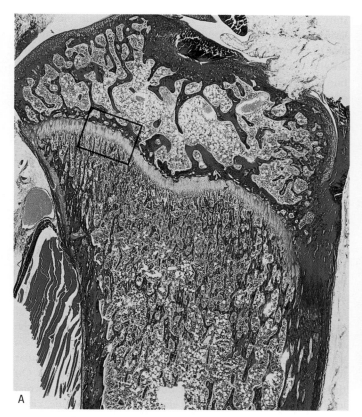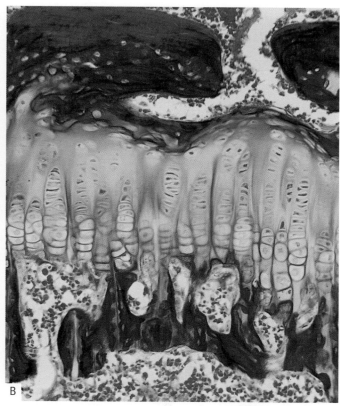

Figure 6.13 (A) Low-power photomicrograph of upper portion of a developing long bone. The pale band across the bone is the cartilaginous epiphyseal plate. (B) The area in the box on (A), at higher magnification. Notice the columns of chondrocytes in the epiphyseal plate, the mottled appearance of the trabeculae below, as a result of the different staining properties of cartilage matrix and the bone matrix.

Internal bone reconstruction does not end with the replacement of primary bone by secondary bone, but continues throughout life. Resorption cavities continue to appear in secondary bone and are filled with third, fourth, and higher orders of Haversian systems. Interstitial lamellae of adult bone represent persisting fragments of earlier generations of Haversian systems. This continuous turnover provides the plasticity that enables bone to alter its internal architecture to adapt to new mechanical stresses.

In histological preparations of bone, all of the Haversian systems look alike, regardless of their age. However, calcification of their lamellae proceeds much more slowly than their deposition, and recently deposited osteons can be distinguished from older ones in historadiograms produced by placing a ground section of bone between an X-ray source and a photographic film. In the resulting image, the recently formed Haversian systems, having a lower calcium content, appear dark, older ones are lighter and interstitial lamellae, which are the oldest, are white (Fig. 6.14).

Repair of fractures

The osteogenic potential of cells of the periosteum and endosteum can be evoked again after they have been quiescent for many years. After a fracture, the blood clot formed between the fragments is soon invaded by cells that form a disorderly mass of collagen fibers and cartilage matrix, described as a **fibrocartilaginous callus**. Quiescent cells of the periosteum are then reactivated and the fibrocartilaginous callus is replaced by a **bony callus**, consisting of a network of trabeculae of membrane bone, bridging the gap between the broken ends of the bone. In the weeks that follow, the lattice of trabeculae uniting the fragments is transformed into compact bone. Subsequent resorption of excess bone formed at the fracture site re-establishes continuity of the marrow cavity and restores the normal surface contours to the bone.

HISTOPHYSIOLOGY OF BONE

The maintenance of normal bone mass depends upon a delicate balance between bone deposition by osteoblasts and bone removal by osteoclasts. The successful maintenance of this balance depends, in large measure, upon the relative numbers of these two types of cells. New osteoblasts arise by further differentiation of fibroblast-like cells of the periosteum, or from stromal cells of the marrow. Their number is regulated by a number of cytokines and hormones.

In tissues in general, monocytes differentiate into macrophages. In bone, proliferation of monocytes and their

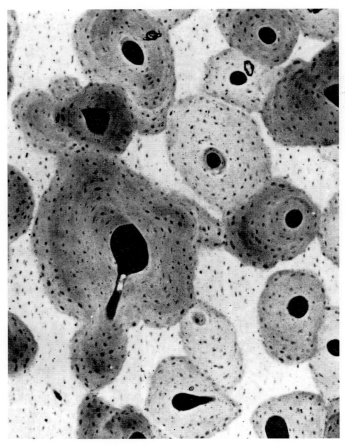

Figure 6.14 Historadiogram of a ground section of bone. The different shades from white to deep gray reflect differing concentrations of calcium. The most recently deposited Haversian systems are incompletely calcified and appear dark gray. Older ones, containing a higher concentration of calcium are lighter, and the interstitial lamellae, which are oldest, are white. (Historadiogram courtesy of R. Amprino.)

further differentiation depends upon two molecules secreted by osteoblasts: **monocyte colony stimulating factor (M-CSF)** and a ligand **Rankl**, which binds to RANK-receptors on the mononuclear precursors of macrophages, inducing their further differentiation and fusion to form multinucleate osteoclasts (Fig. 6.15). Osteoblasts also secrete another important molecule, **osteoprotegerin (OPG)**, which has the opposite effect, preventing the formation of osteoclasts. It accomplishes this by blocking the receptor for RANKL on the precursors of osteoclasts.

There is a need for communication between osteoclasts and osteoblasts after resorption cavities have been formed. A cytokine, **transforming growth factor (TGF)**, is present in bone matrix in a latent form. During bone resorption, this cytokine is taken up by the osteoclasts and liberated in an active form into the extracellular fluid. There it acts upon osteoblasts, increasing their rate of bone deposition to fill the resorption cavities.

Calcium homeostasis

In addition to the rigid support that bones provide in the limbs, and their protection of the brain in the skull, bone is an essential store of calcium that can be mobilized to maintain the normal level of calcium in the blood plasma. The importance of calcium ions in the body cannot be overemphasized. They are required for: activity of many enzymes; maintenance of cell cohesion; regulation of membrane permeability; coagulation of blood; contraction of smooth and striated muscle; and for many other vital functions. Ingenious homeostatic mechanisms have evolved to keep the plasma calcium concentration remarkably constant, in the range of 9–11 mg/100 ml. If it falls below this level, calcium ions can diffuse into the blood from the hydrated shell around the hydroxyapatite crystals of bone matrix. However, this source is only able to maintain a low calcium level in the plasma (7 mg/100 ml). A further increase depends upon increased bone resorption by osteoclasts.

The cells of the parathyroid glands are sensitive to low plasma calcium concentration and respond by increased secretion of **parathyroid hormone (PTH)**. This hormone stimulates the osteoblasts to increase their secretion of M-CSF and RANKL, which induce formation of additional osteoclasts (Fig. 6.15). Calcium ions released by osteoclasts in their absorption of hydroxyapatite crystals diffuse into the blood to restore the normal plasma calcium level. The PTH also acts upon the kidneys to increase the rate of calcium reabsorption from the glomerular filtrate, thus diminishing further loss of calcium in the urine. On the other hand, if the plasma calcium level rises above the normal level, the **C-cells** of the thyroid gland release a hormone, **calcitonin**, which suppresses bone resorption and calcium release by the osteoclasts.

Effects of hormones

The hormones secreted by several endocrine glands affect bone. A deficiency of the pituitary growth hormone, **somatotrophin**, in childhood, may result in dwarfism. An excess of the same hormone, prior to closure of the epiphyses, results in excessive growth, gigantism. In adults, excess secretion of somatotrophin leads to **acromegaly**, a disorder that is characterized by unsightly coarsening of the features as a result of thickening of the bones of the face. These gross abnormalities of bone growth are rare. More common are variations in stature caused by the effects of gonadal hormones (estrogens and androgens) on the time of closure of the epiphyses of long bones. Precocious puberty, in boys and girls, hastens fusion of the epiphyses and diaphyses of the long bones, resulting in premature cessation of growth in height. In aging adults, a decline in the secretion of gonadal hormones alters the balance between bone deposition and bone absorption, resulting in a gradual reduction in bone mass that is detectable in all persons over 50.

Loss of bone mass is accelerated in women after the menopause, when secretion of estrogen declines. This often leads to **osteoporosis**, in which there is a marked reduction in number of trabeculae and a thinning of cortical compact bone. This progressive resorption of bone can often be slowed by administration of estrogen. Nearly one-third of all women who live to age 80 years have had hip fractures or compression fractures of vertebrae.

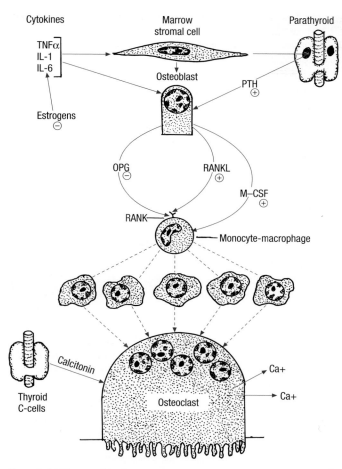

Figure 6.15 Diagram of the factors controlling the balance between bone deposition and bone resorption. Osteoblast secretion of monocyte colony stimulating factor (M-CSF) and a ligand RANKL stimulates mononuclear precursors to proliferate and fuse to form osteoclasts. In other circumstances osteoblasts secrete osteoprotegerin (OPG), which blocks receptors on the precursor cells for RANKL and prevents osteoclast formation. PTH, parathyroid hormone.

Effects of nutrition

Normal development of the skeleton requires an adequate intake of proteins, minerals, and essential vitamins. A gross deficiency of calcium in the diet may lead to rarefaction of bone and increased risk of fracture. A deficiency of **vitamin D** in children may lead to the condition called **rickets** in which there is a disorderly arrangement of cartilage cells in the epiphyseal plates and incomplete calcification of bone in the diaphysis. Such bones are deformed by weight-bearing, resulting in bow-legs. **Vitamin C** is essential for collagen synthesis. A deficiency of this vitamin leads to retardation of growth and slow healing of fractures.

Questions

1   The term osteoid refers to which one of the following?

   a   uncalcified, newly formed bone matrix

   b   woven bone

   c   a Haversian system

   d   material lining the internal circumferential lamellae

   e   structure of the external circumferential lamellae

2   Several zones are present within epiphyseal cartilage. Which zone is located nearest to the marrow compartment?

   a   zone of reserve cartilage

   b   zone of hypertrophy

   c   zone of proliferation

   d   zone of resorption

   e   zone of calcified cartilage

3   Choose the pair that belongs together

   a   periosteum/osteoclasts

   b   osteoid/osteocyte

   c   osteoblast/lacunae

   d   spongy (cancellous) bone/circumferential lamellae

   e   osteon (Haversian system)/compact bone

4   Canaliculi are found in which of the following?

   a   bone marrow

   b   perichondrium

   c   articular cartilage

   d   lamellar bone

   e   elastic cartilage

5   An epiphyseal plate consists of

   a   fibrocartilage

   b   hyaline cartilage

   c   elastic cartilage

   d   spongy bone

   e   compact bone

6   Which statement best defines osteocytes?

   a   they are found in the periosteum and endosteum

   a   they are responsible for bone resorption

   a   they communicate with other osteocytes via gap junctions

   a   they are located in Howship's lacunae

   a   they are not found in spongy (cancellous) bone

7   Osteoprogenitor cells that line compact bone facing marrow are called

   a   osteoblasts

   b   osteocytes

   c   pericytes

   d   endosteal cells

   e   periosteal cells

8   Which type of cell is located in a Howship's lacuna?

   a   osteocyte

   b   osteoblast

   c   osteoclast

   d   chondrocyte

   e   chondroblast

9   Lamellae are always found in which of the following?

   a   spicules of bone

   b   Howship's lacunae

   c   spongy bone

   d   bone marrow

   e   compact bone

10   Which of the following are stimulated by parathyroid hormone to resorb bone, thus releasing calcium into the blood?

   a   chondrocytes

   b   fibroblasts

   c   osteoclasts

   d   pericytes

   e   osteoblasts

11   Compact bone is a vascular structure that is made possible by what system?

12   What is the name of the inner connective tissue lining of compact bone?

13   What is the name of the crystalline structures in the bone matrix?

14   What is located within Howship's lacunae?

15   What type of bone cell is multinucleated?

16   What is the name for the layers that are located along the inner surface of compact bone?

17   What is in the center of the osteon?

18   The processes of osteocytes are located in what structure?

19   What are the oblique channels through which the central canals of osteons communicate with each other called?

20   Trabeculae are located in what type of bone?

Chapter seven

Muscle

Contractility is a property exhibited in varying degree by nearly all cell types, but this ability to convert chemical energy, in the form of ATP, into mechanical force is most highly developed in muscle. The locomotion of animals, the beating of their hearts, and the movements of the stomach and intestines depend upon three different types of muscle: **skeletal muscle**, **cardiac muscle**, and **smooth muscle**, each specialized to exert the kind of force required in their different locations. Contraction of skeletal muscle is rapid, forceful, and under voluntary control. Contraction of cardiac muscle is intrinsically activated, rhythmic and not subject to voluntary control. The contraction of smooth muscle is slow, sustained and involuntary.

SKELETAL MUSCLE

Structure of muscle fibers

The units of organization of **skeletal** or **striated muscle** are not individual cells. They are long, cylindrical, multinucleate syncytia, formed by fusion of multiple individual cells, called myoblasts, during embryonic development. The resulting **muscle fibers**, 0.1 mm in diameter and several centimeters in length, are arranged in bundles (fascicles) large enough to be visible with the naked eye. The striated muscle fibers are not branched and their many nuclei are displaced to the periphery of the fiber by the contractile elements in their interior (Fig. 7.1). The muscle, as a whole, is surrounded by a thin layer of dense connective tissue called the **epimysium**. Thin, branching connective tissue septa extend inward from the epimysium, enveloping each of the bundles of muscle fibers. These septa constitute the **perimysium**.

A delicate network of reticular fibers around the individual muscle fibers is termed the **endomysium**. This network binds the muscle fibers together, but permits some sliding motion between them.

The plasma membrane of skeletal and cardiac muscle fibers is called the **sarcolemma**, and their cytoplasm is referred to as the **sarcoplasm**. The outer surface of the sarcolemma is coated with a thin **external lamina**, that resembles the basal lamina of epithelia but is much thinner. The inner surface of the sarcolemma is coated by a very thin layer of a 400 kDa protein, **dystrophin**, that is not found in other cell types. This is believed to provide internal reinforcement of the membrane, enabling it to resist the stresses developed in muscle contraction, relaxation, and stretching. It may have other functions that are yet to be discovered.

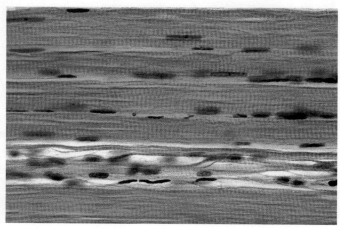

Figure 7.1 Photomicrograph of skeletal muscle, showing its unbranched fibers, and faint cross-striations. The elongated nuclei are at the periphery of the fibers.

In the hereditary disease, **muscular dystrophy**, there is a defect in the gene for **dystrophin**, which normally coats the inside of the sarcolemma. Muscular weakness is evident by the age of 5 years, and by 13 years of age the patient is confined to a wheelchair. The disease is sex-linked, affecting only males.

In longitudinal sections of muscle, examined with the light microscope, the muscle fibers have uniformly spaced cross-striations (Fig. 7.2). This appearance is the basis for the term 'striated muscle' which is often used to distinguish **skeletal** and **cardiac muscle** from the **smooth muscle** which lacks such striations. Within the sarcoplasm of each muscle fiber, there are thousands of **myofibrils** that are also cross-banded. Their dense bands are usually in register across the width of the fiber, and this accounts for the cross-striation of the fiber as a whole (Figs 7.2, 7.3). The column of myofibrils in a muscle fiber occupies the greater part of the sarcoplasm, displacing its many nuclei to the periphery and flattening them against the sarcolemma (Fig. 7.1). The long elliptical profiles of the nuclei are regularly spaced along the length of the muscle fiber. Their number cannot be specified, but in a fiber several centimeters in length, they would number in the hundreds. Their peripheral location is helpful in distinguishing skeletal

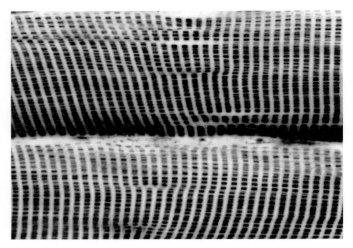

Figure 7.2 A high magnification photomicrograph of two skeletal muscle fibers, stained with iron hematoxylin to reveal the cross-striations more clearly.

muscle from cardiac muscle, in which the nuclei are located in the center of the fiber. All of the common organelles are present. A small Golgi complex and numerous mitochondria are found in the

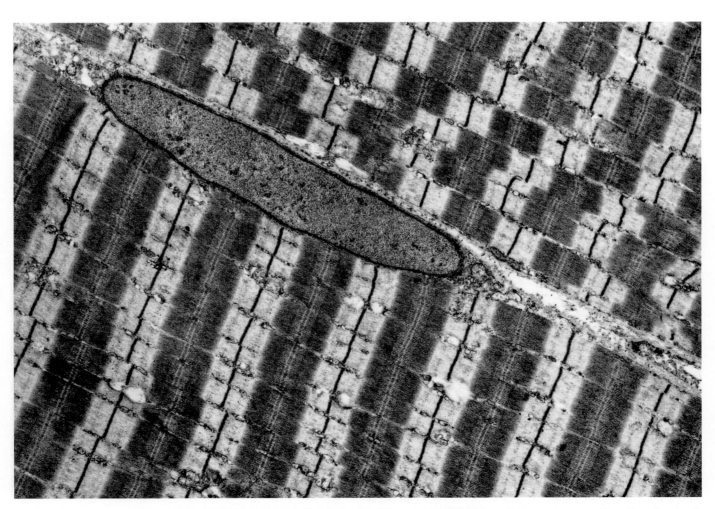

Figure 7.3 Electron micrograph of portions of two skeletal muscle fibers. Note the location of the nucleus immediately beneath the sarcolemma, and the uniform diameter of the myofibrils. Corresponding bands of the myofibrils are normally in register across the fiber. Those of the upper fiber are not, due to distortion in specimen preparation.

juxtanuclear sarcoplasm at the poles of the nuclei. Long mitochondria are also deployed in longitudinal rows between bundles of myofibrils, where they generate the chemical energy necessary for muscle contraction. Lipid droplets are occasionally found among the organelles at the poles of the nuclei, and glycogen particles are distributed throughout the sarcoplasm. In addition to these microscopically visible components, the sarcoplasm also contains an oxygen-binding protein, **myoglobin**, in solution. This protein is largely responsible for the brown color of muscle. Oxygen dissociates from myoglobin, as required, and becomes available for oxidative reactions.

Before the development of the electron microscope, the alternating light and dark bands of striated muscle were named according to their appearance under the polarizing microscope. The dark-staining bands were found to be *anisotropic* and were designated the **A-bands**, and the light bands were *isotropic* and were therefore called the **I-bands**. This terminology has persisted. The relative lengths of the bands depends upon the state of contraction of the muscle. The I-bands are very short in contracted muscle and longer in relaxed muscle. The length of the A-bands remains constant. Each I-band is bisected by a darker narrow transverse line, the **Z-line**, or **Z-disk**. The segments between successive Z-lines are called **sarcomeres** and all morphological changes in the contractile cycle are described with reference to this

subunit of the myofibrils. Each sarcomere includes an A-band and half of the two contiguous I-bands. The A-bands, I-bands, and Z-lines are the only cross-striations visible with the light microscope. These are more clearly seen on electron micrographs, and two additional bands can be identified: a paler-staining **H-band** in the middle of the A-band, bisected by a thin **M-line** at its midpoint (Fig. 7.4).

At high magnification, the myofibrils are seen to be made up of filaments of two kinds, **actin filaments** and **myosin filaments** (Fig. 7.5). Myosin filaments are the major constituent of the A-band of the sarcomere. They are 1.5 μm in length and 15 nm in diameter and are arranged in parallel, with a space of about 45 nm between them. They are held in lateral register by slender cross-links located at the midpoint of the A-band. The transverse alignment of these links is responsible for the linear density identified as the M-line.

Actin filaments are the dominant component of the I-band, and they extend for a variable distance into the A-band, interdigitating with the myosin filaments. Therefore, in cross-sections of myofibrils at the level of the I-band, only punctate profiles of actin filaments are seen, and in sections through the middle of the A-band, only the larger cross-sectional profiles of myosin filaments are found. However, in cross-sections nearer the ends of the A-band, where actin and myosin filaments interdigitate, both

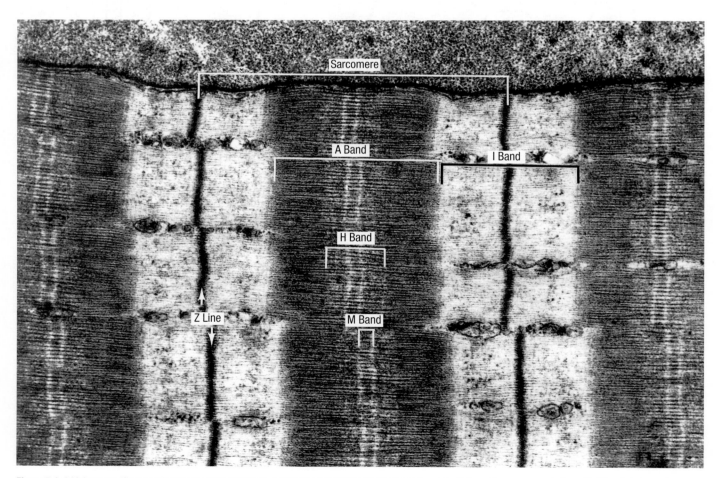

Figure 7.4 A higher magnification micrograph of five myofibrils, labeled to identify the I-band, M-band, and the Z-lines. The sarcomere is the unit of length between two successive Z-lines. It includes the A-band, and half of the two adjacent I-bands.

Skeletal muscle

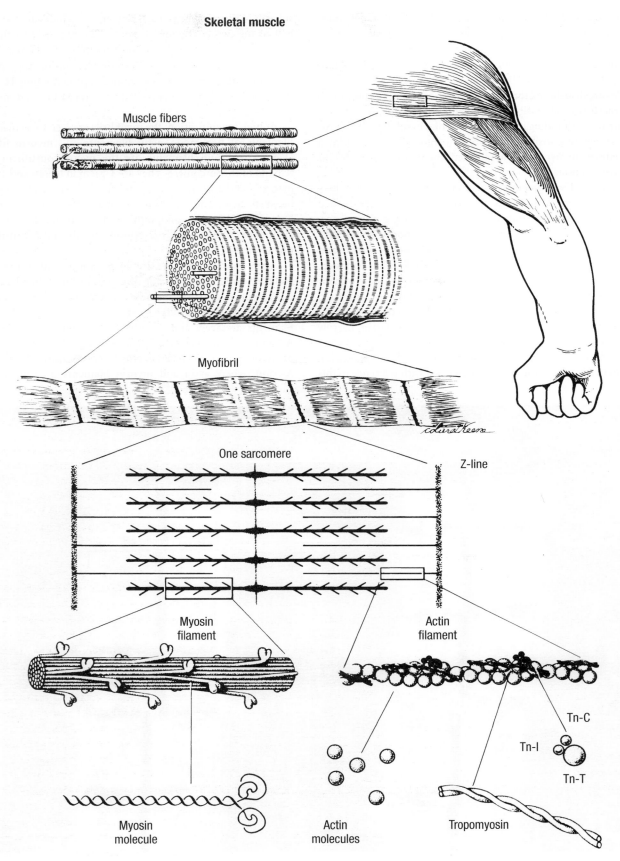

Muscle fibers

Myofibril

One sarcomere

Z-line

Myosin
filament

Actin
filament

Tn-C

Tn-I

Tn-T

Myosin
molecule

Actin
molecules

Tropomyosin

Figure 7.5 Drawing of the structure of skeletal muscle from the gross, down to components of molecular dimensions. The interdigitating myosin and actin filaments of one sarcomere are depicted diagrammatically in the center of the figure. Tn-T, Tn-I, Tn-C are troponin peptides. (Drawing by Sylvia Collard Keene.)

kinds of filaments are found, with cross-sections of the thin actin filaments arranged in a hexagonal pattern around each myosin filament. In longitudinal sections, the space between interdigitating thick and thin filaments is traversed by regularly spaced **cross-bridges** that radiate from each myosin filament towards the surrounding actin filaments.

Information on the substructure of the thick filaments has been obtained by their isolation and mechanical dissociation. Each filament yields about 350 myosin molecules. These, in turn, consist of two polypeptide chains entwined to form the rod-like tail of the molecule (Fig. 7.5). At one end, globular regions of the peptide chains form two diverging heads. The heads of the myosin molecules are the cross-bridges that project from the myosin filaments towards the actin filaments (Fig. 7.5). The actin-binding property of the heads of the myosin molecules is essential for muscle contraction. In forming the thick filaments, myosin molecules assemble in an overlapping antiparallel fashion, with their tails towards the middle of the A-band. A central region of the band therefore consists only of the smooth rod-like segments of the molecules and is devoid of cross-bridges. These regions are in lateral register across the myofibril, forming the H-band in the middle of the A-band of each sarcomere (Fig. 7.4).

Isolated thin filaments have a beaded appearance at high magnification. They arise by polymerization of globular monomers of **G-actin**, 5.6 nm in diameter. The polymers, **F-actin**, form two helically entwined strands, in which each gyre of the helix is about 36 nm in length. A consistent orientation of the subunits of actin gives the thin filaments a definite polarity. The actin filaments on either side of the Z-disk are of opposite polarity. Associated with the actin filaments are long molecules of **tropomyosin** arranged end-to-end in the grooves between the helically entwined F-actin chains. Bound to each molecule of tropomyosin is a complex of three **troponin** peptides designated **Tn-T**, **Tn-I**, and **Tn-C**. Tn-T binds the troponin complex to tropomyosin. Tn-C has a binding site for the calcium that initiates contraction, and Tn-I inhibits the binding of the myosin heads to actin in the resting muscle. These submicroscopic components of the actin filaments have key roles in the mechanism of muscle contraction that will be discussed below.

A more recently discovered muscle protein, called **titin**, is the largest known protein. It is a single chain of 27 000 amino acids with a molecular weight of about 3×10^6 (3000 kDa). These long molecules are nearly a micron in length and span the distance between the M-line and the Z-disk (Fig. 7.6). The portion of each molecule extending into the A-band is believed to be bound to an adjacent thick filament. The portion in the I-band is coiled and has elastic properties. Titin molecules contribute to the stability of the sarcomere by keeping the myosin filaments centered, and the elastic properties of the portion of the molecule in the I-band are probably responsible for the ability of a muscle to spring back to resting length after being stretched. Another protein, **nebulin**, is closely associated with the actin filaments and may have a role in determining their length.

The myofilaments of successive sarcomeres are linked end-to-end at the Z-disk, but it is difficult to observe how because of the density of the disk and the superimposition of its components. The actin filaments appear to end at the edge of the disk. There, each filament is attached to four diverging Z filaments, which course obliquely across the disk to attach to four actin filaments of the next sarcomere. Filaments of one sarcomere are slightly offset with respect to those approaching the disk from the other side. Therefore, in longitudinal sections, the connecting Z filaments form a zigzag pattern across the myofibril. Much of the density of the Z-disk is attributable to α-actinin. Another protein, **zeugmatin**, is localized at the boundaries of the disk. Its exact role has yet to be discovered.

Mechanism of contraction

Studies with the electron microscope have led to a widely accepted **sliding filament hypothesis** to explain muscle contraction. It is assumed that when a muscle contracts, the myosin and actin filaments maintain the same length as in resting muscle, but the thin actin filaments slide more deeply into the A-band, thus shortening the sarcomeres along the entire length of the myofibrils (Fig. 7.7). This accounts for the change in breadth of the H-band in different phases of the contractile cycle, for its length is defined as the distance between the ends of the actin filaments extending into the A-band from opposite ends. It is widest in resting muscle and

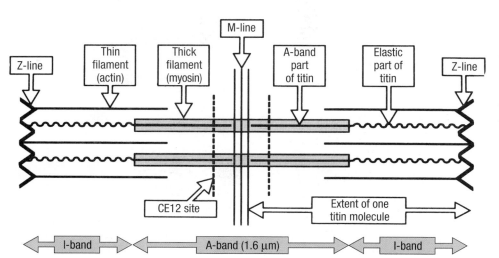

Figure 7.6 Diagram illustrating the probable arrangement of titin molecules within the sarcomere. The elastic portion of the large molecule is shown as a wavy line, only in the I-band, but it extends into the A-band, and attaches to a myosin filament. (Reproduced from J. Trinick *Curr Opin Cell Biol* 1991; 8:112–119.)

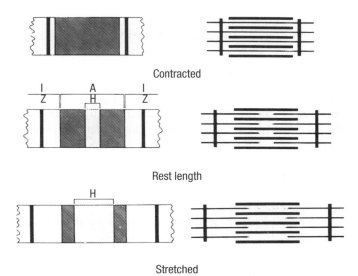

Contracted

Rest length

Stretched

Figure 7.7 On the left, diagram of the changing appearance of the cross-bands in myofibrils of muscle when contracted, at resting length, and stretched. On the right, the position of the actin filaments relative to the myosin filaments in these three states.

becomes narrower in contracted muscle as a result of deeper penetration of actin filaments into the A-band. Sliding of the filaments is initiated by an influx of calcium ions into the sarcoplasm. Calcium storage and release is the function of the sarcoplasmic reticulum, a specialized form of the endoplasmic reticulum unique to muscle fibers.

Sarcoplasmic reticulum

Most of the organelles of muscle fibers do not differ significantly from those of other cells. The only exception is the sarcoplasmic reticulum, which has acquired physiological properties not typical of the endoplasmic reticulum. It is the site of sequestration of calcium during muscle relaxation, and release of calcium into the sarcoplasm to trigger muscle contraction. It consists of a network of membrane-bounded tubules surrounding each myofibril, and it exhibits a repeating pattern related to specific regions of the sarcomeres. The tubules are largely devoid of associated polyribosomes. Their prevailing orientation is longitudinal, but there are lateral branches that form a close-meshed network around the myofibril at the level of the H-band of each sarcomere. Over each junction of an A-band with an I-band, the longitudinal sarcotubules are confluent with a pair of parallel transverse tubules of larger caliber, called the **terminal cisternae** (Fig. 7.8). Thus, along the myofibrils, two pairs of parallel terminal cisternae are associated with each sarcomere (Figs 7.8, 7.9). Between each pair of terminal cisternae there is a slender transverse tubule, called the **T-tubule**. This is not an integral part of the sarcoplasmic reticulum but is a tubular invagination of the sarcolemma that extends inwards from the surface of the fiber, crossing many myofibrils. Where it is continuous with the sarcolemma, its lumen is open to the extracellular space. The two parallel terminal cisternae and the intervening T-tubule form a complex

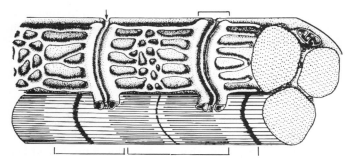

Figure 7.8 Drawing of the sarcolemma and three adjacent myofibrils, illustrating the network of tubules of the sarcoplasmic reticulum around the A-band, and the location of the triads of the reticulum at the A–I junctions. Note the continuity of the T-tubule with the sarcolemma at the arrow.

referred to as the **triad**. To distinguish the terminal cisternae from the longitudinal elements of the reticulum, they are often referred to as the **junctional reticulum**. The lumen of the terminal cisternae contains an amorphous material of low density consisting mainly of **calsequestrin**, a 55 kDa protein that can bind 300 nM of calcium per milligram and is believed to serve as a sequestering agent for storage of calcium within the junctional reticulum.

In cells, in general, the calcium concentration in the cytosol is maintained at a low level by Ca^{2+} ATPases in the plasmalemma that continually pump Ca^{2+} ions out of the cell. Skeletal muscle employs a different strategy to maintain a low concentration of calcium in the sarcoplasm. Special Ca^{2+} ATPases in the membrane of the terminal cisternae, continually pump Ca^{2+} out of the sarcoplasm and into their lumen, where it accumulates in high concentration.

Activation of muscle contraction

Muscle contraction is initiated by generation of an action potential at a **myoneural junction**. This spreads over the sarcolemma

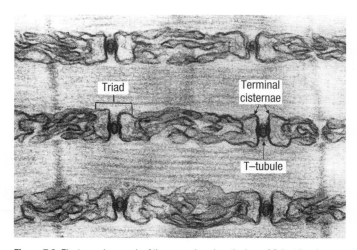

Figure 7.9 Electron micrograph of the sarcoplasmic reticulum of fish striated muscle. The triads are over the ends of the A-band and connected by longitudinal tubules of the reticulum. In mammals, the triads are over the A–I junctions.

and along the T-tubules of the muscle fibers. This triggers events at the interface between the T-tubules and the terminal cisternae, which result in the release of calcium into the sarcoplasm. In resting muscle, binding sites for myosin, on the thin filaments, are blocked by the tropomyosin–troponin complexes. Release of calcium into the sarcoplasm by the terminal cisternae, is followed by its binding to troponin-C in each segment along the actin filaments. This results in a conformational change in the complex that exposes myosin-binding sites on the actin filaments. The heads of the myosin molecules then bind to the neighboring actin filaments and this binding activates myosin-ATPase. The energy released induces flexion of the myosin heads with a force sufficient to slide the neighboring actin filaments deeper towards the middle of the A-band. The myosin heads then detach, and reattach to the next set of binding sites for a new cycle of bridge-making and bridge-breaking (Fig. 7.10). Hundreds of such cycles take place in rapid succession to produce the observed movement of the actin filaments deeper into the A-band. This continues until calcium is taken up from the sarcoplasm and sequestered in the terminal cisternae, and the tropomyosin–troponin complexes again cover the myosin-binding sites on the actin filaments, restoring the muscle to its resting state.

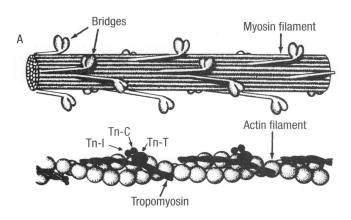

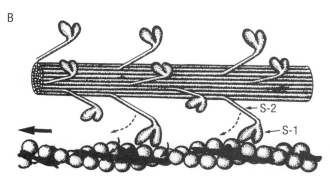

Figure 7.10 (A) Diagram of the structure of the thick myosin filament and a thin actin filament, and its associated tropomyosin–troponin complex. (B) Calcium binding to these complexes causes a change in their configuration that exposes myosin binding sites on the actin filament. Energized by ATP, the heads of the myosin molecules bind and then flex, moving the actin filament towards the middle of the A-band. S-1, head of myosin molecule; S-2, neck of myosin molecule.

Innervation of skeletal muscle

Skeletal muscle is innervated by long processes (axons) of nerve cells located in the spinal cord. At a muscle, the nerve divides into multiple branches that penetrate into its interior via the perimysial septa. Individual axons then branch in the endomysium and form nerve endings (**myoneural junctions**) on a variable number of muscle fibers. A single motor neuron may innervate from one to over 100 muscle fibers. The axon, and the muscle fibers it innervates, constitute a **motor unit**. The activation of a single axon will result in muscle tension proportional to the number of muscle fibers innervated by that axon. In the graded response that is possible in whole muscles, the strength of the contraction depends upon the number of motor units that are activated.

At its junction with a muscle fiber, an axon loses its myelin sheath and branches into several short endings (terminal boutons), each occupying a shallow depression in the sarcolemma. Together, these constitute a **motor end plate** (Fig. 7.11). The axoplasm of each ending contains a large number of small vesicles (40–60 nm) that contain the neurotransmitter **acetylcholine**. In transmission of a nerve impulse, these fuse with the axolemma discharging their content into the **synaptic cleft**, the narrow space between the axon terminal and the sarcolemma of the muscle fiber. The neurotransmitter binds to specific receptors in the underlying sarcolemma. This opens channels that permit the entry of sodium ions into the sarcoplasm of the muscle fiber. This depolarizes the membrane, generating an electrical signal (an **action potential**) that is rapidly propagated over the sarcolemma and along the T-tubules, activating the release of calcium that triggers contraction.

> **Myasthenia gravis** is an autoimmune disease characterized by muscular weakness and fatiguability. For unknown reasons, antibodies are formed against acetylcholine receptors in the sarcolemma at myoneural junctions. The resulting failure in transmission of the nerve impulse at many of these junctions results in inactivation of many motor units and consequent weakness. The disease is most common in women between 20 and 40 years of age. It may be life threatening if the muscles of respiration are seriously involved.

Muscle fiber diversity

The fibers that make up a given muscle are not all identical. They vary in color, diameter, and in cytochemical and physiological properties. Traditionally, three types have been described: **red fibers**, **white fibers**, and **intermediate fibers**. The red fibers (**slow twitch fibers**) are smaller in diameter and have a dark color. The deeper color is attributable to their greater content of myoglobin and to the cytochromes in their unusually large and abundant mitochondria. Lipid droplets are common in their sarcoplasm and the Z-bands are wider than in the other fiber types. They are innervated by slender axons with relatively simple motor endplates. Motor units consisting of red fibers contract relatively slowly, but are more resistant to fatigue than other types because of their greater ability to regenerate ATP. These properties make

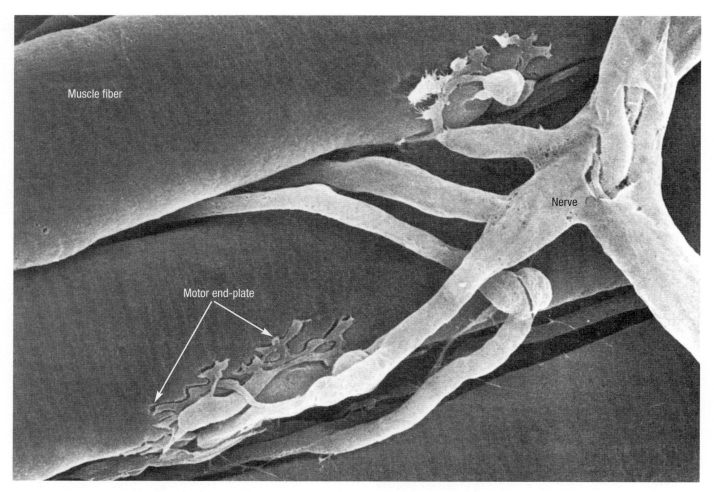

Figure 7.11 A scanning electron micrograph of a motor nerve and two motor end plates on adjacent muscle fibers. (Micrograph courtesy of J. Desaki and Y. Uehara *J Neurocytol* 1981; 10:101.)

muscles that are rich in red fibers well suited for relatively slow activity that requires great endurance, as in marathon runners.

White fibers (**fast twitch fibers**) are the largest of the fiber types. Their subsarcolemmal mitochondria are smaller than those of red fibers, and mitochondria between the myofibrils are relatively few. Their generation of ATP depends on anaerobic glycolysis of glucose derived from glycogen in their sarcoplasm. They are innervated by large axons that have motor end-plates about twice the size of those of red fibers. They contract rapidly and generate a large force, but they fatigue rapidly. They are best suited for brief bursts of intense muscle activity, as in a sprinter. The relative numbers of slow and fast muscle fibers in muscles can be changed by intense athletic training.

As their name implies, the intermediate fibers have characteristics intermediate between the red and white fibers. The disposition of their mitochondria is similar to that of red fibers, except that thick interfibrillar columns of mitochondria are seldom found.

Histochemical reactions reveal other differences in the fiber types. ATPase, succinic dehydrogenase, NADH dehydrogenase activity, and neutral fat content are all low in white fibers, and high in red fibers. Glycogen is abundant in white fibers and sparse in red fibers.

CARDIAC MUSCLE

Structure of cardiac myocytes

Unlike skeletal muscle, cardiac muscle consists of fibers that are not a syncytium but are made up of separate cellular units, **cardiac myocytes**. These are about 80 μm in length, 15 μm in diameter, and are joined end-to-end at junctional complexes called **intercalated disks** (Figs 7.12, 7.13). Although the cell columns so formed are predominantly parallel, the individual myocytes branch and form oblique interconnections with neighboring columns. This results in a complex three-dimensional organization that is quite different from the precise parallel arrangement of the cylindrical fibers in skeletal muscle.

Cardiac myocytes have an ovoid, centrally placed nucleus (Fig. 7.12), surrounded by myofibrils that have a pattern of cross-striations similar to that of skeletal muscle. These diverge around the nucleus, outlining a fusiform central region of sarcoplasm rich in organelles and inclusions. A small Golgi complex is found near one pole of the nucleus. Lipid droplets are common in this region

trally placed single nucleus of the myocytes, and the presence of transverse intercalated disks at intervals along the length of the myofibers. An intercalated disk may extend straight across the fiber, but more commonly, segments of it are slightly offset longitudinally, giving it a staircase-like configuration. The dense transverse portions of the disk are sites of attachment of the myofilaments to the sarcolemma at the ends of the myocytes. The opposing membranes at the junction are highly interdigitated. This is apparent on electron micrographs, but may be partially obscured in histological sections by a dense subsarcolemmal amorphous component of the junction. The intercalated disk is comparable to the zonula adherens of epithelial junctions. Its dense material includes the actin-binding proteins α-actinin and vinculin. In the repeating pattern of cross-striations the transverse portions of the intercalated disks invariably occur at the level of the I-band. Where the transverse segments of the intercalated disk are offset, the membranes of the connecting longitudinal segments have no associated dense material and are unspecialized, except for the presence of occasional gap junctions.

A distinctive feature of cardiac muscle in cross-section is the absence of distinct, polygonal myofibrils of uniform size. The bulk of the cross-section is occupied by a continuum of myofilaments, interrupted here and there by mitochondria (Fig. 7.14). In longitudinal sections, the sarcomeres are normally in register across the whole fiber. The continuity of the cross-striations across the fiber

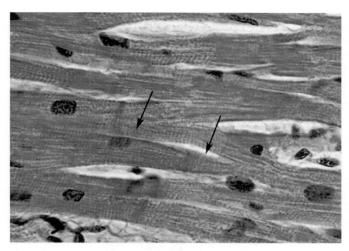

Figure 7.12 Cardiac muscle is distinguished from skeletal muscle, by the branching of the fibers, a centrally located single nucleus, and the presence of transverse intercalated disks (at arrows), between myocytes.

and, in elderly individuals, granular deposits of **lipochrome** pigment may be abundant, constituting up to 20% of the dry weight of the myocardium.

The principal identifying features of cardiac muscle are the cen-

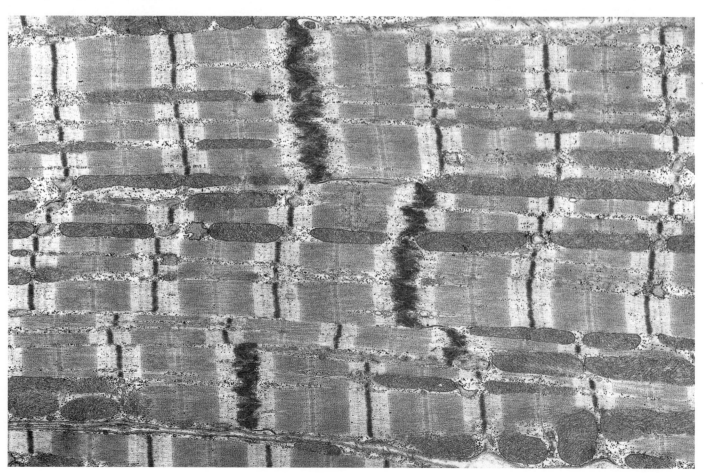

Figure 7.13 A low-power electron micrograph of cardiac muscle in longitudinal section. The cross-banding of the myofibrils is much the same as in skeletal muscle, but cardiac muscle is made up of individual cells that are joined end-to-end at dense intercellular junctions, called intercalated disks. Three are shown in this figure.

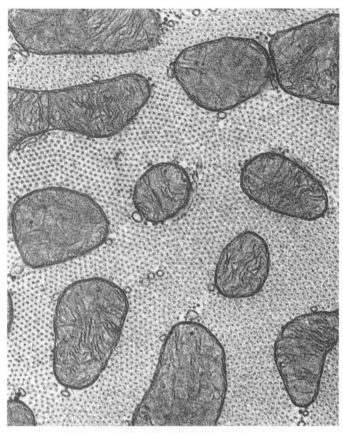

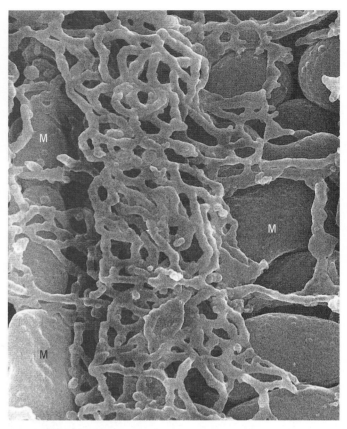

Figure 7.14 High magnification electron micrograph of a small portion of a cardiac myocyte in cross-section. Note that the myofilaments do not form distinct myofibrils. Instead, their profiles are continuous across the myocyte, interrupted only by mitochondria and occasional tubules of sarcoplasmic reticulum.

Figure 7.15 A scanning electron micrograph of a cleft in the column of myofilaments of cardiac muscle, showing the sarcoplasmic reticulum. Note the absence of conspicuous terminal cisternae. Several mitochondria are also visible (M). (Micrograph reproduced from T. Ogata and Y. Yamasaka *Anat Rec* 1990; 228: 227.)

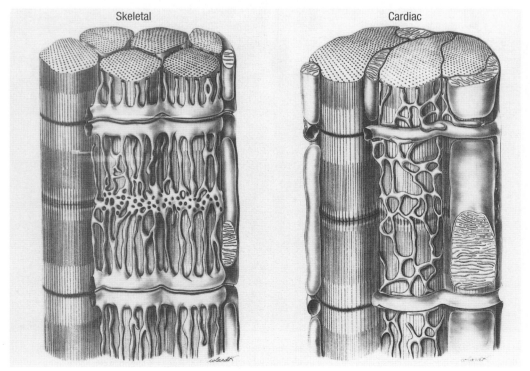

Figure 7.16 Drawing comparing the sarcoplasmic reticulum of skeletal and cardiac muscle. In cardiac muscle there are no triads. The T-tubule is of larger caliber and the terminal cisternae are reduced to small saccular dilations at the ends of certain longitudinal tubules of the reticulum.

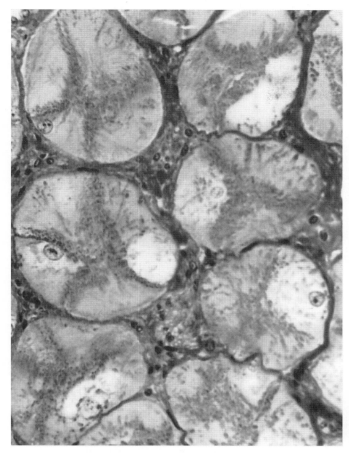

Figure 7.17 Photomicrograph of Purkinje fibers in cross-section. They are atypical cardiac muscle fibers, specialized for conduction rather than contraction. The paler areas are rich in glycogen (not preserved in this preparation).

is interrupted only by longitudinally oriented mitochondria and tubules of the sarcoplasmic reticulum. Rows of **glycogen** particles are occasionally found between myofilaments in the I-bands.

Sarcoplasmic reticulum

The tubules of the sarcoplasmic reticulum are less numerous than those of skeletal muscle. They form a subsarcolemmal network called the **corbular reticulum** that extends into deep clefts in the columns of myofilaments (Fig. 7.15). In skeletal muscle, the T-tubules extending inward from the sarcolemma are slender and located at the A–I junctions. In cardiac muscle, they are of larger caliber and tend to occur at the level of the Z-band between successive sarcomeres (Fig. 7.16). They are not flanked by long terminal cisternae, therefore **triads** are lacking in cardiac muscle. The functional counterparts of the terminal cisternae are relatively small saccular dilatations of certain longitudinal tubules of the

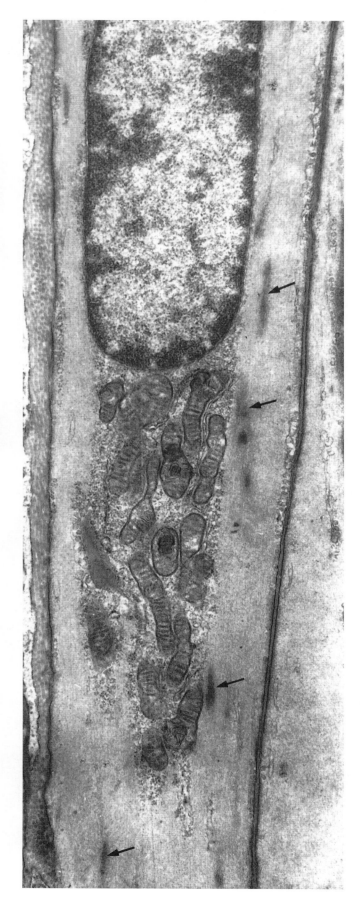

Figure 7.18 Electron micrograph of a portion of a single smooth muscle cell in longitudinal section. The organelles are confined to regions of cytoplasm near the poles of the elongated nucleus. The remainder of the cytoplasm is occupied by actin filaments (not visible at this magnification). Dense bodies scattered throughout the cytoplasm (at arrows) are sites of bonding of the actin filaments to nodal points of the cytoskeleton.

reticulum that establish close contact with the T-tubules. These complexes are referred to as the **dyads**. The transfer of excitation from the T-tubules takes place via rows of transmembrane particles called **spanning proteins** that bridge the gap between the T-tubules and the terminal saccules of the sarcoplasmic reticulum. In addition, there are small expansions of the subsarcolemmal reticulum that are connected to the sarcolemma by spanning proteins. The calcium-binding protein **calsequestrin** can be identified in these junctional saccules, as well as in the dyads.

In cardiac muscle, as in skeletal muscle, contraction is triggered by an increase in calcium concentration in the cytosol. Owing to the absence of long terminal cisternae associated with the T-tubules, cardiac muscle has more limited intracellular calcium reserves. During depolarization of the sarcolemma and the T-tubules, an influx of extracellular calcium is believed to supplement that released from the intracellular reserves in the saccular expansions of tubules of the reticulum, and in subsarcolemmal expansions of the corbular reticulum.

The maintenance of low Ca^{2+} concentration in the cytosol of cardiac muscle is attributed in large part to **antiporter proteins** in the sarcolemma. An antiporter is a membrane protein that cotransports two different ions in opposite directions, one down its concentration gradient and the other against its concentration gradient. In cardiac muscle, a **Na^+/Ca^{2+} antiporter**, instead of a

Ca^{2+} ATPase, is believed to play the principal role in maintaining a low concentration of Ca^{2+} in the sarcoplasm between contractions.

> Certain drugs used in the treatment of congestive heart failure, **ouabaine** and **digoxin**, raise the intracellular Na^+, thereby decreasing the concentration gradient across the membrane. Because the Na^+/Ca^{2+} antiporter functions less efficiently with a lower Na^+ concentration gradient, fewer Ca^{2+} ions are exported. Therefore, the intracellular Ca^{2+} concentration is increased, causing the muscle to contract more strongly.

There are differences in size of the myocytes in different regions of the heart. Those of the atria tend to be smaller than those of the ventricles, and transverse tubules are shorter. Indeed, they are seen only in the largest atrial fibers. It is likely that there is less need for transverse tubules for inward conduction of excitation in fibers of small diameter.

Myocardial endocrine cells

There are specialized myocytes in the right and left atrial appendages that secrete peptide hormones. These are involved in the regulation

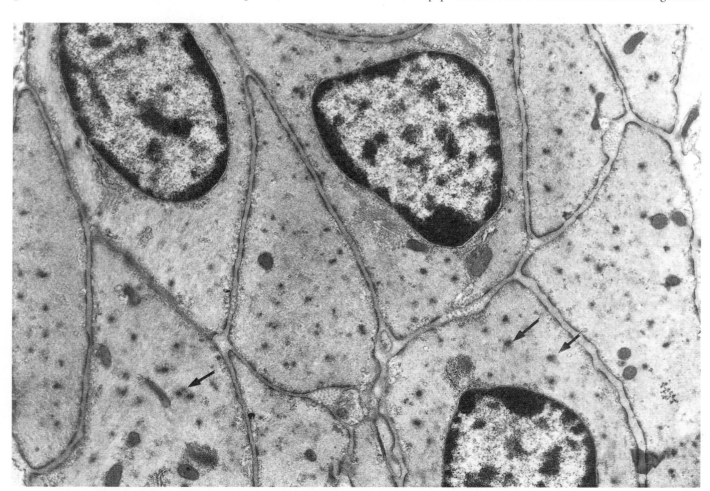

Figure 7.19 Electron micrograph of smooth muscle in cross-section. Dense bodies (at arrows) are rather uniformly spaced throughout the cytoplasm. The cells are separated by intercellular spaces containing a delicate network of reticular fibers.

of blood volume and the electrolyte composition of the extracellular fluid. The **myoendocrine cells** resemble working myocytes in having myofilaments that diverge around a central nucleus. The organelles do not differ significantly from those of myocytes elsewhere. Their most distinctive feature is the presence of many membrane-bounded secretory granules, 0.3–0.4 μm in diameter in the core sarcoplasm that extends in either direction from the poles of the nucleus. The granules contain the precursor of a family of peptides, collectively called **cardiodilatins,** or **atrial natriuretic peptides.** These peptides are released into the blood and cause peripheral vasodilatation and consequent lowering of blood pressure. They also constrict the efferent arteriole of the renal glomeruli, resulting in diuresis (increased urine) and increased excretion of sodium.

Myocardial conduction tissue

The atrial musculature of the heart contains small areas of specialized myocytes, the **sinoatrial node,** that acts as the 'pacemaker' of the heart, determining the frequency of its contractions. This is connected to a second node, the **atrioventricular node,** by

myocytes specialized for impulse conduction. The nodes consist of pale-staining, highly branched **nodal myocytes** that contain relatively few myofilaments, and those are inconsistent in their orientation. The nodes are richly vascularized and contain considerable connective tissue. They are connected by a bundle of impulse-conducting fibers, called **Purkinje fibers.** These are wider than ordinary cardiac myocytes and have relatively few myofibrils, which are arranged peripherally around a clear core of sarcoplasm containing the nucleus and a large amount of glycogen (Fig. 7.17). A bundle of Purkinje fibers emanates from the atrioventricular node and branches throughout the myocardium, transmitting waves of depolarization to the working myocytes via gap junctions. The conducting system will be discussed more fully in Chapter 9, Circulatory System.

SMOOTH MUSCLE

Smooth muscle is very widely distributed in the body. It makes up the greater part of the wall of the alimentary tract and provides the

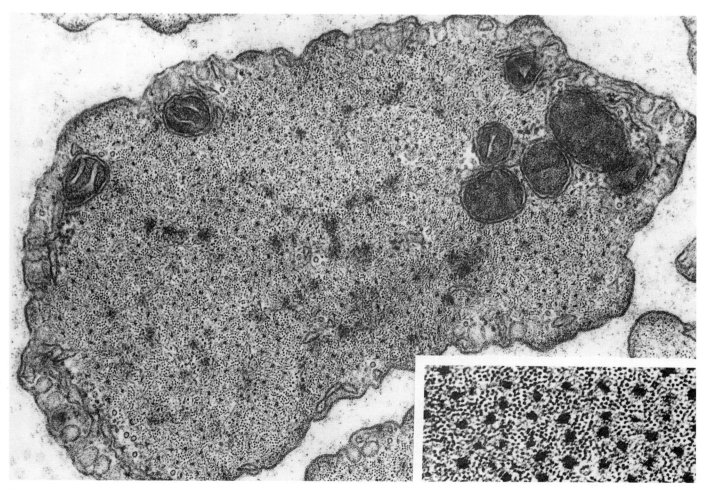

Figure 7.20 High-magnification electron micrograph of a single smooth muscle cell in cross-section. Several mitochondria, multiple dense bodies, and punctate cross-sections of vast numbers of filaments are visible. The latter are seen more clearly at higher magnification in the inset at the lower right. (Reproduced from A.P. Somlyo, E. Devine, and A.V. Somlyo *Vascular Smooth Muscle*, Springer Verlag, Berlin, 1970.)

motive force mixing food and enzymes in the stomach and duodenum and moving the products of digestion through the intestines. Circumferentially oriented smooth muscle in the walls of arteries controls the caliber of the vessel. Smooth muscle also forms the wall of the uterus and provides the sustained contractile force necessary for delivery of a baby.

Microscopic structure

Smooth muscle is made up of long fusiform (spindle-shaped) cells with an elongated nucleus situated in their wider central portion (Fig. 7.18). They vary greatly in length, ranging from 20 μm, in small blood vessels, to 500 μm in the pregnant uterus. Where smooth muscle is organized into bundles or layers, the individual cells are offset so that their wide portions are adjacent to the thin tapering ends of the neighboring cells. Therefore, in transverse sections, smooth muscle appears as a mosaic of polygonal profiles, varying from one to several microns in diameter, with a nucleus found only in the largest profiles (Fig. 7.9). The major cell organelles are confined to the conical regions of cytoplasm at the poles of the elongated nucleus. The rest of the cytoplasm generally appears rather homogeneous under the light microscope, but longitudinal bundles of **myofilaments** can be detected by their birefringence when examined with the polarizing microscope. Each smooth muscle cell is enveloped by a thin **external lamina**, resembling the basal lamina of epithelia. Outside of this, there is a network of reticular fibers that binds the cellular units together so that their contraction produces a coordinated force. Neighboring cells are in contact only at gap junctions, which provide the cell-to-cell communication necessary for integrated contraction throughout the layer of smooth muscle.

On electron micrographs, the juxtanuclear region of the smooth muscle cell contains a small Golgi complex, a few long mitochondria, and short profiles of endoplasmic reticulum. The peripheral cytoplasm, containing the contractile elements, appears rather homogeneous, except for uniformly distributed dense bodies (Figs 7.18, 7.19, at arrows). **Myofilaments** are identifiable only at high magnification (Fig.7.20). A cytoskeleton, consisting of a network of intersecting longitudinal and oblique intermediate filaments can be demonstrated by using labeled antibodies to **desmin**. Myofilaments of **actin**, 4.5 μm in length and 4–8 nm in diameter, form bundles that are oriented longitudinally and obliquely in the cytoplasm. Interspersed among the actin filaments, and parallel to them, are **myosin** filaments 1.5 μm in length and 15 nm in diameter (Fig. 7.20). The ratio of actin filaments to myosin filaments is about 12 to 1 (see inset in Fig. 7.20). The bundles of filaments terminate in the dense bodies located at nodal points in the cytoskeletal network of intermediate filaments, or in dense plaques on the inner aspect of the plasmalemma. Both the cytoplasmic dense bodies and the plaques contain the actin-binding protein α-actinin (Fig. 7.21). The plaques also bind labeled antibodies against a second actin-binding protein, **vinculin**.

Histophysiology of smooth muscle

Contraction of smooth muscle is relatively slow, but it can be sustained for long periods. The cells can shorten to one-quarter of their resting length and can generate a force, per cross-sectional area, comparable to that of skeletal muscle, while consuming far less energy. Contraction is believed to involve a sliding of the actin filaments with respect to the myosin filaments, which results in a shortening of the filament bundles. However, a sliding mechanism of shortening is more difficult to validate in smooth muscle than in striated muscle. Myosin can interact with actin only if its light chain is phosphorylated. Smooth muscle contraction is initiated by an influx of calcium, which binds to a calcium-binding protein, **calmodulin**. The calcium–calmodulin complex binds to **myosin light-chain kinase**, activating this enzyme, which catalyzes the phosphorylation of myosin light chains, enabling them to interact with actin filaments and cause contraction.

Smooth muscle differs in its mode of activation in different

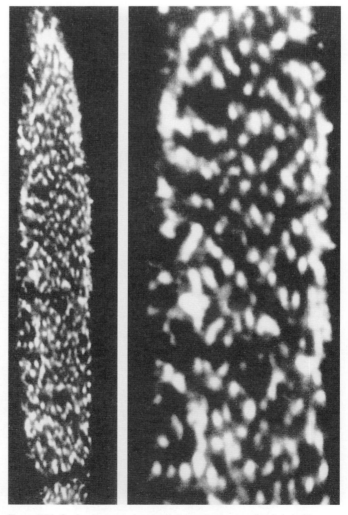

Figure 7.21 Confocal images of contracted smooth muscle cells labeled with fluorescent antibody to the α-actinin of the cytoplasmic dense bodies indicated by arrows in Fig. 7.19. (Reproduced from A. Draeger, W.B. Amos, M. Ikebe and J.V. Small *J Cell Biol* 1990; 11:2463.)

organs. Intestinal smooth muscle, an example of **unitary smooth muscle**, has an autorhythmicity. Intrinsically generated stimuli are conducted, via gap junctions, throughout a large area of smooth muscle that contracts in unison, and waves of contraction (peristalsis) then sweep along the intestine to advance its contents. The type of smooth muscle in large arteries, in the ducts of the male reproductive tract, and in the ciliary body of the eye, is designated **multiunit smooth muscle**. In muscle of this kind, there is little evidence of impulse conduction from fiber to fiber via gap junctions. Instead, each fiber is innervated, and contraction is more rapid than in unitary smooth muscle. Adrenergic and cholinergic nerves to smooth muscle of this type act antagonistically.

Questions

1 Thick filaments are anchored to the Z-disk by a protein known as
   a nebulin
   b titin
   c α-actinin
   d myomesium
   e C-protein

2 In skeletal muscle cells tropomyosin is associated with
   a thick filaments
   b thin filaments
   c intermediate filaments
   d desmin filaments
   e myosin filaments

3 In skeletal muscle the primary function of the sarcoplasmic reticulum is to
   a produce lysosomes
   b package proteins for export to the exterior of the cell
   c synthesize acetylcholine
   d synthesize microtubules
   e sequester and release calcium

4 Which statement best describes an intercalated disk?
   a a specialized region of the sarcoplasmic reticulum
   b site of actin synthesis
   c site of myosin synthesis
   d specialized connective tissue
   e site of attachment between cardiac muscle cells

5 These long cylindrical filamentous bundles, consisting of sarcomeres arranged end to end, fill the sarcoplasm
   a muscle
   b muscle fasciculus
   c muscle fiber
   d myofibril
   e myofilament

6 Invaginations of the sarcolemma surrounding each myofibril and involved in excitation-contraction coupling are
   a sarcoplasmic reticulum
   b transverse tubules
   c tropomyosin
   d troponin
   e sarcomere

7 Which of the following is correct with regards to cardiac muscle?
   a it possesses numerous caveolae
   b it is multinuclear
   c it is connected end-to-end via intercalated disks
   d it is spindle-shaped
   e it requires external stimulation to undergo contraction

8 In longitudinal sections skeletal muscle fibers appear striated; the dark bands in which thin and thick filaments overlap are referred to as the
   a A-band
   b H-band
   c I-band
   d M-line
   e Z-line

9 Endomysium surrounds
   a an entire muscle
   b individual muscle fibers
   c muscle fascicles
   d small bundles of muscle cells
   e individual myofibrils

10 The smallest repetitive subunit of the contractile apparatus of a striated muscle cell, extending between two Z-lines, is a(n)
   a sarcomere
   b myofibril
   c A-band
   d I-band
   e M-band

11 What type of muscle is incapable of regeneration?

12 A T-tubule surrounds what intracellular structures in cardiac muscle cells?

13 What morphologic structure lies within the I-band?

14 What muscle cells, when they die, are usually replaced by connective tissue rather than new muscle?

15 During contraction of smooth muscle, calcium binds to what protein?

16 What type of muscle contains peripherally located nuclei?

17 What is the name of the connective tissue surrounding a single skeletal muscle fiber?

18 What is the name of the functional unit of skeletal muscle that lies between two Z-lines?

19 The sinoatrial node is also known by what other term?

20 What type of muscle is found primarily where unidirectional contraction is needed?

Chapter eight

Nervous System

Dr Jay Angevine

The nervous system has two major divisions: the **central nervous system (CNS)** consisting of the brain and spinal cord, and the **peripheral nervous system (PNS)** made up of **nerves** emerging from the CNS, and small encapsulated aggregations of nerve cells called **ganglia**. The brain contains about 10^{12} nerve cells, **neurons**, each of which has a cell process through which it establishes contacts with hundreds of other neurons. The spaces between neurons are occupied by **neuroglia**, which are supporting cells of several kinds that modulate the activity of the neurons.

A major function of the CNS is to receive sensory stimuli from various parts of the body and to analyze this information and respond by generating signals that are transmitted over peripheral nerves to initiate and integrate muscular, secretory, and other activities in the body. The function of the CNS is not limited to integration of information from the periphery, it is also engaged in less well understood endogenous neural activity that underlies consciousness, memory, reasoning, and regulation of behavior.

NEURON

The typical neuron consists of a cell-body (the **soma**), which has many radiating processes called **dendrites**, bounded by portions of the plasmalemma that are specialized for reception of signals from other neurons. In addition to the dendrites, there is a single, very long cell process, the **axon**, which is capable of generating a **nerve impulse** (action potential) and conducting it over a long distance to stimulate other neurons in the CNS, muscles or secretory cells elsewhere in the body (Fig. 8.1A). As it approaches its end, the axon branches repeatedly in a **terminal arborization**. Each branch of this arborization ends in a small expansion called an **end bulb**, or **terminal bouton**, that makes contact with another cell to form a **synapse**, where the electrical or chemical signals pass from the neuron to a responding cell, the **effector cell**. At these contacts, transmission of the signal from the neuron to its responding cell depends upon compounds that it synthesizes and releases at the synapse to activate the effector cell. These compounds, termed **neurotransmitters**, act rapidly and locally to activate the target cell. Other compounds, called **neuromodulators**, exert influences upon these events more slowly by diffusion through the extracellular fluid.

The size and shape of neurons, as well as the mode of branching of their cell processes, are highly variable. Neurons are, therefore, classified according to the geometry of their processes (Fig. 8.1B). **Unipolar neurons** have an axon but no dendrites. These are rare. Somewhat more common are **pseudounipolar neurons** in sensory ganglia, which have a short process (an axon) with a T-shaped branching, one member of which leads to the CNS and the other goes to an ending in the periphery. **Bipolar neurons** are similar, but have two processes (both axons) emerging directly and oppositely from the cell body. **Multipolar neurons**, in contrast, have one axon and many dozens of dendrites. This latter type is very common in the CNS. The number of synapses on a neuron depends, in large measure, on the number and length of its dendrites. In addition to their classification by shape and number of processes, neurons can be assigned to one of three categories, based on their function: **motor neurons** are involved in stimulating muscles or glands in the periphery; **sensory neurons** receive sensory stimuli from the environment or from the tissues and organs of the body; **interneurons** maintain connections between neurons in the CNS. Of the three types, interneurons are the most abundant.

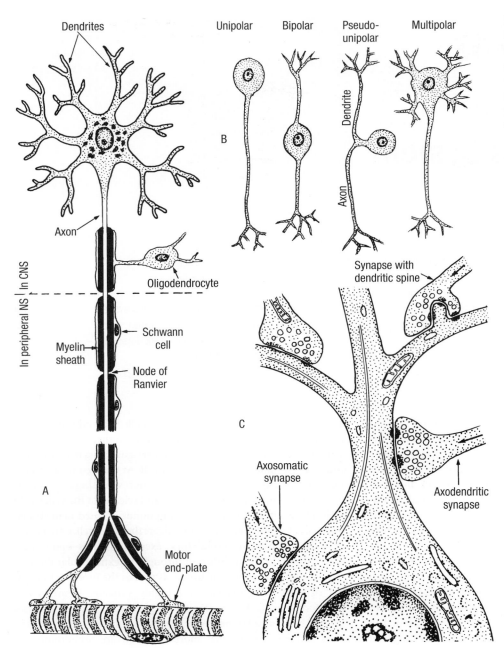

Dendrites

Axon

In peripheral NS | In CNS

Myelin sheath

Axon

Oligodendrocyte

Schwann cell

Node of Ranvier

A

Motor end-plate

B

Unipolar Bipolar Pseudo-unipolar Multipolar

Dendrite

Axon

C

Synapse with dendritic spine

Axosomatic synapse

Axodendritic synapse

Figure 8.1 (A) Drawing of the components of a typical neuron. (B) Types of neurons according to their polarity. (C) Terminology of the synapses on a neuron according to their location. (B) Adapted from A.W. Ham *Histology*, 6th edn J.P. Lippincott, Philadelphia, 1969. (C) Redrawn after R. Bunge in *Bailey's Textbook of Histology*, 16th edn. Williams and Wilkins, Baltimore, 1971.

A typical neuron has a pale-staining nucleus with a conspicuous nucleolus and relatively little heterochromatin. On electron micrographs, the cytoplasm is crowded with organelles and filamentous cytoskeletal elements arranged approximately concentrically around the nucleus. This central region of the cytoplasm is often referred to as the **perikaryon** (Fig. 8.2). In sections stained with basic dyes, the most conspicuous components of the perikaryon are large clumps of basophilic material (**Nissl bodies**), once thought to be unique to neurons. On electron micrographs, each of these is found to be an aggregation of many parallel cisternae of the rough endoplasmic reticulum (rER) (Fig. 8.2). rER is also found in the dendrites, but there it takes the form of tubules or smaller arrays of cisternae. Smooth endoplasmic reticulum (sER) forms a loose network of tubules throughout the perikaryon and continues into the dendrites and axon. In certain neurons, it may

form flat cisternae adjacent to the plasmalemma. The Golgi complex is prominent in all neurons and appears, on electron micrographs, as multiple small arciform stacks of cisternae slightly expanded at their ends. The cisterna at the concave surface of each stack is fenestrated. The function of the Golgi in these cells is much the same as in other cells. It is involved in the concentration of products synthesized on the endoplasmic reticulum. Some of the numerous small vesicles around it contain the neurotransmitter that will be transported along the axon for release at its endings. After severance of a nerve axon, the Golgi complex in the perikaryon regresses to such an extent that it may no longer be detectable with the light microscope. Finally, throughout the perikaryon and the dendrites, there are many slender mitochondria. They also occur along the axon and are especially numerous in the axon terminals. Lysosomes are present in small numbers in the perikaryon.

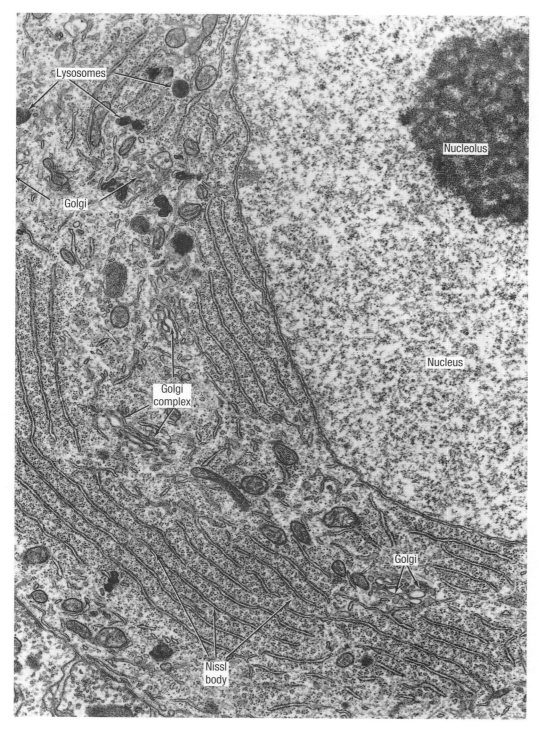

Figure 8.2 Electron micrograph of a portion of the perikaryon of a typical neuron, illustrating its principal organelles. (Micrograph courtesy of Sanford Palay.)

Cytoplasmic inclusions are uncommon in neurons and are largely limited to irregularly shaped granules of lipofuchsin pigment, which represents accumulated end-products of lysosomal activity. In old age, lipofuchsin may accumulate to such an extent as to displace the nucleus and organelles to one side of the cell. In the neurons of a few regions of the brain, coarse granules of the pigment **melanin** are also found in the neurons. Its physiological significance at these sites is unknown.

In specimens prepared for light microscopy by traditional silver impregnation methods, a network of **neurofibrils** can be seen in the perikaryon. Electron micrographs reveal a cytoskeleton not unlike that of other cell types, consisting of actin filaments (3–4 nm), intermediate filaments (10 nm), and microtubules (24–28 nm). The so-called neurofibrils seen by light microscopy were probably bundles of intermediate filaments. The intermediate filaments of neurons are now commonly referred to as **neurofilaments**. The microtubules extend into the axon and continue throughout its length. These are of greater functional significance than those of the perikaryon, for they serve as conveyor belts along which vesicles containing neurotransmitters are transported from their origin in the trans-Golgi network to the axon ending.

> One of the most devastating diseases of the brain is Alzheimer's disease, which is very common in the elderly. It is characterized by an intraneuronal accumulation of loops, coils, and tangles of filaments, consisting, in part, of an abnormal microtubule protein. There are also extracellular plaques composed of similar fibrils in an amorphous material called amyloid. Gradual loss of neurons results in a progressive dementia.

Dendrites

The ability of nerve cells to receive and integrate signals depends, in large measure, on their dendrites. Their extensive branching greatly increases the cell surface available for receiving signals from other neurons. The specific branching pattern typifies each type of neuron. The dendritic tree of spinal motor neurons may receive up to 10 000 synapses, and the exceptionally elaborate dendritic arborization of cerebellar Purkinje cells may have up to 250 000 synapses with axons of other neurons. The main branches of dendrites tend to be smooth-surfaced, but their lateral branches

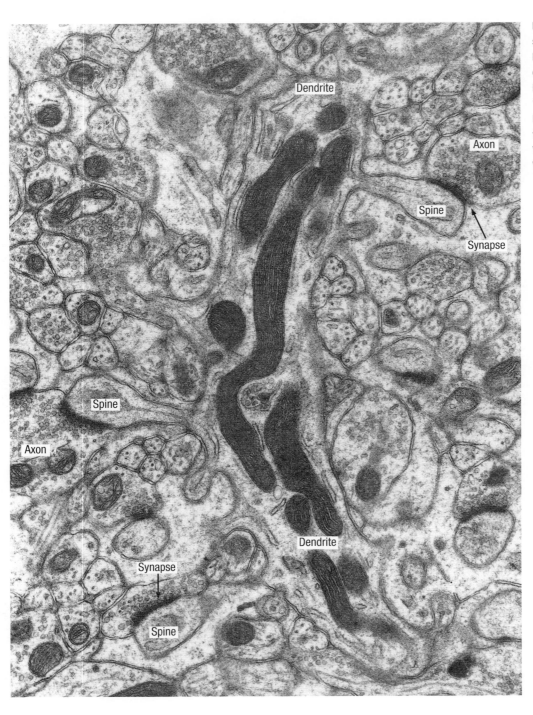

Figure 8.3 Electron micrograph of a small area of the cerebellum. A small branch of the dendritic tree of a Purkinje cell runs vertically across the field. Projecting laterally from the dendrite are 'spines' or 'thorns' with bulbous tips. Note the synapses of granule cells on these. (Reproduced from S.L. Palay and V.C. Palay *Cerebellar Cortex*, Springer Verlag, Berlin, 1974.)

are often quite irregular owing to the presence of numerous small, lateral projections called **thorns** or **spines**. These are preferential sites of synaptic contact and they occupy concavities in the end-bulbs of axons terminating upon the neuron (Figs. 8.1C, 8.3). The capacity of the neurons to integrate input from many different sources is directly related to the degree of branching of their dendrites, and the number of their spines.

In the tapering initial portions of the dendrites, the organelles resemble those of the perikaryon except for the absence of Golgi bodies. With increasing distance from the cell body (the soma), sER and neurofilaments are reduced, but longitudinal microtubules are numerous and mitochondria are aligned parallel to them.

Axon

The axon arises from a conical extension of the cell body, the **axon hillock**. The axon is more slender and usually very much longer than the dendrites of the same cell. Unlike the dendrites, which diminish in diameter as they branch, the axon has essentially the same caliber throughout its length. In spinal motor neurons supplying muscles in the feet, the axon may be as much as 40 in (1 m) in length. Its content, the **axoplasm**, lacks Nissl bodies (rER) but contains short segments of sER and long, slender mitochondria. In cross-section, the neurofilaments are spaced a uniform distance apart throughout the axoplasm (Fig. 8.4). Microtubules are also numerous, but less uniformly distributed, than the neurofilaments.

In addition to its episodic conduction of a nerve impulse along its membrane, the axon is continually engaged in **axonal transport**. Transport is bidirectional: **anterograde transport** from the perikaryon to the ending of the axon, and **retrograde transport** from the axon terminal to the cell body. Anterograde transport is especially important for delivery of the small vesicles, containing the neurotransmitter, to the axon terminal. Microtubules of the axon are polarized with their 'plus-end' towards the axon terminal, and their 'minus-end' towards the cell body. The motor protein involved in anterograde transport is **kinesin**. One end of the molecule is bound to a vesicle and the other end undergoes cyclic interaction with binding sites on the microtubule, resulting in movement of the vesicle from the perikaryon towards the

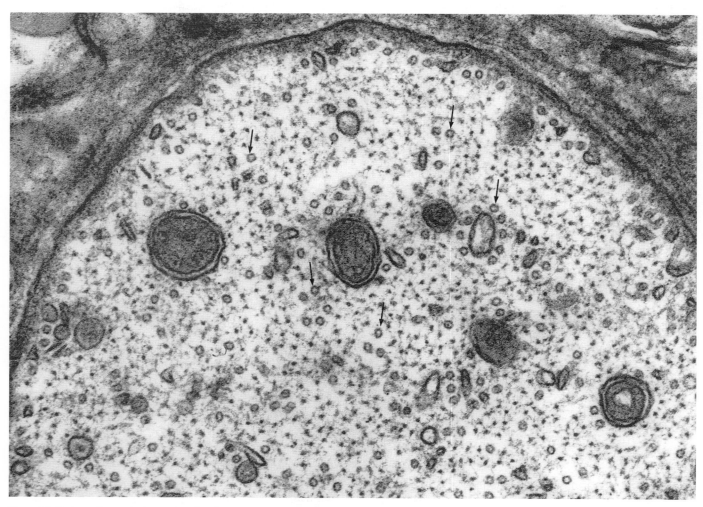

Figure 8.4 Electron micrograph of a cross-section of an axon at a node of Ranvier, showing the very even distribution of neurofilaments, and a less even distribution of microtubules (at arrows). The microtubules serve as tracks along which vesicles of neurotransmitter are moved by the motor protein kinesin. (Micrograph reproduced from R.L. Price *Proc. 47th Annual Meeting, Electron Microscope Society of America*, p. 948, 1989.)

plus-end at about 3 μm/s. Retrograde transport of vesicles or organelles is carried out by the motor protein **dynein**, which moves along microtubules towards the minus-end.

In the PNS, the axons are enveloped in a thin sheath of **Schwann cells**, which are closely applied to the **axolemma**, the limiting membrane of the axon. In the CNS, the axons are similarly ensheathed by **oligidendroglial cells**.

Nerve impulse

An electrical potential (voltage gradient) exists across the plasma membrane of all cells as a result of differences between the intracellular and extracellular concentrations of Na⁺ ions and K⁺ ions. This asymmetry in electrical charge on the two sides of the membrane (the **membrane potential**) remains quite constant in most cell types. In contrast, neurons undergo controlled changes in their membrane potential. Their ability to receive, conduct, and transmit signals depends upon the opening and closing of specific ion channel proteins in their membrane. The limiting membrane of the axon, the **axolemma**, maintains a concentration of Na⁺ ions in the underlying cytosol that is only one-tenth of that in the extracellular fluid, while the internal K⁺ ion concentration is about ten times greater than that outside of the cell. These differences result in an electrical potential of about −90 mV, with

the inside negative to the outside. This is referred to as the **resting potential**.

When a neuron is stimulated, ion channels at the site are opened and there is a sudden influx of extracellular Na⁺ ions that lowers the membrane potential (i.e. makes the inside less negative) and the membrane is said to be depolarized. This is quickly followed by an outflow of K⁺ ions that restores the resting potential. These changes, occupying only about 5 ms, create an **action potential**. Sodium ions diffusing from the initial site towards the axon ending open Na⁺ channels, depolarizing the neighboring region of the membrane and this process continues. Thus, an action potential initiated in the initial segment of the axon is propagated along its entire length. Upon arriving at the axon ending, it initiates discharge of stored neurotransmitter that stimulates another neuron or a non-neural effector cell.

Synapse

The specialized region of contact where neurotransmitter is released from an axon to stimulate another cell is called a **synapse**. In the CNS such contacts are usually with the dendrites of other neurons (**axodendritic synapses**), but they may be with the cell body (**axosomatic synapses**) (Fig. 8.1C). Such contacts with the axon (**axoaxonic synapses**) are uncommon. The

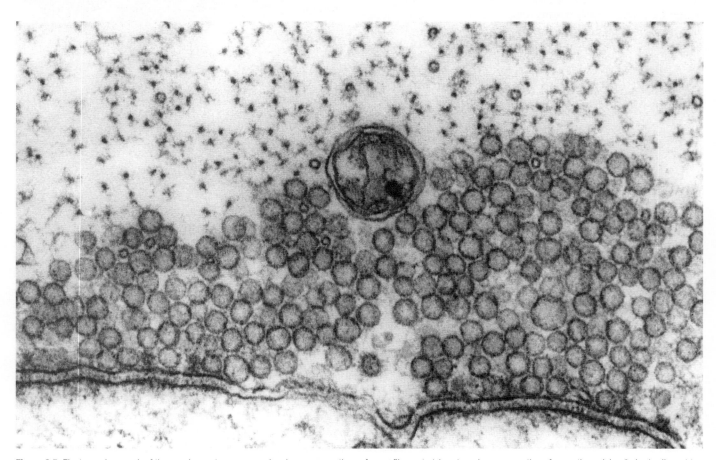

Figure 8.5 Electron micrograph of the axoplasm at a synapse, showing cross-sections of neurofilaments (above), and an aggregation of synaptic vesicles (below) adjacent to the presynaptic membrane and synaptic cleft.

number of synapses in the CNS is of a high order, being estimated at 10^{14}.

In the PNS, the synaptic contact of motor nerves is usually with muscle or glandular epithelial cells. A common neurotransmitter is **acetylcholine**, but a growing number of other compounds serving this function have been identified to date, including certain monoamines, the catecholamines **noradrenaline** and **dopamine**, the indolamine **serotonin**, and at least one amino acid, **aminobutyric acid**.

At a synapse, the **presynaptic** and **postsynaptic membranes** are parallel and separated by a **synaptic cleft**, 12–20 nm in width, which contains a moderately dense material that may contribute to their cohesion. The cytoplasm of the nerve ending contains a few mitochondria and occasional tubules of sER, but its most conspicuous constituents are numerous, small **synaptic vesicles**, 20–40 nm in diameter, clustered near the presynaptic membrane (Fig. 8.5). This membrane is covered on its inner surface with small conical densities of unknown chemical nature. The region of presynaptic membrane bearing these densities and the associated synaptic vesicles are referred to as the **active zone** of the synapse. When an action potential traveling down the axon reaches its terminal, voltage-gated channels are opened, permitting Ca^{2+} ions to enter. This triggers release of neurotransmitter into the synaptic cleft by exocytosis of synaptic vesicles docked in the active zone. The neurotransmitter binds to specific **receptors** in the postsynaptic membrane. This results in a conformational change in the receptors in that membrane, opening ion channels. Entry of ions into the postsynaptic cytoplasm causes depolarization of the membrane and excitation of the target cell. Membrane added to the active zone in exocytosis of synaptic vesicles moves laterally from the release site and is retrieved by endocytosis in clathrin-coated vesicles. These lose their coating and fuse with tubules of sER in the ending.

Synapses may be **excitatory** or **inhibitory**, depending on whether the transmitter depolarizes or hyperpolarizes the postsynaptic membrane. Which of these effects occurs depends on the chemical nature of the neurotransmitter and the type of receptors in the postsynaptic membrane.

Myelin sheath

The axons of many peripheral nerves are invested by a highly refractile layer called the **myelin sheath** (Fig. 8.6). The lipids that make up the bulk of this layer (cholesterol, phospholipid, and glycolipids) are extracted in specimen preparation for light microscopy, leaving behind a delicate network of material called **neurokeratin**. Myelin is preserved by fixation in osmium tetroxide for electron microscopy. It appears as a dense layer of varying thickness, made up of concentric dense and less-dense lines (Figs 8.7, 8.9).

The myelin sheath is an integral part of the investing layer of **Schwann cells**, which are arranged end-to-end, with each completely surrounding the axon. The nature of the myelin sheath is best understood from a study of its formation. The axon initially occupies a deep recess in the surface of the Schwann cell. The borders of the processes surrounding it come into contact and the

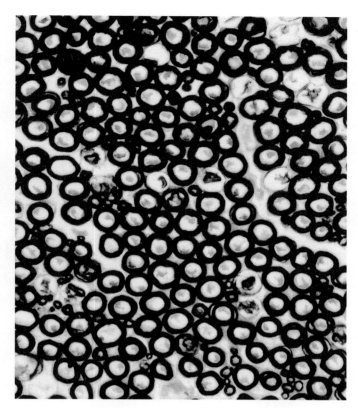

Figure 8.6 Photomicrograph of a cross-section of a nerve showing the myelin sheaths around each axon. The myelin sheaths were blackened by fixation in osmium tetroxide.

apposed membranes are described as the **mesaxon** (Figs 8.8, 8.9). In the subsequent development of the myelin sheath, formation of additional membrane results in lengthening of the mesaxon, which becomes spirally wound around the axon (Fig. 8.8B,C). As the spiral tightens, cytoplasm between successive turns is completely excluded and the inner surfaces of the plasmalemma of successive turns of the spiral come into contact and appear to fuse. Thus the myelin sheath is made up of a coil of Schwann cell membrane around the axon. In cross-sections of the sheath, viewed with the electron microscope, the fused cytoplasmic leaflets of the plasmalemma form a **major dense line**, about 3 nm thick, spiraling around the axon. Alternating with the major dense line is a thinner, less dense **intraperiod line**, formed by the close apposition of the external surfaces of the membrane in successive turns of the spiral. In micrographs of very high resolution, a narrow space (0.2 nm) is visible between these apposed outer surfaces of the membrane. This so-called **intraperiod gap** is continuous through the spiral from the endoneural to the perioaxonal extracellular space.

At intervals along the axon are short gaps in the myelin sheath, called the **nodes of Ranvier** (Fig. 8.10). These are spaces between the successive Schwann cells of the sheath. Small processes of the neighboring Schwann cells interdigitate in these spaces, but do not completely seal off the axolemma from the extracellular fluid around the nerve. The segment of the sheath between successive nodes, called an **internode**, is the length of one Schwann cell, approximately 1–2 mm.

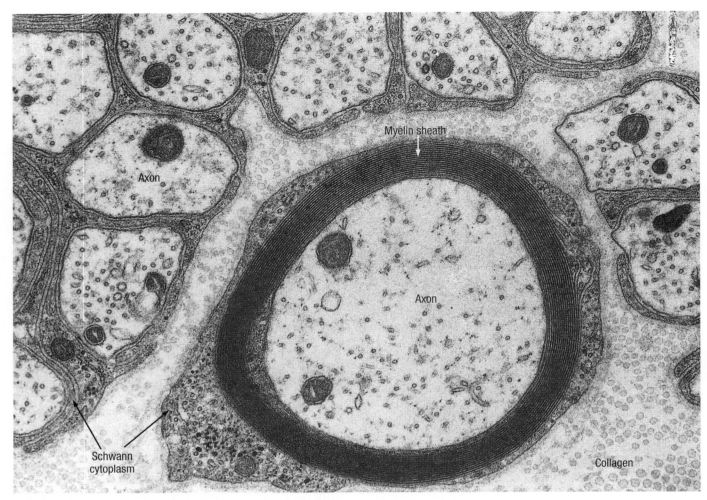

Figure 8.7 Electron micrograph of a myelinated nerve and the axons of several unmyelinated axons (above). Both are surrounded by cytoplasm of Schwann cells.

In longitudinal histological sections, one or more narrow, paler areas can be seen crossing the sheath obliquely. These have traditionally been called **Schmidt–Lantermann clefts**. It is apparent on electron micrographs that these are not clefts, but are sites in which a small amount of cytoplasm persists between the two

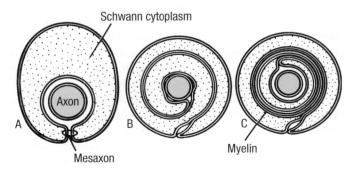

Figure 8.8 Diagram illustrating stages in the development of a myelin sheath. (A) Axon enveloped by a Schwann cell process. (B) Apposing unit membranes of the Schwann cell process (the mesaxon) have come into close contact and have begun to spiral around the axon. (C) A few layers of myelin have formed by contact and fusion of the cytoplasmic surfaces of the spiraling mesaxon. (Redrawn from J.D. Robertson *Prog Biophys* 1960; 10:349.)

leaves of the major dense line (Fig. 8.10B). Thus, these oblique lines represent thin threads of Schwann cell cytoplasm that pursue a spiral course from the cell body nearly to the axon. Their functional significance is not clear. They may provide a path through which metabolites can diffuse into the depths of the myelin, or may simply represent failure to express all of the cytoplasm in the tightening of the spiral during formation of the sheath. The myelin sheath of peripheral nerves begins a short distance from the cell body. The part of the axon between the axon hillock and the beginning of the sheath is called its **initial segment.**

The presence of a myelin sheath greatly influences the ability of an axon to conduct an impulse. It acts as an insulator, with the axon exposed to the extracellular space only at the nodes of Ranvier. The internodal segments of the myelin sheath prevent the interchange of ions necessary to generate an action potential. However, the action potential is regenerated at each node of Ranvier. This is called **saltatory conduction** and is very much faster than conduction in axons lacking a myelin sheath. The speed of conduction varies directly with the diameter of the axon and the number of layers in the myelin sheath. A myelinated axon from the cell body of a motor neuron in the human spinal cord to a muscle in the leg is about 1 m in length, and it takes only 0.01 s for the action potential to reach the muscle and stimulate its

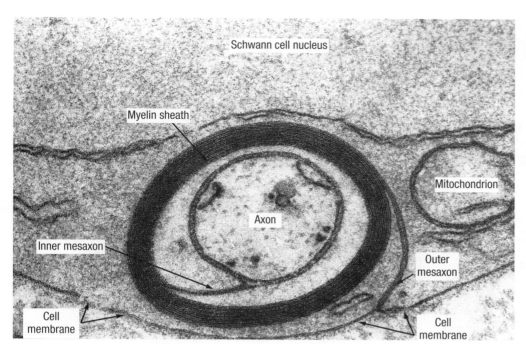

Schwann cell nucleus

Myelin sheath

Mitochondrion

Axon

Inner mesaxon

Outer mesaxon

Cell membrane

Cell membrane

Figure 8.9 Electron micrograph of a recently myelinated nerve showing both the internal and external mesaxons.

contraction. Myelinated axons of varying diameter, and with myelin sheaths of varying thickness, conduct an action potential at rates from 10 m to 100 m/s. Without the myelin sheath they would conduct at about 1 m/s. **Unmyelinated axons** in the PNS are also ensheathed by Schwann cells. These may enclose individual axons or, more often, several axons (Fig. 8.11). The successive Schwann cells along the axons are in close contact, with no gaps corresponding to the nodes of Ranvier of myelinated axons, which accounts for their slower conduction.

Myelin also occurs in major tracts that represent long-distance connections in the CNS. The axons are large and have thick myelin sheaths, and, hence, high conduction velocity. Myelin of the CNS is not made by Schwann cells, but by **oligodendrocytes**,

one of the several types of neuroglial cells (see below). It is the myelin sheaths of nerve tracts that are responsible for the glistening light color of the white matter of the brain.

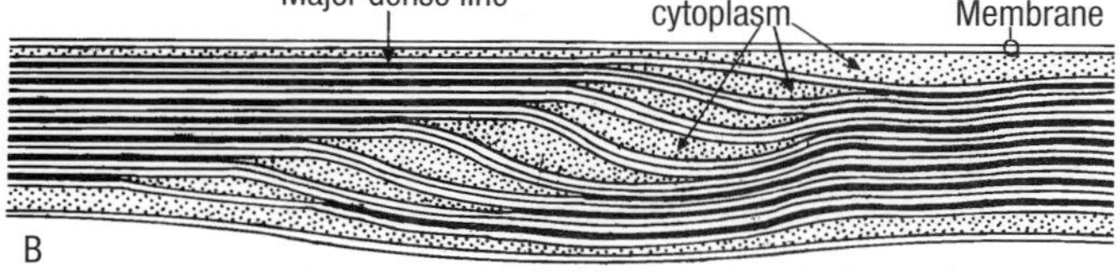

> **Multiple sclerosis** is one of the several diseases of the CNS in which the dominant feature is a destruction of the myelin sheaths. Loss of function depends upon where in the CNS the areas of myelin destruction occur. Disturbance of vision or eye movements is often an early effect, but weakness, loss of position sense, and paralysis of one or more limbs are common sequelae. A conspicuous feature of the pathology is a loss of oligodendrocytes in the areas of demyelinization. The cause of the disease is unknown.

PERIPHERAL NERVES

The nerves of the PNS consist of varying numbers of myelinated and unmyelinated axons originating from neurons located in the brain, spinal cord, or ganglia. They are enclosed in three layers of differing characteristics. The outermost layer, the **epineurium**, consists of dense irregular connective tissue, with the majority of its collagen fibers oriented longitudinally to limit the extent to which the nerve can be stretched. Its cellular elements are fibroblasts, mast cells, and limited numbers of adipose cells. Thinner extensions of this layer penetrate into the nerve as the **perineurium**, a thin sleeve of flattened cells surrounding small bundles of nerve axons. The cells of this layer are joined by tight junctions, making the perineurium an effective barrier to penetration of macromolecules. Within each bundle of nerve fibers there is an **endoneurium** consisting of a delicate network of reticular fibers surrounding each Schwann cell–axon complex.

Nerves are the pathways of communication between centers in the brain and spinal cord with the rest of the body. They contain **afferent fibers**, which carry information from the surface or the

Intraperiod line

Major dense line

Schwann cell cytoplasm

Axon

A

Major dense line

Schwann cell cytoplasm

Membrane

B

Figure 8.10 (A) Drawing of a node of Ranvier of a myelinated nerve, illustrating the major dense lines, and the intraperiod lines, of the myelin sheath. (B) Drawing of a longitudinal section of the sheath, showing the oblique alignment of small fusiform areas of cytoplasm within local dilatations of the lamellae. These correspond to the clefts of Schmidt–Lantermann that are visible with the light microscope.

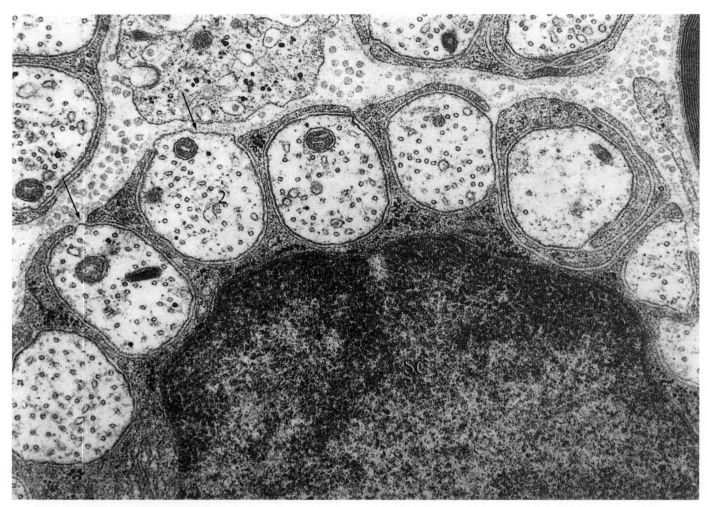

Figure 8.11 Electron micrograph of a Schwann cell of a peripheral nerve with several unmyelinated axons occupying deep recesses on its surface. Most are completely surrounded by Schwann cell, but two (at arrows) are incompletely enclosed. (Reproduced from A. Peters, S.L. Palay, and H. de F. Webster *Fine Structure of the Nervous System*, 3rd edn. Oxford University Press, New York, 1991.)

interior of the body to the CNS, and **efferent fibers**, which carry nerve impulses from the CNS to tissues and organs in the periphery. Afferent nerves from end-organs sensing heat, cold, touch, or pain, are called **sensory nerves**. Efferent nerves to muscles stimulating their contraction, are called **motor nerves**, and the tissues responding to motor nerves are referred to as their **effectors**. Many of the peripheral nerves contain both sensory and motor fibers and are, thus, termed **mixed nerves**.

DISTRIBUTION OF NEURONS

Different regions of the CNS are distinguishable with the naked eye by slight differences in color and texture. The **gray matter** contains the cell bodies of neurons, their dendrites, and the terminations of axons arriving from other regions. The **white matter** is largely devoid of neuronal cell bodies and consists mainly of myelinated axons, the cell bodies of which are in the gray matter or the dorsal root ganglia. Neuroglial cells and their

processes are present in great numbers and variety in both gray and white matter, but they may be distinguished only with special metallic impregnation methods, or with electron microscopy (see below).

Cerebral cortex

The **cerebral cortex** is an outer zone of gray matter over the hemispheres of the brain. It receives and analyzes sensory information from the body and responds by voluntary initiation of motor activity. It is also involved in learning and memory. The cerebral cortex contains over 16×10^8 neurons of many types. It is beyond the province of histology to consider in detail their form and functional connections, but a few cell types will be described. The cells are arranged in six major layers. The most characteristic type is the **pyramidal cell** (Fig. 8.12). Its soma is roughly triangular in section with a large vesicular nucleus and abundant Nissl bodies in the perikaryon. A long apical dendrite extends towards the surface of the brain, with many branches that are sites of axodendritic synapses. An axon arises from its base and descends through the deeper layers of the cortex. The pyramidal cells in the various layers of the cortex differ in size, and in their pattern of dendritic and axonal branching. The dendritic arborization of the smallest is about 10 µm wide, whereas the largest, in the region generating motor activity, is 30–60 µm in width and up to 120 µm in height. Another major cell type is the **stellate cell**, or **granule cell**. These are relatively small, 6–10 µm in diameter, with numerous highly branched dendrites radiating from the cell body and a single relatively short axon (Fig. 8.12). **Horizontal cells**, largely confined to one layer of the cortex, are fusiform, with radiating dendrites and a short axon that divides near the cell body, with the branches running in opposite directions.

> **Amyotrophic lateral sclerosis** (Lou Gehrig's disease) is a progressive loss of motor neurons in the cerebral cortex and spinal cord, resulting in atrophy of the muscles innervated by the neurons affected. The sensory system and cognitive functions are unaffected. There is often tremor, unsteady gait, paralysis of muscles, including those of mastication and facial expression, difficulty in swallowing, and, ultimately, paralysis of the muscles of respiration. Life-expectancy after onset is usually no more than ten years. It is more common in men than women, and its cause is unknown.

Cerebellar cortex

The **cerebellar cortex** (Fig. 8.13) receives informational input from the eyes, ears, and stretch receptors in the muscles. It does not initiate muscular activity, but has an important role in its coordination and in the maintenance of balance and normal posture. Three layers are recognizable. The outer, so-called **molecular layer**, contains relatively few small neurons and many unmyelinated nerve fibers. The middle layer consists of a single layer of large **Purkinje cells** (Fig. 8.14). These have an apical dendrite that ascends into the molecular layer, where it undergoes remarkably elaborate branching in a single plane (Fig. 8.12). The axon extends downwards through the underlying **granule cell layer**. The layer consists of closely packed, small cells with short dendrites and an

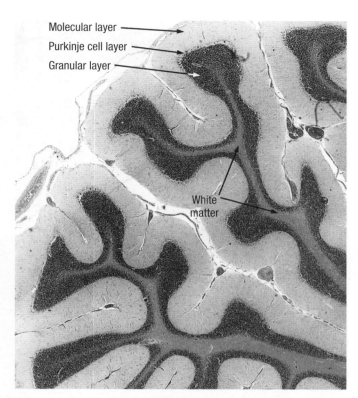

Figure 8.13 Low-power photomicrograph of a small portion of the cerebellum. Each lobule of the highly convoluted organ contains a core of white matter, surrounded by gray matter, containing a layer of granular cells, Purkinje cell bodies, and a layer made up of the dendritic processes of the Purkinje cells.

axon that courses upwards to the molecular layer to form parallel fibers synapsing with the Purkinje cells.

Spinal cord

The **spinal cord** receives motor commands from the brain and relays them via **spinal nerves** that emerge from each segment of the vertebral column to innervate the muscles and other effectors in the periphery. It receives **sensory** input from the body and relays this information back to the brain. Nerve fibers enter and leave the spinal cord at regular intervals via **dorsal** and **ventral roots**, which project laterally from both sides of the cord (Fig. 8.16). There are 31 pairs of roots along its length. Sensory fibers enter the cord through the dorsal roots and motor fibers leave through the ventral roots. A short distance from the cord, the dorsal and ventral roots join to form a sizable **spinal nerve**, containing both motor and sensory fibers that are widely distributed in the segment of the body served by that spinal nerve.

In a cross-section of the spinal cord, there is a central H-shaped area of **gray matter** containing nerve cell bodies and their dendrites (Figs 8.15, 8.16). Around the gray matter are **dorsal**, **lateral**, and **ventral columns** of **white matter** made up of ascending and descending myelinated nerve fibers communicating with other levels in the spinal cord and with nerve centers in the brain.

The cell bodies of sensory neurons entering the cord are located in a fusiform expansion of each dorsal root, called the

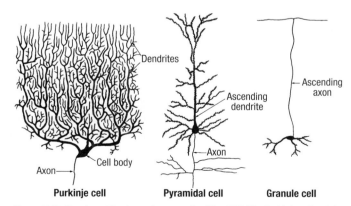

Figure 8.12 Drawing of the form of some cells of the CNS. The Purkinje cells of the cerebellum have a remarkably elaborate arborization of dendrites. Pyramidal cells of the cerebral cortex have many fewer dendrites, but these are covered by very large numbers of spines (not shown here). The granule cells send an axon outwards to synapse with dendrites of the Purkinje cells.

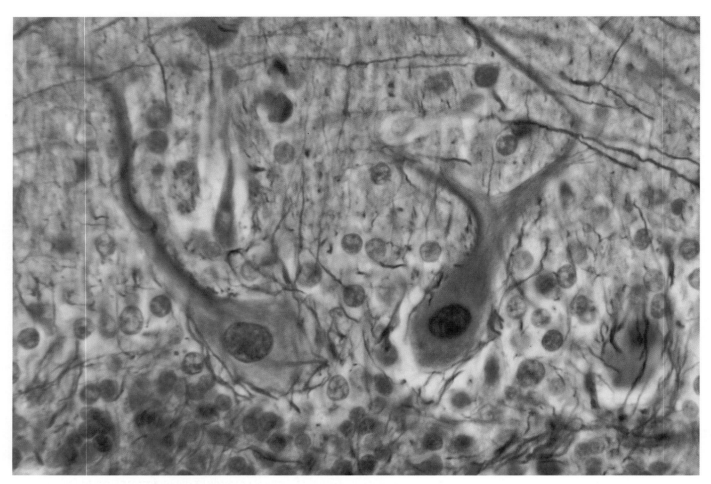

Figure 8.14 Photomicrograph of Purkinje cells of the cerebellum. Only the cell bodies and the initial portion of their dendrites are visible. The elaborate branching of the dendrites is beyond the scope of this field. The closely crowded nuclei at the bottom of the figure are those of the granular cells.

dorsal root ganglion (Fig. 8.16). These are pseudounipolar neurons with a short axonal process that divides into two myelinated branches: a long **peripheral fiber** that courses to distant sensory endings; and a shorter **central fiber** that enters the spinal cord and synapses with neurons in the dorsal horn of its gray matter. The axons of these latter neurons enter the white matter and form ascending and descending tracts in the dorsal column of the spinal cord.

NEUROGLIA

The several types of supporting cells of the central nervous system are collectively called the **neuroglia**. They outnumber the neurons nine to one, and make up more than half the volume of the brain. While the neurons have been very thoroughly studied because of their important role in processing and transmitting information, these other cells were long considered relatively unimportant, as shown by the demeaning term assigned to them, **neuroglia**, from the Greek meaning 'nerve glue'. They have been the focus of more research in recent years, and have been found to do far more than fill the spaces between neurons. They are active and indispensable participants in the physiology of the CNS.

Neuroglia have been difficult to study owing to the elaborate intermingling of cells and cell processes in the brain. Little more than their nucleus can be seen on routine histological preparations,

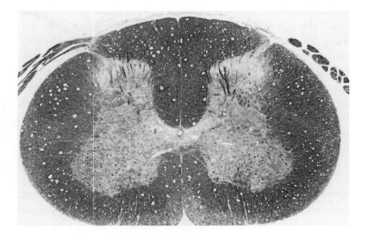

Figure 8.15 Cross-section of the spinal cord stained with Cresyl Violet. Notice the small central canal, the pale-staining, H-shaped gray matter, and the dorsal, ventral, and lateral columns of white matter.

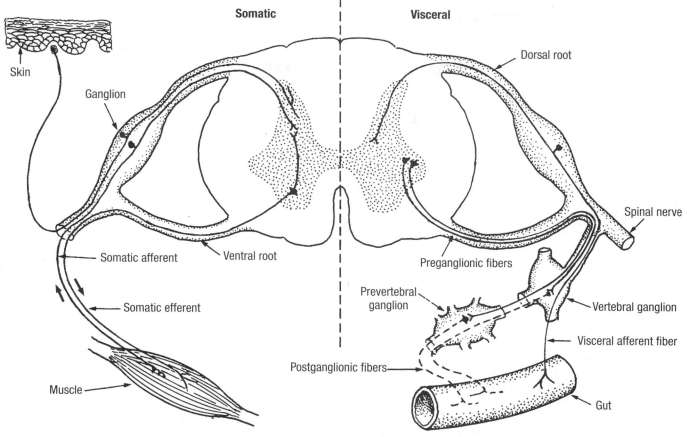

Figure 8.16 Diagram of the spinal cord and dorsal and ventral roots of spinal nerves. The left half of the figure shows somatic nerves, the right half, the visceral nerves. (Redrawn and modified from W. Copenhaver and R. Bunge eds *Bailey's Textbook of Histology*, 16th edn. Williams and Wilkins, Baltimore, 1971.)

and electron microscopy has done little to clarify their relationships to each other and to the neurons. Our knowledge of their shape has depended upon staining techniques, developed in the 1800s that involve their impregnation with silver or gold. There are four types of neuroglia: **astrocytes**, **oligodendrocytes**, **microglia**, and **ependymal cells**.

Astrocytes

Protoplasmic astrocytes, found mainly in the gray matter of the brain, have a stellate form with multiple radiating cell processes that branch repeatedly (Fig. 8.17A). They have an abundant cytoplasm and a spherical nucleus that is larger and paler-staining than that of other neuroglial cells. Some of their processes end in terminal expansions, called **pedicels**, or **vascular feet**, that are applied to the wall of blood vessels. A smaller type of astrocyte is situated close to the cell bodies of neurons as a form of satellite cell. Still others, described as velate astrocytes, have thin veil-like processes that extend between neurons or surround bundles of axons.

Fibrous astrocytes are common in the white matter, but may also occur in the perivascular gray matter. They have an ovoid euchromatic nucleus, pale-staining cytoplasm and long thin

processes that branch less frequently than those of the protoplasmic astrocytes (Fig. 8.17B). On electron micrographs, the cytoplasm of both types of astrocyte has relatively few organelles,

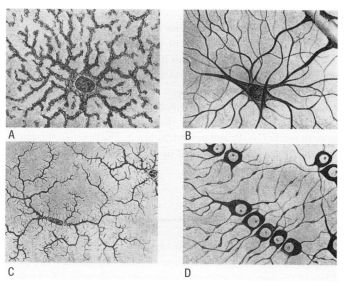

Figure 8.17 Shapes of neuroglial cells of the CNS. (A) Protoplasmic astrocyte. (B) Fibrous astrocyte. (C) Microglia. (D) Oligodendrocyte.

but contains conspicuous bundles of filaments. These are smaller (8 nm) and more closely aggregated than the intermediate filaments of somatic cells. They are also chemically distinct, consisting of **glial fibrillar acidic protein**.

Astrocyte processes associated with synapses are believed to help maintain the neuron's signaling capacity. Potassium ions and glutamate are released at active synapses and, if not quickly removed, they can interfere with subsequent neuronal activity. An important function of astrocytes is the removal of glutamate from the synaptic environment, and its conversion to glutamine, which is returned to the neuron. The astrocytes also contain reserves of glycogen from which glucose can be liberated to contribute to the energy metabolism of the cerebral cortex. Although astrocytes do not respond to electrical stimulation by generation of an action potential, their plasma membrane contains receptors for a number of neurotransmitters. Their long, radiating processes contact other astrocytes via gap junctions, raising the possibility that they may have communication skills that complement those of the neurons.

Oligodendrocytes

Oligodendrocytes are smaller than astrocytes and have fewer processes, which are not highly branched (Fig. 8.17D). Their small, round nucleus stains deeply. On electron micrographs, the relatively dense cytoplasm contains numerous mitochondria and is rich in rER. Microtubules are abundant in the cell body and in the processes. Oligodendrocytes are found close to the perikarya of neurons in the gray matter. In the white matter they are arranged in rows between bundles of axons and are called **fascicular oligodendrocytes**. These are analogous to the Schwann cells of the PNS. Each internodal segment of the myelin sheath in the CNS is formed of apposed membranes of an oligodendroglia cell process wrapped spirally around an axon. Unlike Schwann cells, which ensheath only one axon, a single oligodendrocyte may form segments of the myelin sheath of multiple parallel axons, perhaps as many as fifty.

The **satellite oligodendrocytes** of the gray matter are closely associated with the cell bodies of neurons. Their smooth unspecialized areas of contact give no hint of interaction, but *in vitro* experiments on isolated neurons and their satellite cells, suggest some metabolic interdependence. In addition to the fascicular oligodendrocyte's primary function of myelinization, both kinds of oligodendrocytes produce the neurotrophic factors **nerve growth factor** (NGF) and **neurotrophin-3**. The possible therapeutic use of these in the treatment of Alzheimer's disease and spinal cord injuries is being explored.

Microglia

The **microglia** are small cells of highly variable form distributed throughout the CNS. Their shape depends upon their location. They have short tortuous processes with small spine-like projections. Where they have to fit among the elongated processes of neurons, they may be long and slender. They have a dense ovoid or elongate nucleus and scant cytoplasm. What function, if any, they have in the resting state is unknown, but they become highly motile and are attracted to areas of brain injury, where they become highly phagocytic, engulfing and degrading the residues of damaged neurons, myelin and other particulate material. They are the macrophages of the CNS.

Neutrophils and monocytes that respond to tissue damage and infection elsewhere in the body, are largely excluded from the CNS by a blood–brain barrier (see below) and their role is filled by the microglia. In addition to their garbage collector function, the microglia respond to disturbances of their environment by increased expression of major histocompatibility complexes in their membrane. As in macrophages, these are believed to play a role in antigen presentation. The microglia are probably a major component of the brain's immune system. In carrying out their protective function, however, they produce cytokines and toxic molecules such as superoxide anions, hydroxyl radicals, and hydrogen peroxide, which can damage neurons and oligodendroglia. These products, in excess, may contribute to the generation of amyloid plaques seen in the brain of patients with Alzheimer's disease.

Ependymal cells

The cerebral ventricles are cavities on the medial side of the cerebral hemispheres of the brain, on either side of the midline. These, and a central canal of the spinal cord, are lined by a ciliated cuboidal epithelium made up of **ependymal cells**. Unlike the cells of other epithelia, the ependymal cells have, at their base, one or more processes, like those of fibrous astrocytes, which extend into the underlying gray matter. The beating of the cilia on this epithelium probably contributes to the circulation of the cerebrospinal fluid. If its cells have other functions, they are yet to be discovered.

Repair in the CNS

Nerve cells of adults have long been thought to be incapable of division. Neuroglia retain the ability to divide throughout life and are active in repair of the CNS after injury, proliferating and filling the defects left by the degeneration of neurons. Until recently, restoration of brain function by generation of new neurons was thought to be beyond the realm of possibility. This pessimistic view has now been altered by preliminary trials, in which embryonic stem cells, cultivated *in vitro*, have been implanted in the brain of patients with Parkinson's disease with some evidence of amelioration of their symptoms. At present, the only source of adequate numbers of such stem cells is from excess early embryos obtained in fertility clinics, and there are religious and legal obstacles to their use. However, it has been found, in animal experiments, that stem cells exist in certain regions of the adult brain and can be isolated and grown *in vitro*. Under the right conditions, these cells, as well as stem cells from the bone marrow, can differentiate into either neurons or oligodendroglia. This raises the hope that when the right growth factors and other culture conditions are found to induce their differentiation into the desired cell type, transplantation of cultured neurons to the brain of patients may become more feasible. Whether these neurons will establish the right connections to restore lost neural functions remains to be seen.

AUTONOMIC NERVOUS SYSTEM

The part of the nervous system concerned with reception of sensory impulses and the voluntary generation of motor responses is known as the **somatic nervous system**. Other activities, such as heartbeat, smooth-muscle contraction, and secretion of exocrine glands are regulated automatically and are not subject to voluntary control. These activities are controlled by the **autonomic nervous system (ANS)**. As the name implies, its actions are largely independent, but they are influenced to no small degree by conscious processes of the brain, and vice versa. The system has two divisions, the **sympathetic** and the **parasympathetic** divisions. In the somatic nervous system, a motor neuron acts directly on its effector organ, but in the ANS, two motor neurons in series are involved. The first is located in a center in the brain stem or spinal gray matter, whereas the second is in a ganglion outside of the CNS.

Sympathetic division

The **sympathetic (thoracolumbar) division** of the ANS includes a chain of interconnected ganglia on either side of the vertebral column. As explained earlier, a **ganglion** is an encapsulated collection of nerve cell bodies outside of the CNS. The cell bodies of the preganglionic neurons are situated in the gray matter of the **thoracic** and **lumbar** regions of the spinal cord. Their axons exit the cord through the ventral roots, but soon leave them to enter one of the **paravertebral ganglia** that are interconnected in a chain running parallel to the vertebral column near the junctions of the dorsal and ventral roots (Fig. 8.16). Each preganglionic neuron synapses with multiple postganglionic neurons in the ganglion of the same segment or in ganglia of neighboring segments. The axons of the postganglionic neurons return to spinal nerves and are distributed in peripheral nerves to blood vessels (**vasomotor fibers**), sweat glands (**sudomotor fibers**), hair follicles (**pilomotor fibers**), salivary glands, heart, and lungs. Some preganglionic fibers pass through the paravertebral ganglia without synapsing and travel in **splanchnic nerves** to synapse on nerve cell bodies in the **celiac ganglion** and **mesenteric ganglia** in the abdominal cavity. Postganglionic fibers from these ganglia innervate the gastrointestinal tract, kidneys, pancreas, liver, bladder, and external genitalia. Thus, sympathetic trunks and their ganglia are the avenues of outflow of impulses from the spinal cord to the viscera. The principal neurotransmitter of the sympathetic system is **norepinephrine**.

Parasympathetic division

In the **parasympathetic (craniosacral) division** of the autonomic nervous system, the cell bodies of the preganglionic neurons are located in the brain stem and in several sacral segments of the spinal cord. Their axons do not synapse in the paravertebral ganglia, but extend for long distances to synapse with postganglionic neurons in small ganglia near, or within, their visceral targets. The preganglionic fibers of the cranial component of this division emerge from the CNS in the oculomotor, facial, glossopharyngeal, and vagus nerves, and synapse with postganglionic neurons in the **ciliary, pterygopalatine, submandibular**, and **otic ganglia**. Those of sacral component, derived from the second to the fourth sacral segments, leave via the ventral roots and sacral nerves, and synapse with postganglionic neurons in ganglia associated with the pelvic viscera. In the enteric component that controls the activity of the gastrointestinal tract, pancreas, and gall bladder, the neurons are located in complex networks of ganglia and interconnecting nerves in the walls of these target organs. The two major networks are the **myenteric plexus** (Auerbach's plexus), between the longitudinal and circular layers of smooth muscle in the gut, and the **submucosal plexus** (Meissner's plexus) between the mucosa and the circular muscle layer. The chemical mediator of the parasympathetic division of the autonomic nervous system is **acetylcholine**.

MENINGES

The **meninges** are three layers of connective tissue covering the brain and spinal cord. The outermost is the **dura mater**, the innermost is the **pia mater**, and an intermediate layer between these is the **arachnoid** (Fig. 8.18).

The **dura mater** consists of dense connective tissue adhering rather loosely to the inner aspect of the skull. It was long thought that there was a 'subdural space' between the dura and the underlying arachnoid, but in well preserved specimens examined with an electron microscope, the two are in contact. At their junction, the

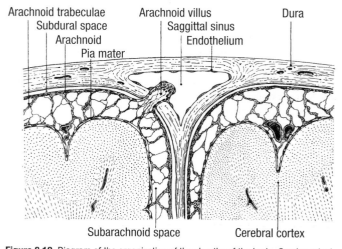

Figure 8.18 Diagram of the organization of the sheaths of the brain. Cerebrospinal fluid, formed in the choroid plexus, circulates in the subarachnoid space and is absorbed into the venous sinuses through the arachnoid villi. Only one is shown projecting into the saggital sinus. The subdural space shown here is now thought to be an artifact. (Reproduced from L.H. Weed *Am J Anat* 1922; 31:191.)

inner layer of the dura is evidently a rather weak plane of cleavage in the meninges and extravasation of blood can create a space where none normally exists. Therefore, the 'subdural hematoma' that often follows head injuries is not beneath the dura, as the name implies, but is an accumulation of blood within a cleft in the dura.

The dura enclosing the spinal cord is separated from the surrounding periosteum by an **epidural space**, which contains very loose connective tissue, a plexus of thin-walled veins, and some adipose cells. The internal and external surfaces of the spinal dura are covered by simple squamous epithelium. The inner epithelium is connected to the sides of the spinal cord by a series of slender **denticulate ligaments**. These attachments help to support the spinal cord.

The **arachnoid** component of the meninges consists of an outer layer of closely apposed cells in contact with the dura, and an inner portion made up of long arachnoid trabecular cells that traverse the **subarachnoid space** to connect the arachnoid to the underlying **pia mater** (Fig. 8.18). This space contains the cerebrospinal fluid. The arachnoid is devoid of blood vessels.

The **pia mater** is a layer of very loose connective tissue, covered, on the side towards the arachnoid, by a thin single layer of squamous cells. Fine elastic and collagenous fibers are interposed between this layer of squamous cells and the underlying neural tissue. The pia mater contains many blood vessels. Macrophages, small groups of lymphocytes, and scattered mast cells, are found among the pia cells and along the blood vessels. The arachnoid and the pia mater are so closely associated that they are often considered to be a single layer, the **pia–arachnoid**.

Questions

1 A typical bipolar neuron has how many axons?
 a one
 b two
 c one afferent and one efferent axon
 d it depends on the number of collateral branches
 e one for each node of Ranvier

2 Choroid plexus is formed where which of the following come into contact?
 a pia and ependyma
 b pia and arachnoid
 c dura and arachnoid
 d arachnoid and ependyma
 e dura and ependyma

3 At axon terminals, neurotransmitters are stored in
 a mitochondria
 b dendritic spines
 c endosomes
 d synaptic vesicles
 e synaptic clefts

4 Nerve cells that make up the majority of cell types within the central nervous system are called
 a motor neurons
 b sensory neurons
 c cholinergic neurons
 d autonomic neurons
 e interneurons

5 With respect to transmission of electrical signals (action potential), the principle conductile portion of a neuron is the
 a synaptic bouton
 b axon
 c dendritic tree
 d axon hillock
 e synaptic vesicle

6 Multipolar neurons are not found in which of the following
 a dorsal root ganglia
 b sympathetic ganglia
 c parasympathetic ganglia
 d enteric ganglia
 e all of the above contain multipolar neurons

7 The so-called Nissl bodies of neurons are composed of aggregations of a large amount of
 a mitochondria
 b Golgi bodies
 c neurotransmitter vesicles
 d rough endoplasmic reticulum
 e myelin

8 Among neurons, a large surface area for synaptic input is provided by the highly branched structure of the
 a Nissl substance
 b axon hillock
 c dendrites
 d axon
 e cell body

9 The space between two adjacent segments of the myelin sheath along an axon is known as the
 a major dense line
 b intraperiod line
 c node of Ranvier
 d cleft of Schmidt–Lantermann
 e mesaxon

10 Along the course of a peripheral nerve fiber, nodes of Ranvier represent spaces between successive
 a oligodendrocytes
 b astrocytes
 c Schwann cells
 d microglia
 e ependymal cells

11 A nerve impulse travels away from the nerve cell body along what cell process?

12 Protoplasmic astrocytes are located in what part of the central nervous system?

13 A unipolar neuron is a misnomer and is more accurately called what?

14 What cell type in the CNS is part of the mononuclear–phagocytic system?

15 Functionally, what type of neuron has its cell body in the dorsal root ganglia?

16 Where in the neuron are neurotransmitters stored?

17 What is the name of the structure that has extrafusal muscle fibers and acts as a transducer in muscle?

18 What is the most rapid form of conduction along an axon?

19 What is the chemical mediator in the parasympathetic division of the autonomic nervous system?

20 What is the name for the group of supportive cells found in the CNS?

Circulatory System

The **circulatory system** (or vascular system) distributes oxygen to the tissues of the body and collects carbon dioxide and other waste products of metabolism from them for elimination by the lungs or kidneys. It consists of a muscular pump, the **heart**, and two separate systems of blood vessels: the **pulmonary circulation**, carrying blood to and from the lungs, and the **systemic circulation**, distributing blood to all other tissues and organs of the body. In both systems, the blood pumped from the heart passes through **arteries** of diminishing caliber to networks of thin-walled capillaries, and then back to the heart through **veins** of increasing caliber.

The initial velocity of blood flowing from the heart into the **aorta** and **pulmonary artery** is about 33 cm/s, but the rate of flow gradually decreases as the total cross-sectional area of the vascular system is increased by repeated branching of the arteries. A further increase in the total cross-sectional area of the system occurs rather abruptly at the level of the arterioles and capillaries, resulting in a decrease in rate of flow to about 0.3 cm/s. This slow flow provides ample time for the exchange of metabolites between the blood and the tissues. The extensive capillary networks of the body present a total surface area of about 700 m² for this exchange. At any given moment, only about 5% of the blood volume is in the capillaries, and 95% is on its way to or from them.

HEART

The heart is the pump of the circulatory system. It consists of four chambers: the **left atrium** discharging its content into the **left ventricle**, and **right atrium** emptying into the **right ventricle** (Fig. 9.1). The right atrium receives venous blood returning from the body and expels it into the right ventricle, which pumps it to the lungs through the blood vessels of the **pulmonary circulation**.

The left atrium receives oxygenated blood returning from the lungs and expels it into the left ventricle, which pumps it through blood vessels throughout the **systemic circulation** (Fig. 9.1). Backflow from the aorta and pulmonary artery, between beats, is prevented by cup-shaped tricuspid valves at their base. Similarly, backflow of blood from the ventricles into the atria is prevented by a **tricuspid valve** in the right atrioventricular canal and a **bicuspid valve** in the left atrioventricular canal. The valve leaflets are thin sheets of dense connective tissue covered by squamous endothelium.

The wall of the heart is made up of three layers: the **endocardium**, the **myocardium**, and **epicardium**. The endocardium is a lining layer of squamous endothelium, underlain by a thin layer of loose connective tissue. Its denser, deep portion is continuous with connective tissue that surrounds bundles of cardiac muscle fibers in the wall of the heart. The myocardium is made up of several layers of cardiac muscle cells of differing orientation. The fibers of the atria converge upon rings of dense connective tissue around the origins of the aorta and the pulmonary artery. Those of the ventricles insert into similar rings of connective tissue encircling the two atrioventricular orifices. These four rings, called the **annuli fibrosi**, together with the **septum membranaceum** in the upper part of the interventricular septum, constitute the **cardiac skeleton**.

A very common cause of heart disease is **rheumatic fever**, which is a complication of streptococcal infections of the pharynx, usually in childhood. Inflammatory lesions of the endocardium cause thickening and adhesion of the valves, with consequent narrowing of the path of outflow of the blood, and backflow between beats, as a result of failure of the valves to close completely. Surgical repair or replacement of the aortic and pulmonary valves is now possible.

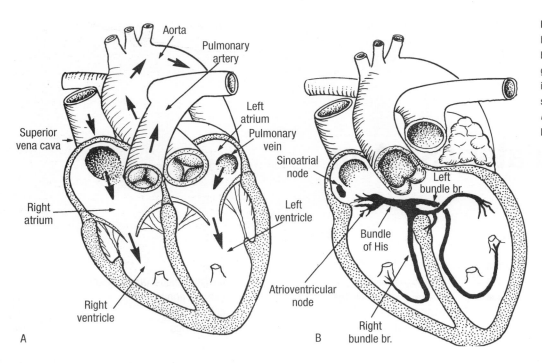

Figure 9.1 (A) Diagram of the posterior half of the heart, showing the path of the blood through the chambers and into the great vessels. (B) Diagram of the impulse-generating and conducting system. (Redrawn from L.C. Junquiera *et al. Basic Histology*, Appleton and Lange, Norwalk, Connecticut, 1992.)

Conducting system

For the heart to pump efficiently, the contraction of the atria, to expel blood into the ventricles, must occur before contraction of the ventricles. However, right and left ventricles must then contract synchronously. Coordination of these events of the cardiac cycle depends on an impulse-conducting system made up of modified cardiac muscle fibers that are specialized for generation and conduction of impulses to activate the myocardium of the atria and ventricles in the correct sequence. The **pacemaker** of the heart is the **sinoatrial node**, located near the junction of the superior vena cava with the right atrium (Fig. 9.1). It consists of muscle fibers that are more slender, and contain fewer myofibrils, than the force-generating muscle fibers of the atrium. The modified muscle fibers of the node undergo spontaneous rhythmic depolarization of their membrane, generating impulses that travel through the myocardium activating the working muscle cells. The node is enclosed in connective tissue and innervated by both divisions of the autonomic nervous system.

Although rhythmic contraction of the heart is independent of the central nervous system (CNS), the heartbeat can be accelerated by nerves of the sympathetic nervous system or slowed by parasympathetic nerves. The electrical depolarization of fibers in the sinoatrial node spreads over **internodal tracts** of conducting **Purkinje fibers** to the **atrioventricular node**, located beneath the endocardium of the interatrial septum. The microscopic structure of this node is similar to that of the sinoatrial node. From there, the wave of depolarization is conducted along a tract known as the **atrioventricular bundle of His**, which penetrates the ring of fibrous tissue around the atrioventricular orifice and divides into **right** and **left bundle branches** that course down either side of the interventricular septum. The conducting fibers are larger than ventricular muscle fibers and have a few myofibrils around a core

of cytoplasm containing the nucleus and a large amount of glycogen. At the apex of the heart, the bundle branches turn back onto the lateral wall of the ventricles and communicate with many working cardiac muscle cells via gap junctions. This arrangement of conducting fibers ensures that the apex of the ventricles begin to contract before their base and facilitates the ejection of blood from the ventricles into the aorta and pulmonary artery.

> Coronary artery disease may result in damage to the atrioventricular bundle of His resulting in **heart block**, a condition in which the coordination of contractions of the atria and ventricles is lost and these chambers contract more-or-less independently and, therefore, inefficiently.

ARTERIES

The walls of the larger blood vessels are made up of three layers: (1) a lining layer, the **tunica intima**, consisting of an endothelium of squamous cells, supported by a thin underlying layer of areolar connective tissue; (2) an intermediate layer, the **tunica media**, composed of circumferentially oriented smooth muscle cells; and (3) an outer layer, the **tunica adventitia**, made up of longitudinally oriented fibroblasts and associated collagen fibers (Figs. 9.2, 9.3). The thickness of the media and adventitia varies greatly in arteries of different size.

At the boundary between the intima and media, there is a fenestrated sheet of elastin called the **internal elastic lamina** (**elastica interna**). This is especially prominent in arteries of medium caliber (Fig. 9.3). A thinner **external elastic lamina** (**elastica externa**) is also identifiable between the media and the adventitia of many arteries. Arteries are classified as: (1) **elastic arteries** (large

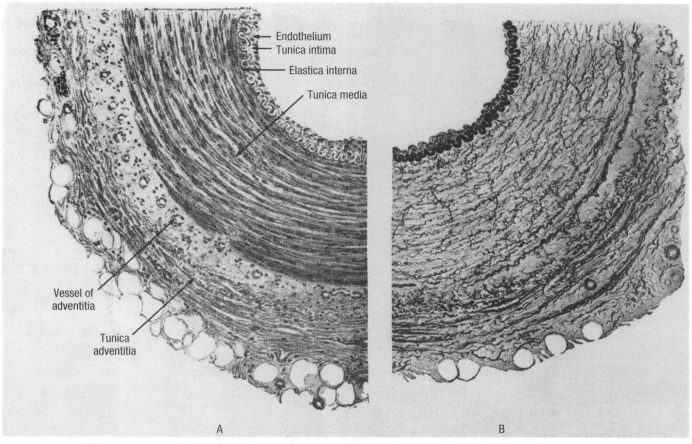

Figure 9.2 (A) Drawing of the wall of a medium-sized artery, in cross-section, showing the tunica intima, tunica media and tunica adventitia. (B) The same vessel stained with orcein to reveal the elastin components of the wall.

conducting arteries); (2) **muscular arteries** (distributing arteries); (3) **arterioles** (small arteries that precede the capillaries). Their identification is based upon their diameter, the thickness of their wall, and the dominant component of the tunica media. This classification is useful, but there is a continuous gradation in the character of the arterial wall from the largest to the smallest, and

for an artery in a transitional region between categories, its assignment to one or the other is rather arbitrary.

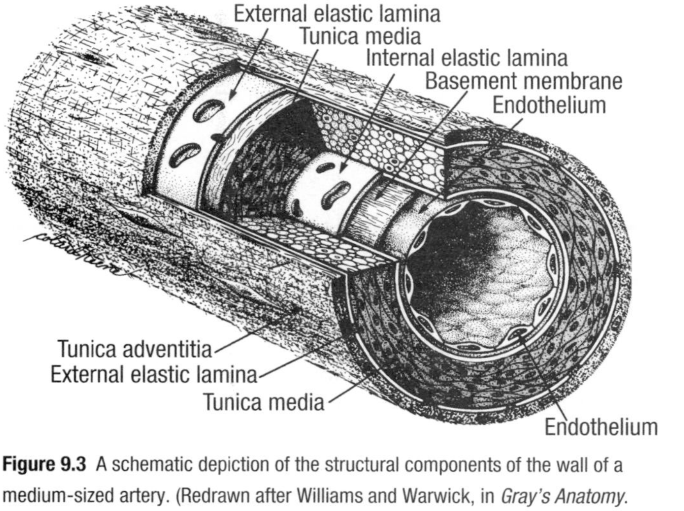

Elastic arteries

The large **elastic arteries** include the pulmonary artery, emerging from the right ventricle, the **aorta**, from the left ventricle, and their primary branches. The tunica intima consists of an endothelium and a layer of fibroblasts and longitudinally oriented collagen fibers between the endothelium and the elastica interna. A conspicuous feature of the endothelial cells of elastic arteries is the presence in their cytoplasm of elongate, membrane-bounded granules, called **Weibel–Palade bodies**. These are sites of storage of **von Willebrandt factor**, a glycoprotein that is synthesized by all endothelial cells, but is stored in visible inclusions only in the endothelium of the large elastic arteries. After an injury, it is released into the blood to participate in the formation of a blood clot to limit blood loss.

In large elastic arteries viewed in cross-section, the most conspicuous feature of their tunica media is the presence of a large number of concentric laminae of elastin (Fig. 9.4). As a result of contraction and shrinkage of the wall during specimen preparation, the elastic laminae often have a wavy outline. The media can be thought of as being made up of units consisting of two

Figure 9.3 A schematic depiction of the structural components of the wall of a medium-sized artery. (Redrawn after Williams and Warwick, in *Gray's Anatomy*. 38th British edn. W.B. Saunders, Philadelphia, 1980.)

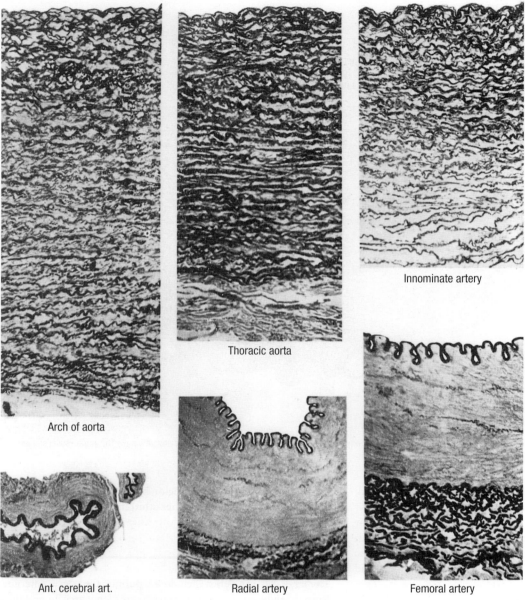

Figure 9.4 Photomicrographs of the wall of elastic arteries (above) and large muscular arteries (below), illustrating the differences in thickness of the walls, and differences in amount of elastin, which appears as black wavy lines in these preparations. (Reproduced from E.V. Cowdry *Textbook of Histology*, Lea and Febiger, Philadelphia, 1950.)

Innominate artery

Thoracic aorta

Arch of aorta

Ant. cerebral art.

Radial artery

Femoral artery

fenestrated elastic laminae separated by a single layer of circumferentially oriented smooth muscle cells. In the human aorta there are 50 to 75 such units. Internal and external elastic laminae cannot be distinguished from the many other laminae. Between the smooth muscle and the flanking elastic laminae of these units, there are circumferentially oriented collagen fibers in an extracellular matrix, rich in proteoglycans. Owing to the unusual abundance of elastin in elastic arteries, smooth muscle makes up a smaller fraction of the media than it does in medium-sized arteries. The relatively thin adventitia contains many longitudinally oriented fibroblasts and collagen fibers.

Diffusion of metabolites from the lumen of these large arteries is inadequate to meet the needs of their very thick tunica media. This deficiency is overcome by small blood vessels in the adventitia, called **vasa vasorum**, from which capillary branches penetrate

for a short distance into the media. Such vessels are not found in the adventitia of smaller arteries.

Muscular arteries

Muscular arteries make up the greater part of the arterial tree, distal to the elastic arteries. Their intima consists of the endothelium and a thin subendothelial layer of areolar connective tissue. There is a conspicuous **internal elastic lamina**. In vessels that have contracted upon immersion in fixative, it has a scalloped or folded appearance (Fig. 9.5). The tunica media consists of several layers of circumferentially oriented smooth muscle fibers and associated reticular fibers. There are no elastic laminae within the media, but varying numbers of slender elastic fibers are found between the

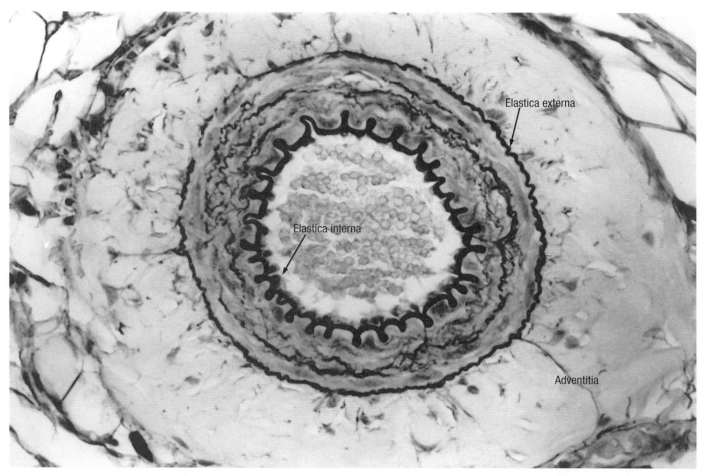

Figure 9.5 Photomicrograph of a small muscular artery, stained for elastin. The elastica interna, the media, and an unusually thick adventitia are clearly shown.

layers of smooth muscle. An **external elastic lamina** is present only in the largest muscular arteries. The tunica adventitia consists of scattered fibroblasts and longitudinally oriented collagen fibers that merge with those of the surrounding connective tissue.

The thickness of the media in muscular arteries varies according to the blood pressure in the system at that level; for example, the coronary arteries of the heart, which are subjected to relatively high blood pressure, have thicker tunica media than other muscular arteries. On the other hand, in arteries of the pulmonary circulation, where the blood pressure is considerably lower, the tunica media is relatively thin. The small muscular arteries and arterioles are a physiologically important segment of the circulation for they provide the major part of the peripheral resistance to blood flow that determines the blood pressure.

Arterioles

Arterioles range in diameter from $200\,\mu m$ to $40\,\mu m$. The tunica intima includes the endothelium and a very thin subendothelial layer of reticular fibers. A very thin, fenestrated elastica interna is present in the larger arterioles, but absent in smaller arterioles. The tunica media consists of one or two layers of circular smooth muscle cells. In the smallest arterioles, there may be a single layer in

which the individual smooth muscle cells are long enough to completely encircle the tube of endothelium (Fig. 9.6). Collagen fibers and occasional fibroblasts form a thin adventitia. In the transition from **terminal arterioles** to capillaries, the smooth muscle layer becomes discontinuous. Single smooth muscle cells, are spaced some distance apart, and completely encircle the tube of endothelium. Such vessels, are often referred to as **metarterioles**. Where metarterioles are continuous with capillaries, the encircling smooth muscle cells act as a **precapillary sphincter**. Their contraction slows or stops flow through a region of the capillary network. Blood may flow, instead, directly to venules through lateral branches somewhat larger than capillaries, that bypass the capillary, bed. Whether these precapillary sphincters remain open or closed depends on the metabolic needs of the local tissues.

Physiology of arteries

The intermittent contraction of the heart results in a pulsatile flow of blood in the large **elastic arteries**. The abundant elastic tissue in their walls enables them to expand slightly during contraction of the heart (**systole**) storing some of the force of the heartbeat. The potential energy so gained is dissipated in the elastic recoil of their wall in the interval between heartbeats (**diastole**). Their recoil thus

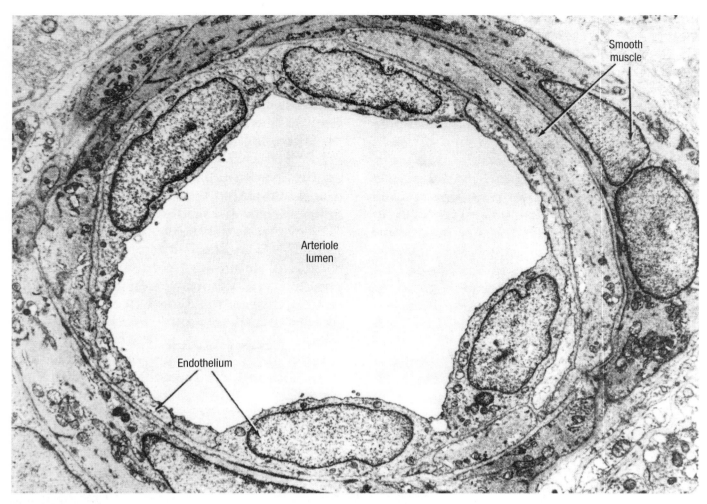

Figure 9.6 An electron micrograph of a small arteriole. Note the single layer of smooth muscle cells around the endothelium.

serves as an auxiliary pump, forcing the blood onwards when no force is being exerted by the heart. This ensures a continuous flow through the capillaries despite the intermittent contraction of the heart.

Impulses continuously generated in the **vasomotor center** of the brain travel via the spinal cord to a chain of sympathetic ganglia, and then via **vasomotor nerves** to the arteries. As a result of these nerve impulses, smooth muscle in the media of medium-sized and small arteries is maintained in a state of partial contraction called **vasomotor tone**. The nerves to the blood vessel walls include both **vasoconstrictor** and **vasodilator** nerve fibers that act upon smooth muscle of the vessels to decrease or increase their caliber. The change in diameter of small arteries can be quite striking (Fig. 9.7). Because the arteries offer the principal resistance to blood flow, a generalized vasoconstriction results in a marked rise in the blood pressure. A change in the caliber of a single distributing artery increases or decreases the flow to the tissue or organ served by that vessel.

Products of tissue injury may also cause local vasoconstriction that limits blood loss. Conversely, if an area of tissue is deprived of oxygen, lactic acid accumulates, causing relaxation of smooth muscle in the walls of small arteries, resulting in vasodilation and consequent increase in blood flow to the area. This so-called

reactive hyperemia is independent of the nervous system and serves to correct any local deficit of oxygen or other metabolites.

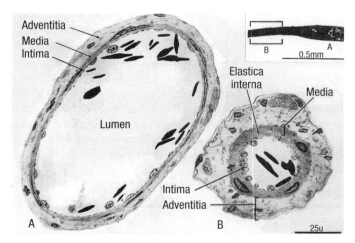

Figure 9.7 A dramatic illustration of vasoconstriction. A microdroplet of norepinephrin was applied to a living vessel, causing vasoconstriction of the segment in brackets in the inset (above). The vessel was then fixed and sectioned. (A) and (B) are cross-sections of the same vessel, less than 2 mm apart. (Reproduced from P.C. Phelps and J.H. Luft *Am J Anat* 1969; 125:399.)

Changes in arteries with age

The walls of large arteries normally continue to undergo developmental changes from birth to age 25 years. There is progressive thickening of the wall of elastic arteries, with development of increasing numbers of elastic lamellae. In muscular arteries, there is an increase in the thickness of the media. From middle age onwards, there is a slow, progressive thickening of the tunica intima of the arteries. There is an increase in collagen fibers and a migration of some smooth muscle cells from the media into the intima. These tend to accumulate droplets of lipid rich in cholesterol esters. These generalized changes in arteries with advancing age are described as **arteriosclerosis**. They are not to be confused with the pathological process of **atherosclerosis**, in which patchy accumulations of lipid-filled smooth muscle cells, macrophages, and collagen fibers form elevated plaques in the intima. Platelets may adhere to the rough surface of the plaques, initiating the formation of a blood clot that occludes the lumen. When this occurs in a coronary artery it causes a 'heart attack' (**myocardial infarction**). When it occurs in an artery in the brain, it causes a 'stroke' (**cerebral thrombosis**).

CAPILLARIES

Capillaries are thin-walled, endothelium-lined tubes of uniform diameter that branch repeatedly to form extensive networks throughout the tissues of the body. Their diameter of 8–11 μm is just large enough to permit unimpeded passage of blood cells. A capillary forming one mesh of the network is only about 1 μm in length, but the total length of the capillaries in the body is estimated to be 4 000 miles, or more. The capillary wall has an extremely thin endothelium with a basal lamina supported by a loose network of reticular fibers (Fig. 9.8). There is no tunica media or adventitia. The endothelial cells are elongated in the direction of blood flow. The nucleus is flattened and thus appears elliptical in cross-sections. The thicker region of the endothelial cell containing the nucleus bulges slightly into the lumen, while the attenuated peripheral portion of the cell is so thin that the adlumenal and ablumenal membranes are separated by a layer of cytoplasm only 0.2–0.4 μm in thickness. The cells have few organelles. The lumenal surface of the endothelium is smooth, but the thin margins of adjacent cells may overlap, with the free edge

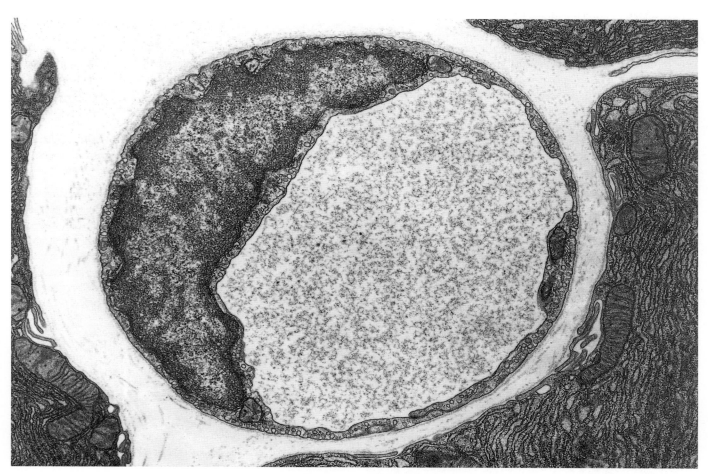

Figure 9.8 A low-power electron micrograph of a capillary. In this example, the entire circumference of the vessel is made up of a single endothelial cell. (Micrograph courtesy of R. Bolender.)

of the uppermost cell projecting a short distance into the lumen. At cell junctions, there are no zonulae adherentes or desmosomes, but freeze-fracture preparations reveal, in the opposing membranes, a few strands that resemble those of the zonula occludens of other epithelia. However, there are discontinuities in these occluding junctions through which a small amount of fluid may be able to pass.

Most capillaries are similar in appearance in histological sections, but with the electron microscope, three types can be distinguished: **continuous capillaries** (somatic capillaries), **fenestrated capillaries** (visceral capillaries), and **sinusoidal capillaries**. Muscle, brain, connective tissues, and lung have continuous capillaries, in which the endothelium is uninterrupted (Figs. 9.8, 9.9A). The pancreas, endocrine glands, and intestinal villi have fenestrated capillaries. In these, the thin peripheral portions of the endothelial cells are traversed by minute circular **pores**, 60–70 nm in diameter, each closed by a thin **pore diaphragm** (Fig. 9.9B). The pores are uniformly distributed with a center-to-center spacing of about 130 nm in some areas, while pores are absent from other areas (Fig. 9.10).

Spaced at intervals along the outside of continuous capillaries are cells called **pericytes**. These have primary processes deployed longitudinally along the capillary wall, and secondary processes extending around the vessel (Fig. 9.11). The endothelium has a thin basal lamina, and there is a thin external lamina that covers the pericytes and merges with the basal lamina between pericytes. The pericyte cytoplasm contains microtubules in the axis of the processes and bundles of filaments in the peripheral cytoplasm that terminate in densities on the inner aspect of the plasmalemma. It was long speculated that the pericytes might be contractile. This has now been verified by the finding that they contain actin, myosin of smooth muscle type, tropomyosin, and a protein kinase similar to one that is involved in contraction of striated muscle.

Sinusoidal capillaries (sinuses) are found in the liver, bone marrow, and spleen. These vessels, have a larger diameter (30–40 μm), and a variable cross-sectional profile. They have multiple discontinuities in their wall that are much larger than the pores of visceral capillaries, and these are not closed by diaphragms. Blood cells easily cross the wall of the sinuses in the bone marrow and spleen. Macrophages are closely associated with the walls of sinuses in the liver and, in some cases, appear to be included in the endothelium.

Physiology of capillaries

The mechanism of exchange across the capillary wall was a subject of lively debate for a long time. This has now been clarified by studies involving intravascular injection of electron-opaque molecules of known dimensions greater than 10 nm. In continuous capillaries, these particles are rapidly taken up in small, flask-shaped invaginations of the adlumenal membrane, called **caveolae**. They are separated from the membrane by closure of their neck and the small vesicles so-formed move across the cytoplasm and fuse with the ablumenal plasmalemma, discharging their contents into the extravascular space (Fig. 9.9A). Fusion of two or three vesicles with one another may form transient transendothelial channels. The term **transcytosis** has been suggested in order to distinguish this activity from pinocytosis in other cell types, where such vesicles do not cross the cell but import substances for use by the cell.

In fenestrated capillaries, injected macromolecules pass freely through the pores. The capillaries of the renal glomeruli are unique in having an unusually thick basal lamina and pores lacking a diaphragm. Fluid and particulate tracers traverse the wall of these capillaries nearly 100 times more rapidly than in continuous capillaries.

Intravenously injected dyes that readily leave the capillaries of most tissues are retained in the lumen of brain capillaries. The

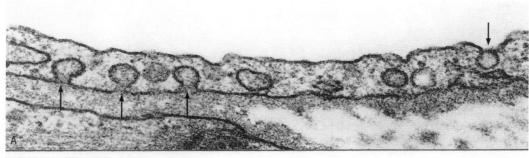

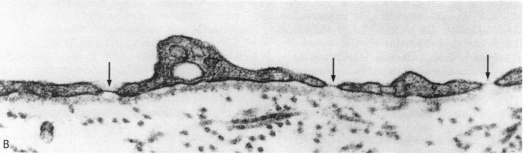

Figure 9.9 Electron micrographs of short segments of endothelium from (A) a continuous capillary, showing transcytosis vesicles, and (B) from a fenestrated capillary. Note the thin diaphragms closing the pores of the fenestrated endothelium (at arrows). (Micrograph courtesy of E. Weihe.)

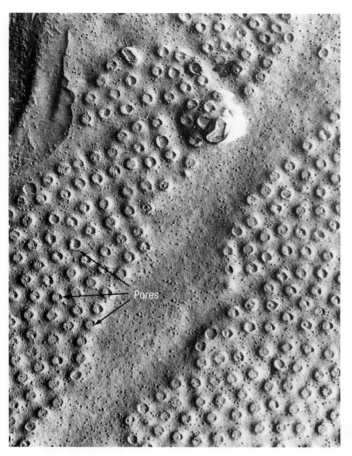

Figure 9.10 Electron micrograph of a freeze-fractured preparation of capillary endothelium, showing areas of closely spaced pores and areas devoid of pores.

endothelial cells of these capillaries are joined by uninterrupted tight junctions. These are believed to be the basis for the so-called **blood–brain barrier**. A blood–ocular barrier and blood–thymus barrier depend on similar properties of their capillaries.

The thin wall of the capillaries permits the exchange of O_2, CO_2, and metabolites between the blood and the tissues. The endothelium has other important functions. It synthesizes and releases **platelet-activating factor** (PAF). After an injury this factor promotes aggregation and adhesion of platelets to form a clot that limits blood loss. It also participates in defense against infections by initiating the migration of neutrophils, monocytes, and T-lymphocytes into the tissues to combat the bacteria. The endothelium also synthesizes and stores an adhesion molecule called **P-selectin**. Upon activation of the endothelium by cytokines diffusing from neighboring infected tissue, P-selectin is incorporated into the adlumenal cell membrane. The extracellular portion of these molecules recognizes, and weakly binds to, an oligosaccharide on the membrane of passing leukocytes, arresting their progress along the capillary. This binding is not strong enough to stop the leukocyte completely, and the flow of blood causes it to roll along the lumenal surface of the activated endothelium until it is stopped by a more stable binding between molecules of an adhesion molecule, **L-selectin**, in its membrane to intercellular adhesion molecules (ICAMs) of the endothelium. The leukocyte is then able to make its way between the endothelial cells and

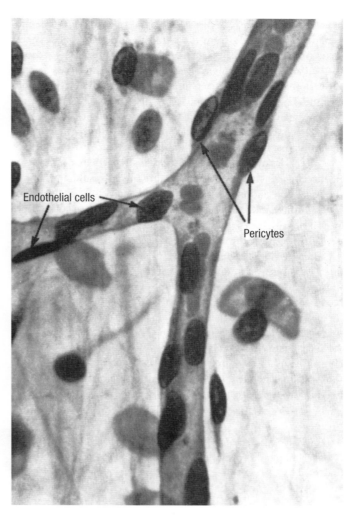

Figure 9.11 Photomicrograph of an unsectioned capillary. The nuclei of the endothelial cells can be distinguished from those of the pericytes.

migrate into the surrounding infected tissue. Thus, leukocyte extravasation is initiated by the endothelium and depends upon successive formation and breakage of bonds between it and the leukocyte membrane.

In humans with the disorder called **leukocyte adhesion deficiency**, there is a genetic defect in the synthesis of an adhesion molecule normally expressed on the surface of T-lymphocytes. In such individuals, binding of these cells to the endothelium is impaired, and they are subject to repeated poorly controlled bacterial infections.

VEINS

The capillary networks are drained by **venules**, thin-walled vessels only slightly larger than capillaries. Their wall consists of endothelium, basal lamina, and occasional pericytes surrounded by a loose network of reticular fibers. Exchange of metabolites between the blood and the tissues continues in the smallest venules, and in cases of acute inflammation these are the principal vessels through which fluid escapes to produce the local swelling (edema). Leukocytes migrating from the blood to attack the bacteria also pass through the wall of small venules. Slightly larger venules (0.2–1.0 mm) have a single layer of smooth muscle cells around the endothelium and collagen fibers are more abundant in the thin adventitia.

The small and medium-sized **veins** have a tunica intima with little or no subendothelial connective tissue. A thin, internal elastic lamina is rarely detectable, and their media consists of one or two layers of smooth muscle and associated reticular and elastic fibers. The principal identifying feature of veins is the thinness of their wall in relation to the diameter of the vessel. The media is much thinner and less compact than that of arteries of comparable size (Fig. 9.12).

A distinctive feature of medium-sized and larger veins is the presence of **valves**. These consist of two semilunar folds of the intima that project into the lumen from opposite sides. Although normally pressed against the lining epithelium by the flow of blood towards the heart, any obstruction of the vessel distal to them causes the free edges of the valve leaflets to come together, preventing retrograde flow of blood. The space between a closed valve cusp and the vessel wall is called the **sinus** of the valve. Just above the arc of attachment of the valve cusps, the vessel wall is thinner. In distended veins, this thinner region bulges slightly, making it possible to locate the site of valves in the intact vessel

with the naked eye. Valves are numerous in veins of the legs, where they are needed to prevent back-flow due to the force of gravity on the column of blood.

Large veins include the vena cava, portal, splenic, external iliac, and azygos veins. These have a thicker subendothelial layer of connective tissue. In general, the media is poorly developed and contains little circular smooth muscle. The relatively thick adventitia of large veins is rich in elastic fibers and longitudinally oriented collagen fibers. Where the vena cava and pulmonary vein enter the heart, strands of cardiac muscle may extend a short distance into their wall.

ARTERIOVENOUS ANASTOMOSES

In many parts of the body, lateral branches of small arteries are directly connected to veins by **arteriovenous anastomoses**. Three morphologically distinct segments are recognizable along their length. The initial segment is similar in structure to the small artery, of which it is a branch. The terminal segment resembles the small vein with which it is confluent. Between these is a contractile intermediate segment with a wall unusually thick for a vessel of its size. It has a subendothelial layer of longitudinally oriented, modified smooth muscle cells. When this segment is contracted, blood flows

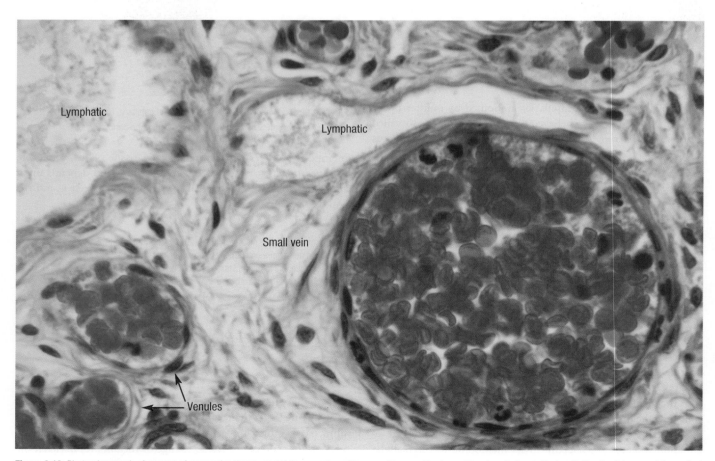

Figure 9.12 Photomicrograph of an area of connective tissue, containing a post-capillary venule, a small vein, and two lymphatic capillaries. Notice the thinness of the wall of the small vein in relation to the diameter of the vessel.

through the capillary bed. When it is relaxed, blood can flow directly from small arteries to small veins, bypassing the local capillaries. Arteriovenous anastomoses therefore play an important role in regulating blood flow to a region. They are abundant in the skin, where they enable the body to conserve heat by diverting the blood away from the superficial network of capillaries.

CAROTID BODIES

The **carotid bodies** are small organs (3×5 mm) at the bifurcation of the common carotid artery that have an important role in regulating respiration, heartbeat, and blood pressure. Although sensory nerves are associated with arteries throughout the body, they are especially abundant in the carotid bodies, which contain chemoreceptors that are sensitive to deficient oxygen, excess carbon dioxide, or elevated hydrogen ion concentration in the blood. The carotid bodies consist of multiple clusters of pale-staining **type I cells (glomus cells)** surrounded by **type II cells (sheath cells)**. These, in turn, are surrounded by connective tissue that contains many fenestrated capillaries. The most distinctive feature of the type I cells is the presence of numerous dense-cored

vesicles (60–200 nm) in their cytoplasm. These contain dopamine and other neurotransmitters. The sheath cells have thin lamellar processes that envelop clusters of two to six type I cells.

The exact location of the chemoreceptor function of the carotid bodies is in dispute, but it is the prevailing view that the membrane of the type I cells contains a heme protein that binds oxygen. In the presence of adequate partial pressures of oxygen, K^+ channels associated with the heme protein are open and Ca channels are closed. In anoxia, the K^+ channels close, Ca channels open, and the type I cells release neurotransmitters that stimulate afferent nerves communicating with regulatory centers in the brain controlling respiration. Similar **aortic bodies**, situated on the arch of the aorta, are assumed to have much the same function as the carotid bodies.

CAROTID SINUS

The **carotid sinus** is a slightly dilated region of the internal carotid artery, where the wall is thinner and contains many sensory nerves. Its nerves are stimulated by stretching and the thinning of the media in this region makes the wall more distensible. The

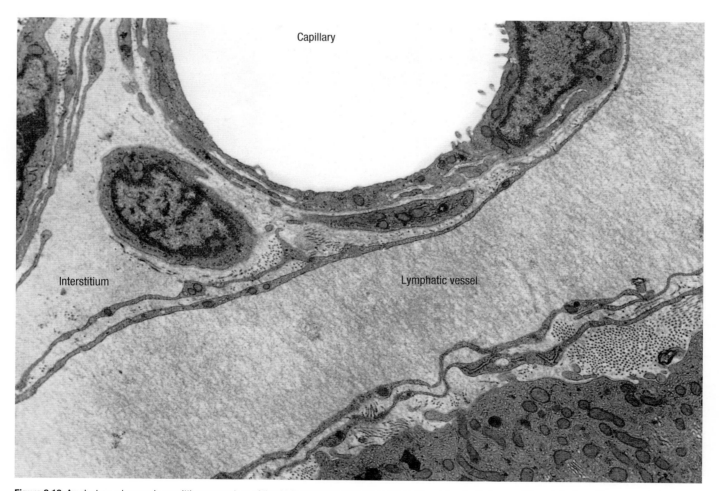

Capillary

Interstitium

Lymphatic vessel

Figure 9.13 An electron micrograph permitting comparison of the thickness of the wall of a blood capillary (above) with the very thin endothelium of the lymphatic capillary (below).

carotid sinus therefore serves as a **baroceptor** that reacts to changes in blood pressure and initiates afferent impulses to centers in the brain. These, in turn, generate efferent impulses that cause vasodilation or vasoconstriction of peripheral arteries and thus maintain blood pressure within normal limits.

LYMPHATICS

In addition to the blood vascular system, the body has a **lymphatic system** made up of very thin-walled vessels that carry excess extracellular fluid from the interstitial compartment back to the blood. Fluid collected in **lymphatic capillaries** in the periphery is conducted through vessels of increasing size to empty into the circulatory system via two main ducts: the **thoracic duct** and the **right lymphatic duct**. These join the blood vascular system at the junction of the subclavian and internal jugular veins. The clear fluid transported in the lymphatics is called **lymph**. Occasional lymphocytes and smaller particulates in the lymph are filtered out in **lymph nodes** that are interposed in the system at intervals along the path of lymph flow. The lymphatic system is not a circulatory system but a drainage system.

Lymphatic capillaries are far more variable in size and in cross-sectional outline than are blood capillaries (Figs.9.13). The endothelium is very thin and there are no tight junctions between cells. A continuous basal lamina is usually absent, but **lymphatic anchoring filaments** extend into the surrounding tissue from small plaques of similar composition on the ablumenal side of the endothelial cells. These filaments help to maintain the patency of these thin-walled vessels. The endothelial cells are not fenestrated. Lymphatic vessels larger than lymphatic capillaries have a somewhat thicker wall, but it is considerably thinner than that of small veins of comparable size. Three layers are not discernible in the wall. At close intervals along their length, the larger lymphatics have bicuspid valves similar to those of veins. Valves are essential to the function of the lymph vascular system which has no pump comparable to the heart. The flow of lymph from the extremities depends, in large measure, on the massaging effect of contraction of the surrounding muscles. The largest lymphatics have some smooth muscle in their wall. They are innervated, and there is visual and cinematographic evidence of their contractility. The presence of smooth muscle may explain lymph flow in organs where there is no muscle-generated movement around them.

The large **lymphatic ducts** have a structure quite like that of veins, but the wall is thinner. It contains smooth muscle fibers oriented both circularly and longitudinally. The adventitia is relatively thin.

Questions

1 The outer surface of the heart consists, in part, of a layer of cells known as
   a endothelial cells
   b mesothelial cells
   c Purkinje cells
   d pericytes
   e myocardial cells

2 The cells found along the outside of the capillary endothelial cells and thought to have contractile function are known as
   a fibroblasts
   b myoblasts
   c smooth muscle cells
   d pericytes
   e mesothelial cells

3 Tight junctions restricting diffusion and pinocytotic vesicles involved in transport are generally characteristics of
   a smooth muscle cells
   b pericytes
   c endothelial cells
   d Purkinje fibers
   e fibroblasts

4 Which of these is the pacemaker of the heart, located in the right atrium close to the entrance of the vena cava?
   a autonomic nerve
   b atrioventricular node
   c atrioventricular bundle of His
   d sinoatrial node
   e Purkinje fibers

5 Layers of smooth muscle cells interposed by fenestrated sheets of elastin characterize the
   a tunica intima
   b tunica media
   c tunica adventitia
   d mesothelium
   e fenestrated capillaries

6 The layer of the blood vessel wall that is characterized by collagen fibers, elastic fibers, macrophages, and longitudinally oriented fibroblasts is known as the
   a tunica intima
   b tunica media
   c tunica adventitia
   d external elastic lamina
   e internal elastic lamina

7 Small vessels needed to maintain the viability of the outer portion of the walls of large veins are called
   a lymph vessels
   b vasa vasorum
   c carotid bodies
   d bundle of His
   e pericytes

8 The annuli fibrosi is a component of
   a myocardium
   b cardiac skeleton
   c pacemaker
   d bundle of His
   e vasa vasorum

9 Prominent inner elastic membranes, often appearing as a wavy structure, as well as an outer elastic membrane are hallmarks of
   a muscular arteries
   b muscular veins
   c elastic arteries
   d large veins
   e capillaries

10 The rhythmic contractions of cardiac muscle are initiated at the
   a sinoatrial node
   b atrioventricular node
   c atrioventricular bundle of His
   d autonomic nervous system
   e Purkinje fibers

11 What type of cell lines blood vessels and the interior of the heart?

12 What layer of the heart wall is most closely apposed to the pericardium?

13 What is the name of the small round cell that lies close to the endothelium of capillaries, contains actin and myosin, and has contractile ability?

14 What is the name of the structure in arteries that lies between the tunica media and the tunica adventitia?

15 What is the name of the modified cardiac muscle cells that contain large amounts of glycogen and participate in the conduction of electrical impulses?

16 What specific specialized physiologic structure is located in the right atrium?

17 What is the innermost layer of a blood vessel called?

18 What is the name for the small blood vessels in the walls of large blood vessels?

19 In general, in large vessels, where are the vasa vasora located?

20 What layer within the wall of a muscular artery is the thickest?

Immune System

IMMUNE SYSTEM DEFINED

The **immune system** consists of four lymphoid organs and a heterogeneous group of motile cell types that are involved in the defense of the body against invasion by bacteria, viruses and other foreign bodies. The organs are the **thymus, lymph nodes, spleen,** and the submucosal **lymphoid nodules** of the gastrointestinal tract. The cells involved are **macrophages, dendritic cells,** and **lymphocytes.** These motile cells are continually patrolling the tissues of the body. Their detection of a foreign body triggers and initiates an **immune response,** in which macrophages and lymphocytes gather at the site in great numbers and cooperate in the destruction of the invaders. Depending upon the nature of the invaders, the response may take one of two courses: (1) a **humoral immune response,** in which B-lymphocytes produce **antibodies** that facilitate phagocytosis and digestion of bacteria by macrophages and neutrophil leukocytes; or (2) a **cell-mediated immune response,** in which T-lymphocytes bind to the surface of parasites, or virus-infected cells, and lyse them by secreting a membrane-disrupting protein and a hydrolytic enzyme.

Types of lymphocytes

As previously stated, there are two principal types of lymphocyte: **B-lymphocytes,** which are generated in the bone marrow; and **T-lymphocytes,** which originate in the thymus. These are similar in appearance (Fig. 10.1) and so cannot be distinguished on the basis of their morphology. However, they can be identified by

using fluorescent antibodies that bind to distinctive proteins on their surface. B-lymphocytes have surface immunoglobulins that can be detected by this immunocytochemical method. There are two or more categories of T-lymphocytes. One of these that serves as a 'helper cell' in the humoral immune response is identified by a surface marker designated CD-4. A second type that is the principal effector cell of the cell-mediated immune response, has a CD-8 surface marker.

To prevent the potentially destructive effects of an immune response on the cells they are intended to protect, the lymphocytes must be able to distinguish the body's own cells (**self**) from foreign

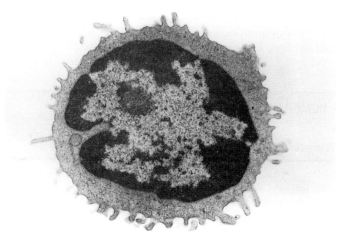

Figure 10.1 Electron micrograph of a typical small lymphocyte. B-lymphocytes can be distinguished from T-lymphocytes only by antibodies to specific proteins on their surface.

cells (**non-self**). An ingenious mechanism has evolved to make this distinction. The plasma membrane of all human cells contains molecules of a large protein called the **major histocompatability complex (MHC)**, which has a configuration and amino acid sequences that are unique to each individual. This complex occurs in two slightly different versions: **MHC-II**, which is largely confined to the surface of macrophages and lymphocytes; and **MHC-1**, which is present on all other cells of the body. As lymphocytes and macrophages migrate through the connective tissues, any cell they may encounter that does not have on its surface the MHC of that individual, will be recognized as foreign. This ability to recognize exogenous proteins, or microorganisms, as non-self is fundamental to the immune responses.

During their development, B-lymphocytes synthesize molecules of **immunoglobulin (IgG)** and display them on their surface. These large Y-shaped molecules (Fig. 10.2) have identical amino acid sequences in the diverging arms of the Y that serve as **recognition sites**, enabling that lymphocyte to bind to any cell surface protein that has a corresponding sequence of amino acids. The B-lymphocyte gene encoding immunoglobulin molecules consists of numerous short segments of DNA at separate sites on the same chromosome, and these must be assembled into a continuous gene for transcription. These segments are combined in many different ways in different B-lymphocytes, and the enzyme involved in their assembly may insert extra coding units of varying length between them. The random nature of this process results in very great variability in the sequence of amino acids on the arms of the immunoglobulin molecules of different B-lymphocytes. Hundreds of thousands of different sequences are represented in the surface immunoglobulins of the B-lymphocyte population. Thus, it is likely that there will be a certain number of B-lymphocytes that have a surface immunoglobulin with an amino acid sequence matching that of a surface protein of an invading microorganism. It is also true, however, that this random rearrangement of gene segments in differentiating B-lymphocytes inevitably results in some bearing immunoglobulins that would recognize and bind to proteins on the body's own cells. These **self-reactive B-lymphocytes** normally undergo apoptosis and only lymphocytes that are not reactive to self are released from the bone marrow. Incomplete elimination of self-reactive lymphocytes may result in **autoimmune diseases** such as multiple sclerosis, rheumatoid arthritis, and juvenile diabetes.

HUMORAL IMMUNE RESPONSES

Primary immune response

Any foreign substance that will induce an immune response is called an **antigen**. The surface immunoglobulins of B-lymphocytes serve as **antigen receptors** enabling the cell to recognize the surface proteins of bacteria as non-self. For reasons that are poorly understood, B-lymphocytes do not bind directly to invading bacteria. These must first be taken up and processed by macrophages or dendritic cells. These cells are mobilized at the site

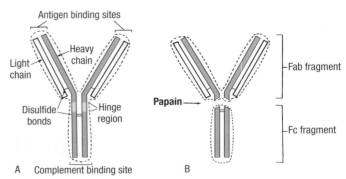

Figure 10.2 Diagram of the structure of an immunoglobulin molecule. (A) It is made up of two longer, heavy chains, and two shorter, light chains in a Y-shaped configuration. The arms of the Y contain the antigen binding sites. (B) Treatment with papain cleaves the molecule into two Fab fragments that bind antigen, and one Fc fragment that binds to complement.

of invasion and avidly phagocytize and digest bacteria. Peptide fragments of the surface proteins of the ingested bacteria are then bound to MHC-II in their cytoplasm, and molecules of the **antigen-MHC complex**, so formed, are inserted into the plasma membrane, where they are exposed to the assembled lymphocytes (Fig. 10.3). Therefore, macrophages and dendritic cells are commonly referred to as **antigen-presenting cells**. Those B-lymphocytes that have a surface immunoglobulin (antigen receptor) with an amino acid sequence matching that of the peptide presented on the surface of the macrophage, bind to it and are activated. The macrophage also secretes a cytokine, **interleukin-I** that attracts **helper T-lymphocytes** (CD-4 lymphocytes) to the site. Those among them having the appropriate antigen receptor also bind to the antigen presented. A cytokine, **interleukin-II**, secreted by the helper T-lymphocytes completes the activation of the bound B-lymphocytes, stimulating them to proliferate to form a clone of B-lymphocytes of the same antigen specificity (Figs 10.4, 10.5). Other cytokines released by the helper T-lymphocytes stimulate raid synthesis and release of antibody by these B-lymphocytes. These activated B-lymphocytes later become widely distributed in the tissues of the body and the antibodies they produce circulate in the blood.

The immune response may not be confined to the site of bacterial invasion. Some macrophages, bearing antigen-MHC complexes on their surface, may migrate from that site, enter lymphatics, and be carried to regional lymph nodes. There they continue, for some time, to present antigen to any of the large resident population of B-lymphocytes that have the appropriate antigen receptor, and these are activated to proliferate and secrete antibody. Physicians commonly palpate for enlarged regional lymph nodes to determine whether the immune response has spread beyond the original site of infection.

Many of the activated B-lymphocytes generated in a primary immune response remain in the connective tissue near the site of bacterial invasion and undergo terminal differentiation into **plasma cells**. These larger cells have a very extensive rough endoplasmic reticulum (Fig. 4.10) and are able to synthesize and release millions of antibody molecules per minute. Their remarkable capacity for immunoglobulin synthesis makes plasma cells the

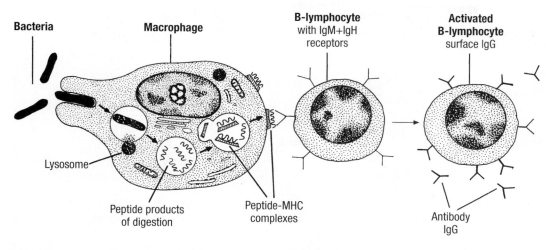

Labels for figure: **Bacteria**, **Macrophage**, **B-lymphocyte** with IgM+IgH receptors, **Activated B-lymphocyte** surface IgG, Lysosome, Peptide products of digestion, Peptide-MHC complexes, Antibody IgG

Figure 10.3 B-lymphocytes do not respond directly to bacteria. Macrophages must first ingest bacteria, digest them, and combine a peptide product of bacterial digestion with MHC-II. This complex is inserted into the macrophage membrane. Presentation of the antigen to lymphocytes, in this form, stimulates them to produce specific antibodies to that antigen.

major effector cell of the humoral immune response. They continue to produce antibody for a week or two and then undergo apoptosis. Other B-lymphocytes generated in the immune response do not differentiate into plasma cells, but enter the blood and circulate for months or years as 'memory cells' prepared for a quick secondary immune response to a future exposure to the same antigen. Of the estimated 8×10^2 lymphocytes in the body, there are probably no more than 1×10^5 that would have surface IgG molecules that would bind to a particular antigen. However, after a primary immune response to that antigen, there are many times that number in the blood, connective tissue and lymphoid organs of that individual.

The importance of cytokines in coordinating the events of the immune response cannot be overemphasized. In addition to interleukin-I and interleukin-II that activate and induce proliferation of responding B-lymphocytes, there is another that enhances the efficiency of macrophages in phagocytosis of bacteria and antigen processing, and another that inhibits migration of the

macrophages away from the site. Others are chemotactic for neutrophils and macrophages, causing them to migrate up the concentration gradient of cytokines diffusing from the site of bacterial invasion. Students will not be burdened here with the names and sources of the 15 or more cytokines that have been identified, but one meriting specification is **interleukin-12**. It is an exceptionally potent stimulator of the immune response, that has now been synthesized and shows promise in the treatment of patients in whom the immune system has been compromised (viz. in AIDS).

Secondary immune response

In adults, many of the B-lymphocytes in the blood, connective tissues, and lymphoid organs, have been generated by clonal expansion in previous primary immune responses. Therefore, they have antigen recognition sites for a number of different kinds of

First encounter

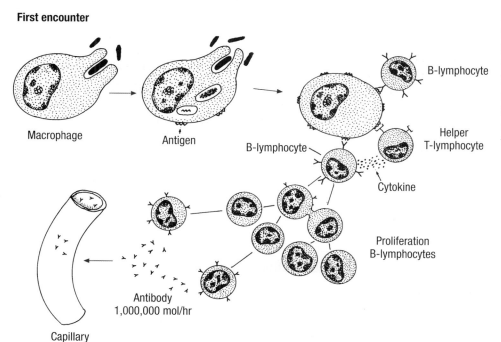

Labels for figure: Macrophage, Antigen, B-lymphocyte, Cytokine, B-lymphocyte, Helper T-lymphocyte, Proliferation B-lymphocytes, Antibody 1,000,000 mol/hr, Capillary

Figure 10.4 In a primary immune response, macrophages digest bacteria and present to lymphocytes a peptide product of their digestion on their surface. B-lymphocytes and helper T-lymphocytes bind to that antigen. Cytokines released by the CD-4 T-lymphocytes stimulate the B-lymphocytes to divide repeatedly, resulting in more B-lymphocytes, all producing antibodies to that antigen.

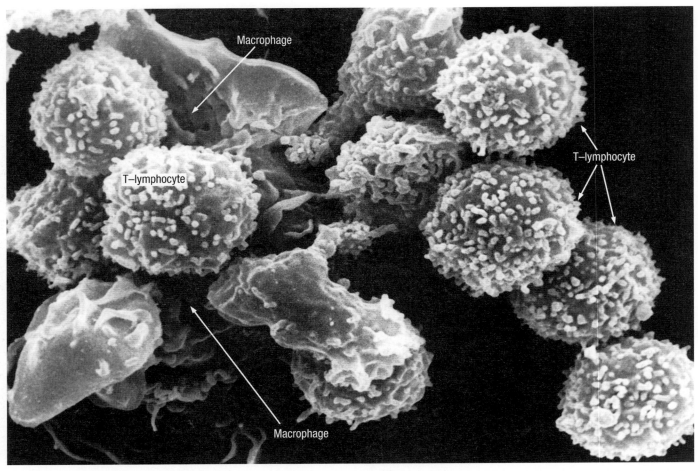

Macrophage

T–lymphocyte

T–lymphocyte

Macrophage

Figure 10.5 A scanning micrograph of B-lymphocytes and helper T-lymphocytes clustered around, and in close contact with a macrophage presenting antigen. (Micrograph courtesy of M.H. Nielsen and O. Werdelin.)

bacteria to which the person was previously exposed. The antibodies that were generated in those immune responses still circulate in the blood. A second exposure to one of those species of bacteria initiates a **secondary immune response**. The diverging arms of the Y-shaped immunoglobulin molecules (antibodies) in the circulation bind to the bacteria, leaving the stem end of the Y projecting outwards (Fig. 10.6). This stem end binds to receptors for this portion of the IgG molecules that are present on macrophages and dendritic cells. The antibody thus serves as an **opsonin**, a molecule that facilitates phagocytosis by binding both to a bacterium and to the surface of a macrophage. This opsonization of bacteria accelerates their antigen presentation and makes a secondary immune response more rapid, and more efficient, than the primary response. The titer of circulating antibody rapidly rises to 10–100 times its previous level.

Vaccination for prevention of infectious diseases consists of injecting a suspension of dead (or weakened) bacteria in order to initiate a primary immune response that will generate antibodies. The body responds to the dead bacteria in the same way as it does to invasion by living bacteria, and a **passive immunity** is induced, without the fever and discomforts that often attend a primary immune response to live bacteria. A 'booster shot' of vaccine induces a secondary immune response.

Classes of immunoglobulins

Different kinds of immunoglobulins are identifiable in the blood and tissue fluid. Seventy-five percent of the antibody produced in humoral immune responses is **immunoglobulin-G (IgG)**. A smaller amount is **immunoglobulin-E (IgE)**, which is formed in response to foreign proteins other than those of microorganisms (e.g. pollens). This class binds to receptors on mast cells and basophilic leukocytes. These respond by releasing histamine, which is responsible for many of the discomforts associated with allergies. **Immunoglobulin-A (IgA)** is found in the secretions of the salivary glands, intestinal glands, and glands of the respiratory tract, and is thought to be responsible for the innate antibacterial properties of their secretions.

CELL-MEDIATED IMMUNE RESPONSE

B-lymphocytes are unable to mount an effective defense against protozoan parasites or viruses. These require a **cell-mediated immune response**, in which T-lymphocytes are the effector cells.

2nd encounter

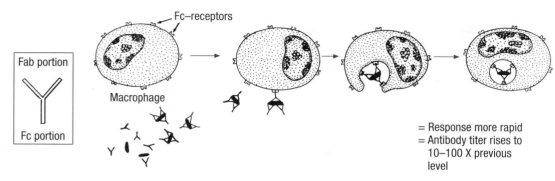

Figure 10.6 In a second encounter, the Fab portions of circulating antibody formed in the primary immune response, bind to the bacteria with their Fc portion projecting outward. This binds to Fc-receptors on the surface of the macrophages. This opsonization of the bacteria enables macrophages to phagocytize and destroy the bacteria more rapidly.

The **cell-mediated immune response** does not depend upon the production of antibodies. It is carried out by cytotoxic T-lymphocytes (CD-8) which directly attack parasites or virus-infected cells. T-lymphocytes do not have surface immuno-globulins, but they do have other protein **antigen receptors**, which are formed by random recombination of multiple gene segments, as described above for immunoglobulins. This results in hundreds of thousands of different amino acid sequences being expressed in the antigen receptors of different members of an individual's CD-8 T-lymphocyte population. The cytotoxic T-lymphocytes circulate in the blood, and migrate through the connective tissues in a continuous search for any cell that their receptors would recognize as non-self. If a cytotoxic T-lymphocyte encounters a parasite, or a virus-infected cell, the lymphocyte binds to that cell, and inserts into its membrane, molecules of a product called **perforin**. The perforin molecules polymerize within the membrane, creating holes in it through which a second product, a proteolytic enzyme, enters and lyses the cell.

Viruses are not directly accessible to T-lymphocytes because they are within host cells that would not ordinarily be identified as non-self. However, in the infected cell's synthesis of new virus particles, directed by the viral DNA, some viral peptides are bound to MHC in the cytoplasm and these are inserted into the membrane of the host cell. Cytotoxic T-lymphocytes recognize the viral peptide as non-self and secrete perforin and proteases to lyse the cell and its enclosed viral particles.

The great benefits of the cell-mediated immune response in our defense against parasites and viruses are partially offset by the problem it creates for the surgeon wishing to transplant a tissue or organ from one individual to another. In a patient with extensive burns, it would be desirable to graft skin from a donor onto the severely burned areas. However, this does not succeed, for patrolling lymphocytes soon recognize the cells of the graft as non-self. They release cytokines that diffuse to the endothelium of the underlying capillaries. These respond by inserting into their membrane, molecules that increase the adhesiveness of their lumenal surface. Lymphocytes in the blood flowing through the capillaries adhere to these sticky areas and migrate through the vessel wall, and up the concentration gradient of cytokines. Lymphocytes accumulate, in large numbers, at the undersurface of the skin graft. The cytotoxic T-lymphocytes among them release perforin and proteases that lyse the cells of the graft, resulting in its rejection (Fig. 10.7). However, if an identical twin

is the donor, his/her cells have an MHC complex identical to that of the graft recipient, and the graft is not rejected because it is recognized as self. In recent years, surgery for heart and kidney transplantation has become routine, but the major challenge remaining is postoperative treatment of the recipient with reagents, which block the immune system and prevent graft rejection.

THYMUS

The **thymus** is a lymphoid organ located in the chest, behind the sternum, and anterior to the heart. Early in life it is quite large and plays an essential role in the development of the immune system. It weighs about 40 g at puberty and then slowly atrophies to 10–15 g late in life, when much of its parenchyma has been replaced by connective tissue and adipose cells. The thymus consists of two lobes, each invested by a thin connective tissue capsule, from which thin septa extend inwards, subdividing the lobes into smaller lobules. Each lobule has a deeply staining and highly cellular **cortex** around a paler-staining **medulla** (Figs 10.8, 10.9).

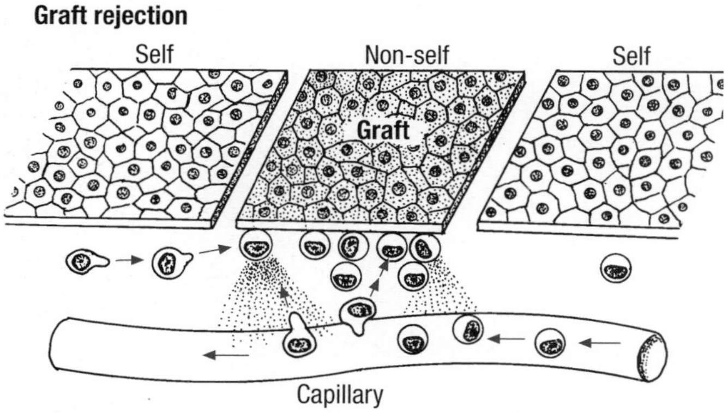

Graft rejection

Figure 10.7 If skin from an unrelated donor is transplanted to a burn patient, T-lymphocytes recognize it as non-self and release cytokines that attract many other T-lymphocytes to migrate through the walls of the underlying capillaries. Their combined cytotoxic immune response results in rejection of the graft.

Microscopic organization

Immediately beneath the capsule of the thymus, there is a continuous layer of cells, called **epithelial reticulocytes**. This layer continues onto the septa separating the lobules. Deeper in the cortex, there is a loose three-dimensional network of atypical epithelial cells, called **stellate reticular cells**. These have long, tapering cell processes that adhere to the processes of neighboring reticular cells, forming a network of interconnected cells throughout the cortex. The interspaces of this network are completely filled with lymphocytes in varying stages of maturation.

In the subcapsular region of the cortex, there are numerous large lymphoblasts, which are often observed in mitotic division. The remainder of the cortex is occupied by lymphocytes generated by division of the lymphoblasts and further differentiation of their progeny. These lymphocytes often occur in large groups, separated by processes of the stellate reticular cells. Macrophages are distributed throughout the cortex and are especially numerous near the corticomedullary boundary. Dendritic cells are also present, but appear to be confined to the medulla.

In the medulla, lymphocytes are less numerous and the epithelial cells are, therefore, more easily seen than they are in the cortex. The cell bodies are ovoid, with a pale-staining nucleus and short, spatulate processes, which do not form close attachments to one another. These cells are sufficiently variable in appearance to suggest, to some investigators, that there may be more than one cell type in the stroma of the medulla. A unique feature of the medulla of the thymus is the occurrence of variable numbers of odd structures, called **Hassall's corpuscles** (Fig. 10.9). These are believed to be formed by several epithelial cells that aggregate, increase in size, and become anucleate and intensely acidophilic. Other viable epithelial cells then wrap around this cluster of dead cells, forming a body consisting of multiple concentric layers. These cannot be associated with involution of the thymus for they are observed in the fetal thymus as well as in that of the adult. Their function, if any, is unknown. In histological section, the presence of Hassall's corpuscles is a feature that helps to distinguish the thymus from other lymphoid organs.

Blood supply

Arteries ramify over the surface of the thymus, sending branches inwards, within the interlobular septa, as far as the corticomedullary boundary. There, arterioles continue into the medulla, but the capillaries derived from them course outwards to form branching and anastomosing arcades in the cortex. The descending portions of these arcades return to the corticomedullary boundary, and postcapillary venules continue into the medulla

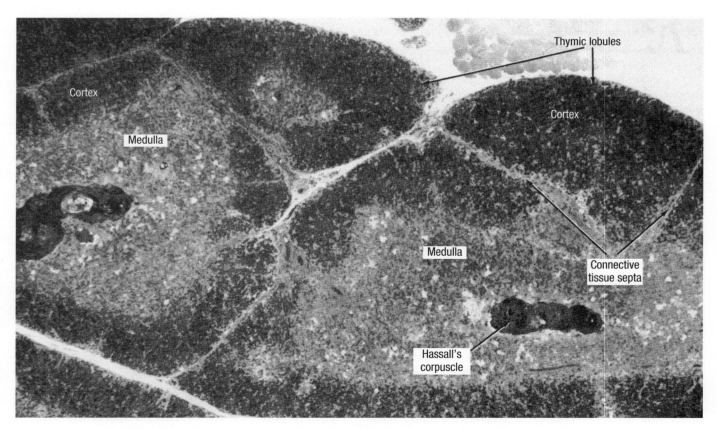

Figure 10.8 A low-power photomicrograph of the thymus, showing portions of three lobules. Notice the deeper staining of the cortex and the presence of a large aggregation of Hassall's corpuscles in the medulla. (Micrograph courtesy of G.B. Schneider and S. Clarke Jr.)

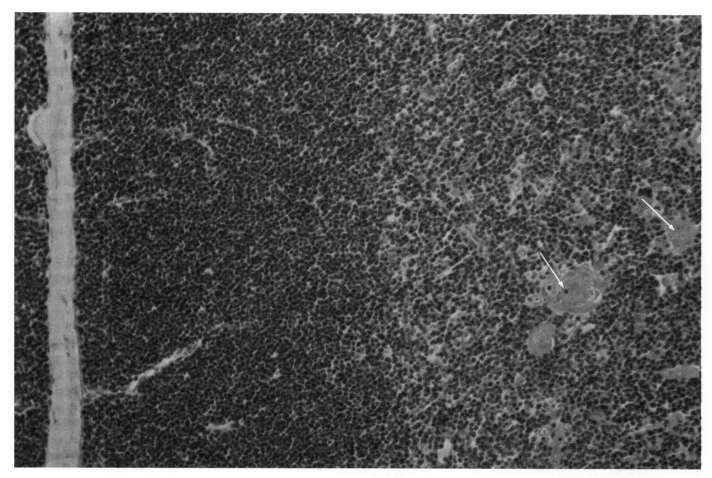

Figure 10.9 Low-magnification photomicrograph of thymus. Closely packed lymphocytes make up the darker staining cortex at the left. Cell density in the medulla, at the right, is considerably lower. Eosinophilic Hassall's corpuscles can be seen at the arrows.

and join to form larger venules, which exit the thymus via interlobular septa. An unusual feature of this vascular pattern is that the medulla contains arterioles, fenestrated capillaries, and venules, but the cortex receives only capillaries.

Electron micrographs reveal that the capillaries of the cortex have an unfenestrated endothelium, supported by a moderately thick basal lamina that is surrounded by a continuous layer of epithelial cells. It was formerly speculated that the continuous endothelium of these capillaries, and their surrounding epithelial cells, might constitute a significant barrier to passage of macromolecules from the blood into the cortex of the thymus. This consideration prompted studies in which electron-opaque tracers were injected into animals. In histological sections of the thymus of these animals, the tracer was abundant outside of the blood vessels of the medulla, but little or no tracer was found outside of the capillaries of the cortex. It was concluded that the continuous endothelium, basal lamina and surrounding epithelial cells of cortical capillaries constitute a **blood–thymus barrier**, comparable to the blood–brain barrier. For three decades or more, the existence of this apparent barrier fostered the belief that the lymphocytes of the thymic cortex develop in an antigen-free environment. In recent years, other experiments have cast doubt upon this conclusion. The unusual vascular pattern of the thymus is no longer believed to be a significant factor in the differentiation of T-lymphocytes.

Histophysiology of the thymus

The thymus has a central role in development of a functional immune system. It provides an environment in which the T-lymphocyte lineage can proliferate, mature, and acquire its antigen-receptor repertoire. In fetal life, monopotential stem cells are carried in the blood, from the bone marrow to the developing thymus. These give rise to the large lymphoblasts that are found in the subcapsular zone. Their proliferation generates large numbers of smaller prolymphocytes, which undergo further differentiation as they move inwards through the cortex. Those near the lymphoblasts do not yet have the surface markers (CD-4 and CD-8) that permit identification of the two categories of T-lymphocytes. Those somewhat deeper in the cortex have both markers in their membrane. In their further differentiation, they lose either one of these. Lymphocytes in the medulla have a single marker, either CD-4 or CD-8. The CD-4 T-lymphocytes will be helper cells in humoral immune responses, and the CD-8 lymphocytes will be effector cells in cell-mediated immune responses.

Clonal selection of T-lymphocytes

In addition to acquiring surface markers during their differentiation, the lymphocytes synthesize, and insert into their membrane, receptors for recognition of antigens. These consist of α-chains and β-chains, which determine both the antigen specificity and the MHC specificity of the receptor. In preparation for the synthesis of the receptors, the genes for the α-chains and β-chains undergo random rearrangements, which result in the expression of a great variety of amino acid sequences in the receptors of the T-lymphocyte population. As previously stated, this random recombination of gene segments inevitably results in some lymphocytes having surface receptors that would recognize and bind to self-MHC. These self-reactive T-lymphocytes contact self-epithelial cells in their passage through the inner cortex, and this triggers their apoptosis (Fig. 10.10). Their residues are phagocytized by the abundant macrophages near the corticomedullary boundary. It is believed that over 70% of the T-lymphocytes that arise from lymphoblasts in the outer cortex undergo apoptosis. Only those that are capable of recognizing, and binding to, non-self peptides associated with the MHC complex, complete their passage through the medulla and enter the blood.

This elimination of self-reactive T-lymphocytes in the thymus is called **negative selection** or **clonal selection** (Fig. 10.10). In rare instances in which this process of selection is not completed, the ability of the lymphocytes to distinguish 'self' from 'non-self' is compromised and may result in an **autoimmune disease**. In such diseases, T-lymphocytes may destroy a single cell type, as in **insulin-dependent diabetes**, where the target is the β-cell of the endocrine pancreas. In other diseases, such as **systemic lupus erythematosus**, the self-reactive T-lymphocytes may be directed against an antigen shared by many cell types.

The reticular epithelial cells of the thymus secrete several hormones and cytokines that mediate interactions between the other cells of this organ. One called **thymotaxin** is believed to attract blood-borne stem cells from the bone marrow to migrate into the fetal thymus. Another, called **thymulin**, stimulates immature T-lymphocytes to synthesize their surface markers. **Thymic humoral factor** stimulates differentiation and clonal expansion of CD-8 T-lymphocytes. A hormone, **thrombopoietin**, promotes lymphocyte differentiation in the thymus, but its effects extend beyond that organ. It also regulates formation of blood platelets by the megakaryocytes of the bone marrow.

LYMPH NODES

Lymph nodes are small kidney-shaped organs, 6–22 mm in diameter, which are distributed along the course of lymphatic vessels draining the various regions of the body. They occur in groups in the axilla, groin, and neck. In the abdomen, they are abundant in the mesentery that supports the intestines. **Afferent lymph vessels** enter each node at several sites on its convex surface (Fig. 10.11), and one or two **efferent lymph vessels** emerge from a shallow depression on its concave surface, called the **hilus**. Lymph nodes filter the lymph passing through them, and their abundant macrophages and lymphocytes mount a vigorous immune response to any antigen carried to them from a site of infection. Physicians routinely palpate the axilla and groin to detect enlargement of lymph nodes that would suggest the presence of an infection, or a malignant tumor, in the region drained by those nodes. Surgeons removing a malignant tumor also remove the regional lymph nodes, to eliminate any malignant cells that may have been filtered out of the lymph flowing from the site of the tumor.

Microscopic organization

In histological sections, the parenchyma of a lymph node is divisible into an intensely staining **cortex** and a paler-staining **medulla**.

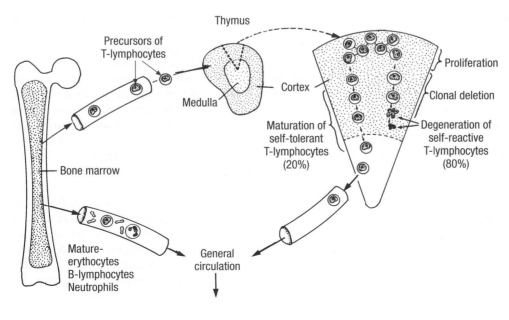

Figure 10.10 Precursors of T-lymphocytes are carried from the bone marrow to the thymus early in life. These give rise to large lymphoblasts in the cortex. Their progeny differentiate and mature as they are slowly moved towards the medulla. Those having receptors that would bind to self, undergo apoptosis in a process called clonal selection. Only those that are unreactive to self enter the circulation.

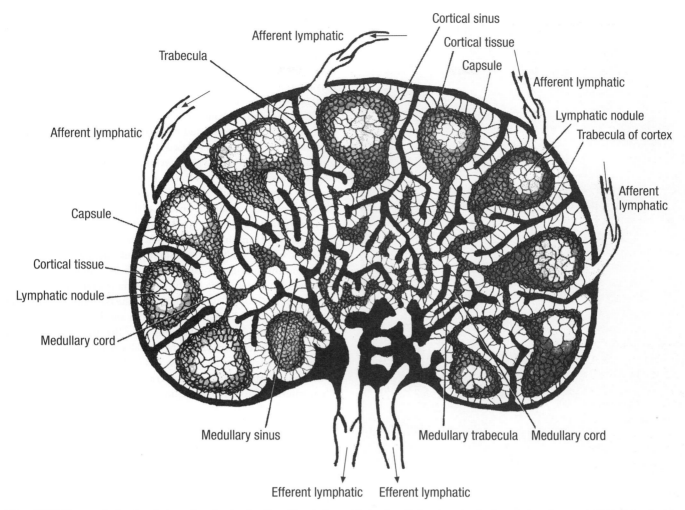

Figure 10.11 Diagram of a lymph node, in section, showing the afferent lymphatics and their valves. Trabeculae extending inwards from the capsule divide the cortex into separate compartments. Notice the subcapsular sinus, confluent with cortical sinuses along the sides of the trabeculae. These form the principal pathways of filtration of the lymph.

It is enclosed in a thin **capsule** of fibroblasts and collagen fibers. Slender branching **trabeculae** of similar composition extend inwards from the capsule, dividing the cortex into a number of compartments that are occupied by lymphoid tissue that is supported by a three-dimensional network of **reticular cells** and associated reticular fibers. Immediately beneath the capsule, there is a narrow space around the lymphoid tissue, called the **cortical sinus**, or **subcapsular sinus** (Fig. 10.11). It is bounded by the capsule, on its outer side, and by a layer of reticular cells and macrophages, on its inner side.

In the deeply staining cortex of each compartment, there are ovoid masses of closely packed lymphocytes, called **lymphoid follicles**. At the outer pole of each follicle there is a cap-like area of very closely packed, small lymphocytes, and a similar dense area is found at the lower pole (Fig. 10.12). In the center of the follicle, between these two denser zones, there is a round paler-staining area, called the **germinal center**, which consists mainly of lymphoblasts and large lymphocytes. From the lower pole of each follicle, a **medullary cord** of less densely packed small lymphocytes extends into the medulla of the node.

Filtration pathway

The afferent lymph vessels pass through the capsule and are confluent with the **subcapsular sinus**. Branches called **cortical sinusoids** pass inwards from the subcapsular sinus along the sides of the trabeculae, and join a network of **medullary sinusoids**. These converge upon a single **efferent lymphatic**, which exits the node at the hilus. The reticular fibers within the lymphoid tissue cross the sinuses and terminate in the trabeculae, or in the capsule. The sinuses are not lined by endothelium, but by a mixture of fibroblast-like cells, macrophages and dendritic cells, which extend slender cell processes across the lumen of the sinuses. Thus, the structure of the sinuses is admirably suited to filter lymphocytes and smaller particulates out of the lymph, as it slowly percolates through the 'obstacle-course' of cell processes crossing the sinuses. Lymphocytes in the afferent lymph migrate into the lymphoid tissue, and any foreign particulates in the lymph are ingested by macrophages or dendritic cells for presentation to lymphocytes.

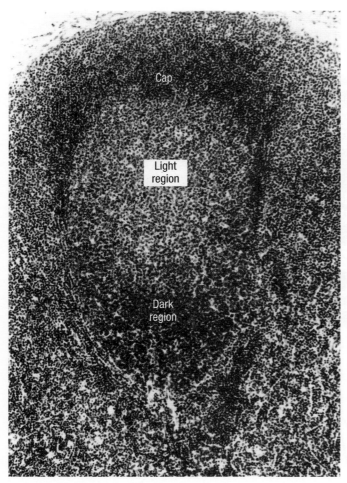

Cap

Light region

Dark region

Figure 10.12 Photomicrograph of a small area of the outer cortex of a mesenteric lymph node. Note the cap or crescent of small lymphocytes at the outer side of a paler germinal center.

Blood supply

The arterial blood supply to the node enters at the hilus and gives rise to straight branches that cross the medulla, giving off few secondary branches, but upon reaching the cortex, they branch into numerous loops of anastomosing arterioles and capillaries. Capillaries are especially numerous around the follicles, but few, if any, of these enter the germinal centers. Blood returns via postcapillary venules between the follicles of the cortex and small veins in the medulla that converge upon a single larger vein exiting the node at the hilus. Of special interest to immunologists are venules in the deeper portion of the cortex that lack a smooth muscle layer and have an unusual endothelium consisting of tall cuboidal, or columnar cells. These vessels are referred to as the **high endothelial venules**. The population of lymphocytes in a lymph node is constantly changing, and the high endothelial portions of the venules are the portal of entry of new blood-borne lymphocytes. The lymphocytes are believed to have a surface glycoprotein that binds specifically to receptors on the high endothelial cells. Having been arrested there, they migrate between the endothelial cells and into the lymphoid follicles.

Histophysiology of lymph nodes

The lymphatic vessels of the body take up excess extracellular fluid from the tissue and return it to the blood. Any particulate matter it may contain is filtered out in the lymph nodes; for example, in coal miners the tracheobronchial lymph nodes are blackened by coal dust that they have inhaled. The filtration efficiency of the lymph nodes has been demonstrated by experiments in which a known number of bacteria were perfused through a lymph node, and the number in the efferent lymph were counted. The filtering efficiency of a single node was found to be over 90%. *In vivo*, those few that emerged would likely be filtered out in the next node of the series of nodes along the course of that lymphatic vessel.

The lymphocytes that make up the greater part of the parenchyma of lymph nodes are not a static population. The lymphocytes of the body are constantly on the move. Some are migrating through the connective tissues in search of microbial intruders. These return to lymph nodes via the lymph. Those circulating in the blood pass through all of the lymphoid organs and may reside for a while in one and then in another. B-lymphocytes binding to the high endothelial cells enter the node and stay for a while in the outer portion of the follicles between the germinal center and the subcapsular sinus. T-lymphocytes tend to migrate to the inner cortex, between the germinal centers and the medulla. Their migration to different regions of the node is thought to be governed by chemotactic cytokines secreted by stromal cells of those areas. If no antigen is presented to them, they may move on to continue their surveillance of other lymphoid organs and may visit several within a week.

After an infection in some part of the body, a late event in the immune response is the migration of the antigen-presenting cells (macrophages and dendritic cells) from the site of the primary response to the cortex of the regional lymph nodes. Presentation of antigen to B-lymphocytes there results in clonal expansion of any that may have a matching IgG receptor. These then produce more antibodies to supplement than those produced at the primary site of infection. Some of the activated lymphocytes migrate into the medulla where they differentiate into plasma cells that continue to produce antibody. Others return to the blood as **memory B-lymphocytes**. These are inactive B-lymphocytes that have participated in a primary immune response, and have specific immunoglobulins on their surface that will enable them to respond more quickly and efficiently in a second exposure to the same antigen. In the germinal centers of the follicles, mitosis of lymphoblasts is continually generating new, naive lymphocytes. Enhanced activity and increased blood flow in lymph nodes draining an infected area cause them to increase in size (swell). If the infection is in an arm or leg, the physician will be able to feel enlarged nodes in the axilla or groin.

SPLEEN

The **spleen** is an intra-abdominal organ about 12 cm in length, 7 cm in width and 3 cm in thickness. It is located in the upper abdomen between the fundus of the stomach and the diaphragm. It contains a large volume of lymphoid tissue and is the largest organ of the immune system. Because it also serves as a filter interposed in the circulation to clear the blood of senescent erythrocytes, it is sometimes described as a hemolymphatic organ. The spleen sequesters circulating monocytes that differentiate into splenic macrophages and these phagocytize and destroy effete erythrocytes. The spleen also stores as many as one-third of the body's blood platelets and returns them to the blood as needed. In some species, the spleen also acts as a reservoir of mature erythrocytes that can be added to the blood in response to unusual demands.

Microscopic organization

The spleen has a thick collagenous **capsule** that is closely invested by the **peritoneum**, the thin layer of squamous epithelium that lines the abdominal cavity and covers its viscera. At a depression on the undersurface of the organ, called the **hilus**, its peritoneal covering is continuous with a fold of the peritoneum, the lienorenal ligament, through which the blood vessels, nerves, and lymphatics enter and leave the organ. Connective tissue trabeculae extend some distance inwards from the capsule and partition the parenchyma, or **splenic pulp**, into compartments. A network of thin intersecting fibrils pervades the entire interior of the organ. Closely associated with this reticulum are reticular cells and numerous macrophages.

Examination of the cut surface of a hemisected spleen, reveals many rounded, gray areas 9.2–0.8 μm in diameter that collectively constitute the **white pulp** of the spleen. These areas are scattered through a mass of dark-red tissue, the **red pulp** of the spleen (Fig. 10.13). In histological sections, the white pulp consists of diffuse, and nodular, lymphoid tissue that resembles the cortex of a lymph node. The red pulp is made up of **splenic cords**, which are highly cellular areas surrounding thin-walled blood vessels called the **splenic sinuses**. The color of the red pulp is due to an

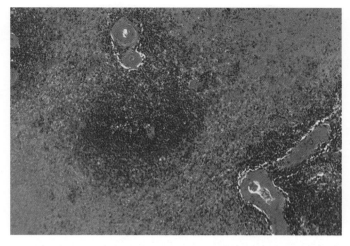

Figure 10.13 A low-power photomicrograph of a section of spleen. The blue areas are white pulp, and the red areas are red pulp. Note the two central arteries of the white pulp.

abundance of erythrocytes in the sinuses, and the many erythrocytes extravasated into the meshwork of stellate reticular cells and reticular fibers surrounding the sinuses.

Blood supply

The functions of the spleen cannot be fully understood without knowledge of some unique features of its vascular system. Branches of the **splenic artery**, called **trabecular arteries**, ramify in the connective tissue of the trabeculae and give off branches, called **central arteries**, that enter the adjacent parenchyma. These are surrounded by a wide **periarterial sheath** of lymphoid tissue resembling that of the cortex of a lymph node. The periarterial sheaths of the organ make up its white pulp (Fig. 10.14).

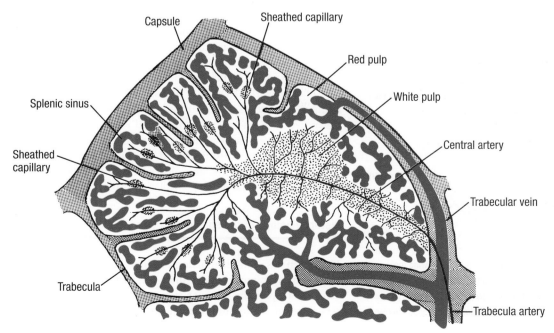

Figure 10.14 Diagram of the organization of a lobule of the spleen. The stippled area around the central artery is the periarterial lymphoid sheath of the white matter. The black areas are the splenic sinuses. An open circulation is depicted here with the capillaries not communicating with the sinusoids.

Capsule
Sheathed capillary
Red pulp
White pulp
Central artery
Trabecular vein
Trabecula artery
Splenic sinus
Sheathed capillary
Trabecula

Upon emerging from the ends of their respective periarterial sheaths, the central arteries branch quite suddenly into several very slender vessels called **penicillar arterioles**. These radiate for a short distance from their abrupt origin, and then each gives rise to two or three small branches. Before the termination of these branches, they pass through a short sheath, called the **ellipsoid**, which consists of three or more layers of macrophages. The endothelium of this segment is atypical in that a basal lamina is lacking. Monocytes evidently pass through the vessel wall and differentiate into macrophages, which reside, for a time, in the ellipsoid and then migrate into the red pulp. The significance of this unusual mode of termination of the penicillar arterioles has long been a subject of controversy. Some histologists, favoring a **closed circulation**, believe these small vessels are in continuity with the venous sinuses of the red pulp. Others, favoring an **open circulation**, believe that they have open ends, permitting extravasation of erythrocytes into the red pulp (Fig. 10.15). The open circulation is now accepted for the human spleen, for it seems unlikely that the spleen could be as efficient as it is in eliminating senescent or damaged erythrocytes if these did not have direct exposure to the abundant macrophages of the red pulp.

Located near the termination of the penicillar arteries are bizarrely structured vessels called **venous splenic sinuses**. They are lined by an atypical endothelium in which longitudinally oriented fusiform cells (stave cells) are separated by narrow intercellular clefts. These endothelial cells are supported by a discontinuous basal lamina in the form of narrow bands, which encircle the vessel like the hoops on a barrel (Fig. 10.16). The normal viable erythrocytes that leave the open ends of branches of the penicillar arteries are believed to return to the circulation by passing between the fusiform endothelial cells of these venous splenic sinuses (Fig. 10.15). Blood flows from the splenic sinuses in short, plump veins that are continuous with **trabecular veins**. These veins converge upon the hilum and there join larger veins that combine to form the splenic vein.

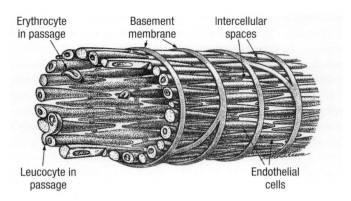

Figure 10.16 Drawing of a splenic sinus. The endothelial cells are fusiform and not in intimate lateral contact, leaving clefts through which leukocytes leave and erythrocytes re-enter the circulation. The basal lamina (basement membrane) of the endothelium is confined to circumferential bands resembling the hoops of a barrel. (Drawing by Sylvia Collard Keene.)

White pulp

The periarterial sheaths of the white pulp consist mainly of T-lymphocytes. Wider, rounded areas of lymphoid tissue, spaced at intervals along the sheaths, consist of tightly packed B-lymphocytes forming lymphoid follicles with one or more germinal centers. In a marginal zone of these **splenic follicles**, lymphocytes are less closely crowded and mingle with many reticular cells, macrophages, and dendritic cells. The blood supply of the follicles is via capillaries from the central artery. In addition, there are thin-walled sinusoidal vessels in their marginal zone. Any blood-borne antigen escaping from these vessels is promptly captured by the antigen-presenting cells of the marginal zone and a local immune response is initiated.

Red pulp

The traditional term, **splenic cords**, is somewhat misleading, for it suggests that they are separate units. Actually, the red pulp is continuous, occupying all areas of the spleen between the periarterial sheaths and splenic follicles of the white pulp (Fig. 10.14). It consists of a network of reticular fibers, with cells of various kinds filling its interstices. These include macrophages, lymphocytes, plasma cells, platelets, and extravasated erythrocytes. Senescent erythrocytes are phagocytized by macrophages, and normal erythrocytes are returned to the blood, through the spaces between endothelial cells of splenic sinusoids, near their site of escape from open-ended branches of the penicillar arterioles.

Histophysiology of the spleen

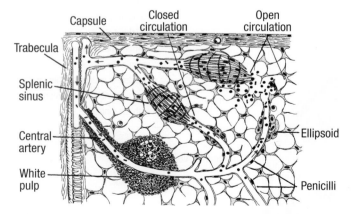

Figure 10.15 A diagram of a small area of splenic parenchyma, showing the meshwork of stellate reticular cells of the red pulp and the perivascular aggregations of lymphocytes that comprise the white pulp. Splenic sinuses are also shown. The alternative interpretations of an open and a closed circulation are also depicted.

The spleen has multiple functions. It filters the blood in much the same way that lymph nodes filter the lymph. This function is dependent upon the reticular structure of the red pulp and its very large population of macrophages. The macrophages seem to be able to monitor the quality of erythrocytes entering the red pulp and destroy any with diminished oxygen-carrying capacity. How they make this choice is not understood. The hemoglobin of the phagocytized erythrocytes is broken down and the iron is transiently stored in the cytoplasm of the macrophages in the form of **ferritin**. It is ultimately recycled to erythroblasts in the bone marrow for use in synthesis of new hemoglobin. Another byproduct of hemoglobin degradation is **bilirubin**, which is transported in the blood to the liver, where it is secreted in the bile.

The spleen also plays a major role in the body's immune responses. Bacteria that enter the bloodstream are filtered out in the spleen and captured by the antigen-presenting cells (macrophages and dendritic cells) in the marginal zone of the lymphoid follicles. These cells secrete cytokines (lymphokines) that mobilize B-lymphocytes and a primary immune response is initiated. In a secondary immune response, the spleen is, for a time, the body's most active organ, per unit weight, in antibody production. However, its activity declines as the response spreads to other lymphoid tissues throughout the body. The spleen is also a major source of new lymphocytes generated in the germinal centers of the white pulp and entering the circulation through the walls of the splenic sinusoids.

Questions

1 The cell-mediated immune response is performed by
   a B-lymphocytes
   b macrophages
   c T-lymphocytes
   d plasma cells
   e monocytes

2 What is the most common antibody produced in humoral immune reactions?
   a IgE
   b IgA
   c IgB
   d IgG
   e IgD

3 When B-cells of a lymph node are activated, they
   a enter the circulation and migrate to the thymus
   b transform into small lymphocytes and undergo a series of mitotic divisions
   c undergo a series of mitotic divisions and then differentiate into plasma cells
   d give rise to 'activated' macrophages
   e become mast cells

4 Aged, abnormal, or damaged erythrocytes are phagocytosed by macrophages in the
   a spleen
   b tonsils
   c lymph nodes
   d thymus
   e liver

5 Periarterial lymphatic sheaths of the spleen
   a are enriched in T-lymphocytes
   b are enriched in B-lymphocytes
   c may be described as the lymph nodules of the spleen
   d constitute the red pulp of the spleen
   e encircle the trabecular arteries

6 Which of the following statements is correct regarding lymph nodes?
   a lymph nodes contain both T-lymphocytes and B-lymphocytes
   b lymphocytes are only found in the cortex
   c medullary sinuses are the sites where blood is filtered
   d secondary lymphatic nodules are prominent in the medulla
   e germinal centers contain mostly T-lymphocytes

7 A unique feature of the thymus is
   a the presence of afferent lymphatics
   b the presence of reticular cells
   c that it has significant immune function in the adult
   d the presence of Hassall's corpuscles
   e the presence of multiple lobes

8 The most common antigen-presenting cells are referred to as
   a macrophages
   b helper T-lymphocytes
   c reticulocytes
   d mast cells
   e plasma cells

9 The principal cell of the humoral immune response is the
   a macrophage
   b B-lymphocyte
   c plasma cell
   d helper T-lymphocyte
   e cytotoxic T-lymphocyte

10 What is the primary cell responsible for tissue graft and organ transplant rejection?
   a cytotoxic T-lymphocyte
   b macrophage
   c B-lymphocyte
   d plasma cell
   e helper T-lymphocyte

11 What lymphoid structure has smooth muscle cells in its connective tissue?

12 One can easily observe an abundance of what type of specialized immune system cell in the medulla of a lymph node?

13 Hassall's corpuscle is the identifying feature of what structure?

14 What lymphoid structure has central arteries?

15 What lymphocyte is the principle agent of the humoral response?

16 What type of lymphocyte performs the cell-mediated response?

17 What do plasma cells secrete?

18 What type of lymphocyte secretes perforin and is involved in graft rejection?

19 What structure is a filter of the blood, a reservoir of erythrocytes, participates in iron recycling, and is a site of production of antibodies?

20 Humoral immune response is associated with a lymphatic cell that has differentiated into what cell?

Chapter eleven

Skin

The **skin** is one of the body's largest organs, accounting for about 16% of the body weight and having a surface area of nearly 2 m². It has multiple functions: it serves as a protective barrier against injury or invasion by microorganisms; its impermeability to water prevents desiccation and makes life on land possible; its sensory organs detect contact, pain, pressure, heat, and cold; and its sweat glands play an important role in maintenance of normal body temperature. Skin varies in thickness from 0.5 to 4.0 mm and is made up of two principal layers: a surface epithelium, the **epidermis**, and an underlying layer of connective tissue, the **dermis** or corium (Fig. 11.1). Beneath the dermis is the **hypodermis**, a layer of looser connective tissue that is not part of the skin but minimizes injury to it by permitting some degree of mobility of the skin over underlying structures. In some regions of the body, it may consist mainly of adipose tissue. At the lips, nose, eyelids, anus, and vagina, the epidermis is continuous with the epithelium lining those structures. Such sites are referred to as **mucocutaneous junctions**.

Associated with the skin are **hair follicles** and two types of small glands, the **sudoriparous glands**, which produce sweat, and the **sebaceous glands**, which produce an oily secretion, the **sebum**. The number of hair follicles and glands varies greatly from region to region. The skin appears relatively smooth over much of its surface, but at low magnification a pattern of shallow grooves and flexure lines are apparent. These are deeper on the thick, hairless regions of the skin over the knees, elbows, palms, and soles of the feet. On the finger pads, the alternating ridges and grooves form the **dermatoglyphs**, the distinctive pattern of arches, loops, and whorls that are the basis of the individuality of our fingerprints.

EPIDERMIS

The epidermis is a **stratified squamous epithelium**. Over most of the body surface, it is 0.07 to 0.12 mm in thickness, but it may reach a thickness of 0.8 mm on the palms and 1.4 mm on the soles of the feet. At birth it is already thicker at these sites than elsewhere, and continuous pressure and friction on these surfaces in postnatal life result in additional thickening.

Thick skin

The epithelium of thick skin is made up of 10 to 20 layers of cells called **keratinocytes**. These arise by continuous division of stem cells that form the basal layer of the epithelium. Daughter cells of those divisions are slowly moved towards the surface of the epithelium by the continual generation of new cells at the base. In their transit towards the surface, they enlarge and differentiate, synthesizing large amounts of a cytoskeletal protein called **keratin**. Keratin polymerizes into 10 nm intermediate filaments that gradually come to constitute 80%, or more, of the cell volume. Near the surface of the epithelium, bundles of keratin filaments completely fill the cytoplasm, replacing the nucleus and organelles. These flake-like, lifeless cells detach, and are continually shed from the surface of the epidermis. The transit time of the keratinocytes from the basal layer to the surface is 20–30 days. The sequence of cytological changes they undergo in their upwards movement is referred to as the **cytomorphosis** of the keratinocytes. Their differing appearance at successive levels in the epithelium makes it

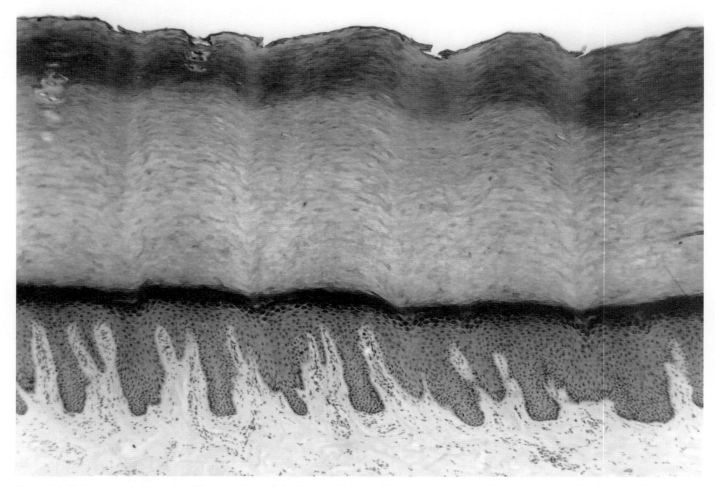

Figure 11.1 Photomicrograph of thick skin of the human finger. Notice the great thickness of the stratum corneum, and the regular spacing of the dermal papillae at the base of the epithelium. The dark horizontal line below the stratum corneum is the stratum granulosum.

possible to distinguish four zones in the epithelium: the **stratum basale** (stratum germinativum), the **stratum spinosum** (stratum Malpighii), the **stratum granulosum**, and the **stratum corneum**. The dermo-epidermal junction of thick skin is highly irregular (Fig. 11.1). It has a scalloped contour, in section, owing to ridges and papillae of dermis that extend into the dermis. The stratum spinosum, between dermal papillae, is therefore much thicker than elsewhere. This irregularity is not seen in the upper layers, which are parallel to the free surface and of uniform thickness.

The **stratum basale** is the single layer of cells resting on the basal lamina. The basal cells are cuboidal, with a nucleus that is large, relative to the size of the cell, and the cytoplasm is intensely basophilic. On electron micrographs, the usual organelles are found in a cytoplasm rich in ribosomes. Intermediate filaments are not uncommonly abundant. The cells are attached to one another by numerous desmosomes (Fig. 11.2), and to the basal lamina by regularly spaced hemidesmosomes. Cells in mitosis are common in this layer.

As the cells generated in the stratum basale move upwards into the **stratum spinosum**, they assume a flatter, polyhedral form, with their long axis parallel to the surface of the epithelium. There

are four to six rows of cells in this zone of the epithelium, and their lateral surfaces have short processes that interdigitate with those of neighboring cells. The cytoplasm is less basophilic, and contains fewer ribosomes, than that of cells in the stratum basale. A prominent feature of these cells is the presence of bundles of keratin filaments that radiate from the perinuclear region and end in the numerous desmosomes along the boundary between adjacent cells (Fig. 11.2). Cells in the upper part of the stratum spinosum, and those in the overlying stratum granulosum, contain membrane-bounded secretory granules 0.1–0.4 μm in diameter, called **lamellar bodies**, or **membrane-coating granules**. These have a distinctive internal structure consisting of alternating electron-dense and electron-lucent lamellae 2.0–3.5 nm in thickness. Pairs of the dense lamellae are continuous at their ends, suggesting that the granules are made up of stacks of flattened discoid vesicles. The granules consist of a mixture of phospholipids, glycoceramides, and cholesterol. They are assembled in a rather diffuse Golgi complex and are released by exocytosis into the intercellular spaces, where they coalesce to form a continuous, dense amorphous layer between cells. Thus, the outermost cells of the stratum spinosum, and those of the stratum granulosum, are

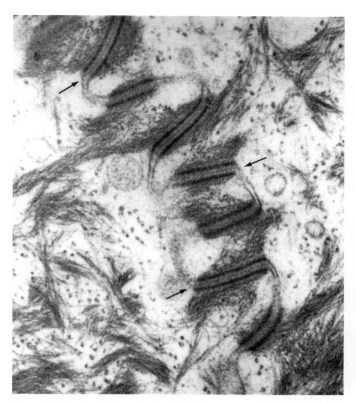

Figure 11.2 Electron micrograph of the boundary between two cells of the stratum granulosum. Desmosomes (at arrows) connect short interdigitating processes of the two cells. Bundles of keratin filaments terminate in the dense plaques of the desmosomes.

thin, clear zone in the lower portion of the stratum corneum. It is made up of one or two rows of flat, translucent keratinocytes. The reason for their translucency is unknown. A stratum lucidum is not found in the epidermis of thin skin.

The epidermis is remarkable for the diversity of products that it synthesizes. The most abundant of these are keratins of several kinds. The keratins are a family of 18 or more polypeptides, ranging in molecular weight from 40 000 to 68 000. They are classified in two groups. The type I keratins are acidic, and type II keratins are basic. The individual molecular species within these two groups are designated by the letter K and a number. The intermediate filaments of the keratinocyte cytoskeleton are assembled from heterodimers of one type I keratin, and one type II keratin. Those in the basal cells of the epidermis are formed of K-5 and K-14 keratins. Upon reaching the stratum spinosum, the cells synthesize two new keratins, K-1 and K-10, which form filaments that assemble into coarser bundles with unusually strong protein–protein interactions between filaments. As the cells move through the stratum spinosum and into the stratum granulosum, they cease to synthesize keratin, and begin to produce several components of **lamellar granules** and, later, the **keratohyalin granules**. They also synthesize **filaggrin**, a basic protein involved in the assembly and binding of intermediate filaments into bundles, and the protein **involucrin**, which is deposited on the inside of the plasmalemma to form a thick envelope around the periphery of the cell. Thus, the cells of the skin are veritable chemical factories.

specialized secretory cells that have the very important function of forming a lipid-rich extracellular layer that is a barrier to transcutaneous water loss.

The **stratum granulosum** of thick epidermis consists of three to five layers of cells that are considerably flatter than those of the stratum spinosum. They contain many lamellar bodies that may occupy as much as 15% of the cell volume. The most distinctive feature of cells in this zone is the presence of irregularly shaped **keratohyalin granules** in their cytoplasm, which stain intensely with basic dyes. These do not have a limiting membrane, and bundles of keratin filaments may be incorporated in their periphery, or may pass through them. Their chemical nature remains unclear, but they are believed to be precursors of a substance that will form an amorphous matrix surrounding the keratin filament bundles in the cytoplasm of the fully keratinized cells of the overlying stratum corneum.

The **stratum corneum** consists of three to five rows of very flat, dead cells, containing no nucleus or organelles. The plasmalemma appears thickened, and the cell body is completely filled with keratin filaments embedded in an amorphous matrix that may be derived from the keratohyalin granules described above. The lowermost cells of the stratum corneum are still firmly coherent, but in the outer rows, desmosomes are no longer present, and the heavily keratinized cells break loose from one another and are desquamated. In the epidermis of thick skin, there may also be a thin **stratum lucidum** between the stratum granulosum and the stratum corneum. As the name 'lucidum' implies, it appears as a

Thin skin

In the thin skin over most of the body, the epidermis is similar, in organization, to that of the palms and soles, but the various strata are less obvious (Fig. 11.3). The stratum corneum is much thinner. A stratum spinosum is always present, and a stratum granulosum is usually identifiable, but it is only two or three cells thick. A stratum lucidum is usually lacking. The contour of the dermo-epidermal junction is less complex than that of thick skin.

Pemphigus vulgaris is a skin disease, largely confined to the elderly, in which numerous fluid-filled blisters form on the face, trunk, extremities, and in the oral cavity. These lesions are due to a loss of cohesion between the stratum basale and stratum spinosum of the epidermis. It is an autoimmune disease resulting from the development of autoantibodies to keratinocyte surface antigens. It was formerly life-threatening, but it can now be controlled by administration of adrenal glucocorticoids.

Pigmentation

Skin color depends upon varying amounts of three components. The tissue has an inherent yellowish color attributable, in part, to its content of **carotene**, a precursor of vitamin A. In addition, a pink tint is imparted to the skin by the oxygenated **hemoglobin** of blood in the underlying capillary bed of the dermis. Shades of brown to black are caused by varying amounts of the pigment, **melanin**,

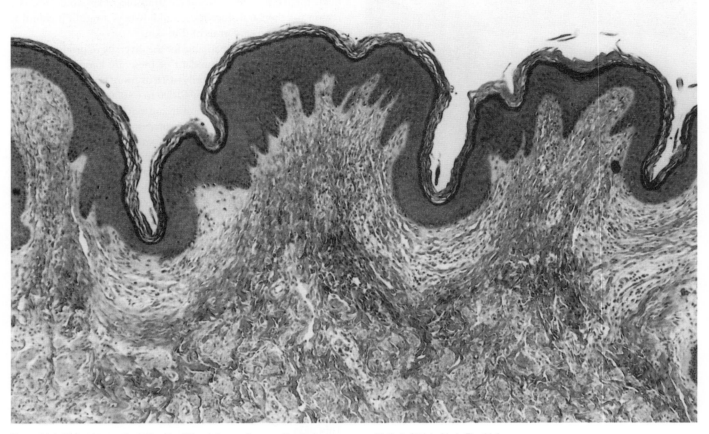

Figure 11.3 Photomicrograph of thin skin of the abdomen. Compare the stratum corneum with that of thick skin in Fig. 11.1.

produced by specialized cells called **melanocytes**, present in varying numbers in the basal layer of the epidermis and, occasionally, in the underlying dermis. Melanin is synthesized from tyrosine, which is transformed into **3-4 dihydrophenylalanine** (dopa), and then to **dopaquinone**, which is converted to **melanin**. The slightly different pigment of red hair consists of a related compound, **pheomelanin**. The melanocytes arise from the neural crest of the embryo, and they have a shape reminiscent of certain cells in the central nervous system. They have numerous branching processes, called dendrites, that radiate from the cell body. These extend between keratinocytes of the stratum basale. Melanin is assembled by their Golgi complex into ellipsoidal granules, 1 μm in length, and 0.4 μm in width, called **melanosomes**. When newly formed, these have a characteristic fine structure consisting of longitudinally oriented parallel filaments with a 10 nm periodicity. This substructure is obliterated, in mature granules, by accumulation of dense melanin pigment on the filaments. Vesicles containing multiple melanosomes are pinched off from the tips of the melanocyte dendrites, and these fuse with the plasmalemma of neighboring keratinocytes, transferring melanosomes to their cytoplasm (Fig. 11.4). This unusual process is called **cytocrine secretion**. A melanocyte, and its surrounding epidermal cells, collectively constitute an **epidermal–melanin unit**. Owing to their continual transfer of melanosomes, the melanocytes may contain less melanin than the keratinocytes of the epidermal–melanin unit.

The number of melanocytes varies in different regions of the body. They may be as few as 1000/mm^2 on the arms and thighs, and as many as 4000/mm^2 on the face and neck. Racial differences in color are not attributable to differing numbers of melanocytes, but to differences in the amount of melanin they produce and transfer. In Caucasians, the melanosomes are largely confined to the cells of the stratum basale. In Negroids, the melanosomes are somewhat larger, more numerous, and are found in keratinocytes throughout the epidermis. The darkening of the skin of Caucasians upon prolonged exposure to the sun, is a result of stimulation of additional melanin synthesis by ultraviolet light.

Limited exposure to sunlight is beneficial, for a precursor of vitamin D in the skin is converted in the liver to the active form of the vitamin. Chronic exposure to excess solar ultraviolet radiation may damage the DNA, leading to **basal cell carcinoma** or to **malignant melanoma**. Melanin pigment is protective against ultraviolet irradiation and, therefore, blacks are at much lower risk of developing these malignancies.

Langerhans cells

The **Langerhans** cell is a solitary cell type widely distributed in the epidermis. It is stellate in form and has a heterochromatic nucleus

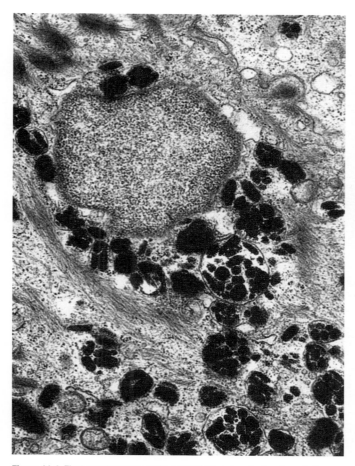

Figure 11.4 Electron micrograph of the perinuclear region of a keratinocyte from stratum spinosum of human skin, showing clusters of melanosomes, received from a melanocyte.

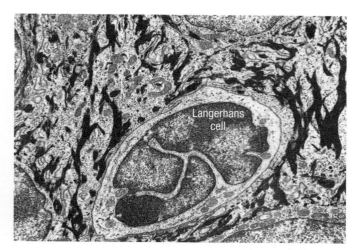

Figure 11.5 Electron micrograph of a Langerhans cell, surrounded by keratinocytes containing dense bundles of keratin filaments. Notice the polymorphous nucleus. The cell processes characteristic of this cell type are not in the plane of this thin section. (Micrograph courtesy of G. Szabo.)

Merkel cells

Small numbers of **Merkel cells** are found in the basal layer of the epidermis over the entire body (Fig. 11.6). They are more abundant in areas such as the fingertips, which have an important role in sensory reception. The naked terminals of myelinated afferent nerves end in apposition to these cells, forming **Merkel cell–neurite complexes**. The long axis of the Merkel cells is usually parallel to the basal lamina and their cell processes extend between overlying keratinocytes, to which they may be attached by desmosomes. The nucleus is deeply invaginated and the cytoplasm contains many dense-cored granules 80–130 nm in diameter, and intermediate filaments of keratins K8, K18, and K19, which differ from those of the surrounding keratinocytes. It is postulated that the Merkel cell–neurite complexes have a mechanoreceptor function sensing pressure, but this has yet to be firmly established. Merkel cells also occur in the epithelium of the oral mucosa.

of irregular shape, surrounded by a pale-staining cytoplasm. On electron micrographs, the cytoplasm is of low density and contains few mitochondria and little endoplasmic reticulum (Fig. 11.5). Langerhans cells contain small membrane-bounded granules of unusual shape, called **Birbeck granules**. These are discoid in form, but appear in section as rodlike profiles 15–50 nm in length and about 4 nm in thickness. Langerhans cells can be distinguished from keratinocytes by their irregular nuclear shape, their lack of bundles of keratin filaments, and the absence of desmosomes binding them to neighboring cells. They are usually located in the upper layers of the stratum spinosum. They may number as high as 800/mm^2 and make up 3–8% of the cell population of the epithelium. They arise from precursors in the bone marrow, and are transported in the blood to the dermis, and migrate from there into the epidermis.

The Langerhans cells participate in the body's immune responses. They have surface markers and receptors similar to those of T-lymphocytes and macrophages. They bind the Fc portion of IgG, IgA, and the C3 component of complement. At sites of allergic contact dermatitis, they are believed to take up antigen and present it to lymphocytes in a form to which they can react by generation of antibodies. Langerhans cells occur in other stratified squamous epithelia, including those of the oral cavity, esophagus, and vagina.

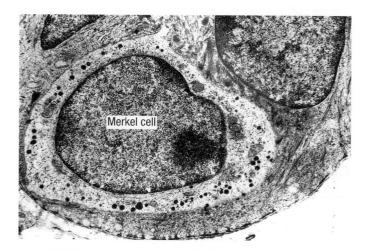

Figure 11.6 Electron micrograph of a Merkel cell near the base of human epidermis. The pale cytoplasm and small dense secretory granules are features characteristic of this cell type.

MUCOCUTANEOUS JUNCTIONS

At the transitions from skin to the mucous membrane lining the mouth and anus, the stratified squamous epithelium has a very thin stratum corneum. Hairs, sebaceous glands, and sweat glands are absent. Owing to the thinness of the stratum corneum, the color of the blood in the underlying capillary bed of the dermis shows through the epithelium, giving mucocutaneous junctions, such as the lips, a red color.

DERMIS

The **dermis** is a tough layer of connective tissue immediately beneath the epidermis, which makes up the greater part of the thickness of the skin. It ranges in thickness from 0.6 mm, in the thin skin of the eyelids, to 3 mm or more, on the palms and soles of the feet. The dermis is usually thinner in women than in men. The interface between the dermis and epidermis is very irregular in contour and varies greatly from region to region (compare Figs 11.1 and 11.3).

In thick skin, the complexity of the dermis is apparent in scanning micrographs of dermis from which the epithelium has been separated by immersion in a calcium-chelating agent (Fig. 11.7). In such preparations, the upper surface of the dermis exhibits a pattern of **primary ridges** separated by deep **primary grooves**, which were formerly occupied by thickenings of the lower zones of the epidermis, inappropriately called interpapillary 'pegs' before

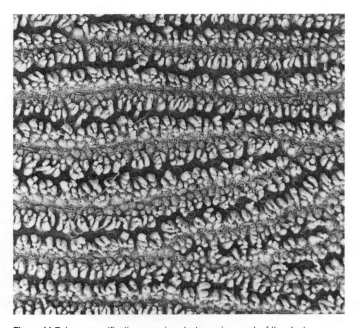

Figure 11.7 Low-magnification scanning electron micrograph of the plantar dermis, after removal of the epidermis. The primary ridges of the dermis are separated by clefts that appear as dark horizontal lines. On each ridge there are two rows of dermal papillae separated by a shallow groove. (Micrograph reproduced from D.K. MacCallum *Anat Res* 1985; 711:142.)

their true form was revealed by scanning microscopy. In the midline of each primary ridge, there is a shallow **secondary groove**, which divides it into two **secondary ridges**. Rows of conical **dermal papillae**, 0.1–0.2 mm in height, project upwards from these secondary ridges, occupying conforming concavities in the underside of the epidermis (Fig. 11.8A,B). The papillae, which number about 80/mm², occur in groups of three to five and share a common base. Regularly spaced, dark circular areas seen in the floor of the primary grooves (Fig. 11.8B) are the openings of channels that were occupied by the ducts of sweat glands, which were pulled out of the dermis in the removal of the epidermis during specimen preparation.

In thin skin, lacking a pattern of dermatoglyphs on its outer surface, the configuration of the dermo-epidermal junction is much simpler than that described above for thick skin. The dermal papillae are shorter, broader, and fewer, and they are not arranged in rows corresponding to ridges on the skin surface, as they are in the thick skin of the palm.

Two layers are identified in the dermis: the superficial **papillary layer**, just described, and a deeper **reticular layer**. In the papillary layer fibroblasts are widely distributed among interlacing thin bundles of type III collagen fibers, and a loose network of elastic fibers. This layer contains many capillaries. The thicker, reticular layer of the dermis is made up of closely packed, coarser bundles of type II collagen fibers. The space between fiber bundles is occupied by amorphous extracellular matrix rich in dermatan sulfate and other glycosaminoglycans. Cell types other than fibroblasts include macrophages, lymphocytes, and mast cells.

SUBCUTANEOUS TISSUE

The **subcutaneous tissue** (or **hypodermis**), deep to the reticular layer of the dermis, is a loose connective tissue in which the bundles of collagen fibers are oriented mainly parallel to the skin surface. In some regions, this layer permits movement of the skin over the underlying structures. In others, collagen fibers of the dermis extending down into the subcutaneous connective tissue are more abundant and the skin is relatively immobile. Adipose cells tend to accumulate in the subcutaneous tissue on the abdomen and buttocks, and may reach a thickness of 3 cm or more. Where this has occurred, this subcutaneous layer of adipose cells is called the **panniculus adiposus**.

SKIN APPENDAGES

Hairs

Hairs develop in deep invaginations of the epidermis, called **hair follicles**. These extend downwards into the dermis, and sometimes a short distance into the subcutaneous tissue (Fig. 11.9). Although humans appear to be largely hairless, the number of hairs on the human body does not differ appreciably from the number on

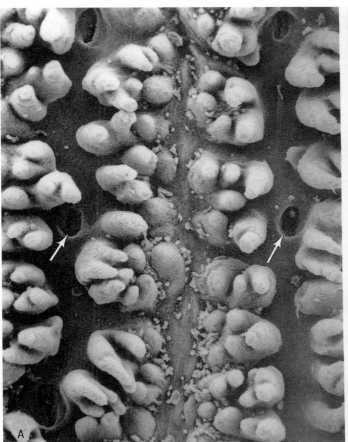 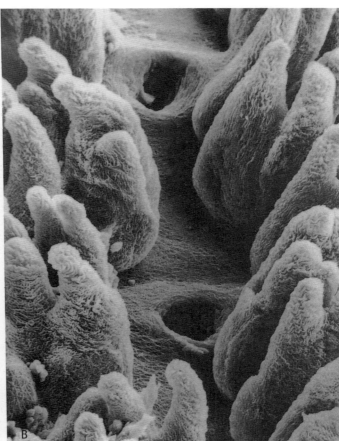

Figure 11.8 (A) Scanning electron micrograph of a primary ridge of the dermis. In the grooves between primary ridges are openings that were occupied by ducts of sweat glands. (B) An oblique view along one of the grooves, at higher magnification, showing more clearly the shapes of the papillae and the openings for the ducts. (Micrograph reproduced from D. MacCallum *Anat Rec* 1985; 711:142.)

other primates. Over much of the body, however, the hairs are very small and colorless and are not noticeable. Hairs are absent only on the palms and soles, the lateral aspect of the feet, the glans penis, clitoris, and the labia minora. There are about 800 hairs/mm² on the face, but on the rest of the body they number only about 60/mm². On the eyelids, no hairs other than the eyelashes project beyond their follicle, but on the head (Fig. 11.10) hairs may grow to well over 1 m in length.

An active hair follicle has a terminal expansion called the **hair bulb**. On its underside, there is a deep recess occupied by a **papilla** of dermal connective tissue (Fig. 11.11). Nutrients diffusing from capillaries of the papilla are essential for normal hair growth and the cells of the papilla have inductive properties that influence the mitotic and synthetic activities of cells in the hair follicle. The epithelial cells of the follicle, adjacent to the papilla, are comparable to those of the stratum basale of the epidermis. Among them are a few large melanocytes whose long dendrites contribute melanosomes to the cells that will form the cortex of the hair. The graying of hair in old age is attributed to a gradual loss in the capacity of these melanocytes to synthesize melanin.

The epithelial cells of the hair bulb around the papilla proliferate and differentiate to form the hair. The cells immediately above the apex of the papilla give rise to highly vacuolated cells that form its **medulla**. Proliferation and differentiation of cells lateral to

these give rise to heavily keratinized cells that make up the **hair cortex**. Lateral to these are cells that form the **hair cuticle**. The cells of this latter layer are initially cuboidal, but higher up the shaft they become highly keratinized, and are transformed into overlapping, flat, shingle-like cells oriented with their free edges directed downwards. Closer to the periphery of the bulb are cells that form an **internal root sheath**, surrounding the proximal part of the hair shaft. The outermost layer of cells in the bulb form the **external root sheath**. This is only one cell thick around the bulb, but becomes several cells thick higher on the hair shaft. This layer of cells is continuous with the stratum basale of the epidermis. In severely burned patients, the epidermis may be slowly regenerated by proliferation of stem cells present in the external root sheath, a short distance above the hair bulb. The hair follicle is surrounded by a condensation of the fibrous components of the dermis. Interposed between these and the epithelium of the external root sheath is an acellular **vitreous layer** (glassy layer), which seems to be an exceptionally thick basal lamina of the epithelium of the external root sheath.

Hair growth is cyclical, and three phases of the cycle are recognized: the **growth phase**, **regression phase**, and **resting phase** (Fig. 11.12). On the human scalp, the growth phase may last for 2–6 years, the regressing phase for 2–3 weeks, and the resting phase for 3–4 months. After the resting phase, the old hair is shed and a

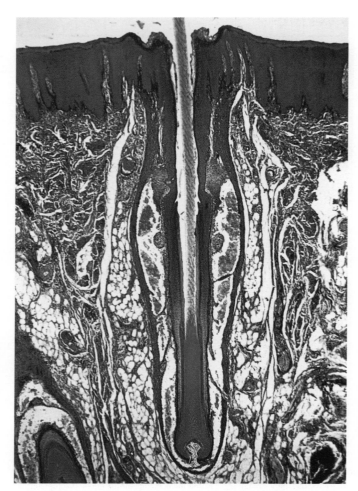

Figure 11.9 Photomicrograph of a hair follicle extending into the dermis. The red-staining layer around the hair shaft is the external root sheath, the blue layer outside of it is the vitreous layer. (Micrograph courtesy of Dr Pietro Motta, University of Rome La Sapienza.)

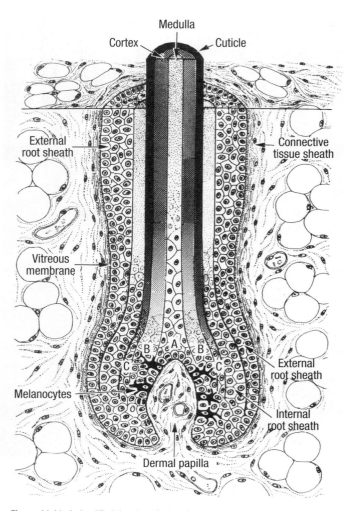

Figure 11.11 A simplified drawing of a hair follicle. The expanded lower end of the bulb contains a dermal papilla. The cells over the papilla (A) give rise to the medulla of the hair. (B) Cells lateral to these form the hair cortex. (C) Those on its sides form the hair cuticle. (Redrawn after L.C. Junquiera *et al. Basic Histology*, Lange Medical Publications, Norwalk, Connecticut.)

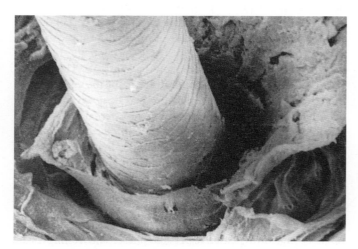

Figure 11.10 Scanning electron micrograph of a hair emerging from the human scalp. Notice the exfoliating cornified epidermal cells around the hair shaft. (Micrograph courtesy of T. Fujita.)

new hair shaft is formed. The bulb of the hair follicle undergoes considerable atrophy during the regression and resting phases (Fig. 11.12B) but is restored at the beginning of the next growth phase.

Bound to the connective tissue sheath of the hair follicle are one or more bundles of smooth muscle fibers, forming the **arrector pili muscle** (Fig. 11.12A). These muscle fibers run diagonally upwards, from the follicle to the papillary layer of the dermis. In animals with a dense coat of hair, their contraction serves to erect the hairs, increasing the efficiency of the fur as a thermal barrier. In the human, their contraction, in response to cold, results in slight depressions of the skin over their sites of attachment to the dermis, and elevation of the site of emergence of the hair. This results in a roughening of the surface commonly described as 'goose-flesh'.

Nails

Nails are plates of closely compacted hard keratin, formed by proliferation and keratinization of epithelial cells in a **nail matrix**,

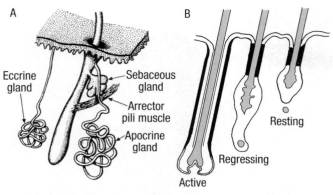

Figure 11.12 (A) Hair follicle and its associated glands, and arrector pili muscle. (B) Hair follicle in various phases of its growth cycle.

which is comparable to the hair matrix but simpler in its organization. The **nail root** and its matrix are located under a fold of skin, called the **proximal nail fold** (Fig. 11.13). The stratum corneum of the epidermis on this fold may extend for 0.3–1.0 mm onto the upper surface of the nail, forming a thin covering called the **eponychium**. Where the surface of **lateral nail folds** turns inwards into the **lateral nail grooves**, their epidermis loses its stratum corneum and continues under the nail plate as the **nail bed**. There, the epidermis consists of a stratum basale and stratum spinosum, with the fingernail replacing the stratum corneum. It is continuous proximally with the **nail matrix** that extends some distance under the proximal nail fold. Growth of the nail from the nail matrix slides the nail over the epidermis of the nail bed, which makes no contribution to its formation. The anterior portion of the nail matrix can be seen through the nail as an opaque, white crescent called the **lunula**.

As in the hair matrix, the cells of the nail matrix synthesize large amounts of keratin. As the cells of the matrix are incorporated into the nail root, they are transformed into extremely flat, anuclear structures consisting of keratin embedded in a hard interfibrillar matrix. Nails grow at a rate of about 0.5 mm per week. Fingernails grow about four times as fast as toenails.

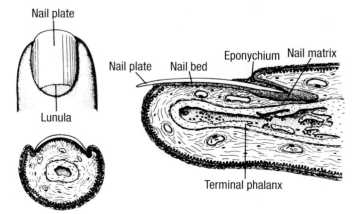

Figure 11.13 Drawing of a fingernail, nail bed, nail matrix and associated structures.

Sebaceous glands

Sebaceous glands are appendages of the hair follicles and are found throughout the dermis, except where hairs are lacking on the palms, soles, and sides of the feet. One or two are associated with each hair follicle (Figs 11.12A, 11.14). The sebaceous glands number 400–800/cm² on the face, forehead, and scalp, but over the rest of the body their numbers are very much lower. The glands are 0.2–2.0 mm in diameter and are located above the origin of the arrector pili muscle. Their duct opens into the follicular canal around the hair shaft. Their secretion, called **sebum**, is a mixture of triglycerides, cholesterol, and waxes. It is thought to maintain the soft texture of thin skin and the flexibility of the hairs.

Sebaceous glands have several small lobules made up of elongated subunits that are continuous with a short duct. These so-called acini have no lumen. The cells near the basal lamina are relatively small, with round nuclei and a cytoplasm containing both rough and smooth endoplasmic reticulum, abundant glycogen, and numerous small lipid droplets. The secretion of the gland is not a liquid. Production of sebum involves loss of whole cells and their content, and is, therefore, an example of **holocrine secretion**. Cells nearest to the duct die and break down, and sebum consists of their lipid content and residues of their cytoplasm. The cells more centrally situated in the acini are in various stages of degeneration, with pycnotic nuclei and coalescing lipid droplets. The ducts of the gland are lined by stratified squamous epithelium, which is continuous with that lining the hair follicle.

At puberty, the level of circulating androgens rises, resulting in increased secretion of sebum. This increase favors the development of **acne vulgaris**, a common skin problem of teenagers. Small papules and cysts (comedones) form on the face and chest due to blockage of the orifice of hair follicles. Bacteria in the cysts release free fatty acids from the impounded sebum, causing inflammation and ultimate rupture of the cyst wall. The condition is self-limiting, but antibiotics may be used to minimize the local inflammatory reaction. Acne is less common in girls, for estrogens tend to decrease sebum production.

Eccrine sweat glands

Eccrine sweat glands are widely distributed throughout the skin. They are coiled tubular glands, with their secretory portion deep in the dermis, or in the hypodermis. Their slender duct ascends through these layers to open at a **sweat pore** on the surface of the skin. The secretory portion of the gland is lined by cuboidal, or low columnar, epithelium containing two cell types, designated **light cells** (clear cells), and **dark cells**, on the basis of their appearance in stained histological sections. Between the epithelium and its basal lamina are **myoepithelial cells** that contract to press the secretion out of the gland. The light cells are pyramidal in form, with their base in contact with the basal lamina between myoepithelial cells (Fig. 11.15). As in other cells involved in transepithelial fluid transport, the plasmalemma at the cell base is elaborately infolded. The egress of their secretion is via intercellular canaliculi that open into

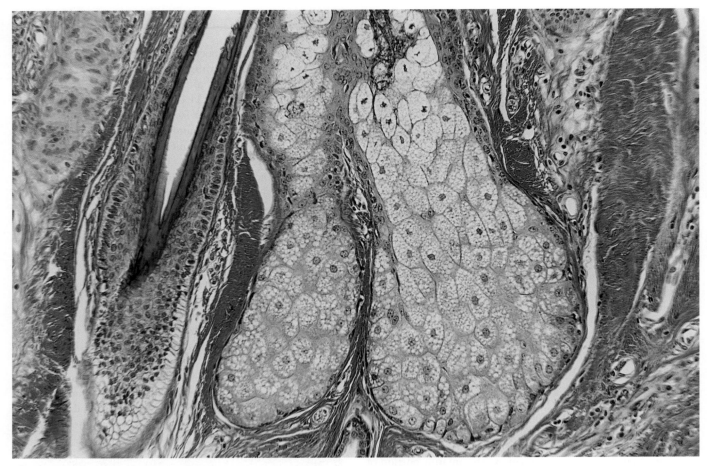

Figure 11.14 Photomicrograph of an oblique section of a hair follicle (at left) and two lobes of its associated sebaceous gland.

the duct. Their cytoplasm is rich in glycogen, but contains no secretory granules. The dark cells have the form of inverted pyramids with a broad adlumenal end tapering down to a slender ablumenal end, that does not reach the basal lamina. They have a small, dark-staining nucleus, a prominent Golgi complex, long mitochondria, and a few cisternae of rER. The apical cytoplasm contains many moderately dense secretory granules. The chemical composition of the granules is not known, but the fact that they stain suggests that their content is glycoprotein in nature. The long duct of the gland is lined by an epithelium consisting of two layers of cuboidal cells. The cells adjacent to the basal lamina have a comparatively large heterochromatic nucleus and abundant mitochondria. Those bordering on the lumen have an irregularly shaped nucleus and relatively little cytoplasm, containing few organelles. There is a conspicuous terminal web beneath their apical plasmalemma.

Because of the wide spacing of the eccrine sweat glands, in histological sections, there is a tendency to underestimate their total mass and their physiological importance. They number between 3 and 4 million, and their aggregate weight is roughly equivalent to that of a kidney. Humans engaged in vigorous physical activity, in a warm environment, may perspire as much as 10 liters a day (Fig. 11.16). This volume of secretion exceeds that of some of the largest exocrine glands.

Apocrine sweat glands

A second kind of sweat gland, the **apocrine sweat glands**, are found in the skin of the axilla, on the mons pubis, and in the circumanal region. These glands are located deep in the dermis, and are larger than the eccrine sweat glands. Their mode of secretion is actually merocrine. Their original designation as 'apocrine' was based on an artifact of specimen preparation, but, unfortunately, the name has persisted. As in sebaceous glands, their duct opens in the canal of a hair follicle. The secretory portion of the tubular gland is lined by cells that are usually cuboidal, but they may be squamous if the gland is distended with secretion. Their apical cytoplasm contains rather large secretory granules. The chemical nature of the secretion has been little studied. It is a slightly viscous fluid that is odorless when secreted, but after modification by bacteria residing on the skin, it acquires an odor that is considered socially offensive. The secretory activity of apocrine sweat glands does not begin until puberty. In women, there is an enlargement of the cells, and of the lumen of axillary apocrine sweat glands, during the premenstrual phase of the cycle, followed by regression during menses. The apocrine sweat glands are innervated by adrenergic nerves, whereas the eccrine glands are innervated by cholinergic nerves.

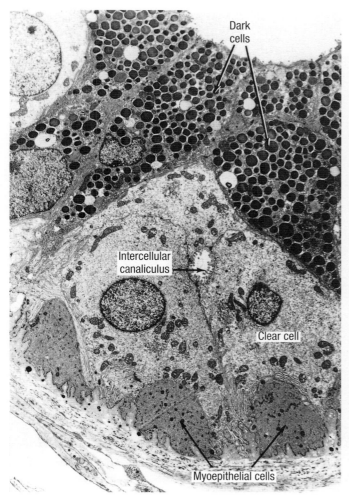

Figure 11.15 Photomicrograph of a portion of the wall of an eccrine sweat gland. Dark-staining cells lining the duct have a mucus-like secretory product. Pale serous cells are more deeply situated in the epithelium. The secretion of the latter is released into intercellular canaliculi, which empty into the lumen.

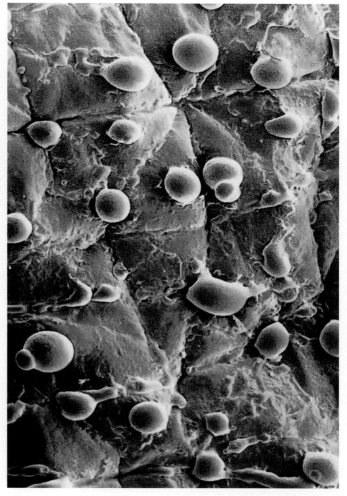

Figure 11.16 Micrograph of skin on the back of the hand after an hour of exercise, showing droplets of sweat emerging from the sudoriporous glands (color added). (R. Wehr and Custom Medical Stock Photo.)

BLOOD VESSELS AND LYMPHATICS

The skin receives its blood from vessels in the subcutaneous tissue. Ascending branches of these ramify to form a plexus, the **rete cutaneum**, at the boundary between the dermis and hypodermis. Ascending branches from this rete form a second plexus, the **rete subpapillare**, in the papillary layer of the dermis. Its branches form a capillary network in each dermal papilla, around the sebaceous glands, and around the sheath of the hair follicle. The capillaries of the dermis drain into a venous **rete subpapillare** and then to a venous rete associated with the rete cutaneum. There are numerous **arteriovenous anastomoses** in the system, which are of physiological importance in controlling blood flow to the skin and thus varying the amount of heat lost to the environment.

A blind-ending lymphatic capillary from each dermal papilla joins a lymphatic plexus below the dermo-epidermal junction. From there, branches descend to a deeper lymphatic plexus associated with the rete cutaneum. Larger lymphatics, possessing valves, arise from this plexus and follow the course of the veins through the subcutaneous tissue.

NERVES

Free endings

Abundant efferent nerves activate the glands of the skin and control blood flow by changing the caliber of its small arteries. There are also many afferent sensory nerves with a variety of endings. Unspecialized **free endings** penetrate the epidermis and terminate in the stratum granulosum. These free endings are thought to sense pain or temperature. The axons of other myelinated nerves end in disk-like expansions, called **Merkel endings**, that are in contact with Merkel cells at the base of the epithelium. Their function is still unknown.

Encapsulated endings

There are also sensory nerves with more complex encapsulated endings. **Pacinian corpuscles** in the dermis and hypodermis are ovoid structures up to 1 mm in length. The axon of a myelinated nerve penetrates into the core of the corpuscle, where it is surrounded by 20–60 concentric lamellae consisting of very thin, flat cells separated by narrow spaces that are filled with a gelatinous material. The corpuscle resembles an onion in cross-section (Fig. 11.17).

Meissner's corpuscles are pear-shaped structures made up of flattened cells oriented transversely, resulting in a ladder-like appearance in section. The nerve axon loses its sheath, enters one pole of the corpuscle, and pursues a spiral or zigzag course among the flat cells in its interior. Meissner's corpuscles are found in occasional dermal papillae (Fig. 11.18). Such endings are probably mechanoreceptors sensing slight deformation of the skin.

Kraus's end-bulbs are small spheroidal bodies in the papillary layer of the dermis. They bear a superficial resemblance to Pacinian corpuscles, but are much smaller and lack concentric lamellae. Their sensory modality is unclear.

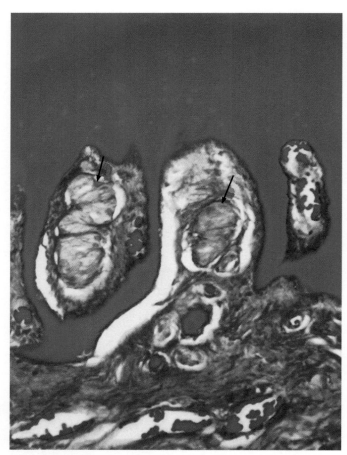

Figure 11.18 A slightly oblique section of thick skin, including the epidermis above (red) and the dermis below (blue). Notice that two of the dermal papillae are occupied by Meissner's corpuscles (arrowed).

HISTOPHYSIOLOGY OF SKIN

The skin has many functions. In humans, it lacks the thick fur, feathers, scales, or spines found on some other creatures, but it still has a significant protective function. The heavy keratinization of the stratum corneum provides some degree of protection against mechanical damage. The lipid-rich intercellular material, in and above the stratum spinosum, prevents loss of fluid and electrolytes and bars entry of toxins from the environment. The rich innervation of the skin, with endings sensitive to touch, pain, heat, cold, and pressure, protects us by initiating evasive action. Skin protects against the harmful effects of excessive solar irradiation by increasing the number of melanosomes that absorb or scatter light. Constantly exposed to large numbers of bacteria, the skin is an effective mechanical barrier to their entry. If they do reach the deeper layers of the skin, the Langerhans cells are there to present antigen to lymphocytes, which respond by producing protective antibodies. Although the number of lymphocytes observed in the epidermis seems small, their total number in this large organ is probably nearly as great as their number in the blood. In bacterial infections of skin, the basal keratinocytes also participate in generation of immune responses by

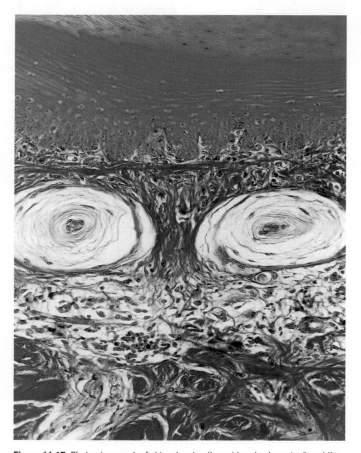

Figure 11.17 Photomicrograph of skin, showing the epidermis above (red) and the dermis below (blue). In the dermis, there are two Pacinian corpuscles. Notice the concentric layers around the nerve ending. (Reproduced from W.A. Ewing *Inside Information. Imaging the Human Body*, Simon and Schuster, New York.)

producing the cytokine interleukin-I, which induces lymphocyte proliferation, and by secreting another cytokine that promotes their activation.

Skin is a major agent of temperature regulation. When the ambient temperature is higher than normal body temperature, evaporation is the only method of heat dissipation subject to physiological control. It depends on enhanced secretory activity of some 3 million sweat glands. An elevated ambient temperature also results in vasodilation of superficial vessels and opening of arteriovenous anastomoses to conduct more of the deep body heat to the surface. In a hot environment, cutaneous blood flow may increase to 2–3 L/m^2 per minute. When exposed to extreme cold, vasoconstriction and closure of arteriovenous anastomoses may reduce flow to 50 ml/m^2 per minute.

Questions

1 The epidermis contains
   a blood vessels
   b lymphatics
   c free nerve endings
   d Meissner's corpuscles
   e all of the above

2 Which of the following is not a layer of the epidermis?
   a stratum corneum
   b stratum reticularis
   c stratum granulosum
   d stratum basale
   e stratum spinosum

3 Myoepithelial cells are most commonly associated with
   a hair follicles
   b Langerhans cells
   c arteriovenous shunts
   d eccrine sweat glands
   e melanocytes

4 Which of the following terms relates most closely to cytocrine secretion in the epidermis?
   a keratinization
   b Langerhans cells
   c cytomorphosis
   d granulocytes
   e melanocytes

5 Which statement best describes the stratum spinosum?
   a it is in contact with the basal lamina
   b it lies between the stratum basale and stratum granulosum
   c it is easily seen because of its granular appearance
   d it is the layer in which the majority of melanocytes are located
   e it contains a heavy concentration of keratohyalin

6 Which of the following cells is part of the immune system?
   a Langerhans cell
   b Malpighian cell
   c Merkel cell
   d melanocyte
   e keratinocyte

7 The majority of the cells of the epidermis are
   a reticular cells
   b melanocytes
   c Langerhans cells
   d fibroblasts
   e keratinocytes

8 The layer of the epidermis that typically appears as a single cell layer of mitotically active basophilic cells is the
   a stratum spinosum
   b stratum granulosum
   c stratum corneum
   d stratum germinativum
   e stratum lucidum

9 The connective tissue counterpart to epidermal ridges are
   a papillae
   b glands
   c epithelial projections
   d rete subpapillare
   e panniculus adiposus

10 Hemidesmosomes are found in which epidermal layer?
   a stratum corneum
   b stratum lucidum
   c stratum basale
   d stratum spinosum
   e stratum granulosum

11 What layer is greatly thickened in palmar and plantar skin?

12 Where are rete subpapillare located?

13 Blood vessels are not found in what layer of the skin?

14 What structure is responsible for raising hair to a vertical position?

15 What layer of the epidermis contains hemidesmosomes?

16 In the epidermis, what cytoplasmic structure contains pigment?

17 What type of cell constitutes the majority of cells of the epidermis?

18 What are epidermal projections into the dermis called?

19 Birbeck bodies are found in what type of skin cell?

20 In what layer of the epidermis do the cells contain a great abundance of irregularly shaped intracellular bodies that stain intensely with basic dyes?

Chapter twelve

Oral Cavity

The digestive tract, or alimentary canal, includes the oral cavity, esophagus, stomach, duodenum, small intestine, colon, rectum, and anus. Each of these is specialized for its particular role in the processing and absorption of nutrients to meet the energy needs of the body. In the **oral cavity**, the food is mechanically fragmented by the teeth, chemically modified by secretions of the salivary glands, and lubricated for its passage through the esophagus to the stomach. The oral cavity is bounded, above by the hard and soft palate, laterally by the cheeks, and below by the tongue and floor of the mouth. It is lined by stratified squamous epithelium throughout, but this epithelium varies from region to region in its thickness and degree of keratinization. On the floor of the mouth and underside of the tongue, it is thin and mobile. Where it is reflected onto the alveolar processes of the upper and lower jaw to form the gingiva (gums), it is thick and firmly fixed to the periosteum of the underlying bone. On the dorsum of the tongue, the inner surface of the cheeks, and on the palate, it is moderately thick and heavily keratinized to withstand the abrasion to which these regions are subjected during mastication of food. There are many small glands in the submucosa of the palate, cheeks, and floor of the mouth that continually secrete mucus to keep the oral cavity moist, and to facilitate movement of food over its surfaces.

TONGUE

The tongue is made up of longitudinal, horizontal and vertical bundles of striated muscle fibers that provide the wide range of mobility required for speech, chewing, and swallowing. The epithelium on the rough upper surface of the tongue is covered with a multitude of small projections called the **lingual papillae**. These are of four kinds: **filiform**, **fungiform**, **circumvallate**, and **foliate**.

Lingual papillae

Filiform papillae are slender, conical projections of the epithelium, 2–3 mm in length, with their tips pointing towards the back of the tongue (Fig. 12.1). They are the most numerous of the lingual papillae, covering most of the upper surface of the tongue. The heavily keratinized cells at their tips are continuously exfoliated.

Fungiform papillae, 0.3–1.0 mm in diameter, have a relatively narrow base and a hemispherical upper portion. They are widely

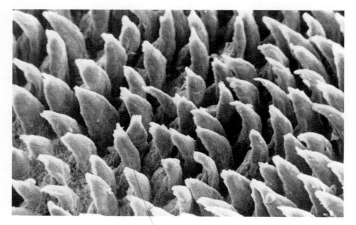

Figure 12.1 Scanning electron micrograph of filiform papillae on the surface of the tongue of a rabbit. The form of these papillae on the human tongue is similar.

scattered among the filiform papillae. They have a connective tissue core and **taste buds** in the epithelium on their sides.

Circumvallate papillae number only 6–14 and are confined to the posterior portion of the tongue. They are 1–2 mm in diameter and are thus considerably larger than the fungiform papillae. Each is surrounded by a circular furrow, or sulcus (Figs. 12.2, 12.3). On its free surface, the squamous epithelium is smooth and unspecialized. That on the sides contains taste buds, estimated to number 60–100 on each papilla. In the underlying submucosa, there are small serous glands, the **glands of von Ebner** (Fig. 12.3). Their ducts open into the sulcus around the circumvallate papilla, and their secretion keeps the sulcus rinsed.

Foliate papillae are well developed in many mammals, but are rudimentary in the human. They are located on the sides of the tongue and consist of several parallel ridges separated by intervening clefts. The ducts of small serous glands in the underlying connective tissue open into the clefts between ridges. Taste buds are numerous on the sides of the ridges.

Taste buds

The taste buds are small neurosensory bodies in the epithelium of the fungiform and circumvallate papillae. There are about 3000 on

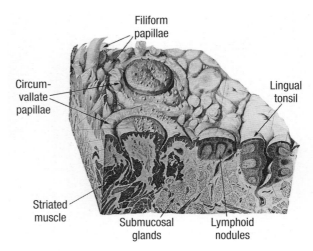

Figure 12.2 Drawing of an area of the surface of the tongue including two circumvallate papillae. Also shown, in section, germinal centers of lymphoid tissue (lingual tonsil). (Drawing modified after H. Braus *Anatomie des Menschen*, Springer Verlag, Berlin, 1924.)

the human tongue. They appear as pale, ovoid bodies, 50–80 μm in height and 39–50 μm in width (Figs 12.3, 12.4.) They consist of 50–75 cells, with tapering apices that converge on a small depression in the surface of the epithelium called the **taste pore**. Three types

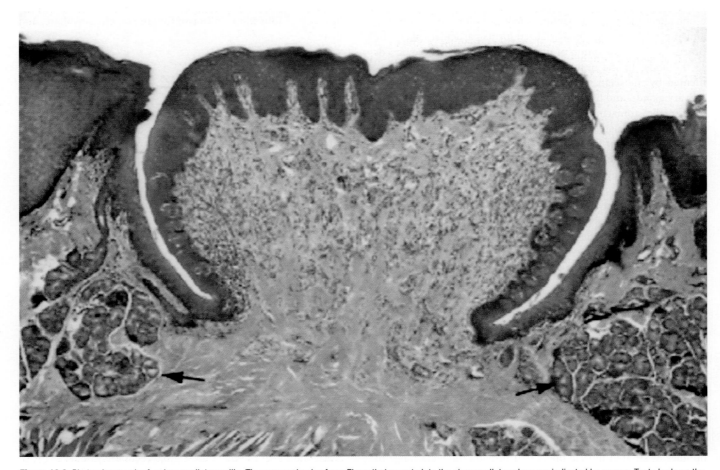

Figure 12.3 Photomicrograph of a circumvallate papilla. The serous glands of von Ebner that secrete into the circumvallate sulcus are indicated by arrows. Taste buds on the sides of the papilla are shown at higher magnification in Fig. 12.4.

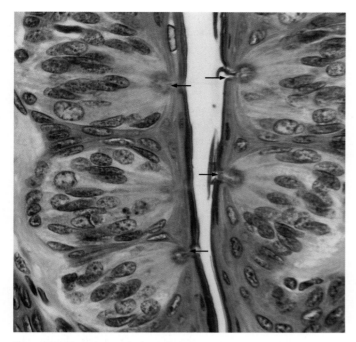

Figure 12.4 Photomicrograph of taste buds in the epithelium on both sides of the sulcus surrounding a circumvallate papilla. Taste pores are indicated by arrows.

of cell are distinguishable by differences in their staining properties. Slender, **dark cells** (**type I** cells) at the periphery of the bud have microvilli that project into the taste pore. Their cytoplasm is rich in fine filaments and contains small secretory granules of unknown chemical nature. The **light cells** (**type II** cells) are less numerous and have a cytoplasm containing some smooth endoplasmic reticulum (sER) and relatively few filaments. Central to these are paler cells (**type III** cells). On electron micrographs of type III cells, the cytoplasm contains longitudinally oriented microtubules and some sER. In the basal cytoplasm are small vesicles, resembling synaptic vesicles. There is a single club-shaped apical process that projects into the taste pore. This unusual apical structure, and the presence of small vesicles near nerve axons that penetrate the epithelium, have fostered the belief that this cell type is the principal taste receptor, but this is disputed. Near the basal lamina are small dark cells, which are interpreted as being stem cells, capable of differentiating into any of the other cell types of the taste bud.

There are four basic tastes: sweet, bitter, sour, and salty. Physiologists have postulated four kinds of taste buds corresponding to these flavors, however, histologists can find only one kind.

Nerve axons form a plexus around each taste bud, sending branches inward between the cells. In the anterior portion of the tongue, gustatory sensation is transmitted over the chorda tympani branch of the **facial nerve** (cranial nerve VII). In the posterior portion of the tongue, the taste buds are innervated by the lingual branch of the **glossopharyngeal nerve** (cranial nerve IX).

LYMPHOID TISSUE

The oral cavity is continuous posteriorly with the **pharynx**, the chamber through which air passes from the nasal cavity to the larynx, and food passes from the oral cavity to the esophagus. On either side, at the transition from oral cavity to pharynx, there are large subepithelial accumulations of lymphoid tissue forming the **palatine tonsils**. A smaller accumulation of lymphoid tissue, on the back of the tongue, constitutes the **lingual tonsil**, and another, on the posterior wall of the pharynx, is the **pharyngeal tonsil**. These form a ring of lymphoid tissue encircling the passage from the oral cavity to the trachea and esophagus. Collectively, these four lymphoid organs have traditionally been referred to as **Waldeyer's ring**.

The stratified squamous epithelium over the pharyngeal tonsil is deeply invaginated to form 15 or more **tonsillar crypts**. A thin connective tissue capsule surrounds the tonsil on its lateral aspects, with thin partitions extending from it into the lymphoid tissue. Mast cells and plasma cells abound in this connective tissue. Infiltrating polymorphonuclear leukocytes become very numerous when the tonsils are infected (tonsillitis). Immediately beneath the epithelium lining the crypts are many closely spaced lymphoid nodules, resembling those in lymph nodes. The space between them is occupied by diffuse lymphoid tissue. The lumen of the crypts contains many lymphocytes, exfoliated epithelial cells, bacteria, and cellular debris. Semisolid masses of this material may accumulate in the crypts, resulting in chronic infection of the tonsils. The pharyngeal tonsils, and other components of the peripharyngeal ring of lymphoid tissue, reach their greatest development in childhood and begin to involute at, or before, puberty.

TEETH

The adult human has 32 permanent teeth, of which 16 are in the alveolar arch of the maxilla, and 16 are in the alveolar arch of the mandible. These are preceded by a set of 20 **deciduous teeth**, which are shed at various times between the ages of 6 and 16 years and are gradually replaced by the four incisors, two canines, four premolars, and six molars that make up the adult dentition. Each of these types of teeth has a distinctive shape, adapted to its specific function. Thus, the chisel-like **incisors** are specialized for cutting or shearing; the pointed **canines**, for puncturing and holding; and the **molars**, for crushing and grinding.

The portion of each tooth that projects above the gum is called the **crown**. The lower portion, the **root** (or roots), fits into a socket of conforming shape in the underlying bone (Fig. 12.5). The bulk of the tooth consists of **dentin**, which is covered over the crown by a thick layer of **enamel**. Enamel is lacking in the root, and the dentin there is covered by a thin layer of **cementum**, which is enclosed by a **periodontal membrane** that binds the root to the surrounding alveolar bone (Fig. 12.5). The crown of a tooth has a small central **pulp cavity** that continues down into each root as the **root canal**. The pulp cavity is occupied by loose connective tissue, supplied with capillaries and nerve fibers that enter through an apical foramen at the tip of each root. Teeth are studied in histological sections of decalcified material, or in thin ground sections, in which the calcium salts are retained.

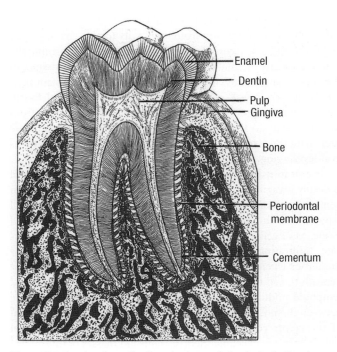

Figure 12.5 Drawing of a section through a human first molar tooth. (Drawing courtesy of I. Schour.)

Dentin

Dentin is an avascular, mineralized tissue, harder than bone but similar in composition. Of its mass, 80% is made up of crystals of **hydroxyapatite**, and 20% is organic matter, mainly type I collagen and glycosaminoglycans. During tooth development, **predentin** is secreted around long apical processes of cells called **odontoblasts**. Subsequent deposition of hydroxyapatite crystals in the predentin around these processes forms the **dentinal tubules**. An **odontoblast process** initially occupies each dentinal tubule, but these may withdraw in old age. In histological sections, dentin has a radially striated appearance owing to the presence of innumerable, parallel dentinal tubules that radiate from the pulp cavity towards the enamel (Fig. 12.5).

The tall columnar cell bodies of the odontoblasts line the pulp cavity, but are less closely adherent than in a typical epithelium. The nucleus is in the lower half of the cell and there is a large supranuclear Golgi complex, abundant rough endoplasmic reticulum (rER), and numerous mitochondria. The apical portion of each cell tapers down to a slender **odontoblast process** that contains mitochondria and numerous small vesicles. The vesicles fuse with the plasma membrane and discharge their content of procollagen into the surrounding matrix. The procollagen is converted extracellularly into tropocollagen which polymerizes into thin, randomly oriented collagen fibers of the predentin.

The frontier between the uncalcified predentin and the outer zone of mineralized dentin is abrupt. In mature dentin, the collagen fibers are obscured by the hydroxyapatite crystals. The latter are randomly oriented, except in the wall of the dentinal tubules, where they are oriented parallel to the long axis of the odontoblast

process. Dentin continues to be formed slowly throughout life and the pulp cavity narrows with advancing age.

Enamel

Enamel is the hardest substance in the body. Ninety-nine percent of its mass is made up of large hydroxyapatite crystals. Viewed with the light microscope, enamel consists of thin **enamel rods** (**enamel prisms**) that radiate from the dentin with a slight inclination towards the occlusal surface (the surface that contacts the opposing tooth). Around each rod is a very thin layer of organic matrix called the **prismatic rod sheath**. Each rod extends through the entire thickness of the enamel. In the small angular spaces between parallel enamel rods, there is **interrod enamel**, which is of similar composition, but its hydroxyapatite crystals are oriented differently from those of enamel rods (Fig. 12.6).

Enamel is produced by a layer of columnar cells called **ameloblasts**. These must be studied before eruption of the tooth, for this layer of cells is no longer present in mature teeth. In sections of developing teeth, the ameloblasts form an epithelium of very tall columnar cells over the outer surface of the dentin. The apex of each cell tapers down to a long conical process, called **Tome's process**. The ameloblasts have a basal nucleus and their cytoplasm contains a large supranuclear Golgi complex surrounded by multiple cisternae of rER. Associated with the Golgi complex, and in the apical Tome's process, there are numerous small, dense, secretory granules that contain **amelogenin** and **enamelin**, proteins of the organic matrix of enamel. The Tome's process of each ameloblast secretes the matrix of an enamel rod. Lateral branches of the process near its base secrete the matrix of the interrod enamel. In subsequent calcification, the hydroxyapatite crystals formed in the interrod matrix are more random in their orientation than those of the rod enamel (Fig. 12.6). When formation of the enamel is complete, the ameloblasts degenerate. Enamel is confined to the crown of the tooth, while the underlying dentin extends down to the tip of the roots.

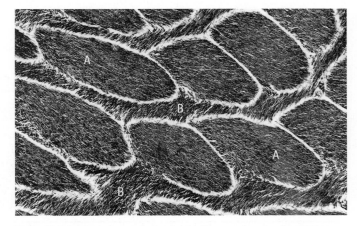

Figure 12.6 Electron micrograph of a slightly oblique section of under-calcified bovine enamel, showing at (A) the enamel rods, or prisms, and at (B) the interrod enamel. Notice the parallel orientation of the hydroxyapatite crystals in the rods and the different orientation of the crystals of the interprismatic enamel. (Micrograph courtesy of E.J. Daniel and M.J. Glimcher.)

Cementum

The dentin of the root of the tooth is covered by a thin layer of **cementum** that meets the enamel of the crown in a sharp line, the **cemento–enamel junction**, which marks the boundary between the crown and the root. Cementum is similar to bone in its composition. Its cells, called **cementocytes**, occupy lacunae with radiating canaliculi, as in bone, but there are no Haversian systems in cementum. On its outer surface is a discontinuous layer of **cementoblasts**, which are comparable to the osteoblasts found on the surface of bone. The cementum maintains close contact, and adhesion, between the root and the tooth socket.

Periodontal ligament

The roots of a tooth are enveloped by a dense layer of collagen, forming the **periodontal membrane** (or **periodontal ligament**). In this layer, interposed between the cementum and the surrounding alveolar bone, the collagen fibers run obliquely from the cementum into the alveolar bone, so that pressure on the tooth applies tension to the fibers inserting into bone. The periodontal ligament firmly anchors the tooth to its socket.

Gingiva

The **gingiva** is a thicker portion of the oral mucous membrane, which is firmly bound to the periosteum on the alveolar ridges of the maxilla and mandible. Around the base of the crown of each tooth, the gingiva is separated from the enamel by a shallow furrow, called the **gingival crevice**. In the depths of the crevice, the epithelium is bound to the enamel by an intervening layer of material resembling that of a basal lamina. The superficial squamous cells of the gingival epithelium are bound to this layer by hemidesmosomes. This seal between the epithelium and the enamel normally prevents entry of bacteria into the periodontal tissues.

> The oral cavity contains a very large and diverse population of bacteria. These adhere to teeth and gums in a thin transparent film called **plaque**. Several kinds of anaerobic bacteria in the plaque cause **dental caries** (cavities), by local destruction of enamel and dentin. This process may progress to painful infection of the tooth pulp. Bacteria may also cause **gingivitis**, a necrotizing infection of the gums immediately surrounding the teeth. This may lead to loosening of the teeth from their sockets.

Tooth development

The structure of teeth is perhaps most easily understood from studies of their mode of development. Tooth formation begins in the sixth week of gestation, when mesenchymal cells of neural crest origin aggregate at 10 sites beneath the epithelium covering the dental arches. These aggregations induce proliferation of the overlying epithelium to form **tooth buds**. At each of these, an invagination of the epithelium expands to form a cap-shaped structure connected to the surface by a stalk called the **dental lamina** (Fig. 12.7A). The epithelium on the underside of this cap thickens and invaginates further into the cap, forming the **inner enamel epithelium**. With further deepening of the concavity of the tooth bud, it takes on a bell shape (Fig. 12.7B). The outer layer of the cap (**outer dental epithelium**) remains relatively thin. The space between the outer and inner layers contains a loose network of stellate cells derived from the epithelium. At this stage the cap, as a whole, is called the **enamel organ**, for it will later form the enamel on the crown of a tooth. The rim of the bell, where the outer enamel epithelium is continuous with the inner enamel epithelium, is called the **cervical loop**. This region will later form the portion of the tooth between the crown and the root. The concavity on the underside of the bell, which is destined to form the pulp cavity of the tooth, is occupied by mesenchyme.

Late in the bell stage, the columnar cells of the inner enamel epithelium begin to differentiate into ameloblasts. This change induces mesenchymal cells, beneath the bell, to differentiate into odontoblasts. These gather on the underside of the basal lamina of the inner enamel epithelium, and begin to secrete dentin (Fig. 12.8). Activation of the odontoblasts induces the ameloblasts

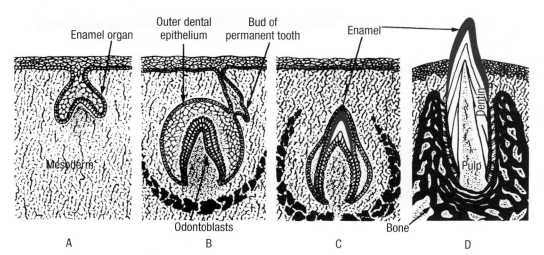

Figure 12.7 Drawing of successive stages in the development of a human deciduous tooth. (A) Early cap stage. (B) Bell stage. (C) Beginning calcification of enamel (enamel, black and dentin, white). (D) Erupted tooth. (Modified after I. Schour and S. Massler.)

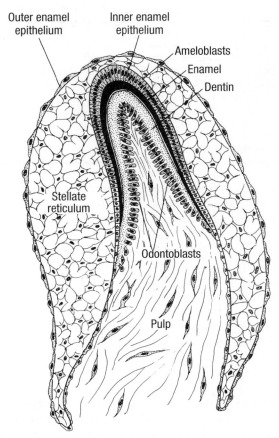

Outer enamel epithelium
Inner enamel epithelium
Ameloblasts
Enamel
Dentin
Stellate reticulum
Odontoblasts
Pulp

Figure 12.8 Drawing of the components of a lower central incisor of a 6.5 month human fetus.

to change their original polarity and begin to secrete enamel matrix at the end resting upon the basal lamina. This end is, thereafter, called the **functional apex** of the ameloblast. Progressive thickening and calcification of both enamel and dentin completes formation of the crown of the tooth. The overlying layer of ameloblasts then degenerates.

Formation of the root of the tooth depends on proliferation of cells in the cervical loop that results in elongation of the juxtaposed inner and outer dental epithelia in this region to form **Hertwig's epithelial root sheath**. As the sheath lengthens, the length of the dental papilla in its interior is increased and cells in its interior differentiate into odontoblasts. These secrete a layer of root dentin that is continuous above with the dentin of the crown. No ameloblasts are formed, hence no enamel layer is formed on the root. When the root has attained its definitive length, the root sheath breaks down and the dentin is exposed to the surrounding connective tissue. Some of its fibroblasts then differentiate into cementoblasts that deposit a layer of cementum on the outside of the root dentin.

SALIVARY GLANDS

The oral cavity contains two categories of salivary gland, **minor salivary glands** (intrinsic salivary glands), which are widely distributed

in the submucosa, and **major salivary glands** (extrinsic salivary glands), which extend beyond the submucosa. Glands, in general, are described as **simple** or **compound**. Simple glands are unbranched tubules that are either composed of secretory cells throughout their length, or have a secretory segment at the end of an unbranched duct. Compound glands are made up of many secretory acini at the ends of a highly branched system of ducts. The acini are described as **serous** or **mucous**. Serous acini consist of rounded aggregations of pyramidal secretory cells around a very small lumen. Their spherical nucleus is displaced towards the cell base by large numbers of secretory granules in the apical cytoplasm (Fig. 12.9). They secrete an enzyme-rich fluid that moistens the oral mucosa and initiates digestion of carbohydrates. Mucous acini may be round, or elongated, and the cytoplasm of the cells is completely filled with closely packed, pale-staining secretory granules (or droplets) that displace the nucleus and flatten it against the basal plasmalemma (Figs 12.9B, 12.10). Their product, **mucus**, has a lubricating function, enabling food to slide over the mucosa with minimal abrasion. In some salivary glands, elongated mucous acini have a crescentic cap of serous cells over their ends, called a **serous demilune** (Figs 12.10, 12.11). The secretion of these cells reaches the lumen via **intercellular canaliculi** between the underlying mucous cells.

The acini of the major salivary glands are at the ends of slender, branching **intercalated ducts** lined by cuboidal epithelium (Fig. 12.10). These are difficult to find in histological sections, for they are smaller than the acini and relatively short. The intercalated ducts are terminal branches of larger **striated ducts**, which are lined by a columnar epithelium (Fig. 12.10). On electron micrographs, the cells of the striated ducts have deep invaginations of the basal plasmalemma. The striations, observed with the light microscope, are caused by vertical alignment of mitochondria in the alcoves between these membrane invaginations. The striated ducts draining separate lobules of the gland converge upon **interlobular ducts** that are lined by stratified cuboidal epithelium. These are branches of the single main duct of the gland, lined by columnar epithelium. Where the duct opens into the oral cavity, this epithelium is continuous with the stratified squamous epithelium lining that cavity.

Major salivary glands

The largest of the major salivary glands are two **parotid glands**, each weighing about 25 g, and located subcutaneously on either side of the face, anterior to the ears. Their long duct opens into the oral cavity opposite the second upper molar tooth, on either side. The **gland** consists almost entirely of serous acini. The ultrastructure of the cells is typical of protein-secreting cells, with abundant rER, a sizable Golgi complex, and apical secretory granules. Interposed between these cells and the basal lamina, are highly branched **myoepithelial cells**. These are sometimes referred to as **basket cells** because the long processes of neighboring cells are adherent at desmosomes, thus forming a loose network around the acinus. The cell body and its processes are rich in actin, and contraction of these cells is believed to expel the secretory product from the lumen of the acini into the intercalated ducts. The striated ducts are unusually conspicuous in histological sections of the parotid.

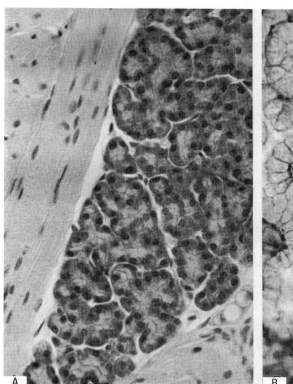
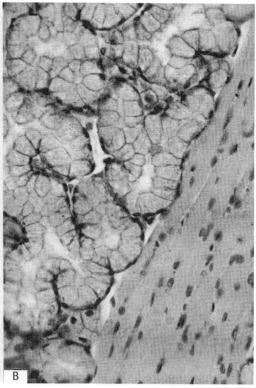

A
B

Figure 12.9 Photomicrographs illustrating the differing appearance of (A) a serous salivary gland, and (B) a mucous salivary gland.

The common childhood disease **mumps** is a viral infection of the cells of the parotid gland, resulting in swelling and tenderness of the gland on one or on both sides. Other salivary glands (sublingual and submaxillary) may also be involved. The disease is self-limiting, with the pain and swelling subsiding in about a week. In postpubertal males, an uncommon complication of mumps is **orchitis**, a painful swelling of one or both testicles, followed by degeneration of the seminiferous tubules resulting in infertility.

The **submandibular glands**, which are approximately 3 cm in diameter, are located beneath the mandible on either side of the midline. Their ducts open onto the floor of the oral cavity on either side of the frenulum of the tongue. These are mixed glands in which seromucous acini, with demilunes, predominate over mucous acini (Fig. 12.12).

The **sublingual glands**, which are the smallest of the major

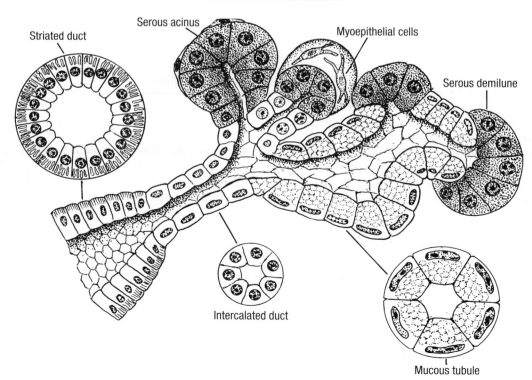

Striated duct

Serous acinus

Myoepithelial cells

Serous demilune

Intercalated duct

Mucous tubule

Figure 12.10 Drawing of the structure of a secretory unit of the submandibular gland. The serous cells have abundant rough endoplasmic reticulum in the basal third of their cytoplasm and small secretory granules in the apical third. The nucleus of the mucous cells is displaced to the cell base by large faintly stained secretory granules. The striated ducts have mitochondria between invaginations of the basal plasmalemma as in other ion transporting cells. Note the myoepithelial cells around the serous acini.

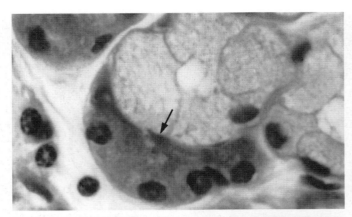

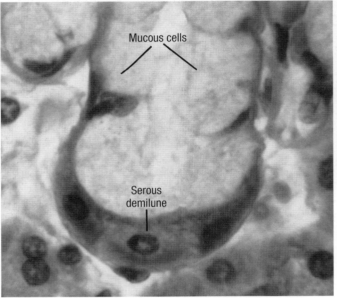

Figure 12.11 Photomicrograph of seromucous acini of human submandibular gland showing the mucous cells capped by a serous demilune (arrowed).

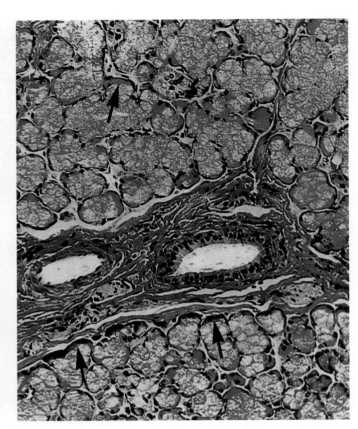

Figure 12.12 Photomicrograph of a canine submandibular gland consisting of seromucous acini. Notice the serous demilunes at the arrows. (Micrograph courtesy of P. Motta, University of Rome.)

salivary glands, are located beneath the floor of the mouth near the symphysis of the mandible. They have a flattened almond shape. The secretory end pieces are, for the most part, elongated acini of mucous cells, but occasional acini with serous demilunes can be also be found. A number of the smaller ducts of the glands open separately onto the floor of the mouth, but there is usually a main duct that opens with, or near to, the duct of the submandibular gland.

Minor salivary glands

Numerous small glands are found in the submucosa on the lateral walls of the oral cavity, and in the floor of the mouth. These are highly branched tubules, some of which are lined by serous cells, while others are lined by mucous cells. The mucous glands greatly outnumber the serous glands. Both of these types of glands open onto the oral epithelium via short ducts lined with cuboidal epithelium. They are believed to secrete continuously to moisten and lubricate the surface of the oral mucosa.

Small glands are also found between the bundles of striated muscle within the tongue. Some of these glands consist of typical serous acini (Fig. 12.13), and others appear to contain only mucous acini (Figs 12.14, 12.15).

Histophysiology of the salivary glands

Between meals, the minor salivary glands secrete continuously at a slow rate of 0.5–1.0 ml/min to keep the mouth moist. When food enters the mouth, the major salivary glands are stimulated by the parasympathetic division of the autonomic nervous system, and the flow of saliva is greatly increased. These glands secrete from 1.0–1.5 L of saliva a day. The watery secretion of the serous cells contains a variety of enzymes, including amylase, lysozyme, and peroxidase. Although saliva is 97–99% water, its solutes have important functions. The enzyme **salivary amylase** breaks down starch to oligosaccharides, initiating digestion of carbohydrates. The enzyme **lysozyme** breaks down bacterial cell walls, and its inhibition of bacterial growth may help to prevent tooth decay. In addition, plasma cells in the interstitial connective tissue of the parotid secrete **IgA**, which is combined with a unique protein produced by the acinar cells to form **salivary IgA**. This secretory immunoglobulin is believed to play an important role in control of the bacterial flora of the oral cavity.

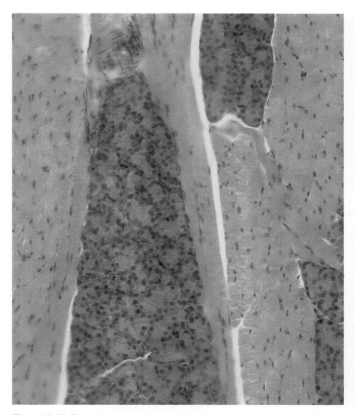

Figure 12.13 Photomicrograph of serous salivary glands between bundles of striated muscle fibers of the tongue.

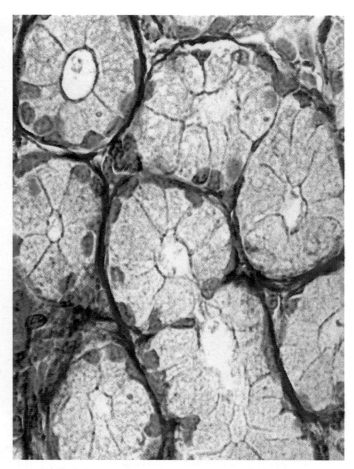

Figure 12.15 Higher magnification of a mucus-secreting salivary gland. Pale-staining secretory droplets occupy much of the cytoplasm, displacing the nucleus to the base of the cell. (Photomicrograph courtesy of Roberto Colombo, University of Milan.)

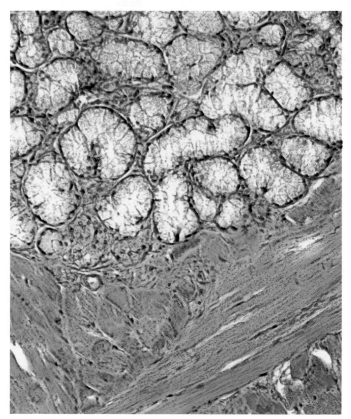

Figure 12.14 Photomicrograph of a mucus-secreting lingual salivary gland. In the lower half of the figure are interlacing bundles of striated muscle fibers of the tongue.

Salivation is controlled primarily by the parasympathetic division of the autonomic nervous system. When food enters the mouth, chemoreceptors send afferent impulses to a nucleus in the brain stem, which activates parasympathetic nerves that stimulate acinar and intercalated duct cells to release **kallikrein**. This causes a vasodilation of blood vessels to the salivary glands, and thus contributes to a dramatic increase in the volume of saliva secreted. Stimulation of sympathetic nerves results in increased output of thick mucous secretion. If the stimulus is quite strong, it causes vasoconstriction, inhibiting release of saliva and leading to a dry mouth.

Questions

1 Von Ebner's glands are associated with
 a   gastric mucosa
 b   circumvallate papillae
 c   esophagus
 d   anus
 e   duodenum

2 Enamel of the tooth is produced by
 a   odontoblasts
 b   fibroblasts
 c   enameloblasts
 d   ameloblasts
 e   macrophages

3 The periodontal membrane contains mostly
 a   collagen
 b   bone
 c   elastic fibers
 d   hyaline cartilage
 e   reticular fibers

4 The part of the oral mucosa that is bound to the periosteum of the alveolar ridge is
 a   cementum
 b   dental lamina
 c   enamel
 d   dental papilla
 e   gingiva

5 Which statement best describes the parotid gland?
 a   it contains both serous and mucous secretory units
 b   it contains only mucous acini
 c   it is a purely serous gland
 d   it contains no excretory ducts
 e   it is a purely mucous gland

6 Which immunoglobulin is most abundant in saliva?
 a   IgE
 b   IgM
 c   IgG
 d   IgA
 e   IgM and IgG are equally abundant in saliva

7 The parotid gland in the human may be distinguished histologically from other salivary glands in that it
 a   consists entirely of serous acini
 b   consists entirely of mucous acini
 c   consists entirely of mixed sero-mucous acini
 d   lacks salivons
 e   none of the above

8 Which phrase best describes circumvallate papillae?
 a   they are slender conical-shaped structures
 b   they are the most numerous of the lingual papillae
 c   they are the fewest of the papillae, numbering only 6 to 14
 d   they are heavily keratinized at their tips
 e   they are located on the anterior one-third of the tongue

9 Lingual salivary glands (von Ebner's glands) empty their secretions into invaginations
 a   at the base of fungiform papillae
 b   at the base of filiform papillae
 c   between the circumvallate papillae
 d   between filiform and fungiform papillae
 e   at the tip of the tongue

10 Dentin is produced by
 a   cementoblasts
 b   fibrocytes
 c   periodontal membrane
 d   ameloblasts
 e   odontoblasts

11 Striated muscle oriented in several planes is typical of what organ?

12 The parotid gland is considered what type of exocrine structure?

13 What type of papillae is associated with von Ebner's glands?

14 What cell secretes enamel?

15 Kallikrein is associated with what secretion?

16 What is the name of the major salivary gland that is composed primarily of mucous elements?

17 What do odontoblasts produce?

18 What structure has two types of epithelial lining, seromucous glands and a core of striated muscle?

19 What type of papilla in the human is the most numerous and does not contain taste buds?

20 What is the most abundant immunoglobulin in saliva?

Chapter thirteen

Esophagus and Stomach

ORGANIZATION OF THE ALIMENTARY TRACT

The gastrointestinal tract (alimentary tract) includes the esophagus, stomach, duodenum, jejunum, ileum, colon, and rectum. Although there are differences in the lining epithelium, and associated glands, along the length of the tract, the basic organization of its wall is much the same throughout, and is shown diagrammatically in Fig. 13.1. The innermost layer, called the **mucosa**, con-

sists of a columnar epithelium and associated tubular glands that extend into an underlying layer of loose connective tissue designated the **lamina propria**. This contains a rich network of capillaries, and a population of migratory cells (macrophages, lymphocytes, and plasma cells) involved in defense of the mucosa against the bacterial flora in the lumen. The lamina propria is bounded below by a thin layer of circumferentially oriented smooth muscle cells, constituting the **muscularis mucosae**. Peripheral to this, a relatively thick layer of connective tissue,

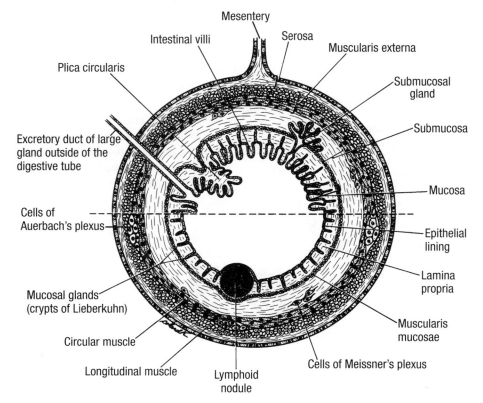

Figure 13.1 Schematic depiction of the structure of the wall of the gastrointestinal tract. The layers mucosa, muscularis and serosa are present in all of its segments. In the upper half of the figure, the mucosa is shown with villi and glands, as in the small intestine. In the lower half of the figure, the mucosa is depicted with glands but without villi, as in the stomach and colon.

Mesentery

Intestinal villi

Serosa

Muscularis externa

Plica circularis

Submucosal gland

Submucosa

Excretory duct of large gland outside of the digestive tube

Mucosa

Cells of Auerbach's plexus

Epithelial lining

Lamina propria

Mucosal glands (crypts of Lieberkuhn)

Circular muscle

Muscularis mucosae

Longitudinal muscle

Lymphoid nodule

Cells of Meissner's plexus

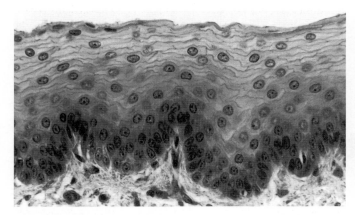

Figure 13.2 Photomicrograph of the stratified squamous epithelium of the esophagus.

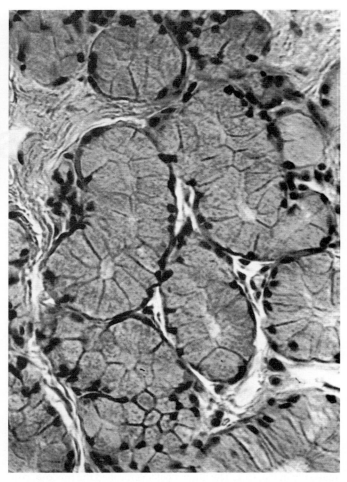

Figure 13.3 Photomicrograph of the tubular submucosal glands of the esophagus. The nuclei are displaced to the base of the epithelium by the large amount of mucus that has accumulated in the apical cytoplasm.

designated the **submucosa**, contains a higher concentration of collagen fibers, and fewer free cells than the lamina propria. Numerous small blood vessels have branches that pass through the muscularis mucosae to join the capillary network of the lamina propria. Peripheral to the submucosa is the **muscularis**, made up of an inner layer of circumferentially oriented smooth muscle, and an outer layer of longitudinal smooth muscle. The muscularis generates waves of contraction (peristalsis) that propel the contents through the gastrointestinal tract. The outermost layer of the wall, the **serosa**, is a thin squamous epithelium (mesothelium) that lines the body cavities and covers all of the viscera within them.

ESOPHAGUS

During a meal, enzymatic digestion of the ingested food is initiated in the oral cavity. It then passes from the oropharynx to the stomach through the **esophagus.** The greater part of this tubular organ is in the thorax, but its terminal 2–4 cm portion emerges from the esophageal orifice of the diaphragm into the abdominal cavity, where it is continuous with the stomach. The esophagus plays no role in digestion. Its mucosa is 300–400 μm in thickness and lined by a stratified squamous epithelium (Fig. 13.2). The very

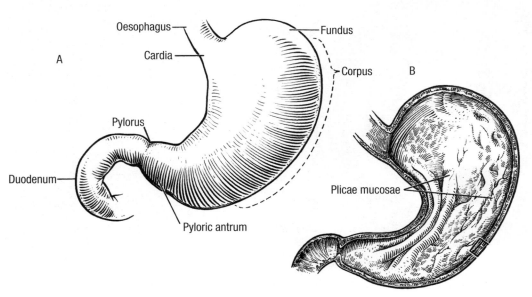

Figure 13.4 (A) A sketch of the regions of the stomach as defined by gross anatomists. (B) Drawing of a hemisected stomach showing the longitudinal plicae mucosae.

thin stratum corneum of the epithelium is not keratinized. Occasional lymphocytes and Langerhans cells can be found among the cells of its stratum granulosum. At the junction of the esophagus with the stomach, there is an abrupt transition from stratified squamous epithelium to the simple columnar epithelium of the gastric mucosa.

In the upper portion of the esophagus, the muscularis mucosae is represented by only scattered fascicles of smooth muscle cells that are predominantly longitudinal in orientation. Lower in the esophagus, these are more numerous and form a thin continuous layer of smooth muscle. The submucosa contains small blood vessels in a moderately dense connective tissue matrix of interlacing collagen and elastic fibers. The elastic fibers maintain the normal surface configuration of the mucosa. When food is not passing down the esophagus, longitudinal folds of mucosa give its lumen a scalloped outline. As a bolus of food slides down the esophagus, these folds are obliterated, and when the bolus has passed, they are rapidly restored by recoil of the elastic fibers in the submucosa.

Two categories of mucus-secreting glands are found in the wall of the esophagus. The **mucosal esophageal glands** are present in small numbers in the upper esophagus and near its junction with the stomach. They are short and are confined to the lamina propria. Longer **submucosal esophageal glands**, extending into the submucosa, are found along the greater part of the length of the esophagus. Both types are branched tubular glands containing only mucus-secreting cells. The apical cytoplasm of the cells is distended with pale-staining secretory granules that deform and displace the nucleus towards the cell base (Fig. 13.3). The function of these glands is to coat the mucosa with a lubricating layer of mucus that facilitates passage of food over its surface.

The muscularis of the wall of the upper esophagus differs from that elsewhere in the alimentary tract. Swallowing is a voluntary act, and this is reflected in the kind of muscle in the wall of the esophagus. In its upper third the muscularis is made up of striated muscle fibers. In the middle third, it is a mixture of striated and smooth muscle fibers, and in the lower third, it is composed entirely of smooth muscle. Swallowing involves: (1) relaxation of pharyngeal muscles that keep the esophagus closed between swallows; (2) contraction of striated muscle fibers in the muscularis of the upper esophagus to propel the bolus of food downwards; (3) peristaltic contraction of smooth muscle in its middle third; and (4) relaxation of myogenic muscle tone in the muscularis at the gastroesophageal junction.

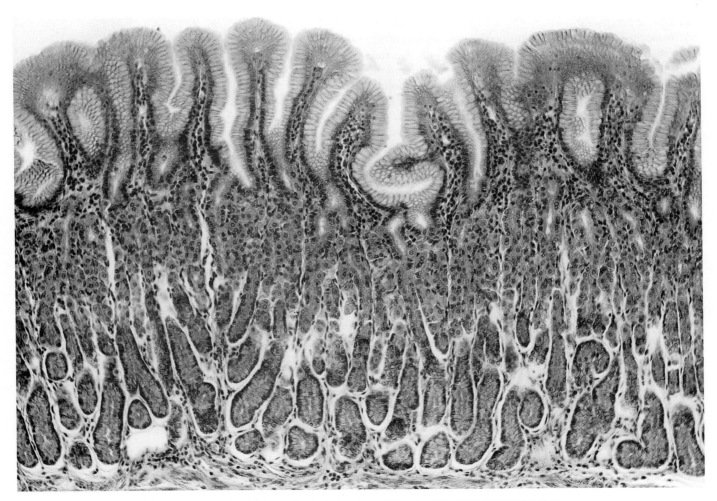

Figure 13.5 Photomicrograph of the gastric mucosa showing the gastric pits, or foveolae, and the long gastric glands that open into them.

Many people complain of 'heartburn' after meals. This is a burning pain in the lower thorax and upper abdomen caused by reflux of highly acidic stomach contents into the esophagus. This condition is diagnosed as **gastro-esophageal reflux disorder**. When it is a frequent occurrence, the hydrochloric acid and peptidases from the stomach may result in chronic inflammation that seriously damages the esophageal epithelium. Gastric reflux is very common in individuals who also have **hiatal hernia**, an abnormally large esophageal aperture in the diaphragm, through which a portion of the stomach herniates into the thoracic cavity. 'Heartburn' is treated symptomatically with any of a great variety of antacids. A large hiatal hernia may require surgical correction.

STOMACH

Gross anatomists have assigned separate terms to five regions of the stomach (Fig. 13.4A). A narrow zone around its junction with the esophagus is called the **cardia**. A dome-shaped region above this is the **fundus**, and a large central segment is the **corpus**. This reduces to a conical region, called the **pyloric antrum**, which narrows to the **pyloric canal** and this terminates in the **pyloris**. There, the smooth muscle of the wall is thickened, forming the **pyloric sphincter**. This remains contracted during the gastric phase of digestion and then relaxes to allow the contents of the stomach to pass into the duodenum.

Histologists are able to distinguish only three regions of the stomach, on the basis of differences in the microscopic structure of the mucosa. These are, a narrow zone 2–3 cm wide around the esophageal orifice, which is referred to as the **cardia**; a **fundic region**, which is coextensive with the fundus and corpus of gross anatomists; and a **pyloric region**, which includes the pyloric antrum, pyloric canal, and pyloris cited by gross anatomists. When an empty stomach is opened, its inner surface presents branching longitudinal folds of the mucosa and underlying submucosa, called **rugae** or **plicae mucosae** (Fig. 13.4B). As the stomach becomes distended with food during a meal, these folds are obliterated, but are restored by recoil of the elastic fibers of the submucosa when the stomach empties. With the pyloric sphincter closed, generation of waves of contraction by the muscularis of the fundic region mixes the food with the gastric secretions, and reduces it to a viscous semi-fluid mass called the **chyme**. In this process, the proteins of the food are broken down by hydrochloric acid and the protease **pepsin**.

Gastric mucosa

The epithelium of the gastric mucosa is invaginated to form countless, closely spaced **gastric pits** or **foveolae**. From the bottom of each of these, several slender **gastric glands** extend downwards (Fig. 13.5). In the mucosa of the fundus, the foveolae occupy one-third, and the glands two-thirds of the thickness of the mucosa. In the cardia and pyloric regions the foveolae occupy two-thirds and the glands one-third of its thickness. The number of foveolae in the human stomach is estimated to be about 3.5 million, and the number of glands 15 million. The narrow

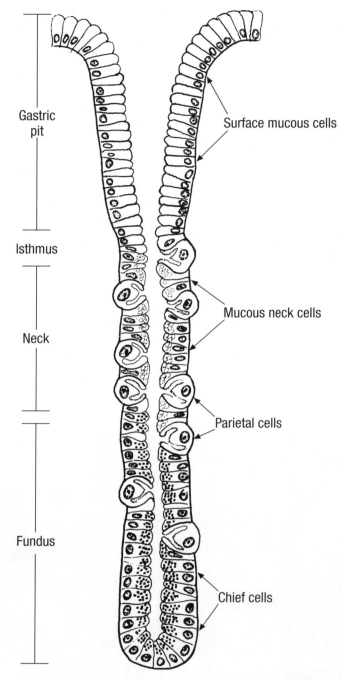

Figure 13.6 Drawing of a gastric pit and contiguous gastric gland presenting the terminology of the different regions and identifying their principal cell types.

spaces between glands are occupied by the loose connective tissue of the **lamina propria**. The epithelium on the surface and lining the foveolae consists of tall, columnar, mucus-secreting cells. These produce a thick blanket of mucus that lubricates the mucosa and protects it from damage by the hydrochloric acid and proteases in the chyme.

The depth of the foveolae, the shapes of the glands, and the relative numbers of the several glandular cell types differ somewhat in the three regions of the stomach. In the cardia, the **gastric glands** are branched and coiled and lined by mucus-secreting cells that are indistinguishable from those lining the foveolae. Among them are a few **enteroendocrine cells** that secrete **gastrin**, a hormone that influences gastric motility and stimulates the secretory activity of the glands. In the fundic region, the gastric glands arise from relatively short foveolae and are long and straight. The glands of this region produce the major portion of the gastric juice. They contain five cell types: **stem cells**, **mucous neck cells**, **parietal cells** (oxyntic cells), **chief cells** (zymogenic cells), and **enteroendocrine cells** (Fig. 13.6). Small undifferentiated **stem cells**, which are few in number and confined to the neck of the gland, are often found in mitosis. The continuous renewal of the gastric mucosa is dependent upon division of these cells. Some of their progeny move upwards and differentiate into the mucous cells of the gastric pits. Others migrate deeper into the glands, where they differentiate into the several cell types found there. Also present in the initial segment of the glands are irregularly shaped cells called **mucous neck cells**. They have a nucleus at the cell base and secretory granules in the apical cytoplasm that have histochemical staining reactions distinct from those of the mucus-secreting cells of the gastric pits. They produce glycoproteins that are more acidic. The physiological significance of secretion of two kinds of mucus by the gastric mucosa is not understood.

The most conspicuous cells of the gastric glands are the **parietal cells** (oxyntic cells), which secrete the hydrochloric acid of the gastric juice. They are large, rounded cells that are most numerous in the upper half of the gland but are interspersed among the other cell types along its entire length (Figs 13.6, 13.7A). The parietal cells have a centrally placed nucleus and an intensely eosinophilic cytoplasm. On electron micrographs, their most distinctive feature is the presence of a deep invagination of the apical plasma membrane, forming a **secretory canaliculus**, that partially encircles the nucleus and extends nearly to the cell base (Figs 13.7B, 13.8). Both the apical plasmalemma, and the portion lining the canaliculus bear numerous microvilli. There are no secretory granules and the Golgi complex is relatively small, but some 40% of the cytoplasmic volume is occupied by large mitochondria possessing numerous cristae (Fig. 13.8). The cytoplasm around the canaliculus contains numerous membrane-limited tubules and vesicles comprising the **tubulovesicular system** of the parietal cell. These might be mistaken for elements of the smooth endoplasmic reticulum (sER), but are actually portions of the plasmalemma that have been detached and taken into the cytoplasm. When the cells are stimulated, they fuse with the membrane of the canaliculus increasing its surface area and thereby enhancing the efficiency of the cell in secreting the **hydrochloric acid** (HCl) of the gastric juice.

A major component of the membrane added to the surface is a specific H^+K^+-ATPase, which serves as a proton pump, moving H^+ ions from the cytoplasm to the lumen, and K^+ ions from the

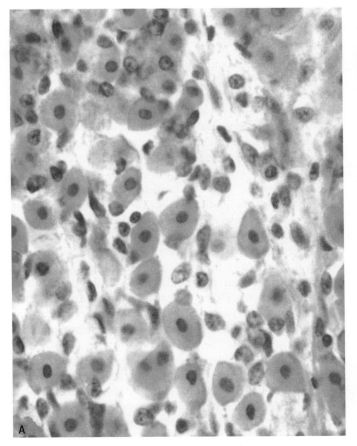
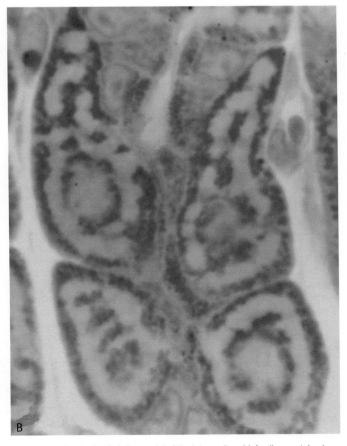

Figure 13.7 (A) Photomicrograph of several gastric glands, showing the large, intensely eosinophilic parietal cells. Only the nuclei of the intervening chief cells are stained. (B) High magnification photomicrograph of four parietal cells, notice the extensive intracellular canaliculi.

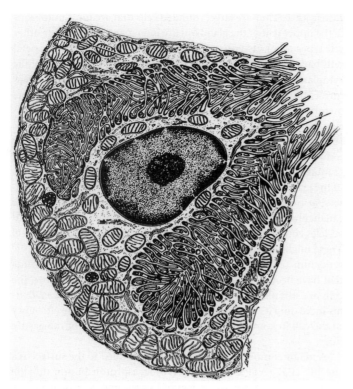

Figure 13.8 Drawing of the ultrastructure of a gastric parietal cell showing the microvilli lining the intracellular canaliculus, and the abundant mitochondria. (Courtesy of S. Ito.)

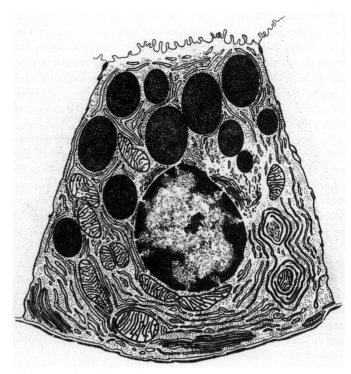

Figure 13.9 Drawing of the ultrastructure of a gastric chief cell (zymogenic cell). Like other protein-synthesizing cells, it has an abundant rough endoplasmic reticulum and apical secretory granules. (Reproduced from S. Ito and R.J. Winchester *J Cell Biol* 1963; 16:541.)

lumen into the cell. For each H^+ ion secreted, a bicarbonate ion (HCO_3) is released into the gastric venous circulation. H^+ ions in the gastric lumen are at a concentration 100 000 times their concentration in the blood plasma. Between meals, the size of the secretory canaliculus is reduced as membrane is withdrawn from its surface in regeneration of the tubulovesicular system of the cytoplasm. In addition to hydrochloric acid, parietal cells secrete **gastric intrinsic factor**, a glycoprotein that is necessary for the intestinal absorption of vitamin B_{12}, a vitamin that is required for erythrocyte production by the bone marrow and is therefore essential for life.

In a third or more of the population, the gastric mucus is inhabited by bacteria of the species *Helicobacter pylori*, which produce toxins causing chronic gastritis. A bacterial enzyme, uricase, breaks down urea to CO_2 and ammonia, and this neutralizes gastric HCl. The mucosal glands compensate by formation of nearly twice the normal number of parietal cells and these produce more HCl. Many of the infected individuals suffer from chronic gastritis, which progresses to formation of a **gastric ulcer**. In the past, it was often deemed necessary to remove the antral portion of the stomach surgically; now treatment is first directed to elimination of this remarkable species of bacteria, which is able to thrive in the highly acidic environment of the stomach (pH 20).

The predominant cell type of the lower one-third of gastric glands, in the fundic region, are the **chief cells** (zymogenic cells). These have a strongly basophilic cytoplasm and conspicuous secretory granules. On electron micrographs, they have the abundant gran-

ular endoplasmic reticulum and prominent Golgi complex characteristic of protein-secreting cells (Figs. 13.9, 13.10). The secretory granules contain **pepsinogen**, the precursor of the proteolytic enzyme **pepsin**. When released into the acidic environment in the gastric lumen, pepsinogen is converted to the active enzyme. These cells also secrete small amounts of a **lipase** that initiates the degradation of lipids to fatty acids, a process that will continue in the small intestine.

Enteroendocrine cells are widely scattered among the exocrine cells of the gastric glands. They are small, ovoid, or pyramidal cells. They were initially recognized in histological sections by their ability to reduce silver salts, and were formerly called **argentaffin cells**. Some have secretory granules that are located at the cell apex. Such cells evidently release their product into the gland lumen to stimulate other cells of the gland (**paracrine** secretion). Others have their granules at the cell base, and their product presumably diffuses into the blood vessels of the lamina propria to be transported to more distant target cells (**endocrine** secretion). The several different types of these cells are not easily identifiable in histological sections, but by taking advantage of improved extraction techniques and immunocytological methods, it has been possible to distinguish 15 types of enteroendocrine cells in the alimentary tract. Their products include a wide variety of amines, polypeptides, and more complex compounds.

The number and type of enteroendocrine cells vary in different segments of the stomach. The so-called **A-cells** (secreting

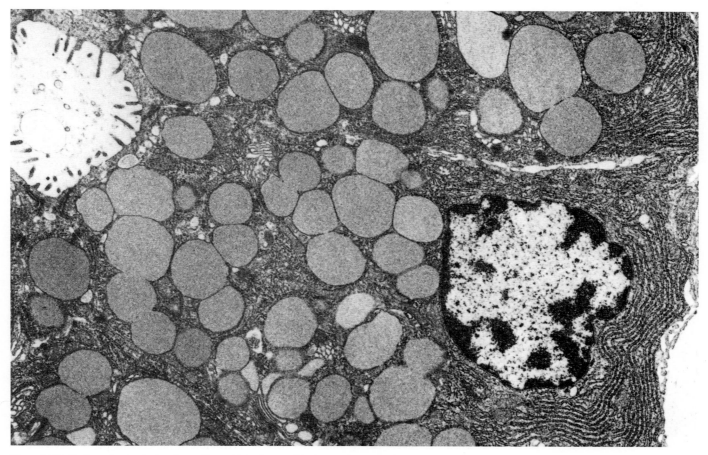

Figure 13.10 Electron micrograph of portions of three chief cells around the lumen of a gastric gland (upper left). Notice the abundance of rough endoplasmic reticulum at the cell base, and the moderately dense secretion granules in the apical cytoplasm. (Micrograph courtesy of S. Ito.)

glucagon; Fig. 13.11), are confined to the upper one-third of the stomach. **EC-cells** (secreting **serotonin**) occur throughout the mucosa, and **G-cells** (secreting **gastrin**) are most abundant in the antrum. **D-cells** (secreting **somatostatin**) are absent from the mid-portion of the stomach, but are widely distributed elsewhere. Their paracrine secretion plays a role in regulating the activity of the A-cells and G-cells.

In the pyloric region, the foveolae are unusually deep, occupying one-half to two-thirds of the thickness of the mucosa. The relatively short **pyloric glands** originating from them are branched, highly tortuous, and have a larger lumen than the glands of the fundic region. Mucus-secreting cells predominate. In addition to mucin, these glands secrete appreciable amounts of the bacteriolytic enzyme, **lysozyme**. Parietal cells are relatively few in the pyloric glands, but enteroendocrine cells are abundant.

Lamina propria

The interspaces between glands of the gastric mucosa are occupied by the **lamina propria**. It is a typical, loose connective tissue containing fibroblasts, and scattered eosinophils, macrophages,

plasma cells, and mast cells. There are also slender vertical strands of smooth muscle cells that extend upwards from the muscularis mucosae into the lamina propria. It is speculated that intermittent contraction of these fascicles of smooth muscle cells may slightly compress the mucosa, promoting discharge of secretion from its glands into the lumen.

Submucosa

The **submucosa** is a denser layer of connective tissue deep to the muscularis mucosae. It contains bundles of collagen fibers, a network of lymphatics, and numerous arterioles from which smaller vessels course vertically to join a network of capillaries around the gastric glands. This network is drained into a plexus of small veins in the submucosa.

Muscularis

The muscularis of the stomach differs from that of the rest of the gastrointestinal tract in having three layers instead of the usual two. Smooth muscle cells of the outermost layer are oriented

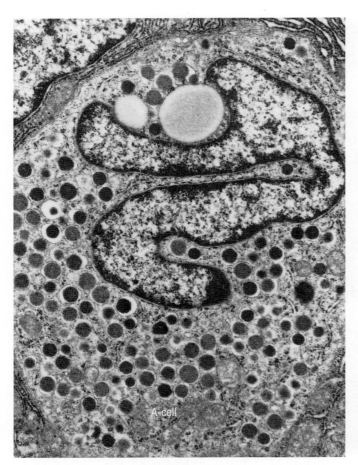

Figure 13.11 Electron micrograph of an enteroendocrine A-cell. It is a small cell with a polymorphous nucleus and many small dense granules in the surrounding cytoplasm.

longitudinally, those of the middle layer are circular, and those in the inner layer are oblique. The outer layer is incomplete. It is present along the greater and lesser curvature of the stomach, but is thin or absent on the dorsal and ventral surfaces of the organ. It thins out and ends before reaching the pyloris. The middle layer of circular fibers is complete and it is greatly thickened around the pyloric canal to form the **pyloric sphincter**.

Histophysiology of the stomach

The principal function of the stomach is the mixing of the ingested food with the gastric secretions. With the pyloris closed, mixing is accomplished by waves of contraction of the muscularis sweeping over the stomach every 20 s. When the gastric phase of digestion is completed, the pyloric sphincter opens and stronger contractions of the muscularis eject the chyme into the duodenum.

Although the enteroendocrine cells are relatively inconspicuous cellular components of the gastric glands, they have an important role in controlling the secretory activity of the gastric mucosa. In the fasting stomach, the pH of its contents is relatively low, and secretion of somatostatin by the D-cells exerts a paracrine inhibitory effect upon G-cells inhibiting their release of the hormone gastrin. Filling of the stomach with food results in a transient rise in the pH of the stomach contents, and this inactivates the D-cells, permitting the G-cells to release gastrin. This, in turn, increases gastric motility and stimulates acid secretion by the parietal cells. The resulting lowering of the pH creates the conditions necessary for activation of the enzyme pepsin, secreted by the chief cells. This enzyme is then able to digest the proteins of the chyme. Upon emptying of the stomach, the pH returns to its fasting level and gastrin secretion by the G-cells is again inhibited.

Questions

1   Regeneration of epithelial cell types in the stomach comes from differentiation of
    a   parietal cells
    b   isthmus mucous cells
    c   mucous-neck cells
    d   body chief (peptic) cells
    e   oxyntic cells

2   Which statement best describes the distal one-third of the esophagus?
    a   it contains a mixture of smooth and striated muscle
    b   it contains only smooth muscle
    c   it contains only striated muscle
    d   it is lined by goblet cells
    e   it is continuous with the oropharynx

3   The parietal (oxyntic) cell of the stomach produces which of the following?
    a   intrinsic factor
    b   lysozyme
    c   serotonin
    d   pepsinogen
    e   none of the above

4   The gastroesophageal junction is characterized by
    a   a transition from a stratified squamous epithelium to a simple columnar mucous epithelium
    b   a transition from a striated muscle coat to a smooth muscle coat
    c   the appearance of Peyer's patches
    d   the appearance of rugae in the esophagus
    e   a transition from a columnar mucous epithelium to a columnar epithelium with a striated border

5   Deep gastric pits and shallow gastric glands are characteristic of
    a   cardiac stomach
    b   fundic stomach
    c   corpus (body) of stomach
    d   pylorus of stomach
    e   none of the above

6   The tubulovesicular system of the parietal cell is
    a   associated with cellular production of NaOH
    b   derived from the plasmalemma
    c   endoplasmic reticulum
    d   enriched in a specific Na+Cl-pump, which exchanges protons across the membrane
    e   the location for the production of pepsinogen

7   The enteroendocrine cells in the stomach include
    a   cells
    b   chief cells
    c   B-cells
    d   parietal cells
    e   mucous neck cells

8   A gastric pit is surrounded by which of the following cell types?
    a   body-chief cells
    b   oxyntic cells
    c   APUD cells
    d   mucous cells
    e   none of the above

9   With regard to the muscularis externa of the esophagus, it would be correct to say that
    a   there is a transition from skeletal to smooth muscle from its oral to gastric end
    b   there is a transition from smooth to skeletal muscle from its oral to gastric end
    c   it consists entirely of smooth muscle
    d   it consists entirely of skeletal muscle
    e   it consists of an equal mixture of skeletal and smooth muscle throughout its length

10 The enteroendocrine cells of the stomach secrete
    a   glucagon
    b   serotonin
    c   gastrin
    d   somatostatin
    e   all of the above

11 What region of the stomach has deep pits and shallow glands?

12 What type of epithelium lines the stomach?

13 What pyramidal-shaped cell type of the stomach stains intensely with eosin?

14 What cell secretes gastric intrinsic factor?

15 What cell in the stomach has a complex system of tubules and vesicles (tubulovesicular system) in its cytoplasm?

16 What is the normal resting pH of the stomach lumen?

17 What is produced by the G-cell (an APUD-type cell) in the pyloris stomach?

18 Where are the gastric glands of the stomach located?

19 What part of the stomach has shallow pits and deep glands?

20 What do chief cells of the stomach secrete?

Chapter fourteen

Intestines

SMALL INTESTINE

The small intestine is the longest portion of the alimentary tract, over 4 m in length. Its function is to continue the digestion of food that began in the oral cavity and stomach, and to absorb the nutrient products of digestion. It is a convoluted tube that is divided, for descriptive purposes, into three segments, which are distinguishable by minor differences in the microscopic organization of their mucosa. The initial segment, the **duodenum**, begins at the pyloris of the stomach and is only 12–15 cm in length. It is firmly fixed to the posterior abdominal wall, and has a C-shaped course around the head of the pancreas. At its distal end, it is continuous with the **jejunum**, which is not fixed but is suspended from the posterior wall on a mesentery. The jejunum, which comprises about two-fifths of the total length of the small intestine, is followed by the **ileum**, which makes up the distal three-fifths. The transition between the three segments is gradual. Throughout its length, the wall of the small intestine is made up of the same four layers previously described for the stomach (see Chapter 13): mucosa, submucosa, muscularis, and serosa.

Surface amplification

The small intestine is organized for absorption of nutrients. The efficiency of this function is enhanced by several structural devices that increase the total area of its surface. The first of these is its great length. A further increase in surface area is achieved by transverse folds of the mucosa and submucosa, the **plicae circulares**, which project into the lumen. These are 8–10 mm in height, 3–4 mm in thickness, and clearly visible to the naked eye. Unlike the transient folds of the mucosa (rugae) seen in the stomach, the

plicae circulares are enduring structures that are not obliterated by distension of the intestine. They are most conspicuous in the first portion of the jejunum. They diminish in number and height more distally and are not found in the ileum. The plicae circulares slow the passage of the intestinal content and probably increase the surface area of the mucosa about three-fold.

The next level of surface amplification is the presence of myriad **intestinal villi**, 0.1–0.5 mm in length and numbering from 15 to 40/mm^2 of mucosa (Fig. 14.1). They are thin foliate

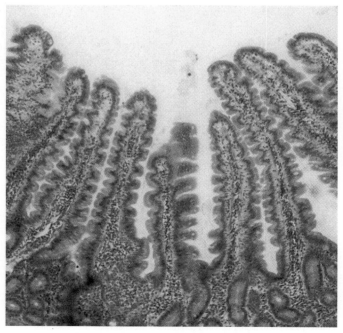

Figure 14.1 Photomicrograph of intestinal villi of the monkey jejunum. Notice the crypts of Lieberkuhn extending downwards between the bases of the villi.

(leaf-like) structures projecting into the lumen, and oriented parallel to the long axis of the intestine. They are longest in the duodenum and proximal jejunum and become shorter and more cylindrical in form in the distal jejunum and ileum. The core of each villus is made up of loose connective tissue containing a subepithelial network of fenestrated capillaries, two or more slender strands of smooth muscle (Fig. 14.2), and a blind-ending lymphatic vessel, called the **lacteal**, which drains into a plexus of lymphatics in the underlying lamina propria (Fig. 14.3). The lacteals and the larger lymphatic vessels of the intestinal wall are an important pathway for transport of absorbed lipids from the intestinal mucosa to the blood vascular system. Intermittent contraction of the smooth muscle in the core of the villi shortens them and moves lymph from the lacteal towards the larger lymphatics in the submucosa. Shortening of the villi during specimen preparation results in an escalloped, or corrugated appearance of the epithelium on their sides (Figs 14.1, 14.4). When the villi are not contracted the epithelium has a smooth surface contour (Fig. 14.3). The intestinal villi achieve an eightfold increase in surface area.

A final surface amplifying device is the presence of 2500, or more, **microvilli** on each cell of the epithelium, resulting in an additional thirtyfold increase in surface area. The total surface area of the intestine is estimated to be 200 m², an area equivalent to the floor space of an average two-story house.

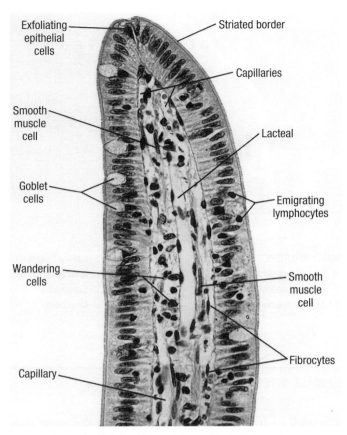

Figure 14.3 Longitudinal section of a villus labeled to show its principal components.

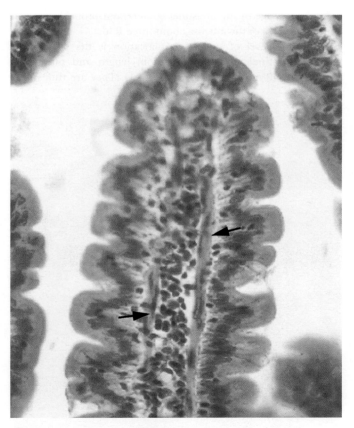

Figure 14.2 Photomicrograph of a contracted intestinal villus. The scalloped appearance of the epithelium is due to shortening by the smooth muscle (at arrows).

Intestinal epithelium

The epithelium covering the intestinal villi comprises **absorptive cells** and mucus-secreting **goblet cells** (Fig. 14.4). Between the bases of the intestinal villi, the epithelium is invaginated to form short **intestinal glands**, also called the **crypts of Lieberkuhn** (Fig. 14.1). These are not involved in absorption, but they produce 1 L/day or more of a watery secretion commonly called the **intestinal juice**. This serves as a solvent for nutrients released in digestion, and as a vehicle for cytokines, paracrine secretions of cells that influence the functions of neighboring cell types. In the duodenum, are longer tubular glands, the **duodenal glands** (Brunner's glands), which form highly convoluted masses in the submucosa.

All of the cells of the intestinal epithelium are short-lived and must be continually replaced. The new cells arise from pluripotential **stem cells** situated in the necks of the intestinal glands (crypts). These undergo frequent divisions, and their progeny slowly move upwards along the sides of the villi as they differentiate into absorptive cells and goblet cells, to replace spent cells that are continually exfoliated at the tips of the villi. Other cells arising from the stem cells move downwards, to replace cells of the crypts that undergo apoptosis. The rapid turnover of the intestinal epithelium can be demonstrated by injecting a rat with tritiated thymidine, which labels the dividing cells in the necks of the

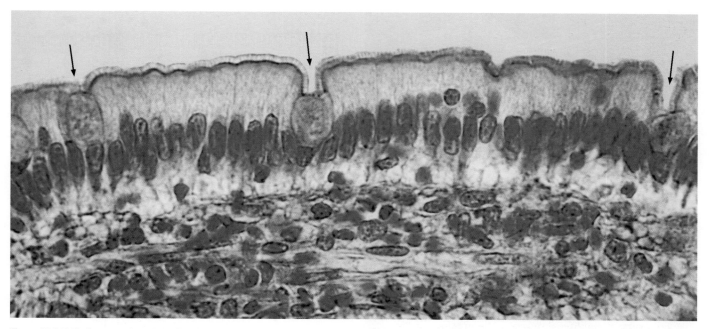

Figure 14.4 Epithelium on an intestinal villus illustrating its columnar absorptive cells with a conspicuous brush border. Scattered goblet cells are indicated by arrows.

intestinal glands. One day later, labeled cells can be found on the sides of the villi, and by the fifth day after the injection, labeled cells are being exfoliated at the tips of the villi. The rate of cell turnover in the human intestine is only slightly slower.

Absorptive cells of the villi are tall columnar cells with a prominent brush-border consisting of microvilli with a core of actin filaments. The microvilli have been observed to shorten from time to time, and this activity may promote movement of absorbed nutrients into the cytoplasm. Exceedingly thin, branching filaments of molecular dimensions project from the tips of the microvilli and intermingle to form a continuous surface coat, called the **glycocalyx** (Fig. 14.5). The filaments comprising the glycocalyx are extensions of integral proteins of the plasmalemma, consisting of a core polypeptide with oligosaccharide side-chains. There is evidence that enzymes hydrolyzing disaccharides and dipeptides are not only present in the apical cytoplasm and microvilli of the epithelial cells but are also released and adsorbed onto the filaments of the glycocalyx (Fig. 14.6). The monosaccharides and amino acids resulting from their activity are then actively transported across the cell, and into the subepithelial capillaries.

There are several inherited **disaccharidase deficiency syndromes**, in which one of the disaccharidases normally associated with the glycocalyx of the intestinal epithelium is lacking. One of the commonest of these is **lactase deficiency**, in which there is intolerance to milk. Drinking of milk, even in small quantity, is followed by bloating, cramping and diarrhea. It is managed by avoidance of milk and dairy products. There are significant racial differences in the incidence of this condition. It is relatively uncommon in Caucasians but its incidence in Blacks and Orientals may be as high as 80%.

After a meal, glucose and amino acids, liberated by intralumenal digestion, are taken up by the intestinal epithelium and transported to the blood in capillaries of the lamina propria.

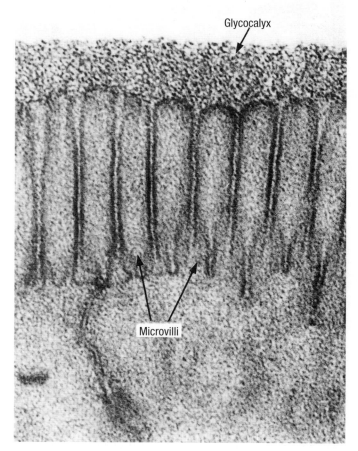

Figure 14.5 Electron micrograph illustrating the thick glycocalyx on the tips of the intestinal villi. (Micrograph courtesy of S. Ito.)

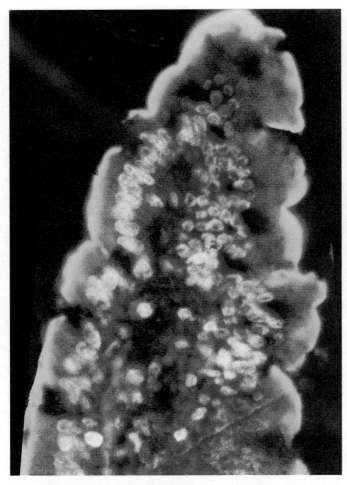

Figure 14.6 Tip of an intestinal villus stained by a fluorescein-labeled antibody to the enzyme lactase. This enzyme and others are concentrated in the brush border and its glycocalyx. Blue, nuclei; yellow, lactase. (Micrograph courtesy of W. Anderson.)

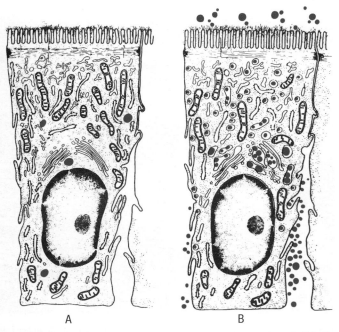

Figure 14.7 Drawings of the ultrastructure of an intestinal absorptive cell, (A) in the fasting state, and (B) after a lipid-rich meal. Note the uptake of lipid in vesicles, their processing in the Golgi complex and release of chylomicrons into the intercellular spaces. (Redrawn after R. Cardell, S. Badenhausen, and K.R. Porter *J Cell Biol* 1967; 34:123.)

Intraluminal digestion of fats depends upon their emulsification by bile, and their degradation by pancreatic lipase to fatty acids and monoglycerides. The apical cytoplasm of the absorptive cells contains abundant smooth endoplasmic reticulum (sER), which has an important role in the absorption of lipids. It contains the enzymes necessary for the synthesis of triglycerides from fatty acids and monoglycerides taken up by absorptive cells of the epithelium. In histological sections of intestine from fasting animals, the absorptive cells are free of lipid inclusions. However, after a meal, when dietary fats are being absorbed, droplets of triglycerides are apparent in the sER (Fig. 14.7). These are transported in vesicles to the Golgi complex, where they are combined with a lipoprotein to form larger bodies called **chylomicrons**. These, in turn, are transported in vesicles to the basolateral cell membranes where their content is released into the intercellular spaces of the epithelium (Fig. 14.7), From there, they move into the cores of the intestinal villi, and enter the lacteals, whence they are slowly carried, via lymphatics of increasing size, to the cisterna chyle, and thence to the bloodstream via the thoracic duct.

The **goblet cells**, scattered among the absorptive cells of the epithelium, secrete mucus. Accumulation of pale droplets of mucus expands the apical portion of the cell and displaces the nucleus into a narrower cell base, resulting in the shape that gives the cell its name. On electron micrographs, rough endoplasmic reticulum (rER), a Golgi complex, and mitochondria can be found in the limited amount of cytoplasm below the mucin droplets. Goblet cells are relatively few in the duodenum, but become more numerous in the jejunum. The mucus that they secrete serves to lubricate the surface of the intestinal mucosa, protect it from abrasion, and prevent adherence and invasion by the numerous bacteria in the intestinal lumen.

Enteroendocrine cells of several types are found scattered among the absorptive cells on the villi and in the glands. They have been described in connection with the stomach (Chapter 13) but are of greater functional significance in the small intestine. They are small cells, usually located at the base of the epithelium. They contain dense argyrophilic granules, which are most abundant on the side of the cell that is near the basal lamina. The several types of enteroendocrine cells secrete different peptide cytokines (or hormones) that modulate various activities of the gastrointestinal tract. Their number and type vary along the length of the tract. The **A-cells** (secreting glucagon) are confined to the upper third of the stomach. The **EC-cells** (secreting serotonin) are the most numerous of the enteroendocrine cells and are found throughout the intestinal tract. **G-cells** (secreting gastrin) are numerous in the duodenum, fewer in the jejunum, and absent in the ileum. **S-cells** (secreting secretin), **I-cells** (secreting cholecystokinin), **D-cells** (secreting somatostatin), and **MO-cells** (secreting motilin) are found in the duodenum and jejunum, but are rare in the ileum. **L-cells** (secreting enteroglucagon) occur throughout the small and large intestines.

Defense mechanisms

A major function of epithelia, in general, is to serve as a barrier to the entry of potentially pathogenic microorganisms from the external environment. The intestinal epithelium is constantly exposed to a vast number of bacteria in the lumen. The epithelium lining the crypts of the small intestine contains cells, called **Paneth cells**, that are specialized for defense against bacterial invasion. They are clustered at the base of the intestinal crypts. They are pyramidal in form and have a moderately basophilic cytoplasm containing numerous large eosinophilic secretory granules. They do not participate in the upwards movement of cells in the glandular epithelium, but remain in the depths of the crypts (Fig. 14.8). Paneth cells have a lifespan of about 30 days and then degenerate, and are replaced by differentiation of daughter cells of dividing stem cells located in the necks of the glands.

On electron micrographs, the cytoplasm of Paneth cells is rich in rER and contains numerous lysosomes. Upon isolation and biochemical analysis, they are found to contain unusual amounts of **lysozyme** and **phospholipase A2**, two enzymes that are capable of digesting bacterial cell walls. Whether these enzymes are confined to the lysosomes, or are also present in the secretory granules, is unclear. It is known that the granules contain several other antimicrobial substances, called **defensins** (cryptidins). The defensins are a family of cationic peptides that kill bacteria by membrane disruption. In the short intestinal glands, the Paneth cells are located near the stem cells, and their secretion no doubt defends these indispensable cells from bacterial damage. Whether defensins reach a concentration in the lumen of the intestine that is sufficient to influence the bacterial flora there, is debated.

Lamina propria

The **lamina propria** of the intestine consists of areolar tissue that surrounds the intestinal glands and forms the core of the intestinal villi. In addition to fibroblasts, it contains many lymphocytes, macrophages, and plasma cells. Very slender strands of smooth muscle pass upwards from the muscularis mucosae into the core of each villus. As previously noted, these are responsible for the intermittent slight shortening of the villi that can be observed in the living intestine.

The constant threat of bacterial invasion has also been countered by the development of special immunological defenses. In addition to the population of lymphocytes, plasma cells, and macrophages normally present in the lamina propria, there are occasional **solitary lymphoid nodules** resembling those of lymph nodes. In the ileum, groups of these coalesce into **aggregated lymphoid nodules** (**Peyer's patches**) that are much larger and extend into the submucosa (Fig. 14.9).

In the epithelium overlying the lymphoid nodules there are specialized cells, called **M-cells**, that are not found elsewhere. They are broad cells with a dome-like apex bearing a limited number of short microvilli. At the cell base, there is a deep invagination of the plasma membrane forming a basal 'pocket' that is occupied by one or two macrophages and numerous lymphocytes (Fig. 14.10). Bacteria are often observed adhering to the apical surface of the M-cells, and it is believed that they are continually taken up from the lumen and their antigens are presented by the macrophages to the surrounding lymphocytes. Having interacted with antigen, these lymphocytes migrate into the underlying lymphoid tissue. From there, some enter the circulation, either directly or via the lymphatic drainage of the intestines, and then return to the lamina

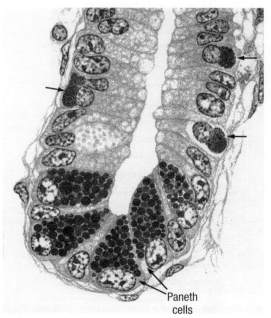

Figure 14.8 Drawing of Paneth cells at the base of an intestinal crypt. Three enteroendocrine cells are shown (short arrows).

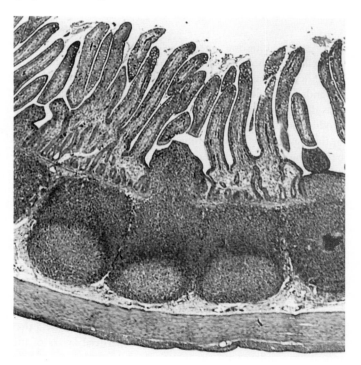

Figure 14.9 Photomicrograph of cat ileum showing the very short crypts and the submucosal lymphoid nodules (Peyer's patches).

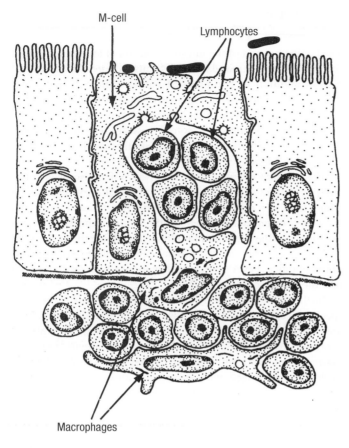

Figure 14.10 Diagram of an M-cell showing a macrophage and several lymphocytes occupying a deep recess in its basal surface. Bacteria adhere selectively to M-cells, which transport antigen to cells in the basal pocket. (Redrawn from M. Neutra and J.P. Kraehenbuhl *Trends Cell Biol* 1992; 2:134.)

propria of the intestine, where they differentiate into plasma cells that release antibodies to the antigen previously presented to their lymphocyte precursors. This so-called **secretory immune system**, depends upon the production of immunoglobulin A (**IgA**), and thus differs from the general immune system of the body which produces antibodies of the **IgG** class. The IgA antibodies produced by the plasma cells in the lamina propria bind to receptors on the base of the epithelial cells and are transported across the cells to be released into the lumen of the intestine, where they are adsorbed onto the glycocalyx. There, they are ideally situated to inhibit bacterial adherence and prevent their penetration of the epithelium. This protective mechanism is referred to as **immune exclusion**.

Muscularis mucosae

The **muscularis mucosae** between the lamina propria and the submucosa is similar to that previously described for the stomach. It is a thin layer of circumferentially oriented smooth muscle that corrects any displacement of the more superficial layers of the mucosa by contact with the intestinal contents. Its contraction also contributes to the movements of villi that can be observed in the jejunal mucosa in the living state. This layer is thin or absent

where aggregated lymphoid nodules underlie the mucosa of the jejunum and ileum.

Submucosa

In the greater part of the length of the intestine, the **submucosa** consists of loose connective tissue containing more collagen and elastic fibers than that of the lamina propria. In addition to fibroblasts, it may contain small clusters of adipose cells. Conspicuous components of the submucosa, in the duodenum, are the **submucosal glands of Brunner** (Fig. 14.11). The ducts of these tubuloacinar glands traverse the muscularis mucosae and open into the gut lumen between the villi. The coiled tubules of the glands are lined by cuboidal cells with a prominent Golgi complex, rER, and pale-staining apical secretory granules. The secretion of Brunner's glands is a clear alkaline mucin (pH 8.2–9.3) with a high

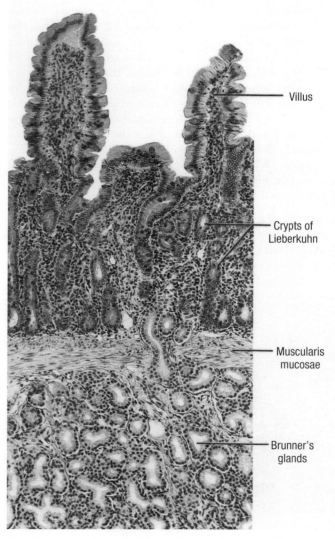

Figure 14.11 Photomicrograph of duodenal mucosa of a macaque. The villi, crypts, muscularis mucosae and Brunner's glands are indicated. Notice the duct of a Brunner's gland crossing the muscularis mucosae to empty into a crypt.

content of bicarbonate. Its principal function is to protect the duodenal mucosa against the potentially damaging effects of the strongly acidic chyme discharged into the duodenum from the stomach. It raises the pH of the intestinal content into the optimal range for activity of the pancreatic enzymes, which are released into this segment of the tract. Brunner's glands form a nearly continuous layer in the submucosa of the initial portion of the duodenum, but they diminish in number, and end at its junction with the jejunum.

Within the connective tissue of the submucosa, there is a network of ganglia and interconnecting nerve bundles that form the **submucous plexus (Meissner's plexus)**. It receives information from chemoreceptors and mechanoreceptors in the mucosa and its efferent fibers innervate the muscularis mucosae and smooth muscle fibers in the core of the intestinal villi.

Muscularis

The **muscularis** of the small intestine consists of outer longitudinal and inner circular layers of smooth muscle. Some thin strands of muscle may pass from one layer to the other. The muscularis of the small intestines is responsible for **peristalsis**, the intermittent, wavelike contractions that travel along the intestine at a rate of a few centimeters per second, advancing the intestinal contents. There are also segmental movements, consisting of alternate constriction and relaxation of short segments. These result in movements that tend to agitate and mix the intestinal contents. In the terminal portion of the ileum, the muscularis is locally thickened, forming the **ileocecal sphincter**, which normally remains partially contracted. Some time after the last meal, there is reflex activation of increased ileal peristalsis and relaxation of this sphincter, permitting the contents of the small intestine to move into the colon.

Between the circular and longitudinal layers of the muscularis, there is another nerve plexus, the **myenteric plexus (Auerbach's plexus)** (Fig. 14.12). Its efferent fibers are largely responsible for the peristaltic movements of the intestine.

LARGE INTESTINE

The **large intestine**, or **colon**, is somewhat shorter and less convoluted than the small intestine. Seven successive regions along its length (1.5 m) are identified by different names: **cecum, ascending colon, transverse colon, descending colon, sigmoid colon, rectum,** and **anus**. The **cecum** is a blind-ending pouch in the lower right quadrant of the pelvis that is continuous above with the **ascending colon**. The ileum joins the cecum on its medial side, and the orifice between the two is closed by the **ileocecal valve**. The ascending colon passes up the right side of the abdominal cavity, and then turns left to become the **transverse colon**, crossing the abdomen below the diaphragm. Turning downwards anterior to the left kidney, it becomes the **descending colon**, which passes down the left side of the abdominal cavity to the rim of the pelvis. There it turns right, as the **sigmoid colon**, this then turns downwards near the midline, as the **rectum**, which is continuous with the **anal canal**.

The ascending and descending portions of the colon are fixed to the posterior wall of the abdominal cavity, while the transverse and sigmoid portions are suspended on a short mesentery. These regional designations are of more value to the surgeon than to the histologist, for the microscopic structure of the colon is much the same throughout its length.

Mucosa

The function of the large intestine is to concentrate the indigestible residues of food by absorbing water and electrolytes, and to move these to the anus for elimination. The surface of the mucosa is quite smooth. There are no folds comparable to the plicae circulares, and no villi. However, it contains large numbers of straight glands (Figs 14.13, 14.14). The epithelium on the

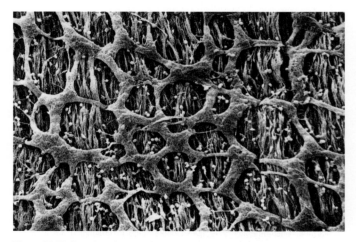

Figure 14.12 Scanning electron micrograph of the myenteric plexus of cat intestine. The overlying longitudinal muscle and connective tissue have been removed by enzymatic digestion. (Micrograph reproduced courtesy of T. Fujiwara and Y. Uehara *J Electron Microsc* 1980; 29:397.)

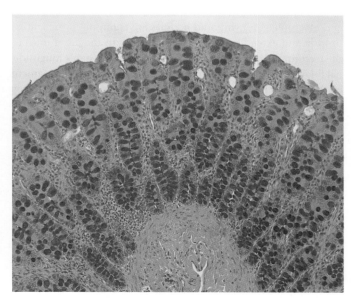

Figure 14.13 Photomicrograph of the mucosa of the colon. There are no villi. The mucosa is made up of straight tubular glands. Notice that the darker-staining goblet cells increase in abundance in the depths of the glands.

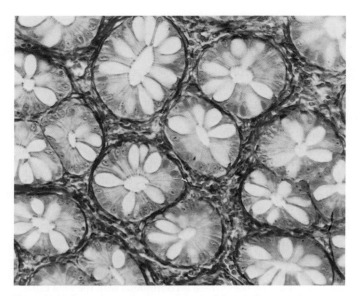

Figure 14.14 Photomicrograph of several glands of the colonic mucosa in cross-section. The mucus of the goblet cells is unstained.

surface, and in the upper one-third of the glands, is composed of columnar absorptive cells and a few goblet cells. In the lower two-thirds, it consists mainly of **goblet cells**, but there are also small numbers of solitary **enteroendocrine cells**. The goblet cells of the colonic mucosa secrete a large volume of mucus that coats its surface and facilitates onward movement of the contents of the bowel, while protecting the surface from abrasion by its increasingly concentrated contents. The lifespan of cells on the surface and in the glands, is about 7 days. They are replaced by the progeny of stem cells, located in the depths of the glands. These divide frequently, generating new cells that rapidly differentiate as they move upwards. The old cells approaching the end of their lifespan are continually lost at **extrusion zones** on the surface, located midway between the openings of the glands.

The lamina propria of the colon contains many lymphocytes and macrophages. Lymphoid nodules are common in the lamina propria and extending into the submucosa. In the distal third of the rectum, the mucosa and lamina propria form stable longitudinal folds called the **columns of Morgagni**. In this terminal segment of the colon, the glands become progressively shorter, and they end along a line a few centimeters above the anal orifice. At this line, there is an abrupt transition from simple columnar epithelium to the stratified squamous epithelium that lines the anal canal. At the anal orifice, this epithelium is continuous with the epidermis of the surrounding skin. In this region, the lamina propria contains a plexus of large veins. These may become abnormally distended and varicose. Some varicosities, covered by mucosa, or by squamous epithelium of the anal canal may project into the anus, forming painful **hemorrhoids**.

Muscularis

The muscularis of the colon differs from that of the small intestine

in that its outer longitudinal layer is incomplete. The major part of its smooth muscle is aggregated into three longitudinal bands called the **taenia coli**. Between these bands, an outer layer of longitudinal smooth muscle is either very thin, or entirely lacking. The taenia coli are normally in a state of partial contraction, resulting in a bulging of the intervening portions of the wall of the colon to form dilations called the **haustra**. These are apparent along the length of the colon up to the rectum. There the smooth muscle of the outer layer becomes continuous and of uniform thickness, and there are no taenia coli or haustra.

The ascending and descending portions of the colon are fixed to the posterior abdominal wall, limiting its movements. It is inactive, much of the time, save for occasional **haustral contractions**, when a local increase in volume of its content stretches the wall and stimulates both circular and longitudinal muscle to contract. These mild local contractions suffice to move the contents from one haustrum to the next. A few times a day, usually after meals, more general contractions sweep along longer segments of the colon to move its contents towards the rectum. At the distal end of the anal canal, the circular muscle is locally thickened to form the **internal anal sphincter**. Immediately distal to this, a ring of striated muscle forms the **external anal sphincter**.

APPENDIX

The **vermiform appendix** is an appendage of the blind end of the cecum. It is a vestigial portion of the intestinal tract of no functional significance. It is 4.0–8.0 cm in length and 0.5–1.0 cm in diameter. All the layers found elsewhere in the intestinal tract are present in its wall but are obscured by many small and large lymphoid nodules that occupy nearly all of the lamina propria and submucosa. Its very small lumen is lined by an epithelium of absorptive cells interrupted by the openings of very short glands made up of goblet cells, and rare enteroendocrine cells. M-cells are common in the epithelium overlying the lymphoid nodules. The lamina propria is crowded with lymphocytes, macrophages, and plasma cells. The narrow lumen of the appendix is small and angular in cross-section and is often filled with dead cells and cellular debris. The appendix is a common site of infection (**appendicitis**), necessitating its surgical removal.

Adenocarcinoma of the colon, resulting from malignant transformation of epithelial cells of the glands, is the second most common cancer of humans. It is treated by resection of a segment of bowel containing the tumor. This is followed by X-irradiation and chemotherapy, if there is a suspicion that the tumor may have metastasized. In the remaining portions of the colon, cell loss continues, but chemotherapy slows, or stops, the division of stem cells that is necessary for their replacement. Consequent atrophy of the epithelium results in diminished water absorption, excess fluid loss, dehydration, nausea, and diarrhea. Chemotherapy is of questionable value in prolonging life of the patient.

Questions

1   Brunner's glands are found in
   a   the colon
   b   the rectum
   c   the stomach
   d   the duodenum
   e   the ileum

2   Peyer's patches are
   a   lymphatic regions in the colon
   b   absorptive regions of the jejunum
   c   lymphatic nodules in stomach mucosa
   d   associated with celiac disease
   e   concentrations of lymphatic nodules in the ileum

3   Plasma cells of the lamina propria secrete
   a   histamine
   b   IgG
   c   heparin
   d   IgA
   e   IgE

4   Cells that transport antigen across the epithelium are the
   a   Clara cells
   b   Paneth cells
   c   G-cells
   d   M-cells
   e   parietal cells

5   In the small intestine, Auerbach's myenteric plexus is located
   a   in the submucosa
   b   in the lamina propria
   c   between layers of muscularis externa
   d   in the serosa
   e   in the muscularis mucosae

6   Which of the following statements about histological features distinguishes the duodenum from the jejunum?
   a   only the duodenum contains plicae circulares
   b   the duodenum contains submucosal glands (of Brunner), whereas the jejunum does not
   c   only the jejunum is usually filled with jujubees
   d   the two structures cannot be distinguished from each other histologically
   e   only the jejunum contains both submucosal glands of Brunner and Peyer's patches

7   A distinguishing feature of the ileum
   a   is the abundance of Brunner's glands
   b   is the presence of the crypts of Lieberkuhn
   c   is the presence of plicae circulares
   d   is the presence of Peyer's patches
   e   the ileum has no distinguishing features

8   The cell producing lysozyme is
   a   body chief cell
   b   parietal cell
   c   goblet cell
   d   Paneth cell
   e   enteroendocrine cell

9   The principal regulators of the exocrine pancreas are secreted by cells of the
   a   stomach
   b   ileum
   c   duodenum
   d   jejunum
   e   all of the above

10   Cell turnover in the small intestine occurs every
   a   6 h
   b   24 h
   c   2 days
   d   4–6 days
   e   none of the above

11   What is the name of the localized thickening of the outer layer of smooth muscle in the large intestine?

12   What type of epithelium lines the small intestine?

13   What is the name of the structure that secretes mucus into the small intestine to help neutralize stomach acid?

14   What is the name of the nerve plexus located between the two smooth muscle layers of the muscularis externa in the small intestine?

15   What specialized cell type is part of the simple columnar epithelium of the small intestine and secretes a surface lubricant?

16   What are wave-like contractions of the muscularis externa called?

17   What is the name of the folds of the mucosa and submucosa seen in the jejunum?

18   What do the enteroendocrine EC cells, found in the crypts of Lieberkuhn, secrete?

19   Where are Peyer's patches located?

20   What is the blind lymphatic capillary in an intestinal villus called?

Liver and Gallbladder

LIVER

The **liver** is a large organ located in the right upper quadrant of the abdominal cavity. Its rounded upper surface conforms to the right dome of the diaphragm. It is an accessory gland of the digestive tract and is the largest gland in the body, weighing about 1.5 kg. It continually secretes **bile**, a fluid that is stored between meals in the **gallbladder**, a sac-like organ attached to its undersurface. After meals, the gallbladder contracts in response to hormones released by enteroendocrine cells of duodenal mucosa, and bile passes through the **bile duct** into the duct of the pancreas, near its opening into the duodenum. Enzymes secreted by the pancreas digest proteins. The function of bile is to emulsify the fats in the chyme and thus facilitate their absorption by the intestinal epithelium.

In addition to the production of bile, the liver has many other functions. Its cells store carbohydrates in the form of glycogen and release glucose into the blood, as needed to maintain the normal concentration of this important energy source. It synthesizes the proteins of blood plasma and releases them directly into the blood as it passes through the organ. It takes up drugs, alcohol and other potentially harmful substances from the blood and detoxifies them by oxidation, or by forming harmless conjugates that pass into the intestinal tract with the bile and are excreted in the feces.

Histological organization

The organization of the liver is quite different from that of other

glands that have a branching system of ducts terminating in rounded secretory units called acini. The parenchyma of the liver

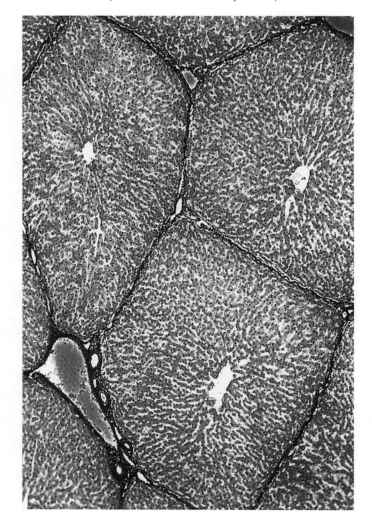

Figure 15.1 Low-power photomicrograph of pig liver. In this species, polygonal liver lobules, with a central vein, are outlined by thin connective tissue septa. This is the classical liver lobule. The absence of these septa, in other species, has led to different interpretations of the functional subunits of the liver. (Photomicrograph courtesy of P. Motta.)

is remarkably uniform in appearance throughout. There is little connective tissue, other than a thin layer called **Glisson's capsule**, which envelops the entire organ. It is possible, however, to discern in histological sections, a repeating pattern of hexagonal units made up of plates of liver cells, **hepatocytes**, arranged radially around a **central vein**. These units were traditionally designated the **liver lobules**. In the pig liver, each of these units is clearly outlined by a thin enveloping layer of connective tissue (Fig. 15.1). In the human, this layer is absent, but the location of small blood vessels associated with each liver lobule helps to define its outer limits. At three of the corners of each hexagonal lobule are small triangular areas of connective tissue containing a small **artery**, a parallel **vein**, and a small **bile duct**. These are commonly referred to as the **portal triads** (Figs 15.2, 15.3). Bile produced by the hepatocytes is released into a network of very small intercellular canaliculi between the cells that make up each radially oriented plate of the lobule. The bile in the canaliculi flows outwards to the small bile duct in the portal triads at the periphery of the classical lobule. The small artery and vein in each triad both have branches that are confluent with the **hepatic sinusoids** that occupy the spaces between the plates of hepatocytes. Blood flows from the vessels of the portal triads through the sinusoids to the **central vein** of the lobule (Fig. 15.2). The hepatocytes of the plates are thus exposed on both sides to a large volume of blood flowing centripetally through the system of sinusoids. The sinusoids are lined by fenestrated endothelium, which is separated from the neighboring plates of hepatocytes by a narrow perisinusoidal space, called the

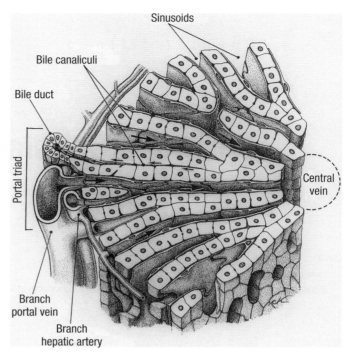

Figure 15.2 Schematic representation of the plates of liver cells arranged radially around the central vein. The flow of blood from the portal triads is inwards to the central vein. The flow of bile is outwards to the bile ductule in the triad. (Modified after A.W. Ham, *Textbook of Histology*, J.B. Lippincott Co., Philadelphia, 1965.)

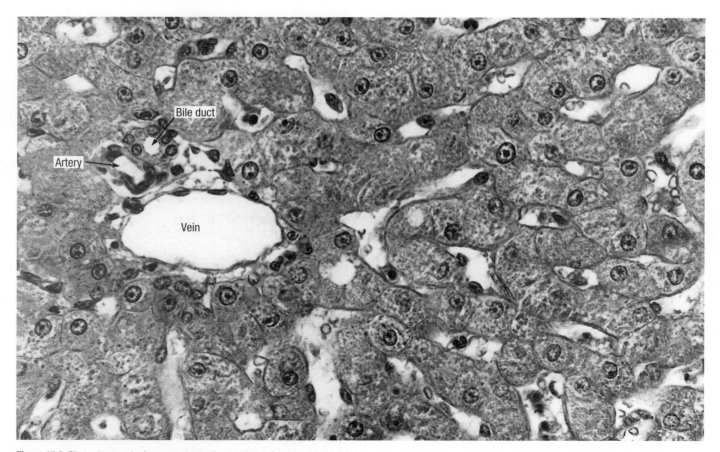

Figure 15.3 Photomicrograph of a portal triad at the periphery of a classical liver lobule. It contains a branch of the portal vein, a small artery, and a small bile duct.

space of Disse (Fig. 15.4). A supporting network of reticular fibers between the endothelium of the sinusoids and the plates of hepatocytes can be revealed by silver-containing stains.

Blood plasma freely enters the space of Disse through the fenestrations in the endothelium of the sinusoids and directly bathes the surface of the hepatic cells. A population of phagocytic cells, called **Kupffer's cells**, adhere to the endothelium and extend processes through its fenestrations into the space of Disse. These belong to the mononuclear phagocyte system of the body referred to earlier (Chapter 4). They function as tissue macrophages, ingesting particulate foreign matter, and they are able to recognize and phagocytize aged or damaged erythrocytes. As long-lived antigen-presenting phagocytes, they can be considered one of the several cell types of the immune system. They are able to incorporate antigen in the major histocompatibility complex (MHC) molecules on their surface and present them to lymphocytes. Like other members of the mononuclear phagocyte system, the Kupffer's cells are derived from stem cells in the bone marrow. The space of Disse also contains a few stellate **fat-storing cells (Ito cells)** that contain many lipid droplets. Their function is poorly understood.

The classical hepatic lobule, described above, was for a long time the most widely accepted unit of structural organization of the liver, but over the years, two alternative interpretations have been proposed. In one of these, a triangular area of parenchyma

around each portal triad, including all cells secreting into its bile ductule, was called a **portal lobule**. It included sectors of three neighboring classical lobules. Its proponents argued that this unit was more consistent with lobules of other glands, having its blood supply radiating from axial vessels, and its secretory product draining into a central duct. However, this interpretation was not widely accepted.

In the past 40 years, the preferred structural and functional unit of the liver has been the **hepatic acinus**. This is an elliptical unit that includes a sector of two neighboring classical lobules (Fig. 15.5). Traversing its center are branches of the terminal arteriole and the portal venule that radiate in three directions from each portal triad. At either end of the acinus is a **terminal hepatic venule** (central vein of the classical lobule). The acinus is commonly considered to have three zones, with zone 1 closest to its axial vessels and so its cells are first to be exposed to the incoming blood (Fig. 15.5). Zone 2, in the middle, and zone 3, at either end of the acinus, receive blood that has already been depleted of some of its solutes by the cells in zone 1. Support for the validity of this interpretation comes from the observation that, after a meal, the cells of zone 1 are first to receive glucose and store it as glycogen, whereas glycogen appears later, and in smaller amount, in zones 2 and 3. In fasting, the cells of zone 1 are first to respond to a low circulating blood glucose level by depolymerizing their glycogen

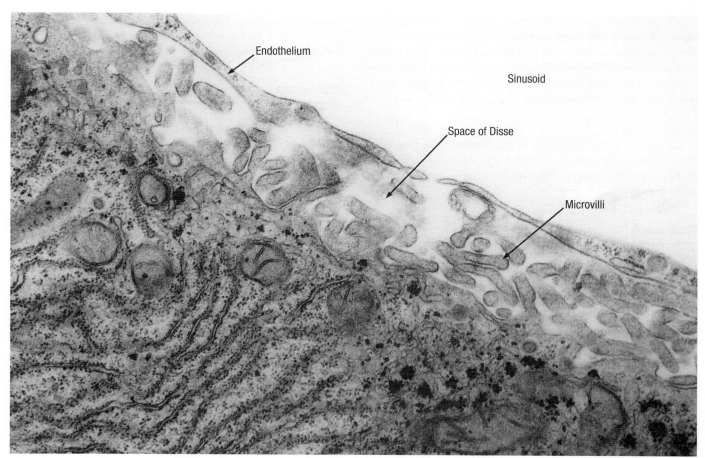

Figure 15.4 Electron micrograph of a portion of a liver cell (at lower left) and the lumen of a sinus (at upper right). Between the fenestrated endothelium of the sinusoid and the surface of the hepatocyte, is the space of Disse. Short microvilli of random orientation can be seen projecting into it from the surface of the hepatocyte. (Micrograph courtesy of K.R. Porter and G. Millonig.)

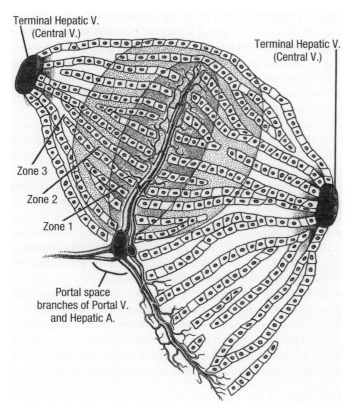

Terminal Hepatic V.
(Central V.)

Terminal Hepatic V.
(Central V.)

Zone 3

Zone 2

Zone 1

Portal space
branches of Portal V.
and Hepatic A.

Figure 15.5 Diagram of the hepatic acinus, consisting of an elliptical area of parenchyma between two central veins. It is transected by branches of the hepatic artery and portal vein. The cells of zone 1 are the first to be exposed to blood-borne oxygen and nutrients. Those in zone 2 are less favored, and those of zone 3 are least favorably situated. (Redrawn after A.M. Rappaport *et al. Anat Rec* 1954; 119:11.)

to add glucose to the blood. The acinus has also been adopted as the functional unit of the liver because it facilitates an explanation of the pattern of cell degeneration seen in hypoxic or toxic damage to the liver.

Blood supply

In order to understand the metabolic functions of the liver, it is essential to be aware of some unusual features of its blood supply. The liver receives blood from two sources: the **systemic circulation** and the **hepatic portal system**. The systemic circulation carries blood from the left ventricle of the heart to the extremities and the abdominal viscera, and venous blood from the lower extremities back to the right atrium of the heart via a large vein, the **inferior vena cava**, located on the posterior wall of the abdominal cavity. The hepatic portal system carries venous blood, which has already circulated through the capillaries of the gastrointestinal tract, to the liver, and which is, therefore, poor in oxygen content but rich in absorbed nutrients. Such a vascular system, in which poorly oxygenated blood is carried from the capillaries of one or more organs, to a system of capillaries (or sinusoids) in another organ, is called a **portal system**.

The liver's processing and metabolism of absorbed nutrients

depends upon its unique position between the portal and systemic circulations. About 75% of its blood flow is supplied by the hepatic portal vein, which undergoes several orders of branching: **interlobar veins**, **conducting veins**, and **interlobular veins**. The latter give rise to **portal venules**, the branches that accompany small branches of the hepatic artery to the portal triads. Terminal branches of these venules course around the periphery of the classical liver lobule as **perilobular veins** and these give off branches, called **inlet venules**, that empty into the sinusoids. The sinusoids, in turn, converge upon the central vein in the axis of each lobule. The wall of the central vein is thin, consisting of endothelium supported only by a loose network of reticular fibers. At the base of each classical liver lobule, the central vein joins a **sublobular vein** which is confluent with **collecting veins**. These join to form large **hepatic veins** that empty into the inferior vena cava, the major vein of general circulation that conducts blood back to the heart from all regions of the body below the diaphragm.

The **hepatic artery** enters the porta hepatis and branches into **interlobar** and **interlobular arteries**. The blood that these carry is distributed mainly to the connective tissue of the organ, but a small volume continues into the **hepatic arterioles** of the portal triads, the lateral branches of which conduct oxygenated blood into the sinusoids. The sinusoids thus receive poorly oxygenated blood from the portal system and well oxygenated blood from the systemic circulation. The cells at the periphery of the classical lobule (zone 1 of the acini) therefore receive oxygen in higher concentrations than those more centrally situated.

Hepatocytes

The liver cells, commonly called **hepatocytes**, make up 80% of the cell population of the liver. In histological sections, they have one, or occasionally two, spherical nuclei with prominent nucleoli. The cytoplasm is acidophilic, but contains conspicuous **basophilic bodies**. In electron micrographs, the latter are found to be parallel arrays of cisternae of the rER (Fig. 15.6). They are important sites for synthesis of albumen, prothrombin, fibrinogen, and lipoprotein of the blood plasma. In some areas of the cytoplasm, the rER is continuous with a network of tubules of sER (Figs 15.6, 15.7). This organelle has an important role in carbohydrate metabolism, bile formation, the catabolism of drugs, and other potentially toxic compounds. It is also the site of synthesis of the very low density serum lipoprotein (VLDL) that is released into the blood as a carrier for cholesterol. Small (30–40 nm), dense globules of VLDL can often be seen in the lumen of the smooth reticulum (Fig. 15.7).

Hepatocytes have multiple, small Golgi complexes located at their periphery near the bile canaliculi (Fig. 15.8). Mitochondria are very numerous and there are many lysosomes and peroxisomes. The peroxisomes participate in oxidative activity in the metabolism of lipids, purines, and alcohol, and in gluconeogenesis (the formation of glucose from molecules other than carbohydrates). The cytoplasm may also contain many small, dense granules of glycogen, which is the storage form of carbohydrate.

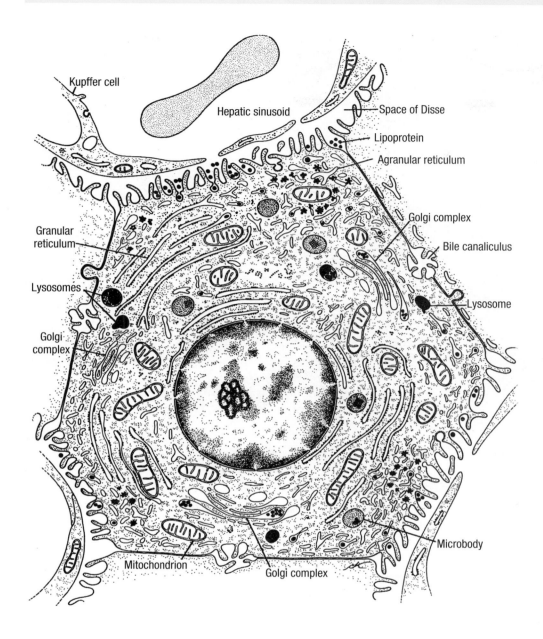

Figure 15.6 Drawing of the ultrastructure of a hepatocyte, showing its relationship to the sinusoids and the location of the bile canaliculi between neighboring cells of the cell plates. Note that Golgi complexes are situated near each bile canaliculus. (Drawing by Sylvia Keene.)

The ultrastructure of the hepatocytes differs significantly in the three zones of the hepatic acinus, reflecting differences in their functions. Gluconeogenesis occurs primarily in zone 1, and glycolysis in zones 2 and 3. The sER is sparse in cells of zone 1, but is well developed in those of zone 3, which are more active in lipid metabolism. The mitochondria of cells of zone 3 are very numerous, but quite small. Those in the periportal region, zone 1, are nearly twice the size of those of zone 3. Glycogen is usually most abundant in zones 1 and 2 (corresponding to the periphery of the classical lobule).

Owing to the arrangement of hepatocytes in plates one cell thick, they have no surface that can appropriately be described as apical or basal. The sides of the cell exposed to the sinusoids are referred to as the **sinusoidal domain** of the plasmalemma, and the sides in contact with neighboring hepatocytes are the **lateral domain**. Midway along the lateral domain of adjoining hepatic cells, the opposing membranes diverge to bound a small intercellular channel 0.5–1.5 μm in diameter, the **bile canaliculus** (Figs 15.6, 15.8). Along either side of its lumen, the closely apposed cell membranes form a junction comparable to the tight junctions of other epithelial cells. These junctions isolate the lumen and prevent intercellular escape of bile secreted into the canaliculi. These minute channels form a network within the cell plates, with a single hepatocyte in each of its polygonal meshes. Although the membrane of the hepatocytes is similar in appearance throughout, cytochemical methods reveal regional functional differences. In the sinusoidal domain, the membrane contains receptors for sialoglycoproteins, mannose-6-phosphate, and other substances taken up from the blood by receptor-mediated endocytosis. The membrane of the lateral domain contains aminopeptidase, phosphatase, and three glycoproteins not found elsewhere in the cell surface. Adenyl cyclase and Na$^+$, K$^+$-ATPase are found in both the sinusoidal and lateral domains.

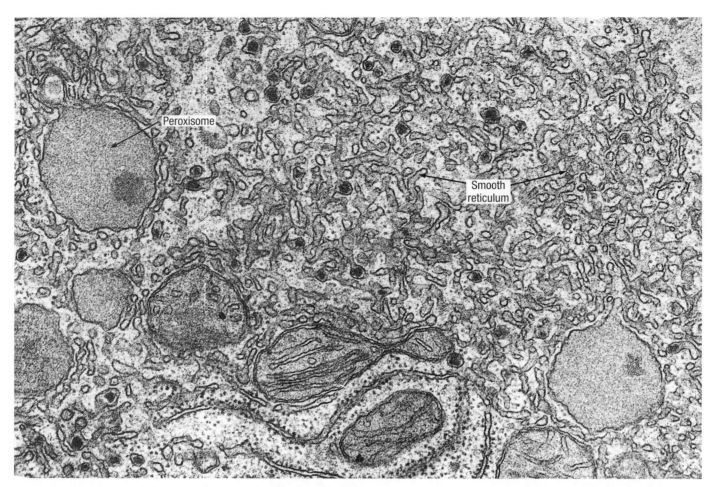

Figure 15.7 Electron micrograph of an area of hepatocyte cytoplasm that is rich in smooth endoplasmic reticulum. Notice that some of its tubes contain small dense droplets of newly synthesized very low density lipoprotein. (Micrograph courtesy of R. Bolender.)

Duct system

At the periphery of the classical lobule (axis of the acinus) the bile canaliculi are confluent with short bile ductules (**canals of Hering**) that drain into interlobular bile ducts of the portal triads. These ducts, lined by cuboidal epithelium, continue into a system of progressively larger ducts that converge to form the **right** and **left hepatic bile ducts** from the corresponding lobes of the liver. These join to form the **common bile duct**, which, in turn, is joined by the **cystic duct** from the gallbladder. The large duct so formed is joined (in the wall of the duodenum) by the **pancreatic duct**. These ducts are lined by columnar epithelium and have a thin submucosa, muscularis, and adventitia. Where they traverse the wall of the duodenum, their intermingling circular muscle is thickened to form the **sphincter of Oddi** (hepatopancreatic sphincter). Between meals, when this sphincter is closed, the bile secreted by the liver flows up the cystic duct into the gallbladder where it is stored and concentrated.

Histophysiology of the liver

The liver has a greater variety of functions than any other organ. Its principal contribution to the digestive process is the secretion of

500–1000 ml of **bile** a day. Bile is a greenish solution containing cholesterol, neutral fats, phospholipids, lecithin, and bile salts. Of these, the bile salts (cholic acid and other derivatives of cholesterol) are the most important. They emulsify dietary fats, reducing them to micelles, which are readily absorbed by the intestinal epithelium. An excretory function of the bile is the elimination of **bilirubin**, a toxic, greenish pigment formed by the Kupffer cells' degradation of the hemoglobin of senescent erythrocytes. Bilirubin is taken up by the hepatocytes, conjugated with glucuronide in the sER, and excreted in the bile. In severe liver disease, interference with this function results in jaundice, a yellowing of the skin and mucous membranes. Determination of the relative amounts of conjugated and unconjugated bilirubin is a clinically useful measure of liver function.

During the elevation of circulating blood glucose after meals, hepatocytes take it up from the blood and polymerize and store it as **glycogen** (Figs 15.9, 15.10). Between meals, glycogen is depolymerized to glucose, which is returned to the blood as needed. The liver is also capable of gluconeogenesis, the synthesis of glucose from compounds such as lactic acid, glycerol, and pyruvic acid. Fatty acids taken up by the hepatocytes are either used by the sER to generate triglycerides, which are stored in lipid droplets, or they are transformed into **VLDL**, which is released into the blood as a carrier for cholesterol. The liver is also the site of synthesis of the

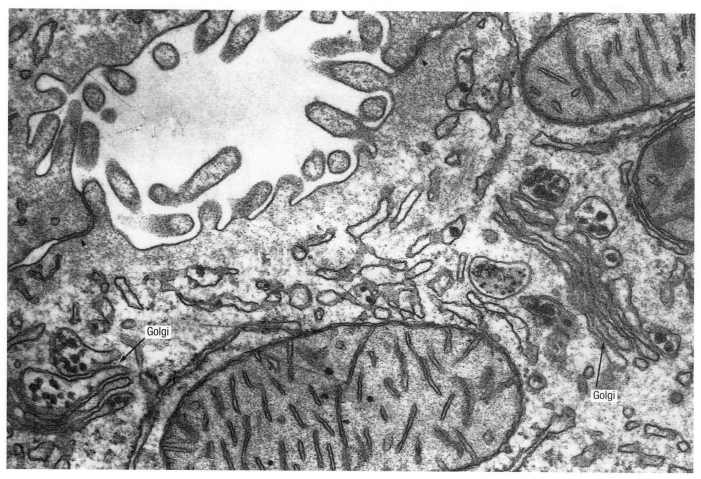

Figure 15.8 Electron micrograph of a bile canaliculus between two hepatic cells. Observe the tight junctions on either side of the canaliculus (at tail-less arrows). Vesicles associated with two small Golgi complexes, near the canaliculus, contain particles of very low density lipoprotein. (Micrograph courtesy of R. Bolender.)

plasma proteins and blood-clotting factors of the blood: **albumen, fibrinogen, thrombin,** and **factor 3**.

The hepatocytes have an accessory role in the immune system of the intestines. A large portion of the IgA antibodies produced by plasma cells in the intestinal mucosa is carried in the lymph to the thoracic duct and then into the general circulation. An immunoglobulin receptor, **secretory component**, is continuously synthesized by the hepatocytes and incorporated into the sinusoidal domain of their surface membrane. IgA is taken up from the blood by receptor-mediated endocytosis and transported to the bile canaliculi, where the secretory component is cleaved off, releasing the IgA into the bile for transport to the gut lumen to defend against intestinal bacterial flora.

> The liver has a remarkable ability to break down drugs and toxins or render them harmless by conjugation with other molecules. However, daily consumption of a pint or more of whisky, or an equivalent amount of wine or beer over a period of 10 years may lead to **cirrhosis of the liver**. Initially the cells become distended with fat as a result of impaired fatty acid oxidation. This progresses to necrosis of hepatocytes and their replacement with connective tissue. The person becomes emaciated, weak, and chronically jaundiced because of increasing amounts of circulating bilirubin.

GALLBLADDER

The **gallbladder** is a pear-shaped, hollow organ occupying a shallow fossa on the undersurface of the liver. It normally measures 10×4 cm and has a capacity of 40–70 ml. It has a fundus, a body, and a narrower neck region, which continues into the **cystic duct**. Its wall consists of a mucosa, a lamina propria, a thin fibromuscular layer, and a serosa which is continuous with that covering the liver. In the empty gallbladder, the mucosa is raised into convoluted folds of varying length that run mainly longitudinally. These are shorter and more widely spaced when the organ is distended. There may also be out-pocketings of the mucosa near the neck of the gallbladder that extend through the lamina propria and between smooth muscle fibers of the submucosa. These are called **Rokitansky–Aschoff sinuses** and may be mistaken for dilated glands. Their lining is continuous with the surface epithelium. They are of no functional significance and may represent pathological changes in the wall of the gallbladder.

The gallbladder epithelium is a single layer of tall columnar cells, having an ovoid nucleus and a faintly eosinophilic cytoplasm. There is a moderately dense population of short microvilli

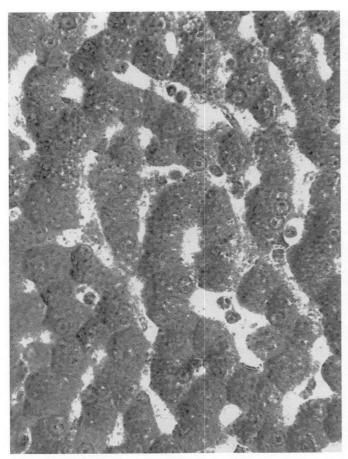

Figure 15.9 Photomicrograph of plates of hepatocytes from an animal fed after a period of fasting. The section was stained with Best's carmine, which is selective for glycogen. The intense red staining is caused by a large amount of glycogen in the cells.

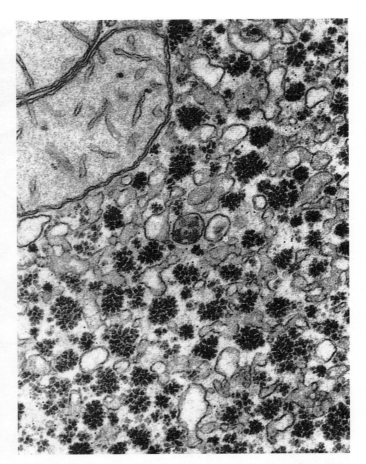

Figure 15.10 Electron micrograph of a small area of cytoplasm from a liver cell of zone 1, after feeding. The many densely stained aggregates of small particles are glycogen.

on the free surface of the cells. Their lateral surfaces are straight in the apical region, but may be interdigitated in their lower portion. While bile is being concentrated by active transport of water across the epithelium, the lower portion of the intercellular clefts may be widened. In the neck region of the gallbladder, the epithelium is invaginated into the lamina propria to form short tubuloalveolar glands lined by mucus-secreting cuboidal cells. The cystic duct continues downwards from the neck of the gallbladder and joins the common bile duct.

Histophysiology of the gallbladder

The main function of the gallbladder is to store and concentrate the bile by absorbing water. Active sodium transport across the epithelium creates an osmotic gradient that draws water out of the bile. Bile contains cholesterol, phospholipids, bile acids, and pigments (primarily bilirubin glucuronide). Release of bile into the duodenum is controlled by endocrine cells of the intestinal epithelium. The presence of lipid in the lumen of the intestine stimulates enteroendocrine cells (I-cells) in the mucosa to secrete a polypeptide hormone, **cholecystokinin (CCK)**, also called pancreozymin. This induces contraction of the smooth muscle in the wall of the gallbladder, adding bile to the chyme to promote lipid absorption.

The most common disorder of the gallbladder is **cholelithiasis** (gallstones), which is estimated to afflict 16 million people over the age of 40 years in the United States. Gallstones are concretions of cholesterol monohydrate, calcium salts, and phospholipid. They may be asymptomatic, or may cause a mild inflammation of the wall of the gallbladder. They cause severe pain only when one of the stones moves into the cystic duct, occluding its lumen. Treatment of cholelithiasis is by surgical removal of the gallbladder, or by cholelithotripsy which breaks up the concretions into small fragments that can easily pass through the cystic duct.

Questions

1 The space of Disse is
   a in the portal triad area
   b between the Kupffer and endothelial cells
   c surrounded by endothelium
   d between the sinusoid and the hepatocyte
   e located only in the area of the portal triad

2 The epithelium lining the gallbladder
   a is pseudostratified columnar
   b is stratified squamous non-keratinized
   c is simple columnar
   d contains goblet cells
   e is ciliated

3 Hepatocytes are involved in
   a synthesis and secretion of fibrinogen
   b bile formation
   c synthesis and secretion of lipoproteins
   d formation of urea
   e all of the above

4 Which of the following statement(s) is/are true of the liver?
   a it can regenerate its parenchyma
   b hepatocytes have at least six surfaces
   c it is both an endocrine and exocrine organ
   d it will metabolize xenobiotics
   e all of the above

5 Glycogen synthesis is associated with which of the following in the hepatocyte?
   a peroxisomes
   b Golgi apparatus
   c smooth endoplasmic reticulum
   d rough endoplasmic reticulum
   e none of the above

6 The portal canal contains all of the following **except**
   a lymphatic
   b central vein
   c bile duct
   d portal vein
   e hepatic artery

7 Which statement is correct concerning liver lobules?
   a the peripheral landmarks of the classic lobule are portal canals
   b the peripheral landmarks of the portal lobule are portal canals
   c the peripheral landmarks of the liver acinus are portal canals
   d the central axis of a portal lobule is the central vein
   e the central axis of a classical lobule is the portal canal

8 Which statement best describes the bile canaliculus?
   a it is formed by specialized fibroblasts
   b it is formed by specialized endothelial cells
   c it develops from an outgrowth of the cystic duct
   d it is continuous with the hepatic duct
   e it is formed by grooves in two opposing hepatocytes

9 Kupffer's cells of the liver are located
   a within sinusoids
   b within the space of Disse
   c along bile canaliculi
   d in portal canals
   e within the bile duct

10 Which statement is true about the gallbladder
   a it is continuous directly with the bile duct
   b cholecystokinin stimulates its contraction
   c scanning electron microscopy shows a smooth apical border on the gallbladder epithelium
   d the gallbladder contains mucus-secreting cells
   e there is little or no folding of the mucosa

11 What is the name of the cell in the liver that actively phagocytoses foreign particles?

12 The canals of Hering are associated with what substance?

13 From what structure does the cystic duct arise?

14 Detoxification of drugs is performed by what cell type?

15 What is the functional unit of the liver?

16 What is the name of the area between the hepatocyte and sinusoid in the liver?

17 What is the name of the vein that drains into the portal canal?

18 Where does the exchange of materials between the blood and liver cells take place?

19 What structure drains its contents into the canals of Hering?

20 This cell is considered a fixed macrophage in the liver and is part of the monocyte-phagocyte system (MAPS).

Chapter sixteen

Pancreas

The **pancreas** is the second largest of the glands associated with the digestive tract. It is flattened from front to back and adheres to the posterior wall of the abdominal cavity behind the antrum of the stomach. It is 12–15 cm in length with a broader **head** and a narrower **tail** region. The head lies within the C-shaped curve of the duodenum and the tail extends transversely towards the spleen, crossing the bodies of the second or third lumbar vertebra. The pancreas is a mixed gland, having an **exocrine portion** and an

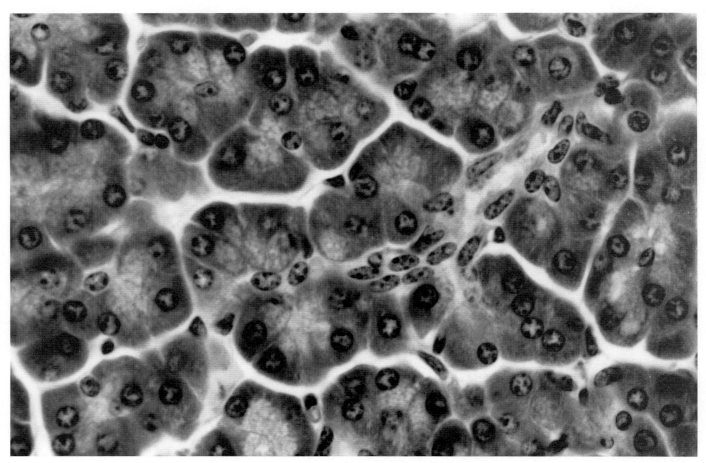

Figure 16.1 Photomicrograph of the exocrine pancreas, showing the glandular acini and one small duct. The basal cytoplasm of the acinar cells is intensely basophilic.

endocrine portion. As in other exocrine glands, the greater part of its volume is made up of secretory acini at the ends of a branching system of ducts. The gland secretes 1.5–3.0 L daily of enzyme-rich fluid into the duodenum for digestion of dietary carbohydrates, fats, and proteins. Scattered through the gland are tens of thousands of small aggregations of endocrine cells called **islets of Langerhans.** These release into the blood the hormones **insulin** and **glucagon,** which regulate the metabolism of carbohydrates.

EXOCRINE PANCREAS

Pancreatic acini

The pancreatic acini are round, or slightly elongated, and are made up of 40–50 pyramidal epithelial cells around a small lumen (Fig.16.1). The acinar cells have a heterochromatic nucleus and an intensely basophilic cytoplasm. The supranuclear portion of the cytoplasm is filled with closely packed secretory granules, commonly called **zymogen granules.** These contain the precursors of several digestive enzymes (Fig.16.2). On electron micrographs, the basal cytoplasm of the acinar cells is crowded with closely spaced cisternae of rough endoplasmic reticulum (rER), and many free ribosomes

(Fig.16.2). Numerous small vesicles are clustered around the cis-face of the Golgi apparatus, and larger vesicles and developing zymogen granules are associated with its trans-face. Mitochondria, lysosomes and occasional lipid droplets are also found in this region of the cytoplasm. The acini are surrounded by a dense plexus of capillaries.

The pancreatic acinar cells synthesize the digestive enzymes **trypsin, chymotrypsin, ribonuclease, carboxypeptidase, decarboxylase, phospholipase, elastase, amylase,** and possibly others. No other cell type produces such a variety of secretory products. In order to protect the gland from self-digestion, resulting from intracellular activation of any of these products, the cytoplasm of the acinar cells contains protease inhibitors and the enzymes are secreted as inactive proenzymes that are normally activated only upon reaching the duodenum.

> Despite intrinsic safeguards against intracellular activation of enzymes, this may occur because of toxins, virus infections, excessive ingestion of alcohol, or as a complication of bile obstruction. These factors may directly activate trypsin, which, in turn, activates the other enzymes leading to *acute pancreatitis*, a potentially lethal disorder. The enzymes liberated destroy cellular membranes, produce edema, cell necrosis, and hemorrhage. Infection is often superimposed upon these effects, leading to abscess formation. Adjacent organs may be secondarily affected. The survival rate of patients with acute pancreatitis is only about 30% with medical treatment alone, but may be nearly twice that with early surgical intervention.

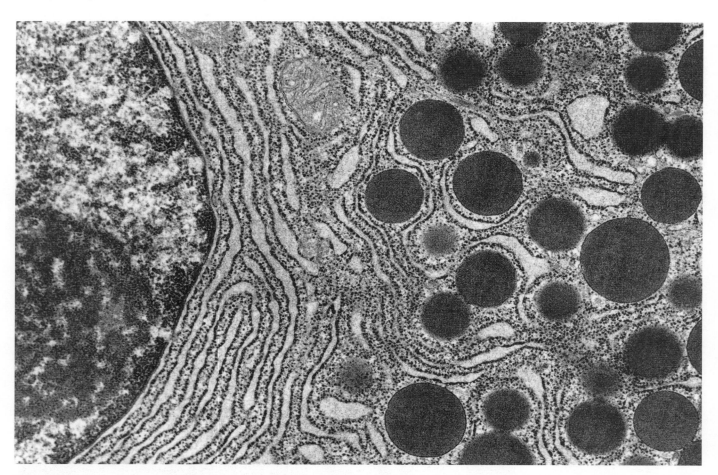

Figure 16.2 Electron micrograph of a portion of a human pancreatic acinar cell, showing a large nucleolus (at left), abundant rough endoplasmic reticulum, and zymogen granules (at right).

Duct system

The pancreas is unique among compound exocrine glands in that the terminal ducts, called **intercalated ducts**, extend a short distance into the acini (Figs 16.3, 16.4). The portion extending into the acinus is made up of pale-staining, low cuboidal cells, called **centroacinar cells**. These contain no secretory granules and have relatively few organelles. The intercalated ducts proximal to the acini, are lined by pale-staining cuboidal cells. The transport of the proenzymes from the acini to the duodenum is not the only function of the pancreatic ducts. Their cells secrete a fluid containing bicarbonate ions in a concentration five to eight times that in the blood. The high concentration of bicarbonate probably prevents proenzymes secreted by the acini from being activated in the duct system. Upon reaching the duodenum, this fluid (pH 8.0) helps to neutralize the acidity of the chyme coming from the stomach. Impairment of ductal secretory function results in serious disease. Furthermore, 90% of cancers of the pancreas are of ductal origin.

The slender intercalated ducts emerging from several acini converge to form **intralobular ducts**. These combine to form **interlobular ducts** in the connective tissue between lobules of the gland. These larger ducts, lined with low columnar epithelium, join a **main pancreatic duct** that runs longitudinally through the

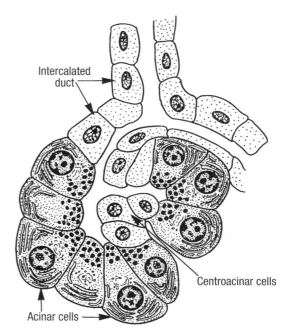

Figure 16.3 Drawing of a pancreatic acinus, showing its centroacinar cells and the intercalated duct.

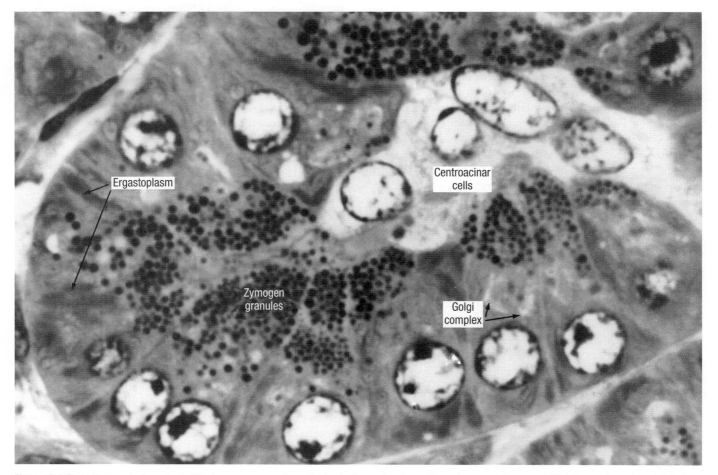

Figure 16.4 Photomicrograph of an acinus of the human pancreas. Several pale-staining centroacinar cells can be seen at the upper right. (Micrograph courtesy of S. Ito.)

entire length of the organ. In the head of the gland, the main pancreatic duct turns downwards, coming into close relationship with the **bile duct**, and the two join to form a short common duct, the **hepatopancreatic duct**, which passes through the wall of the duodenum and opens into its lumen.

Innervation

Small clusters of ganglion cells are located in the interlobular connective tissue of the gland. Small nerves can be observed penetrating the basal lamina of the acini and ending in intimate contact with the base of acinar cells. These are postganglionic cholinergic fibers of the **vagus nerve** (10th cranial nerve). Electrical stimulation of the vagus nerve results in some secretion into the lumen of the acini and small ducts. However, nervous control of pancreatic secretion is thought to be of less importance than its regulation by hormones released by the enteroendocrine cells of the duodenal mucosa. The membrane at the base of the acinar cells contains receptors for three or more of these hormones. Their binding to the cells stimulates secretion by the acinar cells.

Histophysiology of the exocrine pancreas

After opening of the pyloric sphincter and passage of acidic chyme from the stomach into the duodenum, the pancreas secretes into its lumen a large volume of alkaline fluid containing 15 or more digestive enzymes. Its secretion is mainly controlled by hormones of **enteroendocrine cells** in the duodenal mucosa. Passage of acidic chyme into the duodenum stimulates **I-cells** to release the hormone **cholecystokinin**, and **S-cells** to release **secretin**, into the blood. Upon reaching the pancreas, cholecystokinin binds to receptors on the acinar cells, stimulating their release of the highly concentrated proenzymes stored in their zymogen granules. Secretin binds to receptors on the duct cells, causing them to secrete, into the lumen, a bicarbonate-rich isotonic fluid that serves as a vehicle for the proenzymes released by the acinar cells. The alkalinity of this fluid insures that the proenzymes will not be converted to their active form prematurely and damage the pancreas. Upon discharge into the duodenum, the pancreatic juice neutralizes the acidity of the chyme, creating the alkaline environment necessary for maximal activity of the digestive enzymes.

ENDOCRINE PANCREAS

Islets of Langerhans

The endocrine component of the pancreas consists of **islets of Langerhans**, which are widely scattered among the acini of the exocrine pancreas (Fig. 16.5). Each of these is a compact aggregation of a few thousand cells enclosed by a thin layer of reticular fibers. It contains a rich network of fenestrated capillaries. The

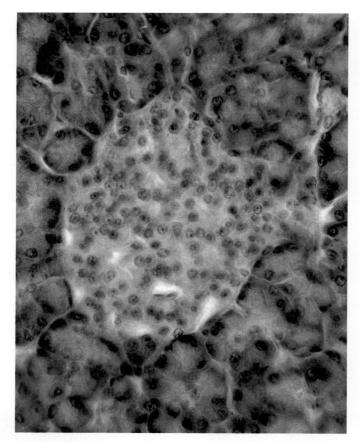

Figure 16.5 Photomicrograph of an islet of Langerhans and surrounding acinar tissue.

islets are most numerous in the body and tail of the gland. Although they are estimated to number over a million in the human pancreas, the islets make up only 1–2% of its volume.

The islets of Langerhans contain four types of epithelial cells: **A-cells** (α-cells), secreting **glucagon**; **B-cells** (β-cells), secreting **insulin**; **D-cells**, secreting **somatostatin**; **F-cells** (PP-cells), secreting **pancreatic polypeptide**. These cell types cannot be distinguished from one another in routine histological sections, but they can be identified by use of fluorescein-conjugated antibodies to their respective products (Fig. 16.6). The only distinctive features that permit their identification on electron micrographs are differences in cell size, location in the islet, and internal structure of the secretory granules. The majority of the A-cells are at the periphery of the islet (Fig. 16.6A), but occasional isolated cells may be found in its interior. The B-cells are the predominant cell type, occupying the central region of the islet and accounting for 70% of its volume. The D-cells and F-cells are few in number and variable in location (Fig. 16.6B).

On electron micrographs, the granules of the four types of cells are subject to great interspecific variation. In the human pancreas, the granules of the A-cells have a dense center surrounded by a narrow clear zone (Fig. 16.7B), and the B-cell granules contain one or more dense crystals of zinc-insulin in a matrix of low density (Fig. 16.7A). Upon release, the contents of the granules diffuse into the blood in neighboring fenestrated capillaries.

Ganglion cells are occasionally found adjacent to a few of the

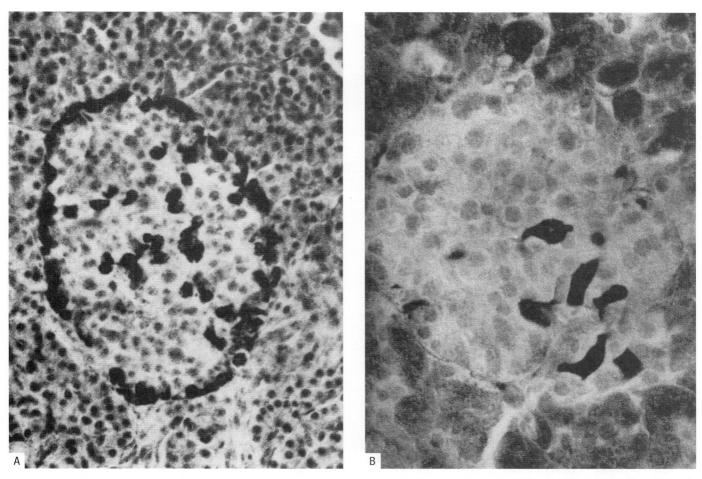

Figure 16.6 (A) Pancreatic islet stained by a method that selectively stains the glucagon-secreting A-cells, located around the periphery of the islet, near capillaries. (B) An islet of Langerhans stained to reveal the somatostatin-secreting D-cells. (Reproduced from C. Hellerstrom *Acta Paediatr Scand* 1977; 270:7.)

islets, and both cholinergic and adrenergic nerves can be found terminating on a very small number of the islet cells, but the autonomic nervous system is believed to play a relatively minor role in islet cell function.

Histophysiology of the endocrine pancreas

The major product of the digestion of carbohydrates is **glucose**, which is an important energy source for cells throughout the body. The hormones of the islets of Langerhans control the level of glucose in the circulation. Following a meal, the rise in the blood glucose level stimulates the B-cells to release **insulin**. This hormone lowers blood glucose by enhancing membrane transport of glucose into muscle cells, connective tissue cells, and white blood cells. It also acts upon the liver to inhibit the breakdown of glycogen to glucose and it inhibits synthesis of glucose from amino acids and fatty acids. The exact mechanisms of these effects are still under investigation.

In the fasting state, the relatively low level of blood glucose activates the A-cells to secrete **glucagon**, which acts upon the liver to increase conversion of glycogen to glucose and its release into the blood. It also stimulates the liver to increase synthesis of glucose from amino acids and fatty acids. Thus, insulin and glucagon have opposite effects, with insulin being a *hypoglycemic* hormone and glucagon a *hyperglycemic* hormone.

The D-cells of the islets, producing the hormone somatostatin, are believed to be involved in inhibition of the release of glucagon by the A-cells during periods of high blood sugar levels. To date, little is known about the function of F-cells, which produce pancreatic polypeptide.

A very common disease of the endocrine pancreas is **diabetes mellitus**, which occurs in two forms. Type I, or insulin-dependent diabetes mellitus (IDDM), develops quite suddenly before the age of 15 years, and is apparently caused by an autoimmune destruction of the B-cells of the islets. These patients produce no insulin, and are dependent upon injections of the hormone. Type II, or non-insulin dependent diabetes mellitus (NIDDM), usually occurs in obese individuals older than 40 years of age. Insulin is produced, but in inadequate amount, and there is also an abnormality of the insulin receptors. This form of diabetes can usually be controlled by diet and correction of the associated obesity.

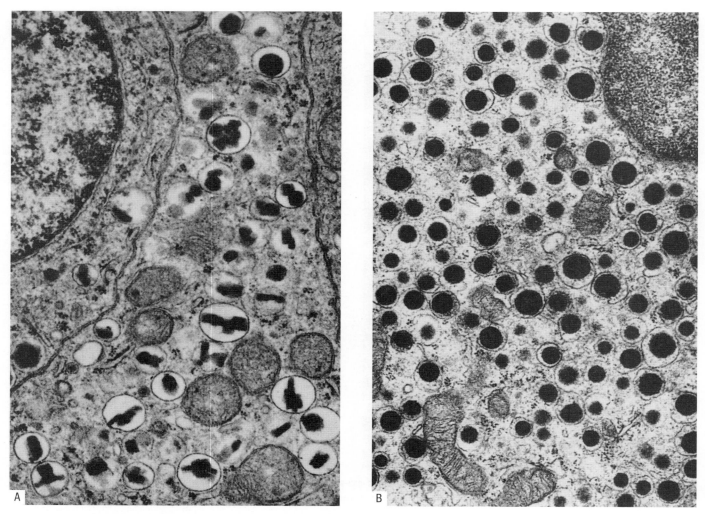

Figure 16.7 (A) Electron micrograph of portions of two human B-cells, showing secretory granules containing crystals of varying form. (B) Cytoplasm of an A-cell, containing granules with a dense core and a less dense periphery.

Questions

1 Bicarbonate production by the pancreas is stimulated by
   a glucagon
   b secretin
   c insulin
   d somatostatin
   e cholecystokinin

2 The pancreas is the only anatomical location for
   a secretory acini
   b intercalated ducts
   c centroacinar cells
   d exocrine secretory units
   e striated ducts

3 Which of the following statements is true about the pancreas?
   a the α-cells are located primarily at the center of the islets
   b delta cells are the primary cell type in islets
   c the α-cells produce insulin
   d the pancreas contains striated ducts
   e intercalated ducts are present in the pancreas

4 Which of the following can stimulate pancreatic exocrine secretion?
   a insulin
   b somatostatin
   c cholecystokinin
   d glucagon
   e blood glucose

5 An increase in concentration of glucose permease is related to all but which one of the following?
   a insulin
   b decreased blood lipid
   c elevated blood glucose
   d a change in the composition of cell membranes
   e a good meal

6 Which of the following statements is true about the pancreas?
   a a fasting state will stimulate β-cell secretory activity
   b D-cells produce glucagon
   c the A-cells produce insulin
   d it contains striated ducts
   e intercalated duct cells can produce bicarbonate

7 Beta cells of the islets of Langerhans produce which of the following?
   a glucagon
   b somatostatin
   c insulin
   d trypsinogen
   e lysozyme

8 Pancreatic acinar cells release proenzymes in response to
   a cholecystokinin
   b aldosterone
   c renin
   d secretin
   e glucagon

9 Glucagon is secreted by which of the following cells of the islets of Langerhans?
   a A-cells
   b B-cells
   c D-cells
   d F-cells
   e all of these cells secrete glucagon

10 Carbonic anhydrase is associated with which of the following cells?
   a centroacinar cells of the pancreas
   b G-cells of the pylorus
   c juxtaglomerular cells
   d mucous-neck cells
   e α-cells of the islets of Langerhans

11 What pancreatic cell secretes somatostatin?

12 In what gland are centroacinar cells found?

13 What type of duct is present in abundance in the parotid gland, but absent in the pancreas?

14 What hormone inhibits secretion of growth hormone from A-cells and B-cells of the pancreas?

15 What hormone causes the release of glucose into the bloodstream?

16 What hormone is secreted by D-cells?

17 What hormone is secreted by the A-cells of the islets of Langerhans?

Respiratory System

The **respiratory system** consists of the **lungs** and the passages that conduct air to and from them. It can be thought of as having a **conducting portion** and a **respiratory portion**. The conducting portion includes the **nose, pharynx, trachea,** and **bronchi.** The respiratory portion is where the vital gas exchange between the inspired air and the blood occurs. It is made up of the terminal branches of the bronchi, called **respiratory bronchioles,** the **alveolar ducts,** and countless **alveoli,** small air-filled sacs that make up the greater part of the parenchyma of the lung. The very thin walls of the alveoli, containing a dense network of capillaries, are admirably constructed to facilitate the diffusion of oxygen from the inspired air into the blood, and the concurrent diffusion of carbon dioxide from the blood into the alveolar air for elimination at the next expiration. Carbon dioxide, formed as a by-product of tissue metabolism, is carried to the lungs in the blood pumped into the **pulmonary circulation** by the right ventricle of the heart. Oxygen-carrying blood, returning from the lungs to the heart, is pumped by the left ventricle into the **systemic circulation** for distribution to tissues throughout the body.

NOSE

The **nose** is made up of a framework of bone and cartilage covered by skin and subcutaneous connective tissue. A cartilaginous median **nasal septum** divides its interior into right and left **nasal cavities** which are continuous posteriorly with the **nasopharynx,** and open anteriorly at the **nares** (nostrils). The surface area of each nasal cavity is increased by three thin scroll-like projections from its lateral wall, called the **nasal conchae.** Four different types of epithelium are found in the nasal cavities. The stratified squamous epithelium of the skin covering the nose continues, for a short distance, into the **vestibule,** a slight dilatation of the cavity just inside the nares. This epithelium bears a few coarse hairs that project into the airway. A few millimeters into the vestibule, stratified squamous epithelium gives way to a narrow band of non-ciliated cuboidal or columnar epithelium. Beyond this, the greater part of the nasal cavities is lined by ciliated pseudostratified columnar epithelium containing occasional goblet cells. Goblet cells increase in number from anterior to posterior. On the lower and middle conchae, the lamina propria is richly vascularized and the flow of arterial blood warms the inspired air as it passes through the nose. The air also acquires some water vapor to prevent desiccation of the delicate alveoli of the lung. There is an extensive venous plexus on the lower part of the septum and on the lower two conchae. These thin-walled veins become engorged, periodically partially occluding the airway, first on one side of the septum and then on the other. This intermittent partial occlusion is thought to enable the nasal mucosa on the closed side to recover from desiccation caused by the airflow. These vessels are also a common site of 'nosebleeds'.

Olfactory epithelium

The roof of the nasal cavity, and a small area of the septum and superior concha, are lined by **olfactory epithelium,** an unusually thick (60–100 μm) pseudostratified epithelium that contains the receptor cells for the sense of smell. It is composed of three types of cells: **sustentacular cells, olfactory cells,** and **basal cells** (Fig.17.1). The tall, columnar sustentacular cells have a striated border of microvilli and a conspicuous terminal web. Their apical cytoplasm contains smooth endoplasmic reticulum (sER), a

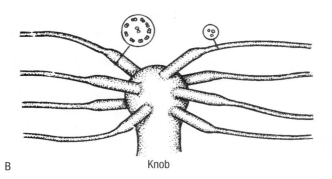

B   Knob

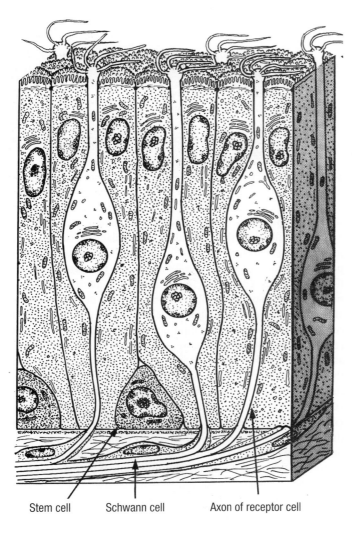

Stem cell   Schwann cell   Axon of receptor cell

A

Figure 17.1 (A) Diagram of olfactory epithelium showing its three cell types, and, below the epithelium, Schwann cells around the axons of the receptor cells. (B) Drawing of the knob at the apical end of the receptor cell dendrite.

cells. Their nuclei are aligned in the epithelium at a level below those of the sustentacular cells. Their apical portion is narrowed to a thin cylindrical process that terminates in a small, rounded expansion, called the **olfactory bulb**, or **knob**, that projects somewhat above the apices of the surrounding sustentacular cells (Fig.17.1). This contains the basal bodies of 6–8 nonmotile **olfactory cilia** that radiate from the olfactory bulb parallel to the surface of the epithelium. These are very long, attaining a length of 70μm. In their initial portion, the axoneme contains the usual 9+2 arrangement of doublet microtubules, but a short distance from the basal body there is an abrupt narrowing of the cilium. In its more slender distal portion, the axoneme is made up of a variable number of single microtubules, instead of the usual doublets. Towards its base, the body of the olfactory cell tapers down to an axon about 0.5μm in diameter. The axon passes through the basal lamina into the lamina propria, where it joins those of other olfactory cells, forming fascicles of unmyelinated axons that are each enveloped by Schwann cells. These axons pass through the **cribriform plate** of the skull and synapse in the **olfactory lobe** of the brain.

At the base of the olfactory epithelium, there are small, basophilic **basal cells**, which are considered to be stem cells, that can divide and differentiate into either sustentacular cells or olfactory cells. The olfactory cells have a limited lifespan and are continually replaced by asymmetric division of stem cells. The ability of this epithelium to renew its sensory neurons (olfactory cells) is exceptional, for regeneration of neurons is rare in other parts of the nervous system. Another unusual feature of this epithelium is that the tips of the olfactory cells are the only place where neurons are directly exposed to the environment.

In the lamina propria of the epithelium are branched tubuloalveolar glands, the **glands of Bowman**, made up of pyramidal cells with apical secretory granules. Their secretion creates a fluid environment around the olfactory cilia that is believed to facilitate access of odors to the sensory receptors on the olfactory cilia.

Histophysiology of the nose

The nose conditions the inspired air for passage to the lungs by warming and humidifying it to prevent desiccation of the delicate alveoli. The moving blanket of mucus on the surface of the nasal epithelium entraps dust particles and carries them to the pharynx where they are swallowed with the mucus. The continuous movement of the mucus towards the pharynx also makes the olfactory receptors accessible to new odors by removing odorants to which the olfactory epithelium has recently been exposed.

How odors are sensed, and how many odors can be distinguished, are questions that have long puzzled physiologists, but recent research has brought us closer to the answers. It has been shown that the human nose is capable of recognizing thousands of different scents. Odors bind to receptors on the unusual cilia of the olfactory cells. Their binding initiates electrical signals that travel along the axons of the neurons to the olfactory bulb of the brain, located in the cranial cavity directly above the nose. Neurons there relay the information to higher sensory centers in the cerebral cortex for interpretation. The existence of specific

supranuclear Golgi complex, mitochondria, and a few pigment granules that give the olfactory epithelium a pale yellowish-brown color. The olfactory cells, the neurosensory elements (neurons) of the epithelium, are located between sustentacular

receptors for particular odors was first suggested by the occurrence of individuals with **specific anosmia**, an inherited inability to detect a particular odor. It is now known that the human genome contains genes that encode 1000 or more different odor receptors. Each sensory neuron in the olfactory epithelium expresses only one kind of receptor and there are hundreds of neurons in the olfactory epithelium expressing that same receptor. These may be scattered through the epithelium, among other neurons bearing a different receptor, but the axons of all those neurons bearing the same receptor converge upon only one, or at most a few, of the thousands of small rounded aggregations of neurons in the olfactory lobe, called glomeruli. Signals relayed by each glomerulus are transmitted to the olfactory cortex, where they are processed to allow odor discrimination.

Most mammals have a **vomeronasal organ** containing a sensory epithelium separate from the main olfactory epithelium. This organ senses the odorants, called **pheromones**, that govern sexual behavior. The neurons of the vomeronasal organ bypass the cognitive centers of the brain and go directly to the areas that control instinctive behavior. An animal in which the vomeronasal organ has been destroyed, can still smell all other odorants, but cannot detect the distinctive odor of the opposite sex, or its pheromones, and does not mate. A rudimentary vomeronasal organ is present in the human nose, but its influence upon sexual behavior seems to have been lost.

Paranasal sinuses

The paranasal sinuses are cavities in the frontal, maxillary, and ethmoid bones, lined by a relatively thin mucosa with a ciliated columnar epithelium. Goblet cells of the epithelium, and of submucosal glands, secrete a blanket of mucus. The beating of the cilia normally moves this mucus towards an opening from the sinus into the nasal cavity. If the sinuses have a specific function, it is not apparent. They are often the site of painful infections, and the inflammatory process may destroy the cilia, resulting in poor drainage and accumulation of pus in the cavity.

LARYNX

Between the oropharynx and the trachea is the **larynx**, a hollow organ with two principal functions: (1) to produce sound, and (2) to close the airway during swallowing to prevent food and saliva from passing down the trachea to the lungs. The wall of the larynx is supported by the **thyroid** and **cricoid cartilages**. These are joined to one another and suspended from the **hyoid bone** by sheets of dense connective tissue. Two pairs of folds of the mucosa lining the larynx project inwards from its wall, on either side. The upper pair are called the **vestibular folds** (false vocal cords) and the lower pair are the **vocal folds** (true vocal cords). The vestibular folds are simple folds of mucosa and lamina propria containing small tubuloacinar mucus-secreting glands and diffuse lymphoid tissue. In the true vocal cords, the mucosa is firmly adherent to a band of elastic tissue in its margin, called the **vocal ligament**

(Fig. 17.2). Within the fold, lateral to the marginal band, is the **vocalis muscle**, originating from the inner surface of the thyroid cartilage anteriorly, and inserting posteriorly into an **arytenoid cartilage**. The two arytenoid cartilages articulate with the upper rim of the **cricoid cartilage** (Fig. 17.2).

In phonation, the arytenoid cartilages are adducted (moved towards the median plane) and sound is produced by vibration of the approximated vocal cords as air is forced through the narrow space between them. Contraction of a muscle between the thyroid and cricoid cartilages increases the tension of the vocal cords and thus influences the pitch of the sound produced. During inspiration, the vocal folds are abducted (moved away from the median plane), widening the interspace between them for passage of air to the lungs. The vestibular and vocal folds are covered by an unkeratinized stratified squamous epithelium. The rest of the larynx is lined by ciliated columnar epithelium, on which the direction of ciliary beat is towards the pharynx.

A thin leaf of fibroelastic cartilage, the **epiglottis**, is attached, by its narrow stem end, to the inner surface of the thyroid cartilage, with its wider upper end projecting upwards and backwards. It is covered on its anterior surface and the upper third of its posterior surface by stratified squamous epithelium. There are small mucus-secreting glands in the underlying lamina propria. The remainder of the posterior surface of the epiglottis is covered by ciliated columnar epithelium. During swallowing, the flexible stem end of

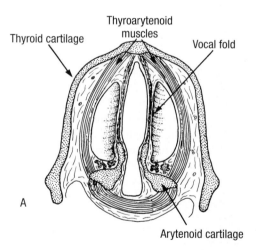

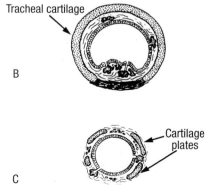

Figure 17.2 (A) Diagram of a cross-section of the larynx at the level of the vocal folds. (B) and (C) Cross-sections of the trachea and a bronchus.

the epiglottis bends and its wider, upper portion is pressed backwards and downwards by the base of the tongue, closing the opening from the larynx, and presenting a smooth upper surface over which the bolus of food slides into the esophagus.

TRACHEA

From the larynx, the conducting portion of the respiratory tract continues as the **trachea**, a flexible tube about 11 cm long and 2 cm in diameter. Its wall is reinforced by 16–20 C-shaped hyaline cartilages separated by interspaces that are bridged by fibroelastic connective tissue. The rings of cartilage in the wall enable it to resist external forces that might constrict the airway, while the fibroelastic segments between rings give the trachea great flexibility. There is also a layer of connective tissue, rich in elastic fibers, outside of the cartilaginous rings. The C-shaped rings are incomplete posteriorly. The gap between their ends is bridged by a fibroelastic ligament covered by a thick band of smooth muscle that mingles, at either end of the band, with the layer of connective tissue around the rings. During the cough reflex, contraction of this muscle can slightly decrease the diameter of the lumen to accelerate the airflow.

The trachea is lined by ciliated, pseudostratified columnar epithelium that has an unusually thick basal lamina. Ciliated cells comprise about 30% of the total cell population, goblet cells 28%, and basal cells 29%. From the upper to the lower trachea, the percentage of ciliated cells increases at the expense of goblet cells. Sparsely distributed at the base of the epithelium are small cells containing dense secretory granules located between the nucleus and the cell base. These small cells (**Kulchitsky cells**) occur in both trachea and bronchi and are believed to be endocrine cells comparable to the enteroendocrine cells of the intestine. They have been less well studied and their product is not known. There are also occasional, so-called, **brush cells**. These are very slender cells having microvilli up to 2 μm in length with an actin filament core that extends some distance down into the cytoplasm. These cells contain no secretory granules and their function remains unknown. The occasional observation of nerve endings at their base has led to the speculation that they might have a sensory function, but physiological validation of this suggestion is lacking. Small pyramidal **basal cells** are stem cells that can divide and differentiate to replace other cell types damaged or lost in the normal turnover of the epithelium. At the boundary between the lamina propria and the submucosa, there is a dense layer of elastic fibers. The submucosa contains numerous mucous glands that have serous demilunes. Their ducts ascend through the elastic lamina to open onto the surface of the epithelium.

LUNGS

The lungs occupy the right and left sides of the thoracic cavity, separated by the heart and mediastinum. Their shape conforms to that of the cavity, but they are separated from its wall by a thin film of fluid that permits sliding movement between the two. The left lung has two lobes and the right lung three lobes, separated by fissures. The filling of the lungs at each **inspiration** depends on enlargement of the thoracic cavity. This is accomplished by descent of the diaphragm caused by contraction of its intrinsic muscle, and expansion of the rib cage by contraction of the intercostal muscles. **Expiration** is the result of elastic recoil of the lungs upon relaxation of the intercostal and diaphragmatic muscles.

BRONCHIAL TREE

In the mediastinum, the trachea branches into right and left **primary bronchi** that enter the lungs through an opening on the medial surface of each lung, called the **hilum**. The primary bronchi branch into **lobar bronchi** to the two lobes of the left lung and the three lobes of the right lung. These divide into **segmental bronchi** to the several **bronchopulmonary segments** of each lobe. Each segmental bronchus, in turn, branches into several smaller bronchi, usually called **bronchioles**. These are the 12th to 15th orders of branching of the airway. Each bronchiole branches into five to seven **terminal bronchioles**, which are the last segments of the conducting portion of the respiratory tract. Their total number is about 65 000. This entire arborization of the bronchi is commonly referred to as the **bronchial tree**.

A common inherited respiratory disease is **cystic fibrosis**, which affects 1 in 3000 newborns in the United States. It is a chronic progressive disease of the respiratory tract, caused by mutation of a gene encoding a protein that channels chloride ions through cell membrane, and thus regulates salt and water balance in epithelia of the lungs and glands associated with the intestinal tract, notably the pancreas. In the lungs there is hypertrophy of the bronchial glands, resulting in plugging and obstruction of the airways by thick mucus. Symptoms can be partially relieved, but there is no treatment for the underlying defect.

Up to the point of their entry into the lungs, the structure of the primary bronchi is similar to that of the trachea. Thereafter, the cartilaginous rings are replaced by small irregularly shaped plates of cartilage distributed around their circumference. These decrease in number and disappear distal to the segmental bronchi. In the smaller bronchi, they are replaced by two thin layers of spirally oriented bundles of smooth muscle. The pitch of the spiral differs in the two layers, so that the bundles cross one another at an angle (Fig. 17.3). The mucosa of the bronchi is not significantly different from that of the trachea, but the submucosal glands gradually decrease in number and end at the level of the bronchioles.

Bronchioles

The bronchioles are tubules 5 mm or less in diameter with no cartilage or glands in their wall. The epithelium is low columnar to cuboidal and consists of ciliated cells, and non-ciliated cells that replace the goblet cells found in more proximal segments of the bronchial tree. The non-ciliated bronchiolar cells, called **Clara**

cells, have a rounded apical end that protrudes into the lumen and bears numerous short microvilli. These cells first appear in small bronchi, but are present in greater number in the bronchioles. There are secretory granules in the apical cytoplasm, and the basal cytoplasm contains long mitochondria and cisternae of rough endoplasmic reticulum (rER). The function of the Clara cells has been a subject of dispute, but it is now believed that they secrete a protective layer of surfactant that coats the epithelium of the lower airway. They also contain **guanylin**, a peptide that is involved in the control of water and electrolyte transport in certain epithelia of the gastrointestinal and respiratory tract.

The smooth muscle present in the wall of the smaller bronchi continues onto the bronchioles, but there some of the fascicles of smooth muscle course circularly and others obliquely so that they appear to form a loose network (Fig. 17.3). They are innervated by parasympathetic nerve fibers, that stimulate bronchiolar constriction, and by sympathetic nerve fibers, that relax the smooth muscle and permit the constricted bronchioles to return to their

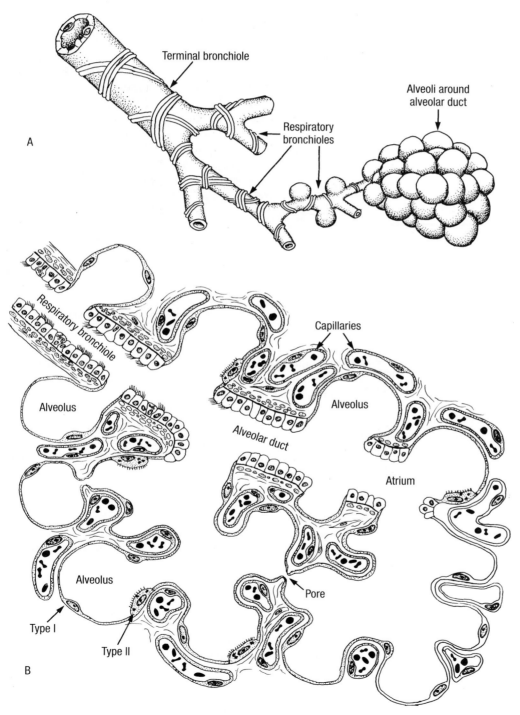

Figure 17.3 (A) Drawing of a terminal bronchiole, respiratory bronchioles and a cluster of alveoli surrounding an alveolar duct. (B) A diagram of the respiratory unit of the lung, in longitudinal section. The alveoli are lined by an epithelium consisting of type I and type II alveolar cells. (Redrawn from *Gray's Anatomy*, 38th British edn, W.B. Saunders Co., Philadelphia.)

full diameter. In persons suffering from asthma, there is excessive bronchiolar constriction, which makes it difficult to empty the lungs during expiration. Sympathomimetic drugs (drugs imitating the action of the sympathetic nervous system) are administered to relax the smooth muscle and open the airway.

Branching of each bronchiole gives rise to from five to seven smaller **terminal bronchioles**. The epithelium, which is pseudo-stratified columnar in the larger bronchi, is gradually reduced in height to simple columnar epithelium in the bronchioles and is further reduced in the terminal bronchioles to cuboidal epithelium. In the terminal bronchioles the thin intersecting fascicles of smooth muscle cells outline sizable polygonal areas of the wall that are free of muscle (Fig. 17.3).

> **Asthma** is hyperirritability of the respiratory tract, expressed in contraction of the bronchial smooth muscle (bronchospasm). This sensitivity has an immunological basis and the symptoms are episodic. Re-exposure to airborne allergen, such as ragweed pollen, stimulates subepithelial mast cells and eosinophils to release histamine and other mediators, which cause immediate bronchoconstriction and labored breathing as a result of the increased airway resistance. Various antihistaminic drugs are helpful in minimizing the severity of the attacks.

Respiratory bronchioles

The transition from the conducting portion of the tract to its respiratory portion occurs in the branching of the terminal bronchioles into the **respiratory bronchioles**. In the human, there are three further orders of branching of the respiratory bronchioles. Their epithelium is initially cuboidal, but becomes non-ciliated, low cuboidal, in subsequent branches. Continuity of their wall is interrupted at intervals by **alveoli**, saccular outpocketings of the wall, lined by squamous epithelial cells thin enough to permit gas exchange, hence the name respiratory bronchiole (Fig. 17.3). With each branching of the respiratory bronchioles, the number of alveoli in their wall increases.

The terminal branches of the respiratory bronchioles are continuous with **alveolar ducts** (Fig. 17.3), in which alveoli are so numerous, and so closely spaced, that the limits of the duct proper are discernible only as thickenings of the edges of narrow septa between alveoli. On the lumenal surface, these thickenings have a few low cuboidal epithelial cells. Alveolar ducts terminate in small spaces, called **atria**, outlined by edges of the several interalveolar septa within a cluster of alveoli.

PULMONARY ALVEOLI

The alveoli (Figs 17.4, 17.5) are where the gas exchange takes place between the blood and the inspired air. In the human lung they number about 300 million, presenting to the inspired air a total surface area of about 140 m² (two-thirds the area of a tennis court). In histological sections they appear as round or polygonal cavities lined by squamous epithelium and bounded by very

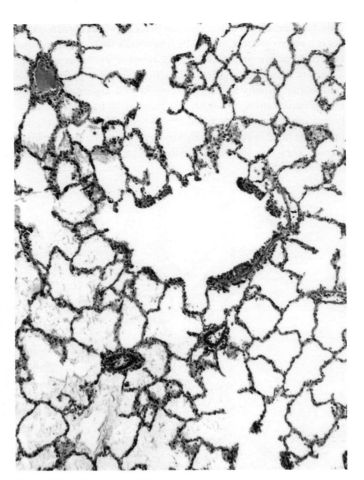

Figure 17.4 Photomicrograph of lung. In the center, a respiratory duct in cross-section. Notice that the continuity of its epithelium is interrupted by the openings of alveolae.

thin **interalveolar septa**. They are about 200 μm in diameter and open on one side to an atrium (Figs 17.5, 17.6). The very thin interalveolar septa consist of the epithelium of adjoining alveoli, separated by a network of capillaries, supported by delicate reticular and elastic fibers. Occasional fibroblasts and macrophages can be found between the two layers of squamous epithelium (Fig. 17.7). Collectively, the capillaries and connective tissue elements of the interalveolar septa constitute the **pulmonary interstitium**.

No connective tissue intervenes between the alveolar epithelium and the endothelium of the capillaries. The air in the alveolus is separated from the blood only by: (1) the unfenestrated endothelium of the capillaries; (2) the alveolar epithelium; and (3) their shared basal lamina. These layers form a blood–air barrier only 1.5–2.0 μm thick, which offers little resistance to diffusion of oxygen and carbon dioxide. The interalveolar septa are traversed by occasional openings, called **alveolar pores** (pores of Kohn) that permit movement of air between adjacent alveoli, if normal access to one becomes obstructed (Fig. 17.8). They may also have a role in maintaining the same air pressure throughout the lung.

The alveolar epithelium contains two types of cells: **type I alveolar cells** (squamous epithelial cells) and **type II alveolar cells**

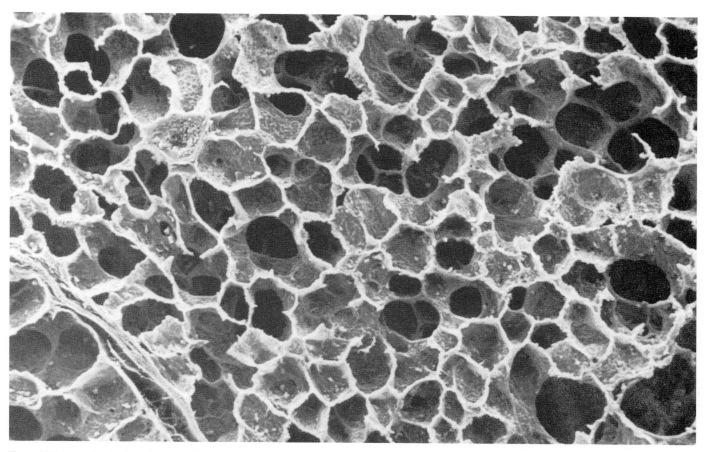

Figure 17.5 A scanning electron micrograph of the interior of the human lung showing the alveolar cavities separated by very thin alveolar septa. (Micrograph courtesy of P. Gehr.)

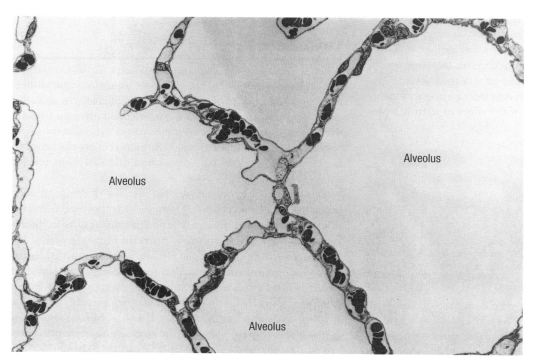

Alveolus

Alveolus

Alveolus

Figure 17.6 Low-power electron micrograph of several alveolae of the equine lung, in section. The black objects are erythrocytes in the capillaries of the alveolar septa. (Micrograph courtesy of P. Gehr.)

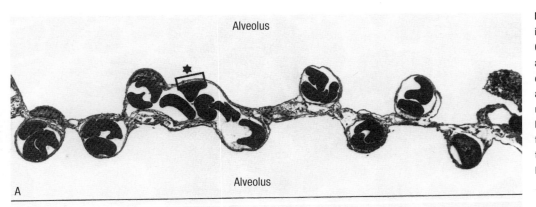

Figure 17.7 Electron micrograph of an interalveolar septum of rabbit lung. Capillaries covered by very thin type I alveolar cells bulge into the lumen, exposing a large surface to the alveolar air for gas exchange. (B) A higher magnification of an area such as that bracketed at the asterisk in (A), showing the layers making up the diffusion barrier to gas exchange. (Micrograph courtesy of P. Gehr.)

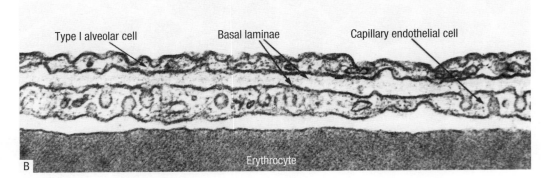

(great alveolar cells). Some histologists prefer the terms **pneumocytes I** and **II** for these cells. The type I cells occupy 95% of the alveolar surface area, and the type II cells occurring singly or in small groups, account for the remaining 5%. The rounded adlumenal surface of the type II cells, covered with short microvilli, projects slightly above the surrounding type I cells (Fig. 17.9). In addition to the usual cell organelles, they contain dense **lamellar bodies** that are atypical secretory granules containing closely spaced, membrane-like lamellae (Fig. 17.10). The secretion of the type II alveolar cells, **pulmonary surfactant**, consists mainly of **dipalmitoyl phosphatidylcholine**. It spreads as a monomolecular layer on the thin film of fluid that normally coats the surface of the alveolar epithelium. It serves to reduce surface tension and facilitate expansion of the alveoli by lowering intermolecular forces in the underlying film of fluid.

Pneumonia is an infectious disease of the lungs affecting some 3 million persons a year in the United States. Its cause is inhalation of bacteria or unintended aspiration of secretions of the nasopharynx, which always contain infectious microorganisms. The ability of the alveolar macrophages to ingest and destroy the bacteria is overwhelmed and an inflammatory exudate accumulates in the alveoli, excluding the inspired air. The resulting consolidation of one or more lobes of the lung is accompanied by fever, cough, and difficulty in breathing. Timely use of antibiotics usually prevents a fatal outcome.

Alveolar macrophages

Macrophages are found in the **interalveolar septa**. Some of these migrate into the lumen of the alveolae and adhere to the epithelial cells, where they phagocytize dust particles and other particulates that have escaped entrapment by the layer of mucus in the upper respiratory tract. In cigarette smokers, these cells are blackened by large accumulations of ingested carbon and tars from inhaled smoke (Fig. 17.11).

The alveolar macrophages are the first line of defense against pulmonary infections. They have surface receptors for IgG and the C3b component of complement, and their ability to ingest bacteria is enhanced by the presence of specific antibody against the species of bacteria reaching the alveoli. When stimulated by the metabolic products of bacteria, they secrete chemoattractants that induce transendothelial migration of polymorphonuclear leukocytes to join them in combating the invading bacteria. Erythrocytes may accumulate in the alveoli of patients with heart failure and are phagocytized by the alveolar macrophages. These can be identified in the sputum by their content of **hemosiderin**, a

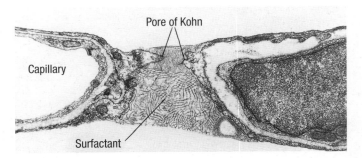

Figure 17.8 An electron micrograph, at higher magnification, showing a small opening (pore of Kohn) traversing the wall between neighboring alveoli. The pore shown here is partially obstructed by an accumulation of surfactant. (Micrograph courtesy of P. Gehr.)

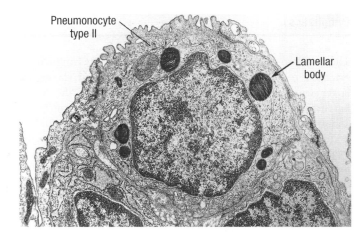

Pneumonocyte
type II

Lamellar
body

Figure 17.9 Electron micrograph of a type II alveolar cell (pneumonocyte) containing several dense lamellar bodies. (Micrograph courtesy of M.C. Williams.)

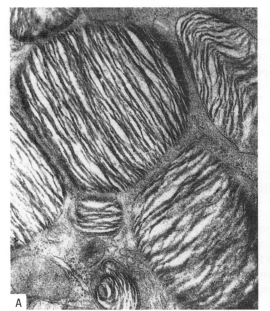

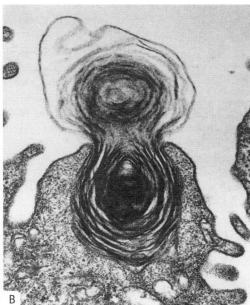

A   B

Figure 17.10 (A) Micrograph of the structure of a lamellar body in the cytoplasm of a type II alveolar cell. (B) A lamellar body in the process of being released into the lumen of an alveolus. (Micrographs courtesy of M.C. Williams.)

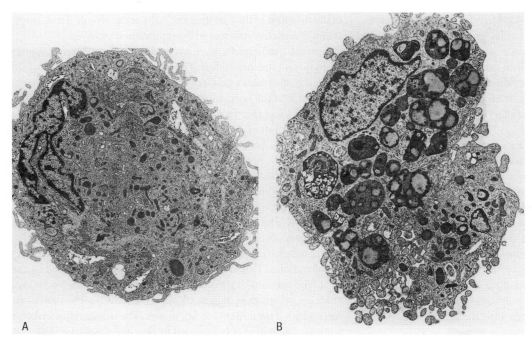

A   B

Figure 17.11 (A) Electron micrograph of an alveolar macrophage from the lung of a non-smoker. (B) Alveolar macrophage from the lung of a smoker. The cytoplasm is crowded with lipochrome pigment deposits representing indigestible residues of inhaled particulate matter phagocytized from the lumen of an alveolus. (Micrographs courtesy of S. Pratt and A.J. Ladman.)

product of hemoglobin degradation. Therefore, such cells are sometimes referred to as **heart-failure cells**. They are also often called **dust cells** because of the accumulation of phagocytized particles from inspired air.

Alveolar macrophages are continually carried upwards in the respiratory tract in the moving surface film and are swallowed upon reaching the pharynx. The rate of clearance of alveolar macrophages from the lungs is estimated to be in excess of 2×10^6/h.

Emphysema is a pulmonary disease in which many of the alveoli beyond the terminal bronchioles coalesce, reducing the total surface area available for gas exchange. This results in inefficient respiration. Owing to destruction of elastic fibers, the walls of the alveoli do not recoil and exhalation is incomplete. Cigarette smoking is a common contributing factor. Smoke inhibits ciliary motility, and impairs alveolar macrophage function. There is mild chronic inflammation of the lungs, and proteolytic enzymes from the polymorphonuclear leukocytes damage the interalveolar septa.

Pleura

The thoracic cavity is lined by a serous membrane, the **parietal pleura**, which is reflected onto the surface of the lung as the **visceral pleura**. The superficial layer of both is a mesothelium similar to the peritoneum that lines the abdominal cavity and covers its viscera. The visceral and parietal layers of pleura are normally separated only by a thin film of fluid, which permits them to slide smoothly over one another in the movements of the lung during respiration. Beneath the mesothelium is a thin layer of connective tissue containing many capillaries and lymphatics.

Blood supply

The lungs receive deoxygenated blood from the right ventricle via the **pulmonary trunk**, which divides into **right** and **left pulmonary arteries** that enter the hila of corresponding lungs. These vessels, in turn, branch into arteries of progressively diminishing caliber that follow the branches of the intersegmental bronchi as far as the respiratory bronchioles. Branches on the alveolar ducts then give rise to capillary networks in the interalveolar septa.

The lung also receives blood and nutrients from **bronchial arteries** that arise from the **aorta** and **upper intercostal arteries**. These supply the pleura, interlobular connective tissue, and the wall of the bronchial tree as far as the respiratory bronchioles, where they anastomose with the small branches of the pulmonary artery. Oxygenated blood returning from the alveolar capillaries is carried by venules in the interlobular septa. These converge to form veins of increasing diameter that run parallel to the arteries. They course along branches of the bronchi and join to form a single large vein draining each lobe of the lung. These, in turn, join to form two **pulmonary veins** that emerge from the lungs at the hila and open into the left atrium of the heart.

Lymphatics

There are two systems of lymphatics in the lungs. The lymph, in an extensive network of pleural lymphatics, is drained via several larger trunks into lymph nodes in the hilum of the lungs. Parenchymal lymphatics originate in the walls of the bronchioles and are drained by a submucosal network of lymphatics and by peribronchial lymphatics to larger vessels that converge upon the hilar lymph nodes. The efferent trunks from the hilar nodes join to form the right lymphatic duct, which is the principal pathway of drainage from both right and left lungs.

Nerves

The lungs receive parasympathetic innervation from the vagus nerve, and sympathetic innervation via nerves from the second to the fourth thoracic sympathetic ganglia. Nerves from these two sources form a plexus around the hilum from which intrapulmonary nerves accompany the ramifications of the bronchial tree and pulmonary artery. These nerves include parasympathetic **bronchoconstrictor fibers** from the vagus, and sympathetic **bronchodilator** fibers from the **thoracic sympathetic ganglia**.

HISTOPHYSIOLOGY OF THE LUNGS

The primary life-sustaining functions of the respiratory tract are the uptake of oxygen from inspired air and the elimination of carbon dioxide from the blood. These functions require expansion of the lungs on inspiration and their recoil on expiration. The abundant elastic fibers in the pulmonary interstitium permit expansion of the alveoli and provide for their recoil. A major additional factor in their recoil during expiration is the surface tension in the thin film of fluid coating the walls of the alveoli. Thus, inspiration is an active process, while expiration is passive.

Several mechanisms have evolved to remove foreign matter taken in with the inspired air. The continual secretion of surfactant in the alveoli creates a gradient that results in movement of the surface film into the bronchioles and upwards to join the blanket of mucus in the upper respiratory tract. This mucus layer is moved upwards at a rate of about 2 cm/min by the cilia of the lining epithelium. The cilia beat constantly at about 14 cycles/s, carrying dust, cellular debris, bacteria, and chemical pollutants to the pharynx where they are swallowed. Another device for removal of particulate matter is the cough reflex, which depends upon sensory nerve endings in the mucosa of the upper respiratory tract. Any irritant in the tract sends afferent impulses to the brain, which trigger an involuntary sequence of events that involves deep inspiration, closure of the glottis, and forceful contraction of abdominal and intercostal muscles. This raises pressure on the air impounded in the lung. The epiglottis is then suddenly opened and the air bursts out, attaining velocities as high as 100 mph (170 km/h). The rush of air carries with it the irritant foreign matter. The sneeze reflex involves a similar chain of events intended to clear the nasal passages.

Questions

1 The respiratory (gas exchange) division of the respiratory system includes all of the following except
   a respiratory bronchioles
   b alveolar sacs
   c alveolar ducts
   d secondary bronchioles
   e alveoli

2 Lamellar bodies are structures seen within
   a type I pneumocytes
   b Clara cells
   c Bowman's cells
   d type II pneumocytes
   e Lambert's cells

3 The major morphologic difference between the epiglottis and the soft palate is that only the epiglottis has
   a respiratory type epithelium
   b a skeletal muscle core
   c simple squamous epithelium
   d a cartilaginous core
   e squamous cell metaplasia

4 The recoil capacity of the whole lung, including the alveoli, is best served by
   a collagenous fibers
   b reticular fibers
   c elastic fibers
   d smooth muscle
   e hyaline cartilage

5 Which of the following are not seen within the alveolar septum?
   a macrophages
   b smooth muscle
   c elastic fibers
   d fibroblasts
   e epithelial cells

6 Which statement is true of Clara cells?
   a they are seen in alveolar ducts
   b they secrete mucus
   c they may be observed in the terminal bronchioles
   d they are located primarily in the lobar bronchi
   e they lie between the goblet and columnar cells of the trachea

7 Bowman's glands are located in the
   a vestibule
   b nasal cavity
   c pharynx
   d larynx
   e trachea

8 Which statement best describes type II pneumocytes?
   a they are squamous
   b they have microvilli
   c they line terminal bronchioles
   d they are the predominant alveolar epithelial cell type
   e they produce mucus

9 The respiratory 'dust' cell relates to the
   a mast cells
   b fibroblast
   c leukocyte
   d type I pneumocyte
   e alveolar macrophage

10 Rings of cartilage are present in
   a the epiglottis
   b secondary bronchi
   c the trachea
   d terminal bronchioles
   e respiratory bronchioles

11 Where are the vocal cords located?

12 What cell type secretes surfactant?

13 What specialized epithelium is located on the superior conchae?

14 What is the name of the muscle located in the wall of the true vocal cords?

15 Terminal bronchioles are part of what subdivision of the respiratory system?

16 The recoil capacity of lungs is attributable to what intra-alveolar structure?

17 What type of nerve is responsible for bronchoconstriction?

18 Type I and type II pneumocytes are located where?

19 Lamellar bodies are observed within what alveolar cell?

20 Where is the Clara cell found?

Chapter eighteen

Urinary System

The urinary system (urinary tract) consists of two **kidneys**, two **ureters**, a **urinary bladder**, and the **urethra**. The kidneys process a filtrate of the blood to form **urine**, the ureters conduct it to the bladder for temporary storage, and the urethra is the passage through which it is voided. By producing urine, the kidneys control the acid-base balance of the body fluids, excrete waste products of metabolism and maintain the normal volume of extracellular fluid by eliminating excess water. The kidneys also have an endocrine function, releasing two hormones: **erythropoietin**, which stimulates production of erythrocytes in the bone marrow, and **renin**, which has an important role in the control of blood pressure.

KIDNEYS

The kidneys are located retroperitoneally on the posterior wall of the abdominal cavity on either side of the vertebral column. They are 10–12 cm in length, 5–6 cm in width, and 3–4 cm in antero-posterior thickness. The medial border of the kidney is slightly concave, and in its center there is a cleft, called the **hilum**, which leads inwards to the **renal sinus**, a deep recess in the interior of the organ that contains the **renal arteries** and **veins**, some adipose tissue, and a funnel-shaped expansion of the upper end of the ureter, called the **renal pelvis**. The renal pelvis divides into two branches, the **major calyces**, and each of these, in turn, has short branches, called the **minor calyces** (Fig. 18.1). In the hemisected kidney viewed with the naked eye, a dark reddish-brown **cortex** is readily distinguishable from a paler **medulla**. The medulla includes 6–10 conical regions called the **renal pyramids**. The broad base of each pyramid is continuous with the cortex, and its apex, called a **renal papilla**,

projects into the lumen of a minor calyx of the renal pelvis. The pyramids are bounded laterally by darker inwards extensions of the cortex, called the **renal columns**. One renal pyramid and its bounding renal columns constitute a **renal lobule**.

The cortex of the kidney is made up of 1.5–3.0 million tubular subunits called **nephrons** (Fig. 18.2). Each has several segments that differ in histological structure and function. These are the **renal corpuscle, proximal convoluted tubule**, the **loop of Henle**, and **distal convoluted tubule**. Each nephron is continuous with a tubule of different embryological origin, the **collecting tubule**, which, in turn, joins a **collecting duct** (Fig. 18.2). A nephron and its collecting tubule and collecting duct, constitute a unit called the **uriniferous tubule**. The kidney cortex contains the renal corpuscles, proximal and distal convoluted tubules, and the collecting tubules. The loops of Henle and the greater part of the length of the collecting ducts are in the medulla.

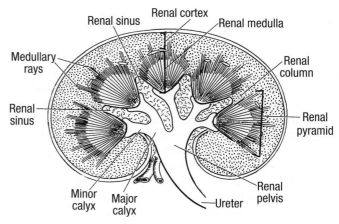

Figure 18.1 Drawing of the regions in the hemisected kidney that are identifiable with the naked eye.

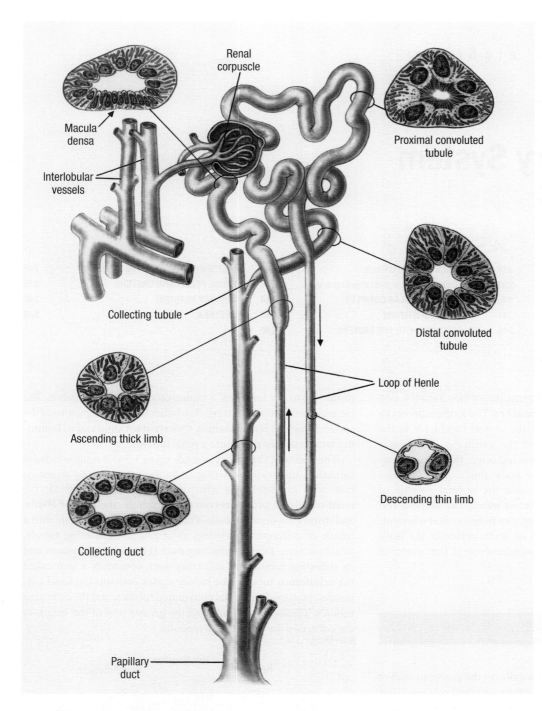

Macula densa

Interlobular vessels

Renal corpuscle

Proximal convoluted tubule

Collecting tubule

Distal convoluted tubule

Loop of Henle

Ascending thick limb

Descending thin limb

Collecting duct

Papillary duct

Figure 18.2 Drawing of a nephron and its collecting duct, which together constitute a uriniferous tubule. The appearance of its successive segments in cross-section is also depicted. (The loop of Henle has been shortened to save page space.)

The **renal corpuscle**, which contains a tuft of convoluted capillaries, collects a filtrate of the blood passing through its capillaries (Figs. 18.3, 18.4). As the filtrate passes through the nephron, its composition is altered by the addition of metabolic wastes and by selective reabsorption of components that need to be conserved. At various levels in the cortex, the distal convoluted tubules of several nephrons are joined via collecting tubules to a straight collecting duct. In these two collecting segments of the uriniferous tubule, water is absorbed from the filtrate to concentrate the urine. The collecting ducts gradually increase in diameter along their course through the pyramid and their terminal segments, the **papillary ducts (ducts of Bellini)**, open into a minor calyx of the renal pelvis.

NEPHRON

Renal corpuscle (glomerulus)

At the blind proximal end of each nephron, there is a thin-walled expansion of the proximal tubule, which is deeply invaginated to form a cup-shaped hollow structure called **Bowman's capsule**. The concavity of this capsule is occupied by a globular tuft of convoluted capillaries called the **glomerulus**. The glomerulus and its double-walled epithelial capsule together constitute a renal

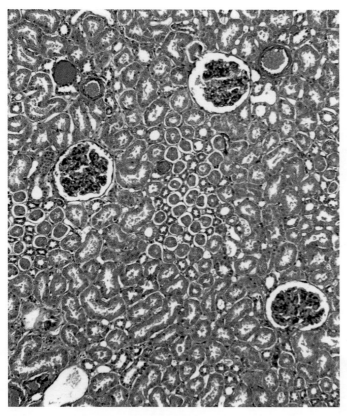

Figure 18.3 Low-power photomicrograph of a histological section, parallel to the surface of the kidney, showing cross-sections of the uriniferous tubules and three renal corpuscles.

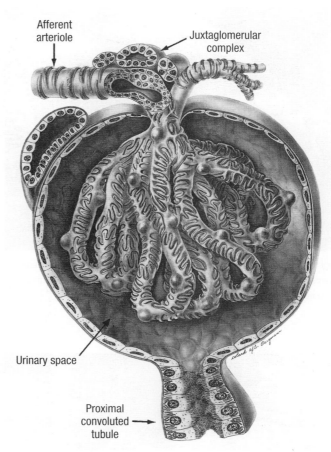

Figure 18.4 A drawing of a renal corpuscle. The glomerulus was formerly described as a cluster of capillary loops as shown here, but these loops are now known to be interconnected to form a network. (Redrawn and modified from W. Bargmann *Zeitchr für Zellforschung* 1929; 8:765.)

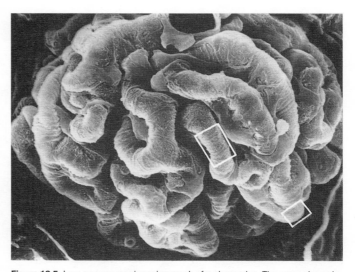

Figure 18.5 Low-power scanning micrograph of a glomerulus. The areas shown in the white boxes are shown at higher magnification in the next two figures. (Reproduced from P. Andrews *J Electr Micros Tech* 1988; 9:115.)

corpuscle (Figs 18.4, 18.5). It has a **vascular pole**, where **afferent** and **efferent arterioles** are continuous with the capillaries of the glomerulus, and a **urinary pole**, where the **capsular space** (between the outer **parietal layer** and the inner **visceral layer** of Bowman's capsule) is continuous with the lumen of the proximal convoluted tubule (Fig. 18.4). At the vascular pole of the renal corpuscle, the visceral layer of Bowman's capsule is continuous with the parietal layer of the capsule. At the urinary pole of the renal corpuscle, the squamous epithelium of the parietal layer is continuous with the cuboidal epithelium of the proximal convoluted tubule (Fig. 18.4).

In the development of the renal corpuscle, the shape of the cells in the visceral layer of Bowman's capsule become so modified that they bear little resemblance to those of any other epithelium. The individual cells, called **podocytes**, have several radiating primary processes that embrace the underlying capillaries, and these primary processes give rise to very numerous secondary branches, called **foot processes** or **pedicels** (Figs 18.6, 18.7). These interdigitate with pedicels of neighbouring podocytes, but are separated from them by narrow intercellular spaces, about 25 nm wide, which permit the plasma escaping from the glomerular capillaries to enter the capsular space. These are referred to as the **filtration slits**. Although the secondary processes of the podocyte are closely applied to the basal lamina of the underlying capillary, the cell body is usually separated from it by 1–3 μm. This permits nearly the entire surface of the capillary loop to be carpeted with the

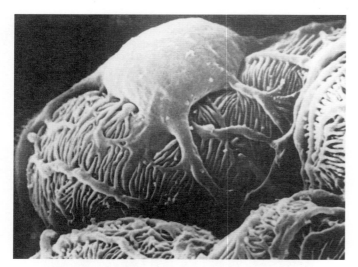

Figure 18.6 Scanning micrograph of a podocyte, showing its primary processes embracing the underlying capillary, and secondary branches (pedicels) forming a labyrinthine system of interdigitating cell processes on its surface.

elaborately interdigitated foot processes. This arrangement maximizes the total area of intercellular clefts available for passage of the filtrate.

The cytoplasm of a podocyte contains a small Golgi complex, a moderate amount of rough endoplasmic reticulum (rER), and abundant free ribosomes. Microtubules and intermediate filaments are plentiful only in the cell body and in its primary processes. In thin sections of a glomerulus, cross-sections of foot processes are seen to be aligned on an unusually thick basal lamina, which is a product of both the capillary endothelium and the podocytes (Fig. 18.8). At the basal lamina, the narrow space between adjacent foot processes is traversed by a **slit diaphragm**, a layer only 4–6 nm in thickness. The slit diaphragm is a unique junction consisting of a zipper-like interdigitation of molecules projecting from the membranes of adjoining foot processes. The 'teeth' of the zipper are molecules of a protein called **nephrin**. These are anchored by another protein (CD2AP) to filaments of the podocyte cytoskeleton. The spaces between nephrin molecules are small enough to exclude plasma proteins, but large enough to permit water, glucose, amino acids and metabolic waste products to pass into Bowman's capsule. Three layers are distinguishable in

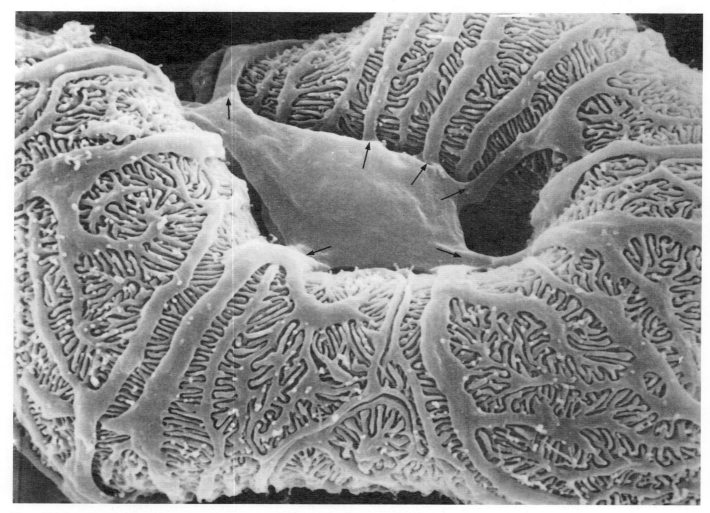

Figure 18.7 Scanning electron micrograph of a capillary loop and a podocyte sending primary branches (arrowed) to both limbs of the loop. Notice the complex pattern of intermingling secondary processes on the surface of the capillary. (Reproduced from P. Andrews *J Electr Micros Tech* 1988; 9:115.)

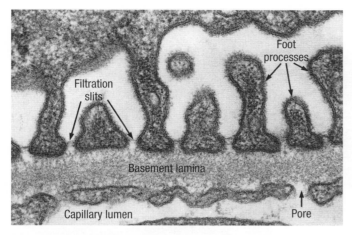

Filtration slits, **Foot processes**, **Basement lamina**, **Capillary lumen**, **Pore**

Figure 18.8 Electron micrograph of a thin section of the wall of a glomerular capillary (below), and cross-sections of podocyte foot processes on the outer surface of the thick basal lamina. (Micrograph courtesy of D. Friend.)

the underlying basal lamina: the **lamina rara interna**, nearest to the endothelium; an intermediate **lamina densa**; and the **lamina rara externa**, adjacent to the podocyte processes. The lamina densa is a meshwork of type IV collagen, and the paler laminae rarae are rich in heparan sulfate and fibronectin. The basal lamina was formerly believed to be the principal barrier in the filter, excluding all molecules with a molecular weight greater than 70 000. The slit diaphragm is now regarded as the size-selective filter.

Children with **congenital nephrotic syndrome** lose large amounts of plasma proteins in their urine. Electron micrographs of their kidneys reveal a disorder of the podocyte processes and absence of slit diaphragms in the glomeruli. It has recently been found that this deficit is attributable to a mutation in the gene encoding nephrin.

The thin squamous cells of the capillary endothelium have numerous pores, 70–90 nm in size. Unlike those of fenestrated capillaries elsewhere, the pores are not spanned by a pore diaphragm. The thicker portion of the endothelial cell, containing the nucleus and organelles, is usually on the side of the capillary away from the capsular space. The spaces between the glomerular capillaries is occupied by the **mesangium**, a connective tissue consisting of **mesangial cells** in an extracellular matrix that is largely devoid of fibrous elements other than fibronectin. The mesangial cells correspond to the pericytes of other capillaries, but have special properties that set them apart. They are phagocytic and may dispose of filtration residues that might otherwise clog the filter. It is speculated that they may also participate in a continual turnover of the basal lamina.

Infections elsewhere in the body may spread to the kidneys, resulting in **glomerulonephritis**. The inflammatory response is largely confined to the glomeruli, with accumulation of neutrophils and lymphocytes around the capillaries. There is a proliferation of mesangial cells and perivascular deposits of immunoglobulins. The basal lamina and walls of the capillaries are damaged and the urine may contain plasma proteins and erythrocytes. The infection usually subsides, but impairment of the kidney function may persist.

Proximal convoluted tubule

Near its origin from the urinary pole of the renal corpuscle, the initial segment of the uriniferous tubule is highly tortuous. In this so-called **proximal convoluted tubule** the cells are cuboidal, or low columnar, and have a spherical nucleus in an eosinophilic cytoplasm. On their free surface, there is a conspicuous **brush border** that results in a 20-fold increase in the area of cell membrane exposed to the glomerular filtrate in the lumen (Fig. 8.9). The tips of the microvilli have a prominent glycocalyx. Opening into the spaces between the microvilli are tubular invaginations of the plasmalemma called the **apical canaliculi**. Numerous small vesicles are found around their ends, suggesting that the canaliculi are involved in endocytosis of macromolecules from the lumen. These vesicles subsequently fuse with lysosomes where the macromolecules are degraded.

The lateral cell boundaries in the proximal tubule are poorly resolved by the light microscope, due, in part, to their elaborate interdigitation with neighboring cells. Their complex shape can only be fully appreciated in three-dimensional reconstruction from serial sections (Fig. 18.10). On a scanning electron micrograph, alternating ridges and grooves are found extending for the full length of the cell (Fig. 18.11). Near the base of the cell, these divide into small lateral processes that pass under adjacent cells. On electron micrographs of thin sections, paired membranes can be seen turning inwards from the plasmalemma, dividing the basal cytoplasm into a number of narrow compartments, which are occupied by long mitochondria oriented parallel to the vertical axis of the cell. Some of these basal compartments that are not open to the overlying cytoplasm are obviously cross-sections of undermining processes of neighboring cells. Interpretation of images of thin-sections is facilitated by referring to the three-dimensional reconstruction (Fig. 18.10).

These specializations greatly increase the surface area of the basal and lateral cell membranes, which are rich in Na^+K^+-ATPase, an enzyme involved in the pumping of sodium out of these cells to create an electrochemical gradient that moves water across the cell to the peritubular capillaries, thus concentrating the urine. The proximal convoluted tubule absorbs about 85% of the water and salt of the glomerular filtrate. It also absorbs glucose and amino acids and excretes creatinine into the urine.

Loop of Henle

From its convoluted juxtaglomerular portion, the proximal tubule continues downwards into the medulla, forming the long **loop of Henle**. In its initial segment, called the **descending thick limb**, the loop has a diameter similar to that of its proximal convoluted portion, but in the outer part of the medulla it abruptly narrows from 60 μm in diameter to about 15 μm and continues as the **descending thin limb** of the loop of Henle. At this junction, the brush border ends and the cuboidal epithelium abruptly gives way to a squamous epithelium bearing a few short microvilli (Fig. 18.12). The thin limb of the loop pumps Na^+ and Cl^- out of the lumen and reabsorbs about 5% of the water of the glomerular filtrate.

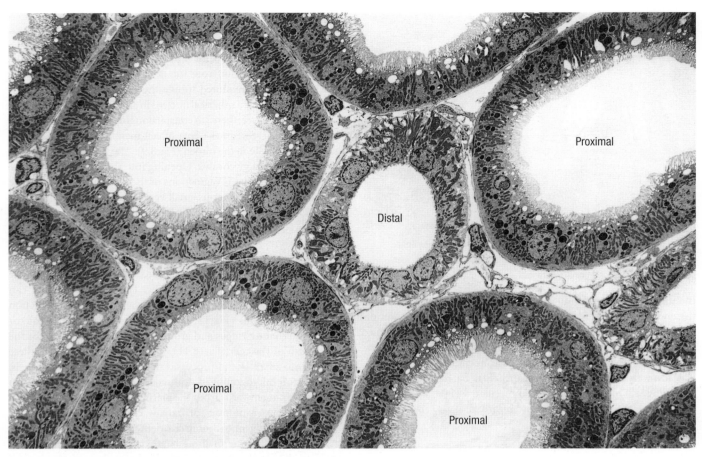

Figure 18.9 Low-power electron micrograph of a small area of the renal cortex, including cross-sections of four proximal convoluted tubules around a distal convoluted tubule. Notice the brush border on the proximal tubule and its absence from the distal tubule. (Reproduced from A. Maunsback *J Ulstrastr Res* 1966; 15:252.)

Two categories of nephrons are distinguished on the basis of the length of their loop of Henle. The **cortical nephrons** have a relatively short loop, in which the descending thin limb is continuous at the bend of the loop with the ascending limb of the distal tubule. The **juxtamedullary nephrons**, which make up a relatively small fraction of the total number, have a very long loop of Henle. In these latter nephrons, the loop extends deep into the pyramid, and the transition of its **thin ascending limb** to the **ascending thick limb** of the distal tubule is in the upper medulla. In short-looped

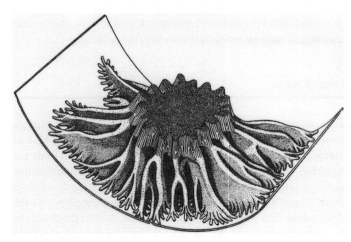

Figure 18.10 Photograph of a three-dimensional model of a cell of the proximal convoluted tubule, reconstructed from serial sections. Notice the fin-like radial processes and their smaller branches at the cell base. (Reproduced from A.P. Evans *et al. Anat Rec* 1976; 191:397).

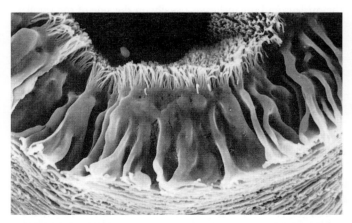

Figure 18.11 Scanning electron micrograph of the ridges on the lateral surfaces of cells of the proximal convoluted tubule. (Reproduced from H. Takahashi-Iwanaga, from *Cells and Tissues: A Three Dimensional Approach*, Alan Liss Inc., New York, 1989.)

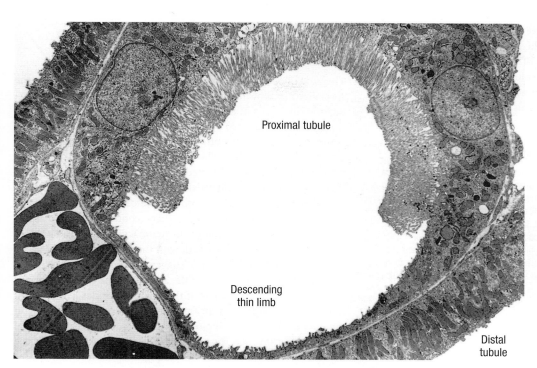

Figure 18.12 Electron micrograph of a slightly oblique section of the abrupt transition from the descending thick limb of the proximal convoluted tubule to the thin limb of the loop of Henle. (Reproduced from J. Oswaldo and H. Latta *J Ultrastr Res* 1966; 15:144.)

nephrons, the squamous cells of the thin segment are polygonal in outline throughout its length. In long-looped nephrons, the cells of the descending limb have long, interdigitating lateral processes. These decrease in number and length towards the bend and increase again in the ascending thin limb. These changes in cell outline along the length of long loops have no obvious physiological significance.

Distal convoluted tubule

The initial portion of the distal tubule, in the outer medulla, is the **ascending thick limb** of the loop of Henle. Continuing outwards into the cortex, it returns to the vascular pole of the renal corpuscle of the same nephron, where it contacts the afferent arteriole of the glomerulus. On the side adjacent to the arteriole, its cells are narrower and the closer spacing of their nuclei results in a darker-staining sector of the wall that histologists call the **macula densa** (Fig. 18.13). Beyond this landmark, the tubule pursues a tortuous course as the **distal convoluted tubule**. The cells of the ascending thick limb are cuboidal and 7–8 μm in height, gradually diminishing to about 5 μm in the distal convoluted tubule. A brush border is lacking, but there may be a few short microvilli. A single, short flagellum, arising from a pair of centrioles in the apical cytoplasm, projects into the lumen. There are small vesicles near the cell apex, but no apical canaliculi. There are a few cisternae of rER, a small Golgi complex, and abundant mitochondria, generally oriented parallel to the long axis of the cell. The nucleus tends to be displaced towards the lumen by deep infoldings of the basal plasmalemma, which bound narrow compartments containing long mitochondria. Closed basal compartments, which represent undermining processes of neighboring cells, are less common in the

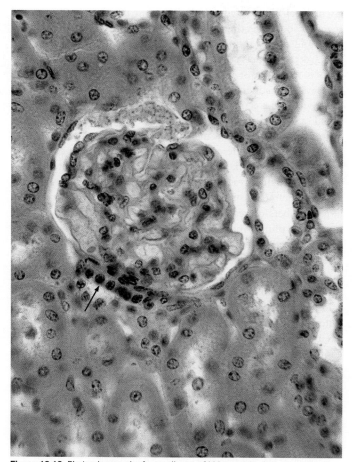

Figure 18.13 Photomicrograph of a small area of kidney cortex including a renal corpuscle. Notice in the epithelium of the adjacent distal convoluted tubule (at arrow), a segment where the nuclei are more closely crowded. This local specialization of the wall is called the macula densa.

epithelium of the distal convolution than they are in the proximal convoluted tubule. The thick ascending limb of the loop actively transports Cl^- out of the tubule, followed by Na^+. The function of the distal convoluted tubule is controlled by **antidiuretic hormone** (vasopressin) of the neurohypophysis. It reabsorbs Na^+ and secretes K^+. This segment absorbs about 8% of the water of the filtrate.

A common congenital disorder is **polycystic disease of the kidney**. In the embryo, the kidneys arise from two sources: (1) a **ureteric bud** that elongates and branches repeatedly to form the ureter, pelvis, calyces, and collecting ducts, and (2) a **renal blastema** that gives rise to all portions of the nephrons other than the collecting ducts. The collecting ducts normally become continuous with the distal convoluted tubules. In polycystic kidneys, this union fails, and the blind ends of the collecting ducts accumulate fluid and form large cysts. In its most severe form, this condition is incompatible with postnatal life. In less severe cases, the patients have enough normal nephrons to be asymptomatic until the 30s to 40s and then gradually develop renal insufficiency.

Collecting tubule and collecting duct

Each distal convoluted tubule is joined by a short transitional segment, the **collecting tubule**, to a **collecting duct**. The collecting tubules of a number of nephrons join the same collecting duct. As these ducts course deeper into the medulla, their epithelium is made up of wide, low columnar cells. At least two cell types are distinguishable. The **principal cells** have short microvilli and a centrally located single flagellum. The nucleus is ovoid and the cytoplasm contains randomly oriented small mitochondria. There are many short invaginations of the basal plasmalemma, but these do not bound basal alcoves containing mitochondria. A darker-staining cell type, the **intercalated cell**, is identified by the presence of numerous small folds, or **microplicae**, on their free surface. The apical cytoplasm contains very large numbers of vesicles ranging from 50 to 200 nm in diameter. Short, plump mitochondria are distributed throughout the cytoplasm. In laboratory rodents, intercalated cells make up 35% of the cells in the ducts of the outer medulla, but diminish in number to 10% towards the papilla. None have been reported in the inner medulla of the human kidney. These cells participate in acid-base balance by resorption of bicarbonate. In animals subjected to chronic bicarbonate loading, the number of intercalated cells increases dramatically. The collecting duct is controlled by antidiuretic hormone and absorbs about 4% of the water in the filtrate.

Some substances excreted by the kidneys have relatively low solubility and in the concentration of the glomerular filtrate by absorption of water, these substances may precipitate, resulting in **nephrolithiasis (kidney stones)**. The concretions formed in the renal pelvis may consist of calcium oxalate, calcium phosphate or uric acid. Attempted passage of a small stone down the ureter is attended by severe pain in the flank and hematuria (bloody urine). If its passage is incomplete, blockage of the ureter may result in progressive loss of kidney function.

JUXTAGLOMERULAR COMPLEX

The **juxtaglomerular complex** has three components: (1) the specialized cells of the **macula densa** in the distal tubule; (2) **juxtaglomerular cells** in the wall of the adjacent afferent arteriole of the glomerulus; and (3) pale-staining **mesangial cells** in the angle between the diverging afferent and efferent arterioles of the glomerulus (Fig. 18.14). The juxtaglomerular cells are modified smooth muscle cells in the media of the afferent arteriole. Rarely, they may also be found in the efferent arteriole. Some retain myofilaments typical of smooth muscle cells and have relatively few dense secretory granules. Others contain many secretory granules and no myofilaments. In the macula densa, the polarity of the epithelial cells is reversed, with the Golgi complex between the nucleus and the cell base, suggesting that they may have a secretory function influencing the activity of the juxtaglomerular cells. The secretory granules of the juxtaglomerular cells contain the hormone **renin**, a protease that cleaves **angiotensinogen** in the blood plasma to **angiotensin-I**. In subsequent passes of angiotensin-I through the circulation, an enzyme on the surface of the endothelial cells of lung capillaries transforms angiotensin-I to **angiotensin-II**, which is a potent vasoconstrictor that raises blood pressure and influences the rate of renal blood flow.

RENAL INTERSTITIUM

The content of the spaces between the renal tubules constitutes the **renal interstitium**. Its volume in the cortex is small, but it increases in the medulla. It includes small bundles of collagen fibers, cells resembling fibroblasts, and cells of the monocyte-macrophage lineage in a matrix of highly hydrated proteoglycans. In the interstitium of the medulla are pleomorphic **interstitial cells**, which differ from the fibroblast-like cells of the cortex. They

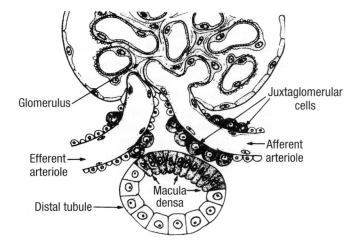

Figure 18.14 Drawing of the juxtaglomerular complex. It consists of modified smooth muscle cells in the wall of the afferent arteriole, the macula densa, and, rarely, modified smooth muscle cells in the efferent arteriole.

are often oriented transversely with respect to the surrounding tubules, with the tips of their long processes adherent to tubules and blood vessels. They contain lipid droplets that vary in abundance in various states of salt and water balance. They were formerly thought to produce prostaglandins, but this is now questioned. There is some evidence that they have an endocrine function in the regulation of systemic blood pressure, but this awaits verification.

BLOOD SUPPLY TO THE KIDNEYS

The kidneys have a very large blood flow, averaging about 1.2 L/min. The **renal artery** as it enters the hilum divides into two main branches, one supplying the anterior and the other the posterior half of the kidney. Arising segmentally from the primary branches of the renal artery are short **lobar arteries** that branch into **interlobar arteries** (Fig. 18.15). These course between the pyramids to the corticomedullary boundary, where they divide into **arcuate arteries** that run parallel to the surface of the kidney. **Interlobular arteries**, arising from the arcuate arteries, course radially towards the kidney surface. Along their course, they give rise to **intralobular arteries** that give off the **afferent arterioles** to the juxtamedullary, midcortical, and superficial renal glomeruli. **Efferent arterioles** from the cortical glomeruli ramify to form a cortical interlobular capillary network. Efferent arterioles of the juxtamedullar glomeruli pass into the medulla, forming vessels somewhat larger than capillaries, called the **vasa recta**. Deep in the medulla, these turn back towards the cortex. These slightly larger, thin-walled, recurrent vessels intermingle with the descending vasa recta, forming **vascular bundles** or **rete** (Fig. 18.16). These bundles of vessels carrying blood in opposite directions constitute an efficient countercurrent system that conserves the osmotic gradient established in the interstitium.

The venous drainage parallels the course of the arteries. Blood from the capsular and cortical capillaries is drained via **stellate**

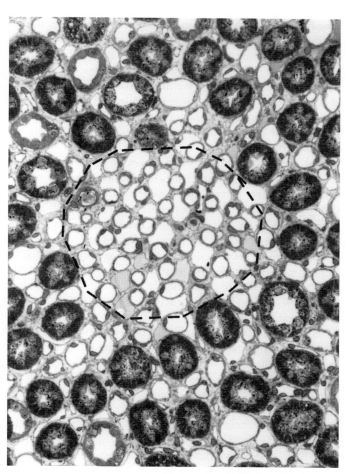

Figure 18.16 Photomicrograph of an area of the renal medulla containing descending thin limbs and ascending thick limbs of the loops of Henle. Outlined in the center of the field is a vascular rete composed of thicker-walled descending blood vessels, and thin-walled ascending vessels.

veins into **interlobular veins**, then to **arcuate veins**, and then to **interlobar veins** that converge to form the renal vein.

HISTOPHYSIOLOGY OF THE KIDNEY

The mission of the kidneys is to filter the blood in order to remove waste products of metabolism, while conserving water, electrolytes, glucose, amino acids, and other essential constituents of the plasma. To accomplish this, the entire blood volume passes through the renal glomeruli about every 45 min. Flow through the renal glomeruli is at a rate of 1.3 L/min, producing filtrate at a rate of 125 ml/min. However, urine is formed at only 1 ml/min, because the other 124 ml are reabsorbed from the filtrate by the tubules of the nephrons and returned to the blood.

Blood circulates through the glomeruli at a pressure sufficient to force fluid through the fenestrated capillary endothelium, the basal lamina and the filtration slits between interdigitating processes of the podocytes. The large plasma proteins remain in the blood and only water and small molecules

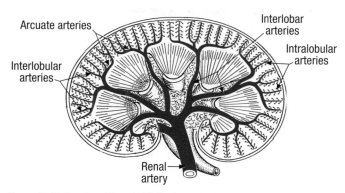

Figure 18.15 Drawing of the arterial blood supply of the kidney. Interlobular arteries radiating from the arcuate arteries give rise to the intralobular arteries, which, in turn, give off the afferent arterioles of the glomeruli. Their branching is more extensive than shown here. In general the veins return along the same paths taken by the arteries.

pass into the lumen of Bowman's capsule. From there, the filtrate flows into the proximal convoluted tubule, where 70–80% of the Na⁺ ions, water, glucose, and amino acids diffuse into the brush border of the epithelium and are actively transported across its cells and into the interstitial fluid. From there, sodium, water, and other small molecules diffuse through the wall of the peritubular capillaries back into the blood. Urea, uric acid and other waste products remain in the filtrate in the lumen of the tubules.

The ability of the kidneys to secrete a concentrated urine depends upon the loop of Henle. Beyond the proximal convoluted tubule the permeability characteristics of the epithelia change dramatically. In its descending limb, the epithelium is permeable to water, but not to salt. The thin ascending limb is permeable to salt, but not to water. Diffusion of water from the descending limb increases the concentration of solutes in its lumen, and at the bend of the loop, the concentration of Na⁺ and Cl⁻ ions in the filtrate is very high. Cells of the thick ascending segment of the loop have a very active salt pump and, as Na⁺ and Cl⁻ ions are pumped out, they contribute to the high osmolarity of the inner part of the renal medulla that is essential for production of a concentrated urine. By losing salt, but not water, in this segment of the loop, the filtrate becomes increasingly dilute (hypotonic) as it moves upwards towards the distal tubule. The distal convoluted tubule and collecting duct have relatively low permeability to both Na⁺ and water. The filtrate ordinarily passes through them without significant change in concentration, and a dilute urine is excreted.

If there is excessive dehydration (e.g. from heavy perspiration), there is a slight increase in osmolarity of the blood. The posterior lobe of the hypophysis responds to this change by secreting an increased amount of **antidiuretic hormone**. This hormone increases the permeability of the epithelium of the distal tubules and collecting ducts to water. This water is then reabsorbed from the filtrate as it passes through the zone of high osmolarity in the renal medulla, resulting in a concentrated urine. Blood loss, or low blood pressure, stimulates the adrenal cortex to secrete more **aldosterone**, which induces the cells of the distal and collecting tubules to synthesize additional membrane channels for reabsorption of more sodium. In the absence of aldosterone secretion by the adrenal cortex, continual loss of sodium in the urine is fatal.

Although elimination of waste products is the primary task of the kidneys, their endocrine function in the control of erythrocyte production, and in regulation of blood pressure, must not be overlooked. Whenever the oxygen-carrying capacity of the blood is diminished (or is inadequate for residence at high altitude), the kidneys release the hormone **erythropoietin**, which stimulates the bone marrow to produce more erythrocytes. In cardiovascular conditions that result in slowing of the rate of blood flow through the glomeruli, the juxtaglomerular apparatus is activated. Paracrine secretion by cells of the macula densa cause dilatation of the afferent arteriole to the glomeruli, and juxtaglomerular cells release **renin**, which converts **angiotensin-I**, produced by the liver, to **angiotensin-II** that acts upon vascular smooth muscle throughout the body causing vasoconstriction and consequent increase in blood pressure.

RENAL PELVIS AND URETERS

The renal pelvis is lined by a thin transitional epithelium that becomes somewhat thicker in the ureters. Beneath the epithelium is a lamina propria rich in elastic fibers. The lamina propria is surrounded by smooth muscle that does not form distinct longitudinal and circular layers, but is made up of bundles of varying orientation. The thickness of the wall gradually increases, and in the lower third of the ureter, an additional layer of predominantly longitudinal smooth muscle is added. Muscle contraction in the renal pelvis and ureter creates peristaltic waves that slowly progress towards the urinary bladder.

URINARY BLADDER

The wall of the urinary bladder is covered by pelvic peritoneum that constitutes its **serosa**. The **muscularis** is made up of three layers of smooth muscle that intermingle to such an extent that their boundaries are indistinct. In the outer layer, smooth muscle bundles are oriented longitudinally along the sides of the bladder and then transversely over its dome. The thin middle layer is discontinuous and its scattered bundles are predominantly circular or oblique. The fibers of the thin inner layer are again mainly longitudinal.

The **mucosa** lining the bladder is loosely attached to the muscularis and has a **transitional epithelium** that is thin in the full bladder, but thicker when the wall is contracted. In the latter state, the epithelium may be six to eight cells thick. The superficial cells are much larger than those more deeply situated in the epithelium, and their rounded free surface bulges into the lumen. In the full bladder, the epithelium is reduced to three or four cells in thickness and the cells are flattened. On electron micrographs, the luminal surface of the cells has a peculiar scalloped appearance (Fig. 18.17). This irregular contour of the surface is caused by the presence of thick plaques within the plasmalemma that are connected by thinner and more flexible interplaque regions. In freeze-fracture preparations, the plaques appear as rounded areas of closely spaced intramembrane particles (Fig. 18.18). In negatively stained preparations of isolated plaques viewed at very high magnification, the plaques are made up of hexagonally packed subunits, each of which appears to be a hexamer of smaller subunits.

In the apical cytoplasm of the superficial cells there are unique discoid vesicles that are lenticular in section (Fig. 18.17). These are made up of pairs of the plaques. They appear to be formed by adjoining plaques of the surface membrane taken into the cell as the bladder empties. They are opened up and reinserted into the membrane to provide for expansion of its surface during bladder distension.

The superficial cells are joined by juxtalumenal tight junctions, and there are desmosomes between cells throughout the epithelium. The occluding junctions and the special properties of the

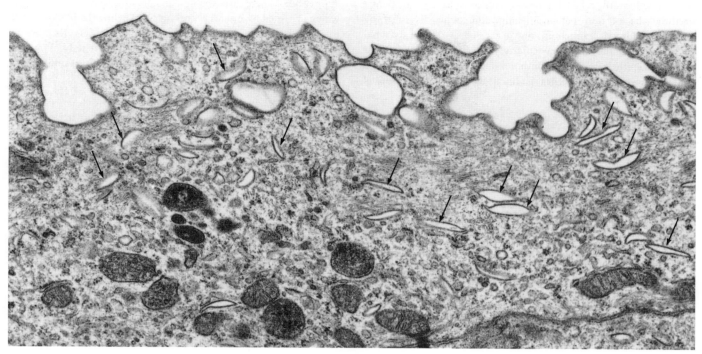

Figure 18.17 Electron micrograph of a portion of a superficial cell of the epithelium lining the bladder. The irregular surface has angular contours owing to the presence of stiff plaques within the plasmalemma. Notice, at the arrows, elliptical cytoplasmic vesicles consisting of pairs of the membrane plaques withdrawn from the surface as the volume of the bladder diminished during urination. (Reproduced from M. Hicks and B. Ketterer *J Cell Biol* 1970; 45:472.)

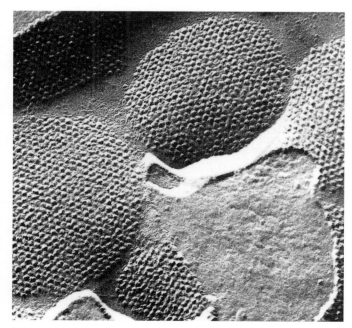

Figure 18.18 Electron micrograph of a freeze-fracture preparation of a small area of the plasmalemma of transitional epithelium, showing three plaques of closely packed particles within the membrane. A fourth plaque has broken out of the membrane. (Micrograph courtesy of M. Hicks and B. Ketterer.)

thick luminal membrane are thought to create a permeability barrier that prevents dilution of the hypertonic urine by movement of water through the epithelium.

URETHRA

The urethra of the male is the terminal portion of both the urinary tract and the reproductive tract. Its initial segment, the **prostatic urethra**, passes through the prostate gland. On its posterior wall, there is a slight elevation, the **verumontanum** (**colliculus seminalis**). In the midline of this elevation is the opening of the **prostatic utricle**, a small blind pouch, of unknown function, that extends into the prostate. On either side of the verumontanum are the openings of the **ejaculatory ducts**. On the posterior and lateral walls of the urethra in this region are the openings of multiple small ducts of the surrounding prostate gland. Distal to the ejaculatory ducts, the epithelium lining the urethra changes from transitional to pseudostratified or stratified columnar epithelium. There is no change in the epithelium in the **membranous urethra**, the portion that passes through the urogenital diaphragm behind the pubic symphysis. In this short segment, the urethra is surrounded by striated muscle of the **external urethral sphincter**, which is voluntarily relaxed to permit outflow of urine. The **penile urethra** (the portion passing through the penis) is lined by stratified columnar epithelium, but in its slightly dilated terminal portion, called the **fossa navicularis**, this changes to stratified squamous epithelium, which continues onto the glans penis.

The short female urethra is lined by stratified squamous epithelium interrupted by areas of pseudostratified columnar epithelium. There are shallow invaginations along its length, which are lined by mucus-secreting cells. Below the bladder neck, the female urethra is enveloped by smooth muscle, forming an involuntary **internal urethral sphincter**. Immediately above the urogenital diaphragm is a voluntary **external urethral sphincter** of striated muscle.

Questions

1 The cells of which structure monitor the concentration of NaCl in the afferent arteriole of the glomerulus?

a   the proximal convoluted tubule

b   the descending loop of Henle

c   the mesangial cells

d   the macula densa

e   the collecting ducts

2 When considering the arterial supply of the kidney, which arteries arise directly from the interlobar arteries?

a   arcuate arteries

b   vasa recta

c   afferent arterioles

d   efferent arterioles

e   interlobular arteries

3 Which statement best describes juxtaglomerular cells?

a   they are modified smooth muscle cells of the afferent arteriole

b   they are derived from the parietal layer of Bowman's capsule

c   they are found in the macula densa

d   they are specialized endothelial cells of the afferent arteriole

e   they are the source of antidiuretic hormone

4 In the kidney, blood is filtered through

a   the parietal layer of Bowman's capsule

b   a slit membrane between the pedicels of the podocytes

c   Bowman's space

d   the intraglomerular mesangial cells

e   proximal convoluted tubule

5 Which of the following is a distinctive feature of the renal cortex?

a   collecting ducts

b   medullary rays

c   arcuate arteries

d   the loops of Henle

e   the area cribrosa

6 A property shared by the calyx of the kidney, the ureter, and the urinary bladder is that they

a   are all lined by simple cuboidal epithelium

b   are all invested by skeletal muscle

c   are all lined by stratified, squamous epithelium

d   are all lined by transitional epithelium

e   all have three layers of smooth muscle

7 Which statement is true of podocytes?

a   they are glomerular endothelial cells

b   they are parietal epithelial cells of Bowman

c   they are mesangial cells

d   they are juxtaglomerular cells

e   they are visceral epithelial cells of Bowman's capsule

8 The proximal convoluted tubule of the kidney is readily distinguished from other tubules of the kidney by the presence of

a   clearly demarcated boundaries between its cells

b   an apical brush border on its cells

c   a clear cytoplasm

d   large apical cilia

e   an intense basophilic staining of the cytoplasm

9 Which statement is true of smooth muscle cells of the afferent arteriole of the glomerulus?

a   they may give rise to mesangial cells

b   they may give rise to the cells of the macula densa

c   they do not participate in the formation of any specialized structure of the kidney

d   they may give rise to juxtaglomerular cells

e   they secrete aldosterone

10 The nephron is best defined as

a   being continuous with the proximal convoluted tubule

b   terminating in the ascending thick limb of the distal tubule

c   being the functional unit of the kidney

d   being located entirely in the medulla

e   being located entirely in the cortex

11 The glomerulus and Bowman's capsule comprise what structure?

12 The afferent arteriole ends in what structure?

13 A brush border is observed in what type of kidney tubule?

14 What type of epithelium lines the ureter?

15 The kidney can be considered to have an endocrine function as it releases which two hormones?

16 Which arteries run along the base of the pyramid and give rise to interlobular arteries?

17 What do the juxtaglomerular cells of the afferent arteriole produce?

18 Blood is filtered through which structure associated with the podocytes?

19 Angiotensin-I results from enzymatic action on angiotensinogen by which substance?

20 What is the name of the structure that contains tubules that look like proximal and distal convoluted tubules and is found in both the cortex and medulla?

Chapter nineteen

Endocrine Glands

Two different systems have evolved for controlling and coordinating the functions of the various organs of the body: the **nervous system** and the **endocrine system**. The nervous system exercises control by generating electrochemical signals that are transmitted over long axons that synapse on the cells that are to be regulated. The endocrine system is made up of glandular cells that secrete **hormones**, signaling molecules that are transported in the blood to distant target cells that have specific surface receptors for them. Their binding to the receptors triggers intracellular biochemical reactions that increase, or decrease, the target cell's activity. Coordination of the nervous and endocrine systems is achieved by pathways of communication between the hypothalamus of the brain and the hypophysis (pituitary gland), which controls the functions of several of the other endocrine glands.

HYPOPHYSIS

The **hypophysis**, or pituitary gland, is located beneath the brain, in a shallow depression in the sphenoid bone, called the sella turcica. It produces several hormones with wide-ranging effects on metabolism, growth, and reproduction. The gland is about 1 cm in length and width, 0.5 cm in depth, and weighs 0.5 g. Its neural and vascular connections with the brain give it a key role in the interactions of the nervous and endocrine systems.

Two major divisions of the hypophysis differ in their embryological origin. The **neurohypophysis** (posterior lobe) develops as a downgrowth from the brain of the embryo, and is composed of nervous tissue. The **adenohypophysis** (anterior lobe) arises as a dorsal evagination of the embryonic pharynx and is composed of glandular tissue. In the adult, three regions of the neurohypophysis are designated by different names. The uppermost portion that is continuous with the hypothalamus of the brain, is called the **median eminence**. A slender stalk extending downwards from the median eminence is called the **infundibulum**. This expands into a wider terminal portion called the **pars nervosa**, or posterior lobe of the hypophysis.

There are also three divisions of the adenohypophysis. A thin layer of glandular tissue enveloping the infundibulum is called the **pars tuberalis**. A bulbous terminal portion that makes up the greater part of the gland is the **pars distalis** (anterior lobe). Several layers of pale-staining epithelial cells located between the pars distalis and the neighboring pars nervosa are called the **pars intermedia** (Fig. 19.1).

Neural control of hypophyseal function depends upon blood-borne **releasing factors**, and **inhibiting factors**, produced in the hypothalamus and carried to the pars distalis in a special arrangement of blood vessels called the **hypophyseal portal system**. A knowledge of the blood supply to the hypophysis is essential to an understanding of its functions.

Blood supply

Inferior hypophyseal arteries arising from the internal carotid arteries on either side of the neck, anastomose to form an arterial ring around the infundibulum. Branches coursing downwards from this ring ramify into a capillary plexus within the pars nervosa (posterior lobe) of the hypophysis. **Superior hypophyseal**

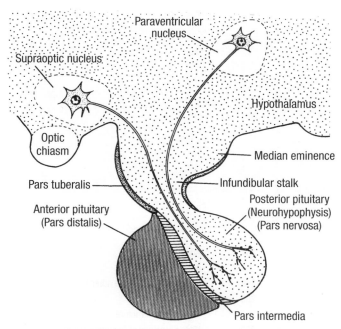

Figure 19.1 Diagram of a sagittal section of the hypothalamus and hypophysis showing the distribution and terminology of the different regions. Two neurons are included to show the origins of the axons that make up the greater part of the pars nervosa.

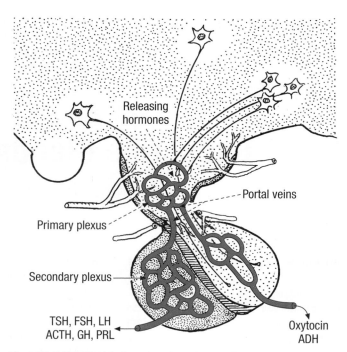

Figure 19.2 Diagram of the hypophyseal portal system. The size of the vessels of the primary and secondary plexuses is greatly exaggerated. They are actually sinusoidal capillaries. There is no connection between the capillary network of the anterior and posterior lobes. ACTH, adrenocorticotrophic hormone; ADH, antidiuretic hormone; FSH, follicle-stimulating hormone; GH, growth hormone; LH, luteinizing hormone; PRL, prolactin; TSH, thyroid-stimulating hormone.

arteries, arising from the right and left carotid, and anterior cerebral arteries anastomose around the median eminence of the hypothalamus, and send branches into it to form a network of capillaries commonly referred to as the **primary plexus**. Vessels emerging from this plexus coalesce into a network of small venules on the surface of the median eminence. These, in turn, merge to form two or three **hypophyseal portal veins** that course downwards along the surface of the infundibular stalk and give rise to an extensive network of sinusoidal capillaries within the pars distalis, called the **secondary plexus** (Fig. 19.2).

Such an arrangement, in which a network of capillaries in one region is connected by veins to a second network of capillaries some distance away, is called a *portal system*, and the connecting vessels are designated *portal veins*. All of the blood supply of the pars distalis is via this **hypophyseal portal system**. Thus, releasing factors generated by neurons in the ventral hypothalamus are carried in the blood to cells in the pars distalis that release their hormones into the general circulation. The hormones of the neurohypophysis (posterior lobe) are produced in the cell bodies of neurons located in the hypothalamus and are transported in their long axons, which extend down into the posterior lobe. In response to action potentials generated by the same cells, their hormones are released at nerve endings near capillaries in the posterior lobe and are carried into the general circulation.

Pars distalis

The pars distalis (anterior lobe) of the hypophysis is composed of irregular cords and clusters of glandular cells in intimate rela-

tion to the thin-walled sinusoids of the secondary plexus. The sinusoids have a fenestrated endothelium. Stellate, fibroblast-like cells with long, branching processes, form a cellular framework throughout the gland, and the secretory cells occupy the spaces within the network. Traditionally, histologists assigned the secretory cells to one, or the other, of two categories: **chromophils**, which contained secretory granules and stained deeply; and **chromophobes**, which had few or no such granules and stained very lightly. The chromophobes were interpreted as undifferentiated or resting secretory cells. The chromophils included **acidophils**, cells which stained with acidic dyes, and **basophils**, which stained with basic dyes. Thus, only two secretory cell types were originally distinguished.

The electron microscope has made it possible to identify more than one cell type within each of these categories. The cell types are distinguishable mainly on the basis of the size and shape of their secretory granules (Fig. 19.3). The different cell types are now identified, with greater precision, by using fluorescein-labeled antibodies to their respective hormones. Of the six hormones secreted by the adenohypophysis, two (**growth hormone** and **prolactin**) are attributable to the traditional acidophils, and four to basophils (**adrenocorticotropin, thyroid-stimulating hormone, follicle-stimulating hormone, luteinizing hormone**). It is now common practice to refer to the cell types of the pars distalis by terms that identify the target organ stimulated by the hormone they secrete. Thus, cells secreting thyroid-stimulating hormone (**TSH**) are called **thyrotropes**; those secreting the gonadotrophic hormones, **FSH** and **LH**, are **gonadotropes**; cells

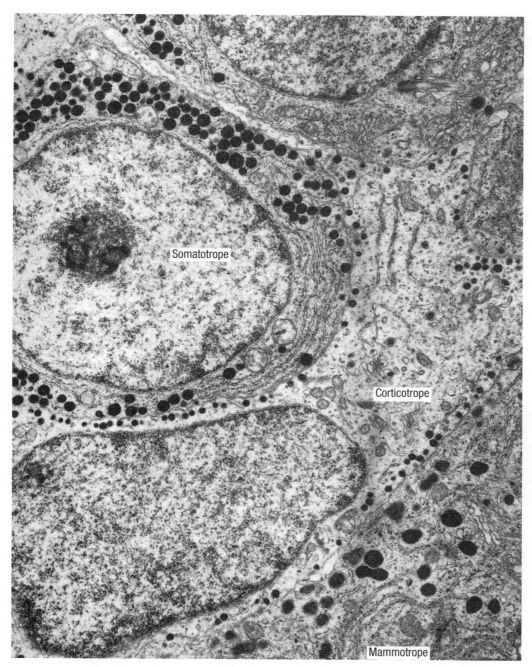

Figure 19.3 Electron micrograph of a small area of the pars distalis that includes a somatotrope, a corticotrope, and a mammotrope, and illustrates the difference in size of the secretory granules of these three cell types. (Reproduced from J. Nakayama, F.A. Nickerson and F.R. Shelton *Lab Investig* 1989; 21:169.)

Somatotrope

Corticotrope

Mammotrope

secreting adrenocorticotrophic hormone (**ACTH**) are called **corticotropes**; those secreting growth hormone (**GH**) are called **somatotropes**; and those secreting prolactin (**PRL**) are **mammotropes** (Table 19.1).

The most numerous cells of the pars distalis during pregnancy are the **mammotropes**. They tend to occur individually in the cell cords of the gland. Their secretory product, **prolactin**, stimulates mammary gland growth during pregnancy, and milk secretion after delivery. During lactation, when mammotropes are most active, they have an extensive rough endoplasmic reticulum (rER) and a prominent Golgi complex. Their ovoid secretory granules are the largest in the pars distalis, measuring up to 700 nm in diameter (Fig. 19.4). In the non-pregnant female, the granules are smaller and less numerous. Mammotropes are also present in small numbers in the male, where their function is not known.

Corticotropes are relatively small cells commonly occurring in groups. They may occasionally form a wall around a small deposit of extracellular glycoprotein. The secretory granules are 200–250 nm in diameter and tend to be located immediately beneath the plasmalemma (Fig. 19.4). The endoplasmic reticulum is tubular or vesicular, and the Golgi complex is small. The product of the corticotropes, **adrenocorticotrophic hormone** (ACTH), or corticotrophin, stimulates release of the hormones of the adrenal cortex.

The **thyrotropes** are elongated cells occurring in small groups. The secretory granules, only 150–200 nm in diameter, are the

Table 19.1 Summary of cell types and functions of the pars distalis of the hypophysis

Cell type	Hormone secreted	Ultrastructure	Physiological action	Releasing hormone
Basophils Gonadotrope	Follicle-stimulating hormone (FSH) Luteinizing hormone (LH)	Rounded cells; usually near sinusoids; 200 nm granules	Stimulates development of ovarian follicles in the female; stimulates spermatogenesis in the male	Gonadotropin-releasing hormone (GnRH)
Thyrotrope	Thyrotropin (TSH)	Angular cells; usually not near sinusoids; 140 nm granules	Stimulates thyroid hormone synthesis, storage and release	Thyrotropin-releasing hormone (TRH)
Corticotrope	Corticotropin (ACTH)	Cells pale, stellate; few large granules at cell periphery; 400–450 nm	Stimulates release of hormones of the adrenal cortex	Corticotropin-releasing hormone (CRH)
Acidophils Somatotrope	Somatotropin	Cells in groups near sinusoids; 300 nm granules	Stimulates growth of long bones; acting via liver-generated intermediates	Somatotropin-releasing hormone (SRH)
Mammotrope	Prolactin	Cells located individually in center of cords; 200 nm granules; 600 nm during lactation	Stimulates the secretion of milk	Prolactin-releasing hormone (PRH)

smallest in the pars distalis and are usually located in the cytoplasm just beneath the plasmalemma. Their product, **thyroid-stimulating hormone** (TSH), also called thyrotropin, stimulates the thyroid gland to release its hormone, **thyroxin**.

The **gonadotropes** are large, round cells close to the sinusoidal capillaries. Their nucleus is often irregular in outline. The rER is tubular in form and moderately abundant, and there is a large Golgi complex. The secretory granules are 200–300 nm in

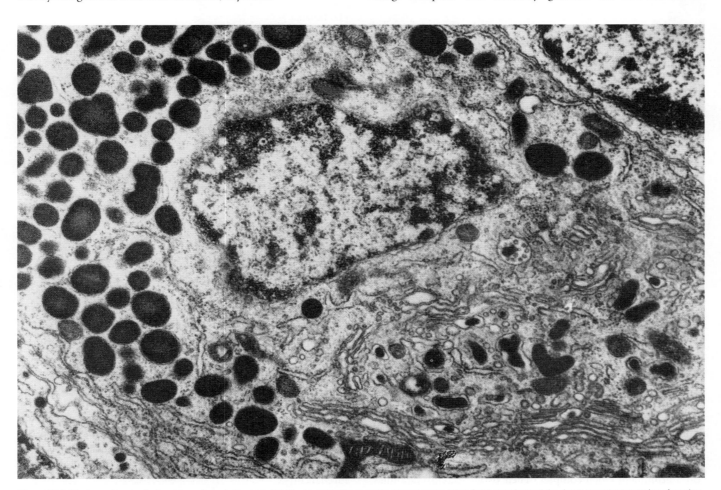

Figure 19.4 Electron micrograph of a mammotrope in the pars distalis of a rodent hypophysis. Note the very large Golgi complex and the dense secretory granules of varying shape. (Micrograph courtesy of M. Farquhar and T. Kanaseki.)

diameter. These cells secrete two hormones: **follicle-stimulating hormone** (FSH) and **luteinizing hormone** (LH). In the female, FSH stimulates development of the follicles in the ovary, and LH stimulates the transformation of follicles into the corpora lutea. Both hormones also affect control of the growth and regression of the endometrium (the tissue lining the uterus). In the male, LH stimulates the interstitial cells of the testes to secrete the male sex hormone, testosterone.

Somatotropes are commonly arranged in groups near the sinusoids. They contain dense spherical secretory granules 350 nm in diameter. They have a large Golgi complex, but the rER is relatively sparse. Their product, **growth hormone** (GH), stimulates increased protein synthesis, and mitotic division of a wide range of cell types. Most of the hormones of the pars distalis act directly upon the cells of their target organs. Growth hormone is exceptional in that its effects on the growth of the body are mediated indirectly by **somatomedins**, which are growth-promoting proteins produced by the liver.

Excess production of growth hormone, before the closure of the epiphyses, results in **pituitary gigantism** in which accelerated growth leads to abnormal stature. In the adult, overproduction of growth hormone by a benign tumor of the pars distalis may cause **acromegaly**, a debilitating condition characterized by overgrowth of bones and soft parts. There is enlargement of the hands and feet, a coarsening of the facial features, enlargement of the tongue and hypertrophy of the larynx. Surgical removal of the tumor to arrest the progressive disfigurement is the treatment of choice.

The great majority of exocrine and endocrine glands contain secretory cells of only one kind, that are activated by the same neurotransmitter. The pars distalis of the hypophysis is unique among endocrine glands in having multiple types of secretory cells, each activated by a different **releasing hormone**. These are molecules released by neurons in the ventral hypothalamus and are carried down to the sinusoids of the pars distalis via the portal venules. The releasing hormones are **somatotropin-releasing hormone** (SRH), **prolactin-releasing hormone** (PRH), **gonadotropin-releasing hormone** (GnRH), **corticotropin-releasing hormone** (CRH), and **thyrotropin-releasing hormone** (TRH).

Pars intermedia

In animals, the pars distalis is separated from the neurohypophysis by a cleft, and this is lined, on the juxtaneural side, by a stratified epithelium of weakly basophilic cells constituting the **pars intermedia**. Its cells secrete **melanocyte-stimulating hormone** (MSH). In the human, this layer of epithelium is present in the fetus. However, in postnatal life, it is no longer a continuous layer. Only isolated groups of its cells can be found invading a short distance into the pars nervosa. There is no compelling evidence for the secretion of significant amounts of MSH, in humans, and no function has been attributed to the small residues of the pars intermedia.

Pars tuberalis

The **pars tuberalis** is a thin sleeve of epithelial cells, only 25–60 μm thick, surrounding the infundibulum. It consists of cords of epithelial cells occupying the spaces between the hypophyseal portal venules coursing downwards to the pars distalis. The cells are cuboidal, or low columnar, and contain small dense granules, lipid droplets, and occasional colloid droplets. They are the only cells in the hypophysis that contain significant amounts of glycogen. No specific hormone is known to be secreted by the pars tuberalis, and its function remains unknown.

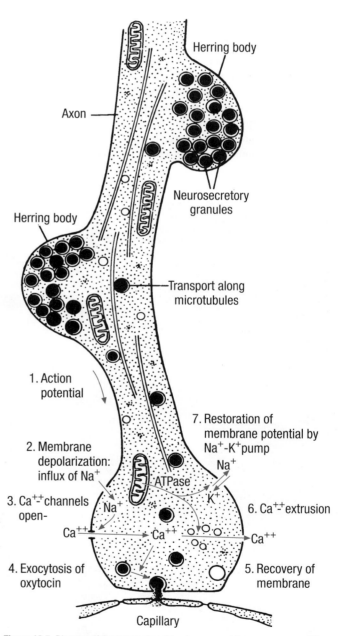

Figure 19.5 Diagram of the terminal portion of an axon of the pars nervosa of the hypophysis. The principal events in stimulus–secretion coupling are indicated. (Reproduced from D.W. Lincoln, *Hormonal Control of Reproduction*, Cambridge University Press, Cambridge, 1984.)

Neurohypophysis

The **neurohypophysis** includes the median eminence of the hypothalamus, the infundibular process, and the pars nervosa. The pars nervosa is made up of tens of thousands of unmyelinated axons of neurons, whose cell bodies are in the **supraoptic nucleus** and **paraventricular nucleus** of the hypothalamus. Glial cells, called **pituicytes**, form a cellular network throughout the lobe, with their long processes in communication via gap junctions. They are highly variable in size and shape and commonly contain lipid droplets and deposits of lipochrome pigment. Some of the pituicyte cell processes wrap around axons near their termination. The significance of this relationship is unclear.

The hypothalamic neurons, whose axons make up the bulk of the posterior lobe, are large cells with an eccentric nucleus, abundant cytoplasm and few dendrites. The rER forms conspicuous parallel arrays (Nissl bodies) and the prominent Golgi complex is the site of assembly of small (120–200 nm) neurosecretory granules that are continuously transported along axonal microtubules into the pars nervosa at a rate of 4–8 mm/h. The granules accumulate and are stored in hundreds of small dilatations along the length of each axon (Figs 19.5, 19.6). Although the individual granules were not resolved by the light microscope, their aggregations were visible with the light microscope and were called **Herring bodies** by earlier generations of histologists. The granules contain the hormones **oxytocin** or **vasopressin** combined with a **neurophysin**, a carrier protein specific for each hormone. The ends of the axons are closely associated with the endothelium of the sinusoids of the pars nervosa. They can be distinguished from cross-sections of more proximal portions of the axon by the presence of many small vesicles that resemble synaptic vesicles. However, these vesicles do not contain a neurotransmitter, but are formed in the retrieval of membrane added to the plasmalemma in exocytosis of the neurosecretory granules.

Histophysiology of the neurohypophysis

An afferent impulse to neurons in the median eminence of the hypothalamus results in a wave of membrane depolarization that travels down the axon. Reaching the ending in the posterior lobe it causes an influx of calcium and an opening of calcium channels. Elevated calcium concentration in the axoplasm triggers exocytosis of the neurosecretory granules. The normal membrane

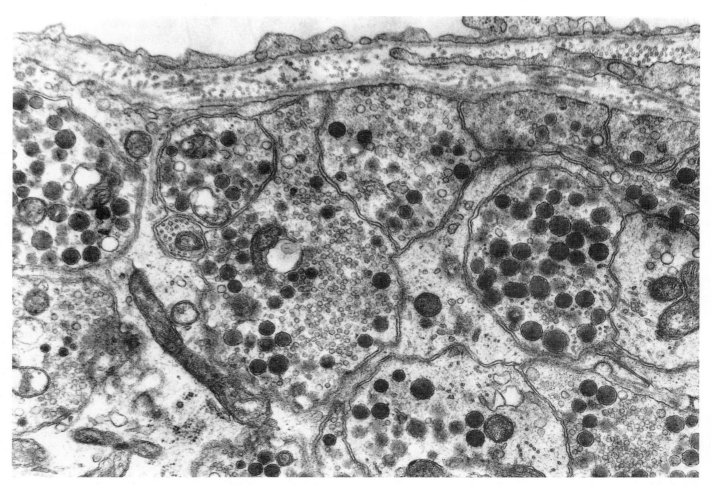

Figure 19.6 Electron micrograph of a small area of the pars nervosa of the rat hypophysis. Several axons of hypothalamic neurons are filled with secretory granules that will be released to permit oxytocin or vasopressin to diffuse into the capillary at the top of the figure. (Micrograph courtesy of P. Orkand and S. Palay.)

potential is restored by pumping out calcium ions, and the excess membrane added to the ending by exocytosis is removed by endocytosis in small vesicles (Fig. 19.5). Prior to exocytosis of the neurosecretory granules, oxytocin or vasopressin are cleaved from their specific neurophysin, and the hormone and its carrier protein both enter the bloodstream. The neurophysins have no known physiological function.

The principal target of **oxytocin**, in the female, is the pregnant uterus. Its concentration in the blood increases in the late stages of labor and stimulates contraction of the smooth muscle of the uterus. After birth of the baby, it is also involved in stimulating the ejection of milk from the lactating mammary gland. Stimulation of the nipple by the suckling infant sends afferent impulses to the brain, which are relayed to neurons of the supraoptic and paraventricular nuclei of the hypothalamus. These respond by releasing oxytocin from their axon terminals into the sinusoids of the pars nervosa. Blood-borne oxytocin then stimulates contraction of myoepithelial cells around the alveoli of the mammary gland, forcing milk into ducts that open onto the nipple.

The principal targets of the other hormone, **vasopressin**, are the collecting ducts of the kidneys and the peripheral arterioles of the vascular system. Whenever the osmotic pressure of the blood rises, it is sensed by osmoreceptor areas of the hypothalamus that stimulate release of vasopressin from their axon terminals in the pars nervosa. The hormone binds to receptors on the cells of certain tubules of the kidney, activating an enzyme that acts upon integral membrane proteins to increase permeability of the apical plasmalemma to water. This increases the uptake of water from the lumen of the tubules, thereby decreasing the volume of urine and increasing its concentration.

Vasopressin is also involved in the control of blood pressure. A sudden decrease in blood volume is a potent stimulus for increased secretion of vasopressin. After a severe hemorrhage, it may be secreted at 50 times the normal level. It acts upon vascular smooth muscle, causing constriction of arterioles. This increases the peripheral resistance to blood flow in the circulatory system, and thereby increases blood pressure.

In the disease called **diabetes insipidus**, the neurohypophysis fails to respond to the normal stimuli for secretion of vasopressin. There is great thirst and excessive intake of water (polydipsia) with very frequent urination caused by the inability of the kidneys to concentrate the urine. Treatment is by injection of vasopressin, or prescription of other drugs with similar effect.

THYROID GLAND

The **thyroid gland** is located in the anterior part of the neck, immediately below the larynx. It has two lateral lobes, connected by a narrow isthmus that crosses the trachea just below the cricoid cartilage. In childhood, its hormones are essential for normal development of the central nervous and musculoskeletal systems. In the adult, its hormones affect the metabolism of many tissues and organs of the body, and are involved in thermoregulation.

Microscopic structure

In most endocrine glands the hormones are stored in intracellular secretory granules. The thyroid is unique in having an organization that permits extracellular storage of the secretory product. The gland is made up of spherical **thyroid follicles**, ranging from 0.2 to 0.9 mm in diameter. These consist of a simple cuboidal epithelium surrounding a central cavity that contains a gelatinous substance called **thyroid colloid** (Figs 19.7, 19.8). The gland is enclosed in a connective tissue capsule, from which septa of looser connective tissue extend into the gland surrounding groups of thyroid follicles. Each follicle is supported by a meshwork of reticular fibers, and is surrounded by a very dense network of capillaries.

The follicular epithelium is cuboidal, or low columnar, depending upon its state of activity. The cells are polarized towards the lumen of the follicle and joined by typical junctional complexes. There are a few short microvilli on their apical surface. The rER is extensive, and its cisternae are often somewhat dilated. There is a prominent juxtanuclear Golgi complex with many associated vesicles containing newly synthesized **thyroglobulin**. These vesicles move to the cell apex and release their content by exocytosis into the lumen of the follicle. Extracellular storage of the product necessitates two-way traffic across the epithelium. On electron micrographs of cells activated by thyroid-stimulating hormone (TSH), one observes at the cell apex, large vacuoles containing colloid being

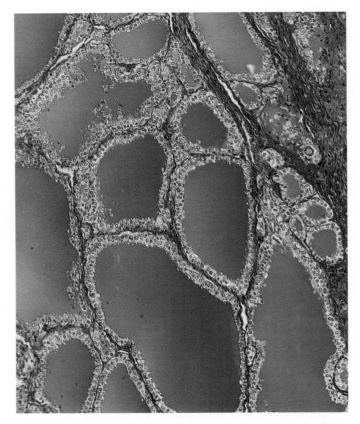

Figure 19.7 Photomicrograph of a thyroid gland. Notice the variation in size of the follicles. The red area in the large follicle at the bottom of the figure is a staining artifact.

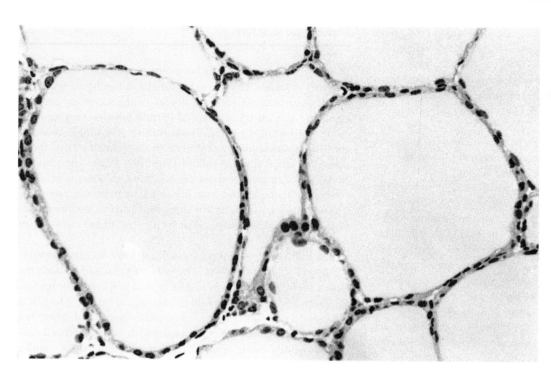

Figure 19.8 Photomicrograph of a monkey thyroid gland. The follicles have a low cuboidal epithelium and there is very little interstitial connective tissue between the follicles.

taken up from the lumen by endocytosis. Similar vacuoles are also seen in transit towards the cell base for exocytosis (Fig. 19.9). Two compounds, **thyroxine** (T_4) and **triiodothyronine** (T_3), collectively called thyroid hormone, are derived from the thryoglobulin and released into the blood flowing through the dense network of capillaries surrounding each follicle (Fig. 19.10).

Pale-staining **parafollicular cells** are found singly or in small groups at the base of the follicular epithelium. These are always separated from the lumen of the follicle by overarching processes of the neighboring thyroid follicular cells. The nucleus is round or ovoid and the cytoplasm contains tubular and cisternal profiles of the endoplasmic reticulum. Small electron-dense secretory granules are congregated near the cell base. These contain **thyrocalcitonin** (calcitonin), a polypeptide hormone which, in some animal species, is an important regulator of blood calcium. In those species, it lowers the concentration of calcium in the blood by suppressing bone resorption. In the human, it is probably physiologically significant only in childhood, when the bones are growing and bone turnover is rapid. In the adult, its hypocalcemic effect is minimal.

In **hyperthyroidism** (Grave's disease) there is thyroid enlargement (goiter), and excess production of thyroid hormones. The height of the epithelium of the follicles is increased and there are papillary thickenings of their wall. Excess hormone results in restlessness, sleeplessness, tremor, and a noticeable prominence of the eyeballs (exophthalmos). Treatment is by radioactive iodine or subtotal thyroidectomy.

Histophysiology of the thyroid

The principal hormones of the thyroid are **thyroxine** and **triiodothyronine**. They are stored in the colloid as constituents

of a very large secretory glycoprotein, **thyroglobulin** (600 000 mol. wt.). After synthesis of its protein moiety on the endoplasmic reticulum, carbohydrate is added in the Golgi complex and the thyroglobulin is packaged in vesicles for exocytosis. The cells also synthesize a peroxidase that is located mainly in the apical plasma membrane, where it oxidizes iodine taken up

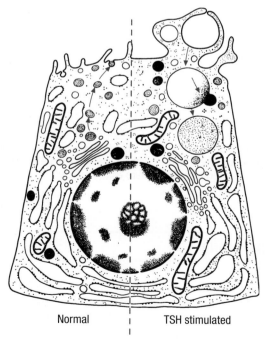

Normal   TSH stimulated

Figure 19.9 Drawing showing (on the left) normal secretion of thyroglobulin into the lumen of the follicle, and (on the right) the uptake of colloid by endocytosis after stimulation with thyroid-stimulating hormone (TSH). Lysosomes then fuse with the vacuoles and thyroxine is released from their content of thyroglobulin.

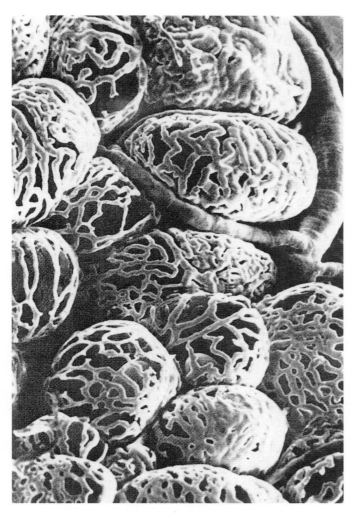

Figure 19.10 Scanning micrograph of a monkey thyroid in which the blood vessels were injected with a plastic and the soft tissues then digested away. It shows the very rich capillary network around each follicle. (Reproduced from H. Fujita and T. Murikami *Arch Histol Jap* 1974; 36:181.)

at the cell base. The iodine binds to tyrosine groups of the thyroglobulin to form **iodinated thyroglobulin**, which is a substance stored in the colloid. In the intracellular degradation of colloid after its uptake from the lumen of the follicle, the principal products are thyroxine (tetraiodothyronine T4) and triiodothyronine (T3), and these are released at the cell base. The circulating thyroid hormones stimulate enzymes concerned with glucose oxidation in other organs, thereby increasing metabolic rate, oxygen consumption, and heat production. Both overactivity and underactivity of the thyroid cause severe metabolic disturbances.

In some regions of the US, where there is little iodine in the soil, residents are apt to develop an enlargement of the thyroid (colloid goiter). In the absence of iodine, the thyroid cells make thyroglobulin but cannot iodinate it to make a functional hormone. The follicles accumulate excess colloid, resulting in an enlargement of the gland as a whole. This form of hypothyroidism is now prevented by the widespread use of iodinated table salt.

The primary control of thyroid function is mediated by TSH of the hypophysis. Blood-borne TSH binds to receptors on the basolateral membrane of the thyroid follicular cells. These cells respond by accelerated iodine uptake, increased production of cyclic AMP, and enhanced synthesis and release of thyroid hormones.

> Deficient secretion of TSH in an adult results in **myxedema**, a severe form of hypothyroidism. There is weakness, drowsiness, and slowing of mental activities. There is also a thickening of the skin and subcutaneous tissue causing undesirable alterations in the facial features. If deficiency of TSH develops in childhood, it causes **cretinism**, which is characterized by retarded bone growth, respiratory distress, and mental retardation.

PARATHYROID GLANDS

The parathyroid glands are small ovoid bodies adhering to the posterior surface of the thyroid gland. There are usually four, and they measure about 5 mm in length, 4 mm in diameter, and 2 mm in thickness. Each weighs only 20–50 mg. Accessory glands and ectopic glands located lower in the neck or in the mediastinum are not uncommon. The parathyroids are endocrine glands secreting **parathyroid hormone** (PTH) which acts upon bone, intestines, and kidneys to maintain the necessary concentration of calcium in the blood and extracellular fluid. Calcium is an essential element in mammalian physiology. It is involved in muscular contraction, glandular secretion, blood coagulation, and in the activation of many key enzymes in intermediary metabolism.

Microscopic structure

Each parathyroid gland is enclosed in a thin capsule from which thin trabeculae of loose connective tissue extend inwards, carrying the blood vessels, nerves, and lymphatics. The parenchyma of the gland consists of branching and anastomosing cords of epithelial cells, supported by a delicate framework of reticular fibers. Rarely, the epithelial cells may form isolated small follicles resembling those of the thyroid. They contain a colloidal material of unknown nature. The glands slowly increase in size from birth through adolescence, attaining their maximum size at age 20 years. The connective tissue stroma of the gland, in older individuals, contains variable numbers of adipose cells, and in the elderly these may occupy 60%, or more, of the gland.

The parenchyma of the human parathyroid gland consists of two epithelial cell types: **chief cells** and **oxyphil cells** (Fig. 19.11). The chief cells are 5–8 μm in diameter and have a centrally placed nucleus in a slightly eosinophilic cytoplasm. On electron micrographs they are found to be joined by occasional desmosomes. In contrast to other glands, in which all cells normally exhibit the same degree of activity, parathyroid chief cells appear to go through their secretory cycle independently. Both active and inactive cells are found within the gland. In the active cells, the cytoplasm contains long mitochondria, parallel cisternae of rER, a prominent Golgi complex, and small deposits of glycogen.

Conspicuous dense bodies of varying shape are common and are interpreted as lipofuchsin pigment deposits. Numerous small granules 200–400 nm in diameter are secretory granules containing the polypeptide, **parathyroid hormone** (PTH). Inactive cells contain relatively little endoplasmic reticulum, a small Golgi complex, and only a few secretory granules. The inactive cells outnumber the active cells.

Cells of the second type, the **oxyphil cells**, are up to 10 μm in diameter. They are clearly larger than the chief cells, and they stain more deeply with eosin (Fig. 19.11). They are few in number and occur singly or in small clusters. The Golgi complex is small, the endoplasmic reticulum is sparse, and there are no secretory granules. They have an extraordinary number of mitochondria and these have closely spaced cristae, suggesting a high degree of metabolic activity. The small amount of cytoplasm between the closely packed mitochondria is rich in glycogen.

Histophysiology of the parathyroids

The concentration of calcium in the body fluids is maintained within a narrow range of 8.5–10.5 mg/100 ml. Whenever the concentration falls below this range, the cells of the parathyroid glands are stimulated to increase their secretion of PTH to as much as 5–10 times the basal rate. The hormone acts upon osteocytes, causing them to mobilize bone mineral from the matrix immediately around them, a process called **osteocytic osteolysis**. If this does not quickly correct the low blood calcium level, the osteocytes release a cytokine that causes coalescence of precursor cells to form increased numbers of osteoclasts, which erode bone and thus release its calcium. This process, called **osteoclastic osteolysis**, is slower, taking many hours to reach effective levels of calcium release.

In addition to effects upon bone, PTH acts upon the distal convoluted tubules of the kidney to increase their reabsorption of calcium from the glomerular filtrate, thus reducing the loss of calcium in the urine. Parathyroid hormone also indirectly influences the rate of absorption of calcium from the lumen of the intestines. Uptake of calcium is dependent upon vitamin D, but the form of vitamin D absorbed in the diet is relatively inactive. It must be converted to its active form in the kidneys. This conversion process is stimulated by PTH.

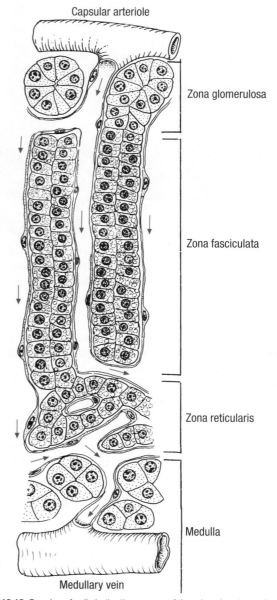

Figure 19.12 Drawing of cells in the three zones of the adrenal cortex and outer medulla. The zona fasciculata is usually longer than depicted here.

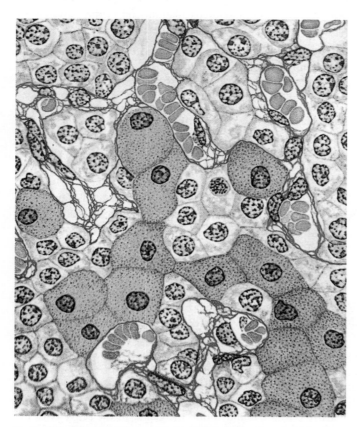

Figure 19.11 A drawing of the parathyroid gland, illustrating the pale chief cells and the larger, more deeply stained oxyphil cells. (Drawing by Esther Bohlman.)

Rare tumors of the parathyroid glands result in **hyperparathyroidism**, in which excess parathyroid hormone leaches calcium from the bones. They become soft and deformed by weight-bearing. Effects on the nervous system result in slowing of the reflexes and weakening of skeletal muscles. Elevated levels of calcium in the blood may lead to the deposition of calcium salts in the kidneys (kidney stones). **Hypoparathyroidism** may result from injury to one or more parathyroid glands or their accidental removal in the course of a thyroidectomy. There is increased excitability of nerves, muscle spasms (tetany), and convulsions. Spasms of the laryngeal muscles and respiratory paralysis may be fatal.

ADRENAL GLANDS

The adrenal glands are located at the cranial pole of each kidney. They are relatively flat, triangular organs, less than 1 cm thick and ranging in width from 2 cm at the apex to 5 cm at their base. On the cut surface of a transected adrenal, a thick yellow **cortex** is readily distinguishable from a gray **medulla** in the interior of the gland. The cortex and medulla are both endocrine glands, but they differ in their embryological origins and their function. The gland is enclosed by a connective tissue capsule that sends thin septa into the interior of the organ.

Blood supply

The adrenal glands have an exceptionally high rate of blood flow, and an unusual pattern of blood vessels. Each adrenal is supplied by three arteries that ramify over the surface, giving rise to branches that pass through the capsule and form a dense **subcapsular plexus**. Short cortical arteries arising from this plexus branch into a very extensive network of fenestrated sinusoidal capillaries around the groups and columns of cells in the cortex. These cortical sinuses are confluent with a plexus of veins in the medulla. This plexus is drained by veins that converge to join the **suprarenal vein** emerging from the hilus of the gland. In addition to the short branches of the subcapsular plexus and their branches, there are longer cortical arteries that pass through the cortex unbranched and form a network of capillaries in the medulla. The adrenal medulla thus has a dual blood supply, receiving blood indirectly via the cortical sinuses and directly via the long cortical arteries.

Adrenal cortex

Three concentric zones are distinguishable in the adrenal cortex: a thin **zona glomerulosa** immediately beneath the capsule; a broad

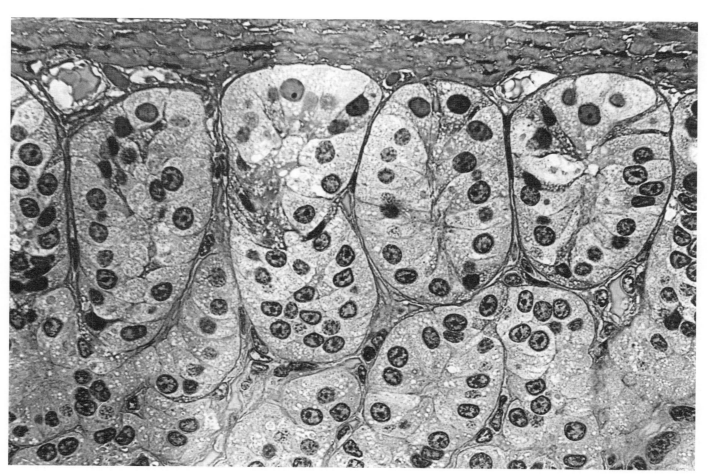

Figure 19.13 Photomicrograph of the zona glomerulosa of the adrenal cortex, showing the acinar arrangement of the cells.

intermediate **zona fasciculata**; and an inner **zona reticularis**, adjacent to the medulla (Fig. 19.12). In histological sections, the transition from zone to zone is gradual, but the three zones have very distinctive vascular patterns, and their boundaries are more apparent in preparations in which the blood vessels have been injected with a contrast medium.

The zonation of the cortex is reflected in its production of different hormones in the three zones. **Aldosterone** is produced exclusively in the zona glomerulosa. **Cortisol** is secreted mainly by the zona fasciculata, and the zona reticularis is the principal site of production of **dehydroepiandrosterone**. When isolated from their natural location, cells of all three layers produce the same product. This has led to the interpretation that products of the outer zone, carried in the blood downstream to the next zone, influence the nature of the product synthesized in that zone. Moreover, the synthesis of a key enzyme by cells of the medulla has been shown to be dependent upon their exposure to glucocorticoids reaching them in blood from the cortex. Thus, the unusual vascular pattern of the gland has physiological significance.

Zona glomerulosa

The columnar epithelial cells of this zone form closely spaced arcades, separated by thin connective tissue septa extending inwards from the capsule (Fig. 19.13). Cells have spherical, heterochromatic nuclei and an acidophilic cytoplasm, containing occasional angular basophilic areas. On electron micrographs, these are found to be stacks of cisternae of rER. There is also a conspicuous network of smooth endoplasmic reticulum (sER) throughout the cytoplasm, and a few lipid droplets. Desmosomes and occasional gap junctions are found on the cell boundaries.

Zona fasciculata

In preparations for the light microscope, this middle zone is made up of pale-staining polyhedral cells arranged in long columns oriented radially with respect to the medulla. Sinusoidal capillaries, of the same orientation, run between the columns (Fig. 19.12). The cells have a highly vacuolated appearance, owing to the extraction of abundant lipid droplets during specimen preparation (Fig. 19.14). On electron micrographs, the nucleus is seen to have a prominent fibrous lamina and a large nucleolus. Lipid droplets are present in great numbers in the cytoplasm, and the mitochondria have atypical tubular or vesicular cristae. Smooth endoplasmic reticulum occupies a large part of the cytoplasm between lipid droplets. An extensive network of tubules of sER is a feature common to steroid-secreting cells.

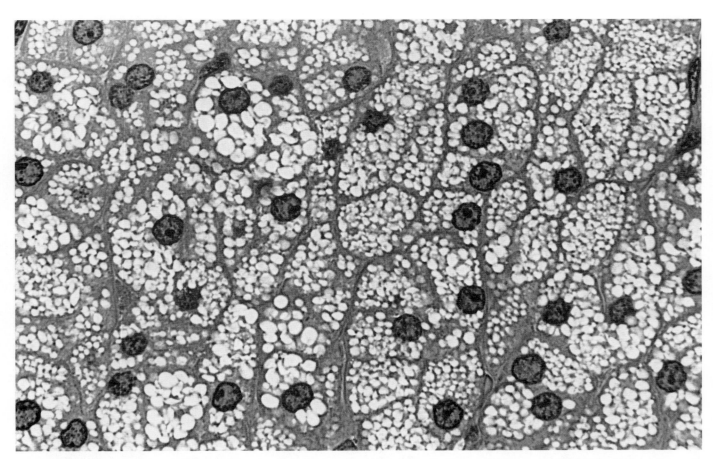

Figure 19.14 Photomicrograph of the zona fasciculata of the adrenal cortex. The cells are filled with round, clear areas that were occupied by lipid droplets before these were extracted during specimen preparation.

Zona reticularis

In this inner zone, the parallel columns of cells of the zona fasciculata give way to a three-dimensional network of anastomosing cell cords (Fig. 19.15). The cells are somewhat smaller, and stain more deeply, than those of the outer zones. On electron micrographs, lipid droplets are fewer and the sER is less extensive. Large aggregations of lipochrome pigment are common. Near the medulla, there are variable numbers of so-called 'dark cells', which have a shrunken nucleus and dense cytoplasm. Their nuclear changes, the paucity of their organelles, and large accumulations of lipochrome pigment suggest that cell degeneration may be common in this zone.

Adrenal medulla

The medulla is composed of large cells in clusters or short cords close to the capillaries and venules. In adrenals that have been fixed in a solution containing potassium dichromate, these cells contain many very small granules. These are more apparent on electron micrographs (Fig. 19.16). This staining by dichromate is called the **chromaffin reaction**. It results from oxidation and polymerization of **catecholamines** in the secretory granules. Cells exhibiting this staining are termed **chromaffin cells**. Catecholamines serve as neurotransmitters for cells of the sympathetic nervous system. The adrenal medulla can be thought of as a modified sympathetic ganglion made up of postganglionic neurons that lack dendrites and axons. The specific catecholamines of the adrenal medulla are **norepinephrine** and **epinephrine**. These are secreted in response to stimulation by preganglionic fibers from splanchnic nerves. Two kinds of cells giving the chromaffin reaction can be distinguished in the adrenal medulla. On electron micrographs, the granules of cells that store norepinephrine have a dense core and a less dense outer zone. Cells that store epinephrine have granules with a more homogenous content, of lower density.

Histophysiology of the adrenal glands

The principal function of the adrenal glands is to maintain the constancy of the internal environment of the body and to make appropriate physiological changes in response to acute stress, injury, or prolonged deprivation of food and water. The adrenal cortex secretes three classes of steroids: **mineralocorticoids**, **glucocorticoids**, and **androgens**.

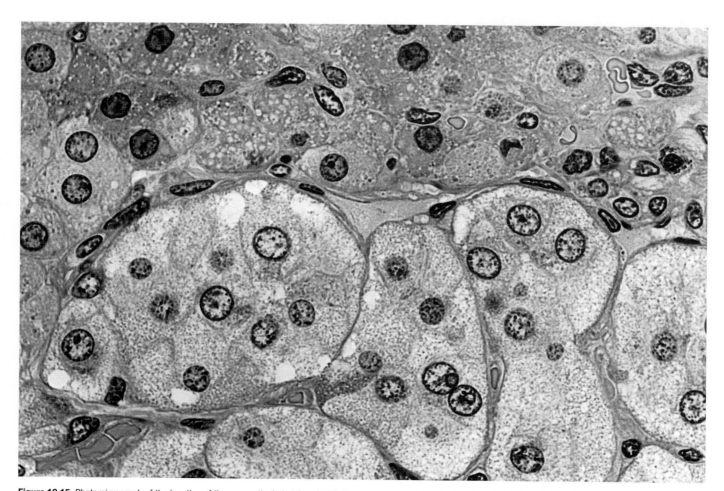

Figure 19.15 Photomicrograph of the junction of the zona reticularis (above) with the clusters of cells of the adrenal medulla below. Catecholamine granules are not visible in the latter with the light microscope unless first exposed to dichromate in the chromaffin reaction.

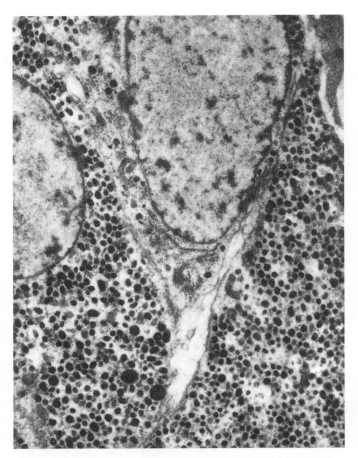

Figure 19.16 Electron micrograph of cells of the cat adrenal medulla, showing the very numerous small granules containing catecholamines. (Micrograph courtesy of R. Yates.)

The principal mineralocorticoid is **aldosterone**, which is secreted mainly by the zona glomerulosa. It controls body fluid volume by influencing the rate of reabsorption of sodium by the kidneys. Its secretion is stimulated by: (1) a fall in sodium concentration in the blood plasma; (2) release of **adrenocorticotrophic hormone (ACTH)** by the hypophysis; or (3) by **atrial natriuretic hormone**, which is produced by specialized cardiac muscle cells.

The principal glucocorticoid is **cortisol**, which is secreted by the zona fasciculata in response to stimulation by adrenocorticotrophic hormone. It has many effects: it decreases protein synthesis, thereby increasing the circulating level of amino acids; it acts on the liver to enhance gluconeogenesis; and it mobilizes fatty acids and glycerol from adipose cells. In addition to these metabolic effects, it has anti-inflammatory effects: it stabilizes lysosomal membranes, reducing release of damaging proteolytic enzymes at sites of inflammation; and it decreases capillary permeability, minimizing local swelling. These attributes make cortisol a valuable medication.

Small amounts of **androgens** are secreted by the zona reticularis. The principal adrenal androgen is **dehydroepiandrosterone**, which is far less potent than testosterone and has little physiological significance.

The adrenal cortex is under hormonal control (by ACTH),

while the secretory activity of the medulla is under nervous control. Centers in the hypothalamus relay impulses to the adrenal medulla via splanchnic (visceral) nerves that end among its cells. Their activation leads to secretion of **epinephrine** and **norepinephrine**. Secretion of these, occurring in response to acute fear or stress, results in an increase in heart rate, and a surge of glucose, which is released into the blood by the liver as an energy source. Thus, the release of adrenal hormones and transmitters in threatening circumstances prepares the body for combat or flight.

Chronic infectious disease, or an autoimmune process, may cause a progressive degeneration of the adrenal glands, leading to **Addison's disease**, adrenocortical insufficiency. Inadequate secretion of adrenal hormones results in low blood pressure (hypotension), fatiguability, weakness, and abnormal pigmentation of the skin. Patients with a small tumor of the pars distalis of the hypophysis, secreting excessive amounts of ACTH, exhibit **Cushing's syndrome**: high blood pressure (hypertension), obesity, osteoporosis, an increase in body hair (hirsutism), and purplish striations of the skin of the abdomen. Similar signs and symptoms may result from a tumor of the adrenal glands, producing excess cortical hormones. Excision of the hypophyseal or adrenal tumor usually brings relief.

PINEAL GLAND

The **pineal gland** (or **epiphysis cerebri**) is a small organ projecting from the roof of the diencephalon, in the midline of the brain. The gland is a conical gray body 5–8 mm in length and 3–5 mm at its greatest width. The gland is invested by the pia mater, the delicate inner layer of connective tissue that covers the brain. Thin septa extend inwards from this layer to surround cords, or clusters of cells in its interior.

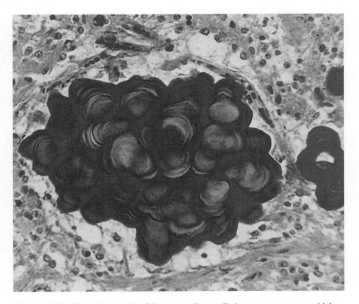

Figure 19.17 Photomicrograph of the concretions called corpora arenacea which are often found in the human pineal gland.

Microscopic structure

The parenchyma consists of pale-staining cells, called **pinealocytes**. Their nucleus is often deeply indented and may be quite irregular in outline. The cytoplasm is slightly basophilic and contains both rough and smooth endoplasmic reticulum, a small Golgi complex, and many mitochondria. It may also contain a few lipid droplets. When stained by silver-impregnation methods, the pinealocytes can be shown to have one or more long processes that terminate in bulbous expansions. The majority of these end on, or near, capillaries (Fig. 19.17). Their ends contain clusters of small vesicles that are often associated with a **synaptic ribbon**, a dense rod or lamella extending inwards from the plasmalemma. Such structures are also found at synapses in sensory cells of the retina and inner ear. In the pinealocytes, they are multiple and may be found on the cell body as well as at the ends of the cell processes. Their function remains a mystery. The pinealocytes secrete the hormone **melatonin**, which is apparently released at the rate it is produced and not stored in secretory granules.

Cells of a second type, called **interstitial cells** or **astroglial cells**, are found among the pinealocytes and around capillaries. These resemble the astrocytes of the brain in having a long cell process containing abundant intermediate filaments. The pineal of humans contains peculiar extracellular concretions called **corpora arenacea** ('brain sand'), which consist of calcium phosphate and calcium carbonate in an organic matrix (Fig. 19.18). Their calcium content makes them radio-opaque, and they are useful to the radiologist in localizing brain tumors that may displace the pineal from its normal midline position.

Histophysiology of the pineal gland

The pineal is a gland that modulates gonadal function. Its biosynthetic activity exhibits a diurnal rhythmicity related to the periods

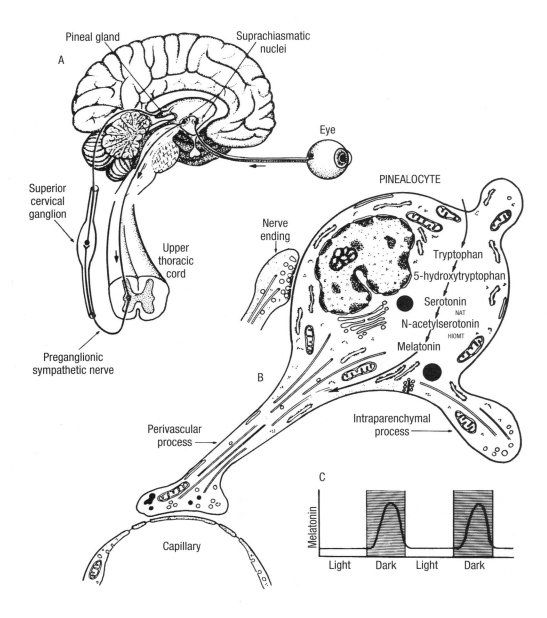

Figure 19.18 (A) Diagram showing the path of information transfer from the eyes to the pineal. (B) Upon stimulation of a pinealocyte, tryptophan is taken up and converted to melatonin, which is released into the blood. (C) A graph of the light–dark cycle of melatonin concentration in the blood. (Reproduced from R.J. Reiter in *Groot's Endocrinology*, W.B Saunders, Philadelphia, 1989.)

of light and dark. The plasma concentration of its hormone, **melatonin**, increases in the dark phase of the cycle. Information as to day or night is transmitted from the eyes to nuclei in the hypothalamus, and from there to the pineal (Fig. 19.17A). Release of the neurotransmitter norepinephrine by the nerves controls the secretory activity of the pinealocytes. Their hormone, melatonin, acts upon the hypophysis to suppress its release of gonadotrophic hormones.

In species that are seasonal breeders, the gonads regress in the winter and regain reproductive competence in the spring. It is the pineal that mediates this response of the reproductive system to changing day length. Increased secretion of melatonin during the longer nights of fall and winter leads to regression of the testes. Longer days of sunlight in the spring, decrease pineal secretion, permitting the testes to respond to gonadotrophic hormones, with resumption of spermatogenesis.

In the course of evolution, humans became continuous breeders. There is no evidence that reproductive activity of humans is subject to pineal regulation. With the invention of the electric light-bulb, day length may have become physiologically irrelevant.

ISLETS OF LANGERHANS

The **islets of Langerhans**, secreting the hormones **insulin**, **glucagon**, **somatostatin**, and **pancreatic polypeptide**, could appropriately be included in this chapter on the endocrine glands, however, they do not constitute a separate organ. They consist of spherical aggregations of endocrine cells widely distributed within the parenchyma of the pancreas, and they were described and their function was discussed in Chapter 16 (Pancreas).

Questions

1 Large lipid droplets are typical of which one of the following?
  a median eminence
  b pineal gland
  c zona fasciculata of the adrenal cortex
  d somatotropin cells of the pituitary
  e adrenal medulla

2 Aldosterone is secreted by the
  a zona reticularis
  b chromaffin cells
  c chromophobes
  d zona glomerulosa
  e pituicytes

3 The pars intermedia secretes
  a FSH
  b TSH
  c LH
  d ACTH
  e MSH

4 Somatostatin is produced by which one of the following?
  a pars distalis of the pituitary
  b pineal gland
  c adrenal cortex
  d parathyroid
  e thyroid

5 Synthesis of which one of the following is controlled by hypothalamo–hypophyseal feedback?
  a insulin
  b calcitonin
  c melatonin
  d thyroxin
  e FSH

6 Pituicytes are found in which one of the following?
  a median eminence
  b pars distalis
  c pars nervosa
  d pars intermedia
  e anterior pituitary

7 Large numbers of fat cells are typical of the aging stage of which one of the following endocrine glands?
  a thyroid
  b parathyroid
  c spleen
  d adrenal
  e pineal gland

8 Paraganglia are closely related by their origin and functions to which one of the following?
  a adrenal medulla
  b adrenal cortex
  c follicular thyroid
  d adenohypophysis
  e gastrointestinal endocrines

9 Pituitary acidophils produce which one of the following?
  a somatotropin
  b somatostatin
  c ACTH
  d FSH
  e oxytocin

10 Large aggregations of lipochrome are typical of which one of the following?
  a zona glomerulosa of the adrenal
  b adrenal medulla cells
  c follicular thyroid cells
  d parathyroid cells
  e zona reticularis of the adrenal

11 What organ secretes insulin?

12 Where are pituicytes located?

13 What hormone is an antagonist to parathormone?

14 What pituitary cell secretes TSH?

15 Neurohypophyseal secretions are synthesized in which two structures?

16 What hormone stimulates growth of long bones?

17 What are the principal targets of oxytocin?

18 What organ secretes melatonin?

19 Which hormone is secreted by thyroid parafollicular cells?

20 What is the name of the adrenal cortical region adjacent to the adrenal medulla?

Male Reproductive System

The external genitalia of the male consist of two gonads, the **testes**, suspended in a skin-covered, fibroelastic sac, the **scrotum**, and a copulatory organ, the **penis**. The excurrent ducts from the testes, the **ductuli efferentes**, join a long, highly convoluted duct that

forms the **epididymis**, an elongated organ adherent to the posterior surface of each testis (Fig. 20.1). The **spermatozoa** produced in the testes are stored in the epididymis. At the lower pole of each epididymis the coiled epididymal duct is continuous with a long

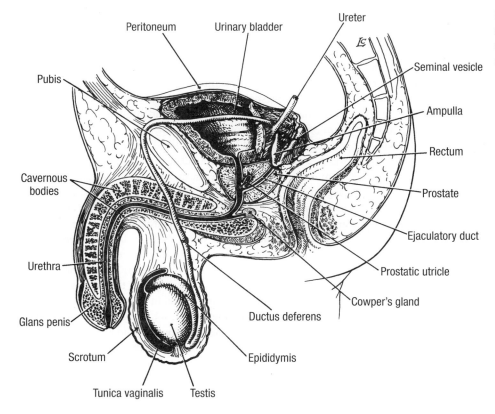

Figure 20.1 Diagram of the male reproductive system. Midline structures are shown in saggittal section. Bilateral structures such as the testis are depicted in the round. (Drawing after C.D. Turner.)

straight **ductus deferens** that ascends from the scrotum and passes through the inguinal canal to enter the pelvis, where its terminal portion, called the **ejaculatory duct**, passes through the **prostate gland** to open into the urethra immediately below the bladder. The ducts of two accessory glands of male reproduction, the **seminal vesicles** and **prostate gland**, deliver their secretions into the ejaculatory duct. The ducts of the small **bulbourethral glands** open into the urethra below the prostate. The **semen** that is discharged at ejaculation consists of millions of spermatozoa in a semifluid medium made up of the secretions of the accessory glands.

TESTES

The testes are ovoid in shape, 4–5 cm in length, 2.5 cm in width, and 3 cm in anteroposterior diameter. They develop early in embryonic life in the abdominal cavity and later descend into the scrotum. As they descend, they carry with them an outpocketing of the peritoneum, called the **tunica vaginalis propria testis**, which forms an independent serous cavity around the anterior and lateral surfaces of the testis. Like the peritoneum, this closed cavity is lined by mesothelium. The limited amount of mobility permitted within this cavity, and within the elastic scrotum, helps to prevent damage to the organ. Descent into the scrotum provides a testicular environment with a temperature a few degrees lower than that of the abdominal cavity. This lower temperature is a necessary condition for development of the spermatozoa.

The testis is enclosed in a thick, fibrous capsule, the **tunica albuginea**. On its posterior surface, a dense connective tissue extends inwards from the capsule to form the **mediastinum** of the testis, through which its blood vessels enter and its ducts leave the organ. Thin, fibrous **septula testis** radiate from the mediastinum to the tunica albuginea, dividing the interior of the organ into about 250 pyramidal compartments, the **lobuli testis**. Each lobule contains from one to four tortuous **seminiferous tubules**, 150–200 μm in diameter and 30–70 cm in length (Fig. 20.2). The majority of these form highly convoluted loops that return to the mediastinum, but a few may end blindly. At the apex of each pyramidal lobule, there is an abrupt transition of its seminiferous tubules to the **tubuli recti**. These converge upon a plexus of epithelium-lined spaces within the mediastinum testis, called the **rete testis** (Fig. 20.2). A number of slender **ductuli efferentes** arising from the rete testis emerge from the testis and conduct spermatozoa to the long, convoluted **ductus epididymidis**, where they are stored and undergo further maturation.

The interstices between the seminiferous tubules of the testis are occupied by a loose reticular connective tissue, containing a dense network of peritubular capillaries, lymphatic vessels, mesenchymal cells, and occasional macrophages. Within this stroma are clusters of **Leydig cells** (Fig. 20.3), which constitute the endocrine component of the testis, secreting the male sex hormone **testosterone**.

Seminiferous tubules

The total length of the seminiferous tubules in the two testes of the human is well over 200 m, enabling them to produce astronomical

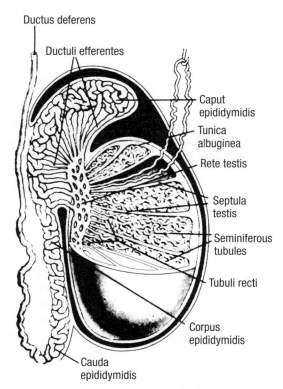

Figure 20.2 Cut-away diagram of the testis and its excretory duct. Septa divide the organ into compartments occupied by convoluted seminiferous tubules. (Reproduced, with modifications, from W.J. Hamilton *Textbook of Human Anatomy*, McMillan and Co, London, 1927.)

numbers of spermatozoa. Each tubule is bounded by a thin sheath. In rodent testes, the sheath includes an epithelioid layer of flat, polygonal cells, called **myoid cells**. These contain longitudinally and transversely oriented bundles of actin filaments and associated proteins that generate rhythmic contractions of the sheath, which result in slight constrictions that can be observed to move along the length of the seminiferous tubules of the living animal. In the human testis, all of the sheath cells are fusiform and appear to be fibroblasts. No myoid cells are identifiable and no contractions of the seminiferous tubules have been observed. The tubules are lined by a thick pseudostratified **seminiferous epithelium**, which is made up of multiple ill-defined layers of differentiating germ cells interposed between uniformly spaced tall **Sertoli cells** (Fig. 20.4). The stem cells of the germ-cell lineage, called **spermatogonia** rest upon the basal lamina. Immediately above them are pairs of spherical **primary spermatocytes** and larger groups of **secondary spermatocytes**. Above these are large clusters of small round **spermatids**. Spermatids, more advanced in their differentiation, undergo dramatic shape changes, taking on a form approaching that of a spermatozoon, and they come to occupy deep recesses, of conforming shape, in the apex of a neighboring Sertoli cell. Their tapering head, containing a greatly condensed pyriform nucleus, is directed downwards, and a portion of the cell body and the long flagellum project into the lumen of the seminiferous tubule (Fig. 20.4). Thus, the seminiferous epithelium consists of two distinct cell populations: (1) non-proliferating supporting cells (Sertoli cells); and (2) dividing stem cells

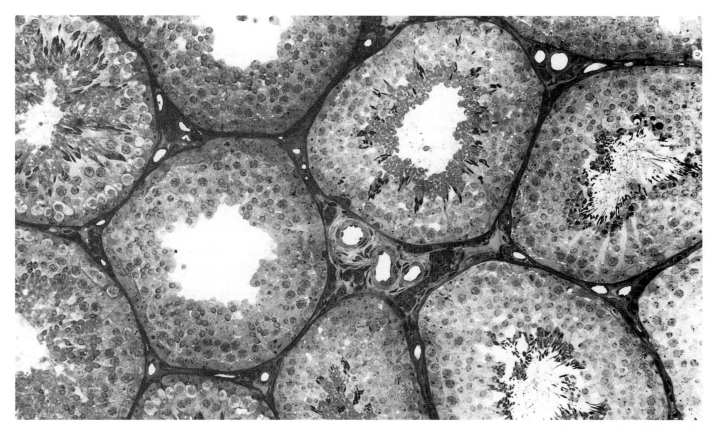

Figure 20.3 Photomicrograph of several seminiferous tubules in cross-section. Notice their thick lining epithelium and the interstitial tissue between them, containing blood vessels and clusters of Leydig cells.

(spermatogenia) and their proliferating progeny that move upwards in the epithelium as they differentiate into spermatozoa.

The Sertoli cells provide mechanical support for the germ cells and, by changes in their shape, they no doubt contribute to the upward movement of the differentiating germ cells and the release of the spermatozoa into the lumen. Unlike other columnar epithe-

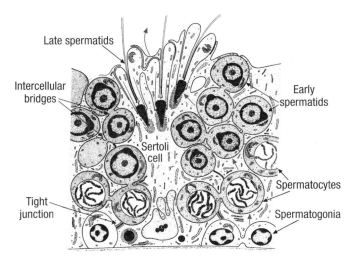

Figure 20.4 Drawing of a short segment of seminiferous epithelium showing spermatogonia, groups of spermatocytes and spermatids along either side of a tall Sertoli cell. The heads and cell bodies of more advanced spermatids occupy deep concavities in the apex of the Sertoli cell.

lial cells, which usually have straight sides, the sides of Sertoli cells are highly irregular, with multiple shallow concavities that conform to the rounded shape of the adjacent spermatocytes and spermatids. Their ovoid nucleus contains a large nucleolus that is usually flanked by two dense masses of heterochromatin. Electron micrographs reveal a conspicuous Golgi complex but few small vesicles are associated with its cisternae and there are no secretory granules. Rough endoplasmic reticulum (rER) is sparse but smooth endoplasmic reticulum (sER) is abundant in the basal cytoplasm. A few lipid droplets and occasional aggregations of lipochrome pigment may also be found in this region. There is a well developed cytoskeleton including a meshwork of actin filament in the cell cortex and bundles of longer actin filaments that traverse the cytoplasm in various orientations. Numerous intermediate filaments are oriented more-or-less parallel to the long axis of the cell, and microtubules of similar orientation are also abundant at certain stages of the spermatogenic cycle. The bundles of actin filaments and the microtubules are no doubt involved in the shape changes of the Sertoli cells that contribute to upwards movement of the germ cells and the release of spermatozoa into the lumen of the seminiferous tubules.

Blood–testis barrier

Most epithelia have zonulae occludentes between their cells, just below their free surface. The seminiferous epithelium is exceptional in having occluding junctions nearer to the base of the epithelium. They occur between lateral processes of neighboring Sertoli cells that arch over the intervening spermatogonia. These occluding junctions divide the epithelium into two compartments: a **basal compartment** containing the spermatogonia and an **adlumenal compartment** containing the later stages of germ cell differentiation. These junctions constitute a **blood-testis barrier** that prevents large molecules from entering, or leaving, the adlumenal compartment. The barrier may be necessary for maintenance of a special environment for germ cell differentiation in that compartment.

SPERMATOGENESIS

The term 'spermatogenesis' encompasses the entire sequence of proliferative events and cytological changes undergone by the germ cells in their development from stem cells to mature spermatozoa. Stem cells with pale-staining nuclei, called **type A spermatogonia**, are situated on the basal lamina. In the initial phase of spermatogenesis, these undergo multiple mitotic divisions. Half of the daughter cell population goes on to differentiate into **type B spermatogonia**, and the others maintain the stem cell population (Fig. 20.5). Division of each type B spermatogonium produces two **primary spermatocytes**, which are large spherical cells located above the spermatogonia (Fig. 20.4). These immediately enter prophase of the first meiotic cell division. **Meiosis** occurs only in the development of the germ cells of both sexes and consists of two successive divisions that reduce the normal somatic chromosome number from 46 (44 + XY in the male) to 23 (22 + X or 22 + Y in spermatozoa).

Five stages of **meiotic prophase** can be distinguished by the changing appearance of the chromosomes and chromatids in the nucleus of the primary spermatocytes. These stages are called **leptotene, zygotene, pachytene, diplotene**, and **diakinesis**. Prophase of the first meiotic division is a slow process extending over 20 days. Therefore, most of the spermatocytes seen in histological sections will be in one or another of the stages of meiotic prophase. In the leptotene stage, the chromosomes appear as long, thin filaments. These later begin to shorten and thicken. In the zygotene stage, homologous chromosomes come together in pairs, in register along their length; a process called **synapsis**. In pachytene, shortening of the chromosomes continues, and in diplotene, each of the paired chromosomes have duplicated, resulting in tetrads of four parallel **chromatids**. Adjacent chromatids of the paired chromosomes exchange segments, a process called **crossing-over**. In diakinesis, the homologous chromosomes shorten further and begin to separate, but they may adhere briefly at sites of crossing-over. Prophase ends with the dissolution of the nuclear envelope and migration of the chromosomes to the equatorial plate.

In **metaphase** the chromosomes become connected to centrosomes at opposite poles of the cell by microtubules of the mitotic spindle, and in **anaphase**, the pairs of chromosomes, each consisting of two chromatids, separate and migrate to the poles. In **telophase** the cytoplasm constricts, separating two haploid (i.e. containing half the number of chromosomes found in the somatic

cells) secondary spermatocytes. These proceed quickly through prophase of the second meiotic division. The chromosomes gather on the equatorial plate, and at anaphase, the two chromatids of each chromosome separate and migrate to opposite poles. At telophase, the second meiotic division is completed. The two meiotic divisions thus result in four haploid spermatids that develop into haploid spermatozoa. Because of the separation of the members of the XY pair during meiosis, half of the spermatozoa have a chromosome complement of 22 + X, and the other half, 22 + Y. The ova of the female are all 22 + X. Their fertilization by an X-bearing spermatozoon results in a girl, and fertilization by a Y-bearing spermatozoon results in a boy.

Failure of the chromosomes to separate normally in meiotic division during spermatogenesis, or oogenesis, may result in male offspring with one or more extra X chromosomes (47XXY, 48XXXY), a condition called **Klinefelter's syndrome**. These men are tall, have small firm testes with no spermatogenesis and after puberty they exhibit gynecomastia (breast development) as a result of excess secretion of female hormones, and lower than normal blood levels of testosterone. This is the commonest abnormality of sexual development with an incidence of 1 in 500 male births.

Telophase of the cell divisions in spermatogenesis is atypical in that the daughter cells do not completely separate, but remain in

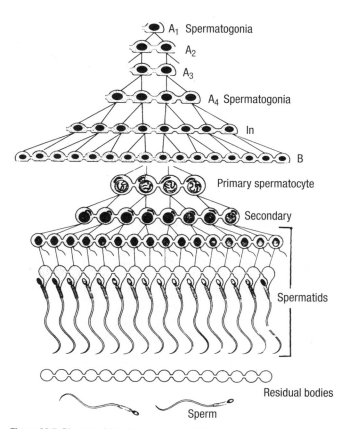

A₁ Spermatogonia
A₂
A₃
A₄ Spermatogonia
In
B
Primary spermatocyte
Secondary
Spermatids
Residual bodies
Sperm

Figure 20.5 Diagram of the clonal expansion of the male germ cells. Only the type A spermatogonia complete cytokinesis. In subsequent generations, cytokinesis is incomplete and chains of daughter cells remain connected by intercellular bridges. The lower half of the figure shows the further stages of proliferation and differentiation of the cells derived from a single type B spermatogonium.

continuity through a narrow intercellular bridge. Therefore, a pair of conjoined type B spermatogonia gives rise to a group of four conjoined primary spermatocytes. The two subsequent divisions produce chains of eight secondary spermatocytes and 16 spermatids that differentiate without further division to yield 16 spermatozoa (Fig. 20.5).

Spermiogenesis

The term **spermiogenesis** refers to the sequence of postmeiotic changes by which spermatids are transformed into spermatozoa. For descriptive purposes, this process is divided into a **Golgi phase**, an **acrosome phase**, and a **maturational phase**. The spermatids are initially small, closely spaced spherical cells, 7–8 μm in diameter, located above the spermatocytes. In the Golgi phase, small membrane-limited proacrosomal granules appear in their juxtanuclear Golgi complex. These coalesce into a large granule within a sizable **acrosomal vesicle** which adheres to the nuclear envelope (Fig. 20.6A, B). The Golgi complex remains close to the outer aspect of the acrosomal vesicle and continues to form vesicles that fuse with it, contributing to an increase in the volume of the vesicle and the size of the acrosomal granule in its interior. The

area of the membrane of the vesicle adhering to the nuclear envelope spreads laterally from the point of initial contact, and the vesicle assumes a hemispherical shape (Fig. 20.6B). This marks the end of the Golgi phase.

In the acrosome phase, the granule remains at the pole of the nucleus, while the surrounding vesicle continues to expand, forming a thin fold that extends laterally and posteriorly until it forms a cap over the entire anterior half of the nucleus (Fig. 20.6C). The substance of the granule then becomes distributed throughout the interior of the cap formed by the acrosomal vesicle. This completes the development of the **acrosome**.

Concurrent with these changes, there is a condensation of the chromatin, and the ovoid nucleus takes on a narrower shape (Fig. 20.7). In the course of these events, the cell as a whole changes its orientation so that the acrosome is directed towards the basal lamina of the epithelium. The cell elongates and the centrioles move to the posterior pole of the nucleus, and become fixed to the nuclear envelope. One member of the pair is oriented transversely; the other is parallel to the long axis of the nucleus. The triplet microtubules in the wall of this centriole serve as templates for assembly of tubulin to form nine doublet microtubules that rapidly elongate to form the **axoneme** of the sperm flagellum.

In the cytoplasm of the elongating spermatid, microtubules increase in number and become arranged in a cylindrical array, termed the **manchette**. This extends backwards from the posterior rim of the acrosome. In the formation of the manchette, the bulk of the spermatid cytoplasm is shifted posteriorly and the plasma membrane at the anterior end becomes closely applied to the outer membrane of the acrosome. After this shape change, the microtubules of the manchette depolymerize.

Where the plasma membrane is continuous with the flagellar membrane, a dense material accumulates on its inner surface to form a dense ring called the **annulus**. As the flagellum continues to elongate, the annulus moves along it and the mitochondria of the spermatid assemble behind it and become arranged in a tight spiral around the initial portion of the axoneme, forming the

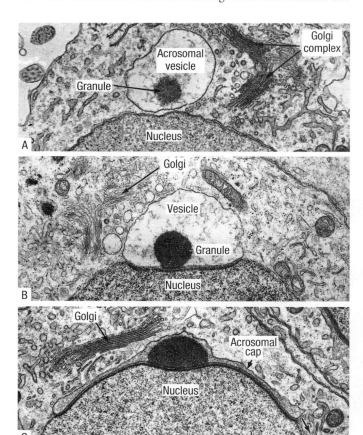

Figure 20.6 Electron micrographs of three successive stages in the formation of the acrosome. (A) The acrosomal vesicle and granule are adjacent to the Golgi complex, as in development of a secretory granule. (B) The vesicle adheres to the nuclear envelope. (C) The vesicle spreads laterally over the anterior pole of the nucleus to form the acrosomal cap.

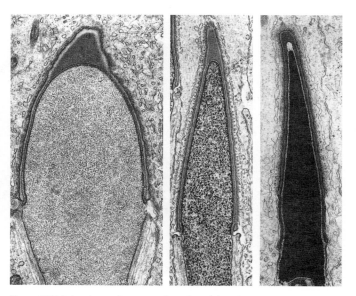

Figure 20.7 Later stages of acrosome formation and condensation of the spermatid nucleus.

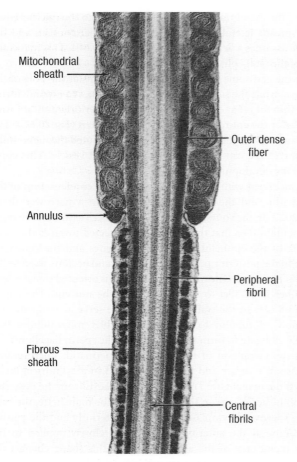

Figure 20.8 Longitudinal section of a portion of a sperm tail showing the mitochondrial sheath of the mid-piece, the annulus, and the outer dense fibers and fibrous sheath of the principal piece.

mitochondrial sheath of the sperm flagellum (Fig. 20.8). While these events are in progress, a thick **outer dense fiber** is assembled adjacent to each of the nine doublets of the axoneme, and peripheral to it (Figs. 20.8, 20.9). Posterior to the annulus, semicircular rib-like structures form in the thin layer of cytoplasm between the flagellar membrane and the outer dense fibers. These are joined together by their continuity with dorsal and ventral longitudinal columns of the same material. The circumferential ribs and their connecting longitudinal columns constitute the **fibrous sheath** of the developing sperm tail (Fig. 20.9).

Spermiation

The release of spermatozoa from the semeniferous epithelium is called **spermiation**. During their development, the spermatids are slowly moved towards the surface of the epithelium by proliferation of spermatocytes below them and by active movements of the Sertoli cells (Fig. 20.10). When they have reached the stage of development described above, they consist of a condensed nucleus capped by an acrosome, a flagellum enclosed in a mitochondrial sheath proximally, and a fibrous sheath, distally. They also have a retort-shaped appendage of excess cytoplasm on one side. At this stage, the heads of the spermatids occupy conforming recesses in the apical surface of the Sertoli cells, with their flagella projecting into the lumen of the seminiferous tubule (Fig. 20.10C). Their appendages of residual cytoplasm remain connected by intercellular bridges. In the process of spermiation, the slender stalk connecting them to the residual body is broken and they are extruded from the Sertoli cell as free spermatozoa in the lumen of the seminiferous tubule (Fig. 20.10D). The residual cytoplasm of the spermatids is retained in the apical cytoplasm of the Sertoli cell and is subsequently degraded by lysosomal enzymes.

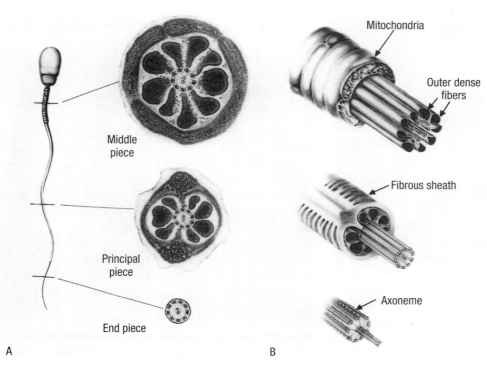

Figure 20.9 Electron micrographs of the midpiece, principal piece, and end piece of a sperm tail in cross-section. (B) Drawings of the three-dimensional organization of the three segments of the sperm tail.

A   B

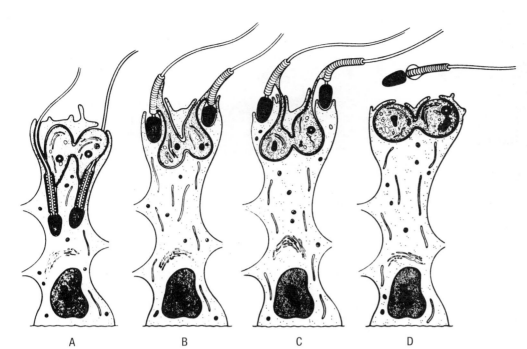

Figure 20.10 (A) Late stage spermatids occupying deep concavities in the apex of the Sertoli cell. (B) The axial elements of the future spermatozoa and their residual cytoplasm are moved closer to the lumen. (C) The spermatozoa are pushed into the lumen, still connected to their residual cytoplasm by a narrow stalk. (D) The stalk gives way, and the spermatozoa are then free in the lumen. The residual bodies are retained and degraded by lysosomal enzymes of the Sertoli cell.

A   B   C   D

SPERMATOZOON

The mature spermatozoon has a **head** and a **tail**. The head consists of the condensed nucleus, capped by the acrosome. The tail includes: (1) a **connecting piece**, consisting of nine cross-striated fibers that are continuous distally with the outer dense fibers of the flagellum; (2) a **mid-piece**, 5–7 μm in length, made up of the axoneme surrounded by the mitochondrial sheath; (3) a **principal piece**, about 45 μm in length in which the axoneme is enclosed in the fibrous sheath; and (4) the **end piece**, 5–7 μm long, consisting of the terminal part of the axoneme distal to the termination of the fibrous sheath. It is enclosed throughout by the plasmalemma.

Spermatozoa are produced in enormous numbers. The human ejaculate of 2–5 ml of semen contains 40–100 million spermatozoa/ml; men with fewer than 20 million spermatozoa/ml are usually infertile. It is not surprising that some mistakes are made in the assembly of these complex cells. Spermatozoa of abnormal structure, or non-progressive motility, are not uncommon in the normal ejaculate.

CYCLE OF THE SEMINIFEROUS EPITHELIUM

At any one site in the seminiferous tubule the development of the clusters of conjoined germ cells is synchronous, but from segment to segment along the tubule, different associations of cell types, representing different stages of germ cell differentiation, can be identified. Therefore, in cross-sections of the testis, neighboring tubules have a different appearance (Fig.20.11). For each species, there is a specific number of recognizable cell associations. In the guinea pig, there are 12 and cells of the same stage are found around the entire circumference of the tubule. If cross-sections of enough tubules are examined, all 12 associations can be found. At any point along the length of a seminiferous tubule, the cell types change with the passage of time, ultimately passing through all 12 stages and then repeating the sequence. The **cycle of the seminiferous epithelium** is defined as the series of changes occurring in a given area of epithelium between two successive appearances of the same cell association. In the human, there are only six different cell associations (Fig.20.11). These do not extend around the entire circumference of the tubule as they do in the guinea pig, but occupy small, wedge-shaped areas of the epithelium. Thus, one may find three different associations of cells in the same cross-section. The duration of one cycle in man is 16days and the total duration of spermatogenesis is 64days.

INTERSTITIAL TISSUE

The angular spaces between the seminiferous tubules are occupied by clusters of **Leydig cells** in a very loose connective tissue containing: blood and lymphatic vessels; occasional fibroblasts; macrophages; and rare mast cells. Collagen fibers are few (Fig.20.12). In some mammals, notably the opossum, boar, and stallion, the Leydig cells are far more numerous, filling nearly all of the extravascular space of the interstitium.

Leydig cells are the principal endocrine cell type of the testis, secreting the male sex hormone, **testosterone**, and other androgenic steroids. They first appear in the interstitial tissue at puberty, increase to a maximum at the age of 30 years, and then slowly decline in number with advancing age. Where they are closely packed, they are irregularly polyhedral and 14–20 μm across. Binucleate cells are common. There is a prominent Golgi complex, but no secretory granules, for they secrete continuously

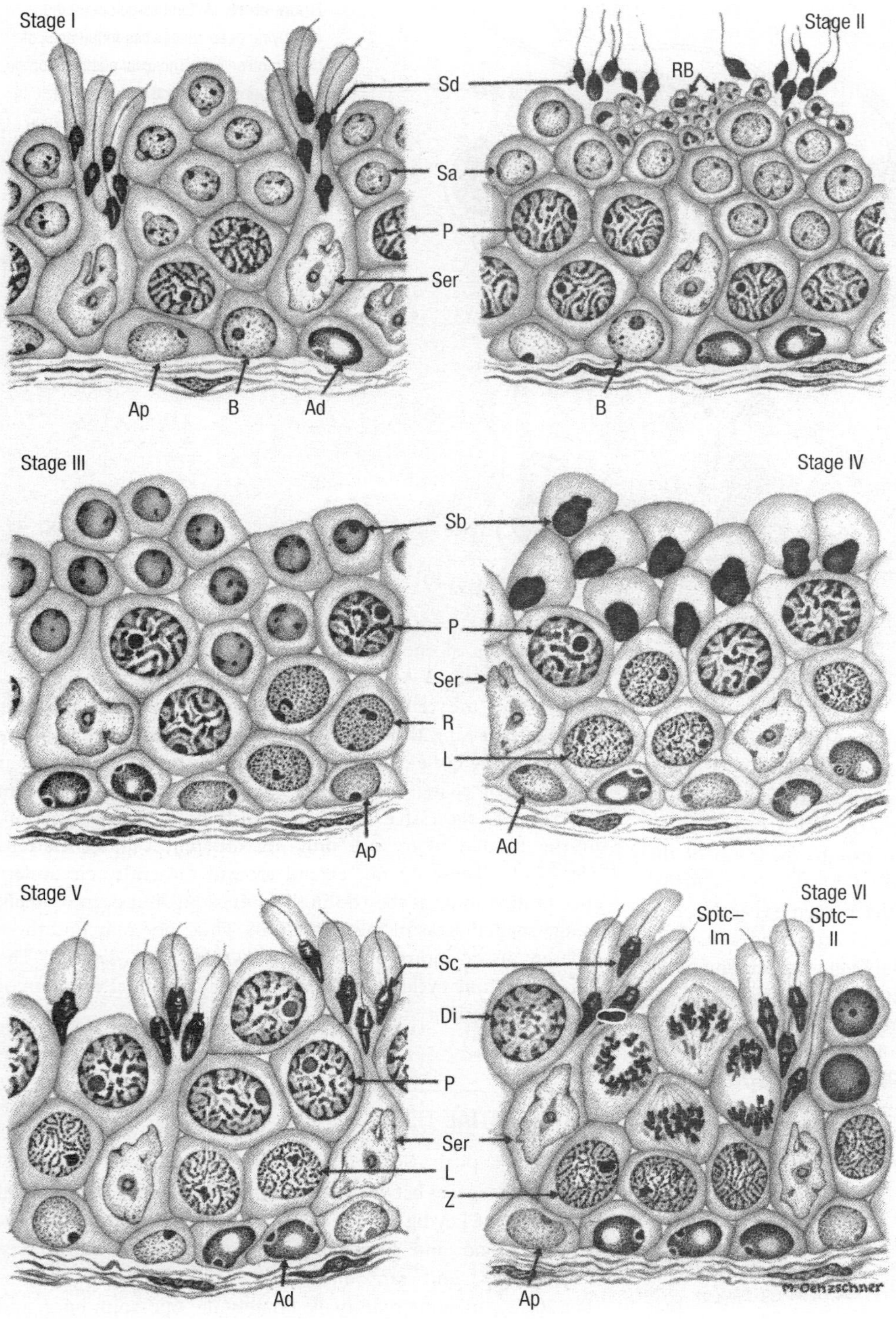

Figure 20.11 Drawings of the six stages of the cycle of the human seminiferous epithelium. Labels: Sertoli cell (Ser); A and B spermatogonia (Ad and Ap); type B spermatogonia (B); resting spermatocyte (R); leptotene spermatocyte (L); pachytene spermatocyte (P); dividing primary spermatocyte (sptc-Im); spermatids in various stages (Sa, Sb, Sc, etc); residual bodies (RB). (Reproduced from Y. Clermont *Am J Anat* 1963; 122:35.)

without intracellular storage of their product. The cytoplasm contains abundant mitochondria and variable numbers of lipid droplets. There are occasional cisternae of rER, but the most conspicuous feature of these cells is an extensive sER throughout the cytoplasm. This is a feature common to all steroid-secreting cells. Deposits of lipochrome pigment are common and increase with age. A feature unique to the human Leydig cell is the presence, in the cytoplasm, of conspicuous crystals 3 μm or more in diameter

and up to 20 μm in length, called the **crystals of Reinke**. Such crystals occur in most men, from puberty to senility, but their number is highly variable. They have the solubility properties of protein. Their significance is unknown.

The **testicular arteries** arise from the abdominal aorta and pass downwards, through the inguinal canal, to enter the scrotum, where they ramify over the surface of the testes. Branches that enter the parenchyma at its mediastinum form a rich network of

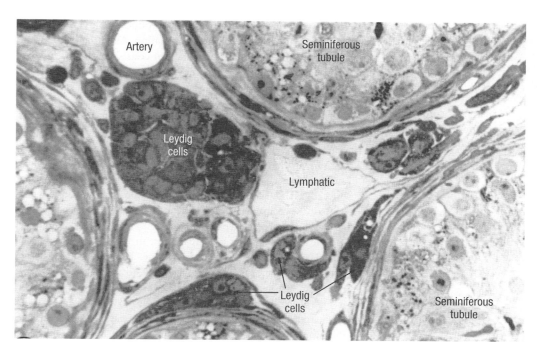

Figure 20.12 Electron micrograph of interstitial tissue of a mammalian testis. Clusters of Leydig cells are found near blood vessels. Very thin-walled lymphatic vessels are also present.

capillaries in the interstitial tissue between the seminiferous tubules. Also present in the interstitium are very thin-walled lymphatic capillaries (Fig. 20.12). Leydig cells are not always intimately related to the blood or lymphatic capillaries, but their hormone, **testosterone**, diffuses into both.

HISTOPHYSIOLOGY OF THE TESTIS

The normal functioning of the testis depends on the maintenance of a temperature about 3°C below normal body temperature (37°C). This is the reason for their descent into the scrotum. Cooling of the testis depends, in part, on perspiration and evaporative heat loss from the surface of the scrotum. An equally important mechanism of temperature control depends upon a special arrangement of the blood vessels supplying the organ. In the upper scrotum and spermatic cord, a plexus of veins, draining blood from the testis, closely surrounds the testicular artery. A countercurrent heat-exchange system is thus created, in which the cooler venous blood returning from the testis pre-cools the arterial blood flowing to the testis. In a cold environment, the **cremaster muscle**, a network of smooth muscle around the testes, draws them up to a warmer site nearer the inguinal canal.

Spermatozoa can be thought of as a holocrine secretory product of the seminiferous epithelium. In the human, the number produced daily is very large, 5.6×10^6/g of testicular tissue. However, this number is low compared to other species (e.g. rabbit, 25×10^6/g of testis; boar, 23×10^6/g of testis—taking into account the weight of the boar testes, the daily production would be 16.2×10^9).

Spermatogenesis depends on gonadotrophic hormones

secreted by the hypophysis. **Luteinizing hormone (LH)** binds to specific receptors on the Leydig cells. This stimulates production of cyclic AMP and activation of kinases. Free cholesterol is released from lipid droplets in the cytoplasm of the Leydig cells, by an esterase. Mitochondrial enzymes cleave off the side-chain of cholesterol to yield **pregnenolone**, and enzymes of the sER carry out several steps in its transformation to **testosterone**. It is calculated that a single Leydig cell can produce 10 000 molecules of testosterone per second. **Follicle-stimulating hormone (FSH)** stimulates Sertoli cell synthesis of androgen-binding protein, which binds to testosterone produced by the Leydig cells. There is a feedback control of hypophyseal FSH release by a hormone, **inhibin**, produced by the Sertoli cells.

Testosterone circulating in the blood is essential for maintenance of the function of the prostate, seminal vesicles, and bulbourethral glands. It is also responsible for establishment of the male secondary sex characteristics: pattern of pubic hair, growth of beard, low-pitched voice, and muscular body build.

EXCURRENT DUCTS

Tubuli recti and rete testis

The several seminiferous tubules in each lobule of the testis converge upon the **rete testis**, an epithelium-lined plexus in its mediastinum. As they approach the rete, they narrow and are joined to the rete by short **tubuli recti**. The tubuli recti and rete testis are lined by a cuboidal epithelium that does not appear to be secretory. There are microvilli on its free surface and many of the cells have a single long cilium.

Ductuli efferentes

From the rete testis, 12 or more **ductuli efferentes** conduct the spermatozoa to the ductus epididymidis. They are highly coiled and ultimately join to form the single ductus epididymidis. They are lined by an epithelium made up of clusters of columnar ciliated cells alternating with groups of shorter non-ciliated cells. The latter have invaginations of their apical membrane, suggesting that they take up fluid from the lumen by endocytosis. The action of the cilia on the taller cells moves fluid and spermatozoa towards the epididymis (Fig. 20.13).

Epididymis

The epididymis is an organ about 7cm long, running along the posterior surface of the testis from its upper to its lower pole. It consists of a single, highly convoluted tube, the **ductus epididymidis** (Fig.20.2). If freed of connective tissue and straightened out, it would be approximately 6m in length. At its lower end, it is continuous with the **ductus deferens**. The epididymis is the site of accumulation, storage, and maturation of spermatozoa. When the spermatozoa leave the testis, they are physiologically immature and non-motile, but after 5–7days in transit through the epididymis, they acquire motility. Products of the epididymal epithelium contribute to their maturation. The duct is lined by a pseudostratified columnar epithelium consisting of two types of cells: **principal cells** and **basal cells** (Figs 20.14,20.15). The principal cells are very tall in the first part of the duct, but decrease in height along its length, becoming cuboidal at its lower end. Each cell has a tuft of very long microvilli on its free surface (Fig.20.15), which because they are as long as cilia but immobile, they are commonly called **stereocilia**. There are numerous shallow invaginations of the membrane between stereocilia, and many vesicles and multivesicular bodies in the apical cytoplasm, indicating that the cells take up fluid from the lumen by pinocytosis. Ninety percent of the volume of fluid leaving the testis is absorbed in the ductuli efferentes and epididymis.

The nucleus of the principal cells, in the lower third of the cytoplasm, is highly irregular in outline. The supranuclear Golgi complex is exceptionally large. There is no visual evidence of its involvement in concentration of a secretory product. However, it has been established that these cells do incorporate amino acids and carbohydrate into a glycoprotein that is released into the lumen and is believed to influence sperm maturation. Large granules throughout the cytoplasm were formerly considered to

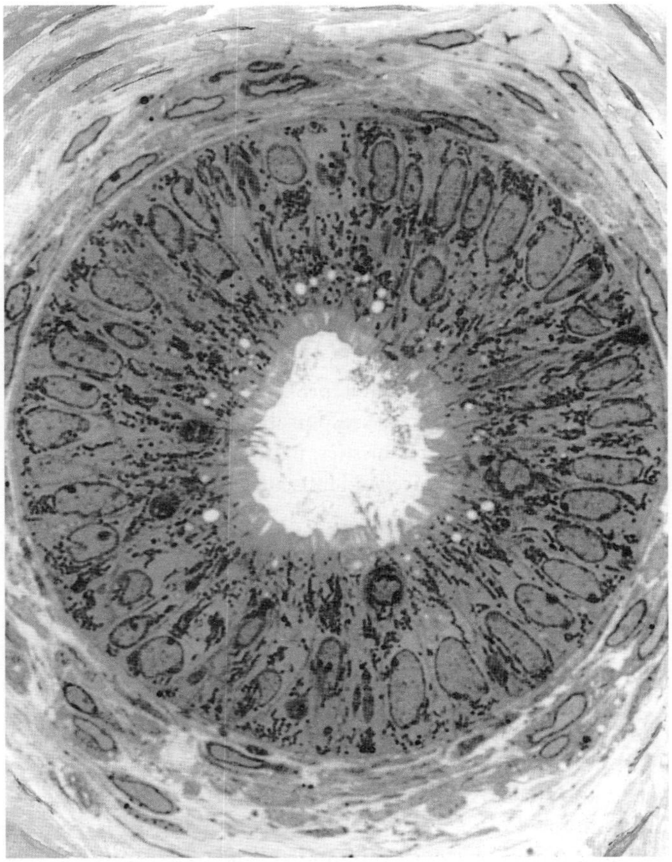

Figure 20.13 Cross-section of a ductulus efferens, showing its columnar epithelium with a prominent brush border and groups of ciliated cells. (Courtesy of A. Hoffer.)

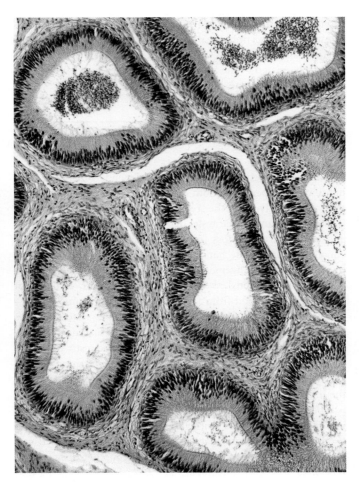

Figure 20.14 Photomicrograph of the cross-sections of the highly convoluted ductus epididymidis lined with pseudostratified columnar epithelium. Notice, at the top of the figure, masses of spermatozoa in the lumen.

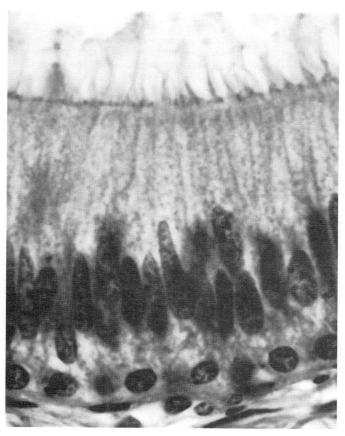

Figure 20.15 Photomicrograph of epididymal epithelium. Notice the two rows of cell nuclei, and the long stereocilia projecting into the lumen.

be secretory granules, but these have now been identified as lysosomes. The small rounded, or pyramidal, basal cells resemble the stem cells of renewing epithelia, but there is no evidence that they have such a role in this epithelium. Their function is unknown.

Ductus deferens

In the transition from the ductus epididymidis to the **ductus deferens** (**vas deferens**), the lumen widens and the wall thickens. The pseudostratified epithelium and its lamina propria form longitudinal folds that give the lumen an irregular cross-sectional outline. The surrounding muscular coat is about 1 mm in thickness and consists of inner and outer longitudinal layers separated by a middle layer of circular smooth muscle. The ductus deferens ascends to the pelvis in the **spermatic cord**, which contains the testicular artery, nerves, and the pampiniform plexus of veins. In the pelvis it expands into a fusiform **ampulla**, in which the mucosa has highly branched folds. Out-pocketings between the folds extend a short distance into the muscularis and are lined by pale-staining low-columnar secretory cells. The tapering distal portion of the ampulla is joined by the duct of the seminal vesicle. The confluence of the two ducti deferentes forms the **ejaculatory duct**, a tube nearly 2 cm long that opens into the prostatic urethra. The mucosa of the ejaculatory ducts forms short folds projecting into the

lumen. These are covered by a simple columnar epithelium, but near their termination the epithelium becomes stratified and resembles the transitional epithelium that lines the bladder and urethra.

ACCESSORY GLANDS

Seminal vesicles

The seminal vesicles are a pair of glands about 5 cm long situated behind the neck of the urinary bladder and lateral to the ampulla of the ductus deferens. They have an external layer of connective tissue, investing a muscularis that is thinner than that of the ductus deferens and consists of outer longitudinal and inner circular smooth muscle. Each vesicle is a convoluted tube with numerous diverticula along its length that result in a lumen of labyrinthine complexity (Fig. 20.16). Thin folds of the mucosa branch into secondary and tertiary folds that bound narrow compartments. These open into a wider central portion of the lumen that is lined by pseudostratified epithelium. The cells have sparse microvilli and some have a single cilium. They

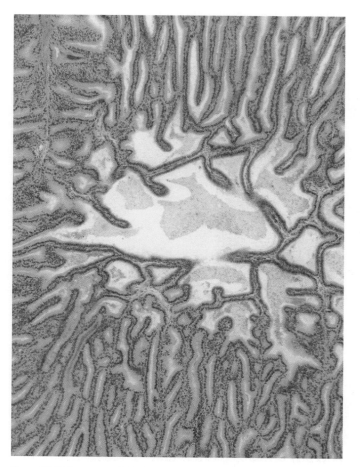

Figure 20.16 Low-power photomicrograph of the many elaborately branching tubules of secretory cells around the lumen of a seminal vesicle.

have a well-developed rER and abundant secretory granules that resemble those of goblet cells. The secretion of the seminal vesicles, discharged at orgasm, makes up a large fraction of the volume of the ejaculate. It contains fructose, which serves as an energy source for the spermatozoa.

Prostate gland

The prostate is the largest of the accessory glands of the male reproductive tract. It surrounds the urethra at its origin from the urinary bladder. It has a fibrous capsule, from which fibroelastic septa extend deep into the gland. Its parenchyma consists of 30 or more highly branched tubuloalveolar glands. Their ducts empty separately into the prostatic urethra. The epithelium is simple columnar, but may be cuboidal in the cystic dilatations of the glands (Fig.20.17A). The cells have abundant granular endoplasmic reticulum, a large Golgi complex, and numerous secretory granules. In older individuals, ovoid dense bodies of glycoprotein, called **corpora amylacea (prostatic concretions)**, are often found in the lumen of the glands (Fig.20.17B). Their significance is not known. The abundant stroma of the prostate contains smooth muscle cells that contract during ejaculation, adding its secretory product to the semen. The prostatic secretion contains **acid phosphatase**, **amylase**, and **fibrinolysin**. It appears to promote sperm motility.

For reasons that are not understood, the cells of the prostate begin to proliferate in men over 45 years, leading to **prostatic hyperplasia**. New nodules of hyperplastic glandular tissue project into the prostatic urethra, narrowing its lumen. This causes difficulty in starting to urinate, dribbling after voiding and incomplete emptying of the bladder. Eighty percent of men in their seventies have this condition. It is treated surgically by transurethral prostatectomy. The third commonest cancer of men over 45 years of age is **adenocarcinoma of the prostate** which is treated by radical prostatectomy, radiation and chemotherapy.

Bulbourethral glands

The paired **bulbourethral glands (Cowper's glands)** are distal to the prostate and partially embedded in the muscle of the urogenital diaphragm. They are compound tubuloalveolar glands less than 1 cm in diameter, each opening via a single duct into the beginning of the penile urethra. The capsule and the septa within the gland contain both smooth and striated muscle. The nuclei of the cuboidal epithelium are irregular in outline and displaced to the cell base by large numbers of secretory granules. The ducts are lined by epithelium resembling that of the urethra. The secretion contains galactose, galactose amine, and sialic acid. It is a clear viscous fluid that is thought to have a lubricating function. The bulbourethral glands are the first to be activated during sexual arousal, resulting in the appearance of droplets of clear fluid at the urethral meatus of the erect penis.

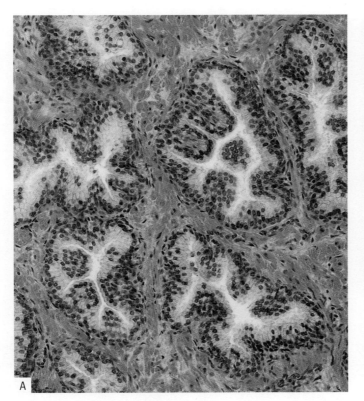

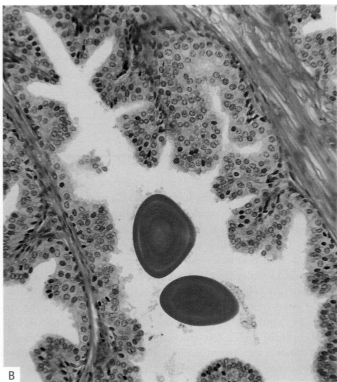

Figure 20.17 (A) Photomicrograph of a section of the prostate gland. Notice the large amount of stroma between the secretory elements of the gland. In addition to abundant collagen fibers, it contains numerous smooth muscle cells that contract to expel the secretion into the prostatic urethra. (B) A view at higher magnification to show two corpora amylacea in the lumen of one of the tubuloalveolar secretory units of the gland.

PENIS

The penis is made up of three cylindrical bodies of erectile tissue: two **corpora cavernosa** dorsally, and a single **corpus spongiosum** ventrally (Fig. 20.18B). The corpus spongiosum is expanded at its distal end into the acorn-shaped **glans penis**, which forms a cap over the ends of the two corpora cavernosa. The glans is covered with a fold of skin, the **prepuce** or **foreskin**. The penile urethra runs through the center of the corpus spongiosum for its entire length. In the shaft of the penis, the three corpora are enclosed in a thick connective-tissue sheath called the tunica albuginea, which also forms a partition between the two corpora cavernosa. The tunica is separated from the skin by a layer of loose connective tissue.

The erectile tissue of the corpora is a sponge-like mass of endothelium-lined vascular spaces that are fed by **afferent arteries** and drained by **efferent veins**. Dense fibrous trabeculae, containing smooth muscle cells, extend inwards from the tunica albuginea, branching and rejoining to form an elaborate framework around the vascular spaces. A **central artery** in each corpus gives off multiple **helicine arteries** that course in the trabeculae and open into the vascular spaces. These are drained by a number of veins on the inner aspect of the tunica albuginea that penetrate the tunica to join branches of the **deep dorsal vein** of the penis. In the flaccid state, the vascular spaces contain little blood and appear as narrow clefts.

Histophysiology of the penis

Erection of the penis is under control of the brain and autonomic nervous system. In the non-aroused state, the autonomic nervous system controlling the diameter of the penile arteries actively limits the amount of blood flowing to the penis. A state of arousal triggers stimuli from the brain that cause release of neurotransmitters (nitric oxide or acetylcholine) from the nerves to the blood vessels of the penis. These relax the smooth muscle in the wall of the penile arteries, permitting more blood to flow into the endothelial-lined chambers of the corpus spongiosa. Their filling compresses the veins that normally drain blood from the penis, resulting in stiffening and erection of the penis. After orgasm, the sympathetic nervous system again restricts flow of blood into the penis and it becomes flaccid (Fig. 20.18). During the dreaming phase of sleep, the nucleus coeruleus of the brain inhibits the sympathetic neurons, resulting in nocturnal erections in the absence of sexual arousal.

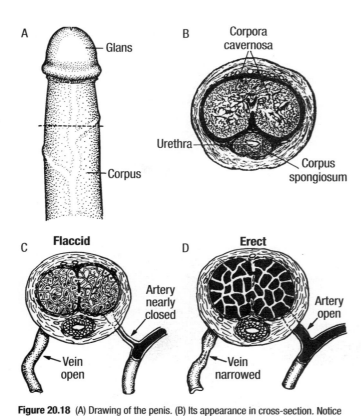

Figure 20.18 (A) Drawing of the penis. (B) Its appearance in cross-section. Notice the two corpora cavernosa and the corpus spongiosum around the urethra. (C) Cross-section of the flaccid penis showing its partially occluded artery. (D) Cross-section of the erect penis with the artery open and the vascular spaces of the corpora cavernosa distended with blood.

Erectile dysfunction is a consistent inability to acquire and maintain an erection that is adequate for sexual intercourse. It may be caused by anxiety, depression, neurological diseases, vascular problems, drugs, and some medications prescribed for other complaints. It may also be caused by accidental surgical interruption of nerves during prostatectomy. Some degree of erectile dysfunction affects 40% of men over 40 years, and 70% of men over 70 years. In some cases it can be temporarily corrected by an oral medication, sildenafil citrate (Viagra).

Questions

1   Fluid particularly rich in fructose is secreted by which one of the following?

   a   seminal vesicle

   b   prostate

   c   testis

   d   Cowper's glands

   e   epididymis

2   Which statement best describes spermiation?

   a   it refers to the release of spermatozoa from the seminiferous epithelium

   b   it is a term for the cycle of the seminiferous epithelium

   c   it is another term for ejaculation

   d   it refers to the release of spermatozoa from the epididymis

   e   it is another term for fertilization

3   Concretions are often found in which one of the following?

   a   epididymis

   b   seminal gland

   c   prostate

   d   ampullar region of the vas deferens

   e   rete testis

4   Which statement is true of the epididymis?

   a   it is the site of capacitation

   b   it is lined by low columnar cells with motile cilia

   c   it has an unusually thick (and, therefore, characteristic) muscular wall

   d   it connects directly with the seminiferous tubules

   e   it is the site where spermatozoa become motile

5   The largest stereocilia occur in which one of the following?

   a   efferent ductules

   b   epididymis

   c   vas deferens

   d   ampulla (of the vas deferens)

   e   penile urethra

6   Inhibin is produced by

   a   Leydig cells

   b   Sertoli cells

   c   spermatogonia

   d   epididymal epithelial cells

   e   primary spermatocytes

7   The final steps of maturation of the spermatozoon take place in the

   a   ampulla of the oviduct

   b   uterus

   c   epididymis

   d   rete testis

   e   seminiferous tubules

8   Which hormone(s) is (are) primarily and directly responsible for secondary sex characteristics?

   a   FSH

   b   LH

   c   aldosterone

   d   testosterone

   e   LH and FSH

9   The ejaculatory duct is formed

   a   as a result of thickening of the prostatic urethra

   b   by the progressive thickening of the ductus deferens

   c   by the joining of the ductus deferens and the seminal vesicle ducts

   d   when the penile urethra and ductus deferens meet

   e   as the ducts from Cowper's gland join the urethra

10   Helicine arteries are located in the

   a   prostate

   b   seminal vesicle

   c   testes

   d   Cowper's gland

   e   penis

11   What structure drains the seminal vesicles and the ductus deferens?

12   What is the name for the process by which spermatozoa are released from the seminiferous epithelium?

13   The penile urethra is located within what structure of the penis?

14   Fibrolysin is produced by what gland?

15   What is the name of the cell that acts in a supportive capacity for the spermatogenic series?

16   What structure is known for its uniquely thick muscular wall relative to its lumen?

17   What type of epithelial cell lines the epididymis?

18   What does the Leydig cell secrete?

19   What gland secretes the acid phosphatase found in the ejaculate?

20   The midpiece of the spermatozoa contains the axoneme and which other organelle?

Chapter twenty-one

Female Reproductive System

The principal organs of the female reproductive system are the ovaries, the oviducts, the uterus, and the vagina. The uterus and ovaries arise early in embryonic life, but their development is not completed until gonadotrophic hormones of the anterior lobe of the hypophysis initiate puberty. In the female, puberty involves widespread changes in the body, including increased muscle mass, an increase in adipose tissue over the hips and buttocks, development of breasts, appearance of axillary and pubic hair, and activation of the ovaries and uterus. Maturation of these organs is followed by the first menstrual flow, **menarche**, at about 13 years of age. Thereafter, the ovaries and uterus undergo a regular sequence of changes every 28 days called the menstrual cycle. These cycles continue until the onset of **menopause**, at about age 50 years, when they become irregular, and within a few years, menstruation ceases. Around the middle of each cycle, a single ovum is released from one of the ovaries and passes into the oviduct, where it may, or may not, encounter a spermatozoon for its fertilization. The survival of the species is insured by the unusually long reproductive life of the human female. Over this 35 years or more, as many as 400 ova may become available for fertilization, and 30 pregnancies are, theoretically, possible. Fortunately, there are occasional anovulatory cycles and only a few of the many ova released from the ovary are fertilized.

OVARY

Each ovary is a slightly flattened organ, 3 cm in length, 1.5 cm in width and 1 cm in thickness, suspended from the broad ligament

of the uterus in a fold of peritoneum called the **mesovarium** (Fig. 21.1). At the junction of the mesovarium with the ovary, there is a transition from flat squamous mesothelium to a low cuboidal **germinal epithelium** covering the ovary. Its basal lamina rests upon a pale-staining layer of connective tissue called the **tunica albuginea**. Beneath this is the cortex of the ovary, which contains many large germ cells called **oocytes**. Deeper in the cortex are oocytes that are enveloped by one or more layers of smaller cells to form **ovarian follicles** (Fig. 21.2). These are in different stages of development and vary greatly in size. Deep to the cortex is the medulla, the connective tissue core of the ovary, made up of collagen fibers, fibroblasts, occasional smooth muscle cells, and numerous tortuous arteries and veins, from which branches radiate into the cortex. The cortex and medulla grade into one another without a clear line of demarcation.

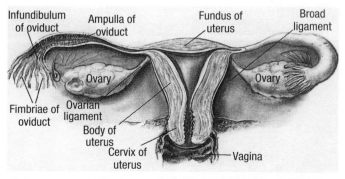

Figure 21.1 Drawing of the female reproductive organs. The vagina, uterus and one oviduct have been hemisected to show the shape of their lumen and the thickness of their wall.

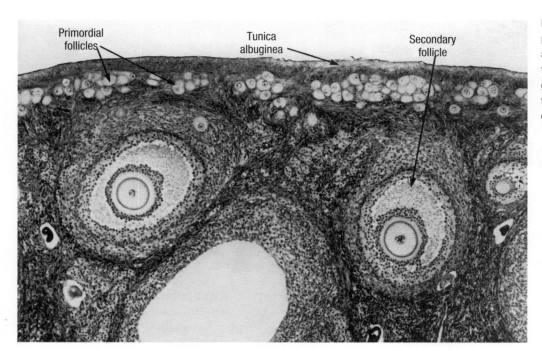

Figure 21.2 Photomicrograph of a portion of an ovary, showing the tunica albuginea, and numerous primordial follicles immediately beneath the germinal epithelium, and two secondary follicles deeper in the cortex of the organ.

Oocytes

Oocytes arise in the early embryo from precursors called **oogonia** (primordial germ cells), which first appear in the yolk sac and later migrate into the germinal ridge, from which the ovaries develop. There they proliferate by mitotic division until they number in the millions. They then enter prophase of the first meiotic division, but proceed no further. At this stage they are called **primary oocytes** (Fig. 21.2). Although great numbers of these later undergo atresia (degeneration), both before and after birth, as many as 400 000 are present in the ovaries of a young woman, where they form a conspicuous layer immediately beneath the tunica albuginea (Fig. 21.2).

In the postnatal ovary, the primary oocytes are large, spherical cells, about 25 μm in diameter, each enveloped by a single layer of squamous epithelial cells. An oocyte and its cellular investment constitute a **primordial follicle** (Fig. 21.3A). The nucleus of the oocyte has a prominent nucleolus, and, by the use of appropriate stains, the meiotic chromosomes can be seen as thin meandering threads in the nucleoplasm. A large number of mitochondria are aggregated near the nucleus. There is a small Golgi complex and the endoplasmic reticulum is represented by tubular profiles with relatively few associated ribosomes.

Development of follicles

In the years approaching puberty, some of the primordial follicles undergo further development to become **primary follicles**, in which the oocyte is surrounded by two or more layers of cuboidal cells (Fig. 21.3B). In each menstrual cycle after puberty, several primary follicles enter a phase of rapid growth, with further enlargement of the oocyte and proliferation of the surrounding follicular cells, now called **granulosa cells**. Proliferation of the granulosa cells results in a rapid increase in diameter of the follicle (Fig. 21.4). Glycoprotein is secreted into the space between the oocyte and the innermost granulosa cells and condenses to form a highly refractile layer, called the **zona pellucida** (Figs 21.4, 21.5, 21.6). The granulosa cells and the oocyte are in communication via gap junctions between filiform processes that extend from each into the zona pellucida.

Small fluid-filled spaces appear among the proliferating granulosa cells, and when the growing follicle reaches a diameter of

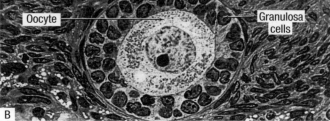

Figure 21.3 Photomicrograph of early stages of follicular development. (A) A primordial follicle. (B) A primary follicle with two rows of granulosa cells.

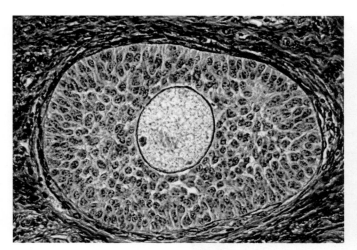

Figure 21.4 A more advanced primary follicle in which the granulosa cells have greatly increased in number and a zona pellucida is beginning to form around the oocyte.

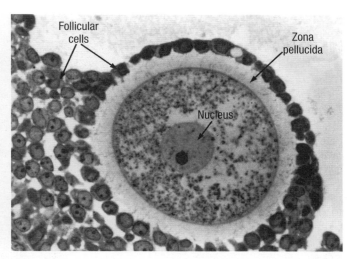

Figure 21.6 Photomicrograph of a human oocyte in a secondary follicle. The surface of the surrounding zona pellucida is now covered by a single layer of granulosa cells on the side projecting into the antrum. (Micrograph courtesy of L. Zamboni.)

about 200 μm, these spaces coalesce to form the **antrum**, a single, fluid-filled cavity that displaces the oocyte to one side. The oocyte is located in the **cumulus oophorus**, a thickening of the granulosa cell layer that projects into the antrum. At this stage of development the follicle is called an **antral** or **secondary follicle** (Fig. 21.5). The clear **liquor folliculi** within the antrum is a transudate of blood plasma, but it contains a much higher concentration of steroids and gonadotrophic hormones.

While these events are occurring within the follicle, stromal cells gather around it to form a highly cellular layer with ill-defined outer limits, called the **theca folliculi**. This layer is separated from the granulosa cells by a thick basal lamina. As development progresses, two zones become distinguishable in the theca, a richly vascularized **theca interna** and a less vascular **theca externa**. In their differentiation, the cells of the theca interna acquire an extensive smooth endoplasmic reticulum (sER) and other characteristics of steroid-secreting cells. They synthesize

androgenic steroids that diffuse into the follicle and are converted to **estradiol** by the granulosa cells. The fibroblast-like cells of the theca externa do not synthesize steroids.

The ovary of a woman of reproductive age contains a very large reserve of primordial follicles, many quiescent primary follicles, and five or six developing antral follicles. In each menstrual cycle, one member of the cohort of follicles that has reached the antral stage becomes dominant and continues to enlarge. Continuing its growth and accumulation of liquor folliculi, the dominant follicle attains a diameter of up to 20 mm and bulges from the surface of the ovary. The other members of the cohort of antral follicles undergo **follicular atresia**, a normal process of regression and ultimate degeneration. Of the hundreds of thousands of primordial and primary follicles in the ovary of a young woman, fewer than 500 will complete their maturation and release an ovum during her reproductive lifespan.

At mid-cycle (days 13–14) the dominant follicle, now 15–20 mm in diameter, bulges 1 cm or more above the surface of the ovary. At this stage of follicular development, the oocyte that began meiotic division during embryonic life, but was arrested in prophase, resumes division. The nucleus moves near the oolemma and the chromosomes assemble on the metaphase plate of a spindle, oriented tangentially to the cell surface. The spindle then rotates 90° and at anaphase, a small rounded mass of protoplasm around its outer pole projects above the surface of the oocyte. Telophase of this division results in two daughter cells of vastly unequal size: a tiny spherical cell with little cytoplasm, called the **first polar body**, and the huge **secondary oocyte**, which proceeds quickly to metaphase of the second meiotic division (Fig. 21.7), where it is again arrested. While these events are occurring, fluid-filled spaces appear among the granulosa cells at the base of the cumulus oophorus and their coalescence results in detachment of the oocyte. The oocyte then floats free in the liquor folliculi, with a few granulosa cells still adhering to its zona pellucida.

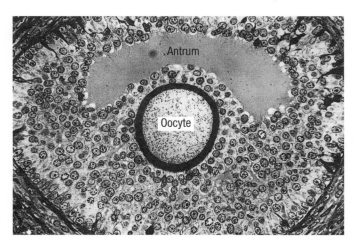

Figure 21.5 A secondary follicle in which the oocyte and surrounding granulosa cells are beginning to form a cumulus oophorus projecting into a fluid-filled cavity called the antrum.

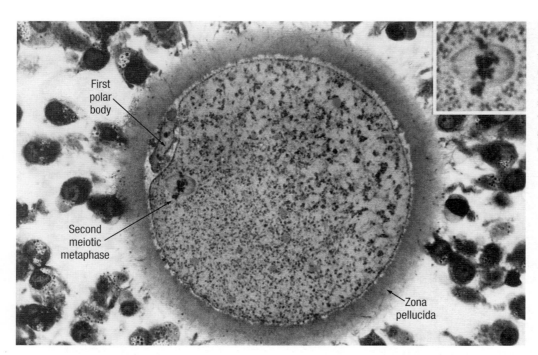

Figure 21.7 Photomicrograph of a human oocyte at the completion of the first meiotic division. The first polar body can be seen between the oocyte and the zona pellucida. The chromosomes and spindle of the second meiotic division are visible in the cytoplasm. These are seen at higher magnification in the inset. (Micrograph courtesy of L. Zamboni.)

Ovulation

Ovulation is the release of an ovum from the ovary. It has been observed directly in anesthetized animals and humans. A pale, translucent, oval area, called the **stigma** or **macula pellucida**, appears on the bulging surface of the mature follicle. Its blanching is the result of local cessation of blood flow in the capillaries of the theca interna. This is followed by a further thinning of the theca and the overlying tunica albuginea. The thinning is believed to result from a rearrangement of the cells and enzymatic digestion of the collagen fibrils of the theca and tunica albuginea. Through this thin area, a small translucent vesicle then bulges outwards. Within a minute or two of its formation, it ruptures and the ovum and adherent cumulus cells pass through the opening, followed by a gush of follicular fluid. The ovum then passes into the oviduct for transport to the uterus.

Corpus luteum

After ovulation, the wall of the follicle collapses and becomes extensively infolded. Blood vessels and stromal cells invade the previously avascular layer of granulosa cells. The granulosa cells, and those of the theca interna, then hypertrophy (enlarge). They develop smooth reticulum, accumulate lipid droplets, and become plump, pale-staining **lutein cells** that form clusters surrounded by a minimal amount of connective tissue. By these changes, the follicle is transformed into a more-or-less spherical **corpus luteum**.

In the corpus luteum of the human ovary, two kinds of lutein cells are distinguishable. Those arising from the granulosa cells are called **granulosa lutein cells**, while smaller, more deeply staining

cells, arising from cells of the theca interna are **theca lutein cells**. Both types of lutein cells have an abundance of sER, mitochondria with tubular cristae, and lipid droplets in their cytoplasm; characteristics typical of steroid-secreting cells (Fig. 21.8). Despite their similar ultrastructure, the two types of lutein cells have different functions. The principal steroid secreted by the granulosa lutein cells is **progesterone**, whereas the theca lutein cells secrete mainly **estradiol** and **estrone**.

In a cycle in which the ovum is not fertilized, the corpus luteum regresses within about 9 days. Its lutein cells undergo apoptosis, and invading macrophages phagocytize and digest their residues. Degeneration of the corpus luteum results in decreased hormone production. This causes increased production of follicle-stimulating hormone (FSH) by the hypophysis and this initiates further development of another follicle for the next cycle. A pale-staining fibrous scar, at the site of the corpus luteum, called a **corpus albicans**, persists for several months. The sequence of events in the ovary, during a cycle in which the ovum is not fertilized is reviewed in Fig. 21.9.

In a cycle in which the ovum is fertilized and successfully implanted in the uterus, the corpus luteum persists and grows further under the influence of **gonadotrophic hormones** secreted by the placenta of the developing embryo. For the first 2 months of pregnancy, the hypertrophied corpus luteum is the major source of the steroid hormones needed to maintain pregnancy.

Histophysiology of the ovary

The cyclic activity of the ovary is dependent on two gonadotrophic hormones of the hypophysis: **follicle-stimulating hormone (FSH)** and **luteinizing hormone (LH)**. Formation of primary follicles appears to be independent of hormones, but their further development to antral follicles, and beyond,

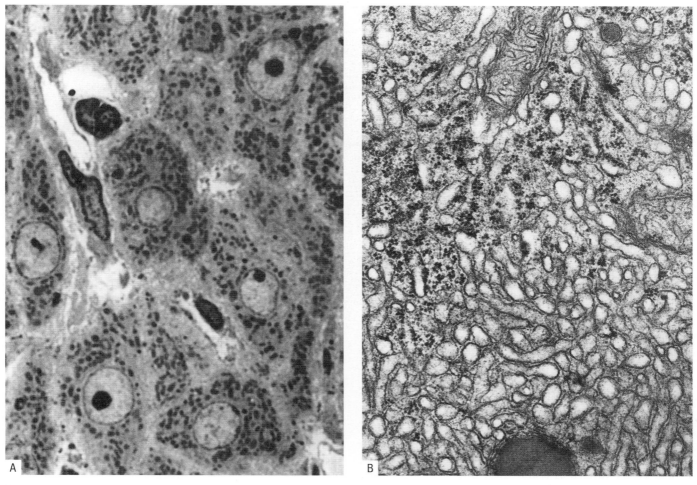

Figure 21.8 (A) Photomicrograph of cells of a corpus luteum. Note their euchromatic nucleus and large number of mitochondria. (B) Electron micrograph of a small area of cytoplasm showing their abundant smooth endoplasmic reticulum.

requires FSH, which stimulates proliferation of granulosa cells and activates an enzyme that is essential for steroid synthesis. Cells of the theca interna secrete androgenic steroid precursors

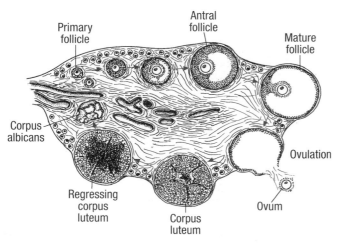

Figure 21.9 A diagram of the ovary illustrating the successive stages in the development of a follicle and the corpus luteum in a cycle in which the ovum is not fertilized.

that diffuse into the follicle, where the granulosa cells convert them to estradiol. Proliferation of granulosa cells and their synthesis of an increasing amount of estradiol, raises the concentration of this hormone in the blood. These increased levels, in turn, act upon the hypothalamus and hypophysis, stimulating a mid-cycle surge of LH that induces ovulation. Thereafter, the granulosa cells reduce their production of estradiol and secrete increasing amounts of progesterone, the hormone that prepares the uterine mucosa for reception of the ovum. The elevated level of LH triggering ovulation is also responsible for the transformation of the postovulatory follicle into a corpus luteum.

THE OVIDUCTS

The **oviducts** are two tubes, about 12 cm in length, extending laterally from the uterus, in the upper border of the broad ligament (Fig. 21.10). The oviduct receives the ovum, provides an appropriate environment for its fertilization, and transports it to the uterus. Four regions of the oviduct are distinguished. The

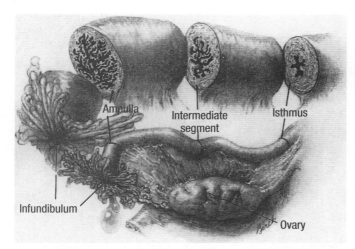

Figure 21.10 Drawing of the ovary and oviduct, and above, an oviduct transected at successive levels to show the pattern of mucosal folds in its interior. (Reproduced from M.J. Eastman and H. Hellman (eds) *William's Obstetrics* 13th edn, Appleton, Century and Crofts, New York, 1961. Labeling added.)

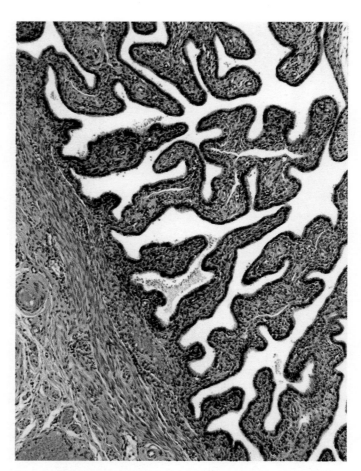

Figure 21.11 Photomicrograph of the elaborately branched folds, or folia, of the mucosa projecting into the interior of the oviduct.

portion traversing the wall of the uterus is its **interstitial segment**. The slender medial third is the **isthmus**. Lateral to this, it expands slightly to form the **ampulla**, and this is continuous with the funnel-shaped **infundibulum**, which opens into the peritoneal cavity near the lateral pole of the ovary. Radiating from the opening (osteum) of the infundibulum are numerous slender tapering processes, called the **fimbriae** of the oviduct (Fig. 21.10).

The wall of the oviduct consists of a moderately thick layer of smooth muscle covered by a thin serosa of mesothelium. In its interior, the mucosa forms long, branching longitudinal folds that project into its lumen. In the four segments of the oviduct, these vary in their length and degree of branching. In the interstitial segment and isthmus, they are simply low ridges. Farther laterally, they increase in length and number, and in the ampulla they become elaborately branched thin folia (leaflike structures). In cross-sections at this level, the lumen is a labyrinthine system of narrow spaces between the numerous branching folia (Fig. 21.11).

The oviduct is lined by a simple columnar epithelium. Its cells are tall in the infundibulum and ampulla, but gradually decrease in height towards the uterus. They are of two types: ciliated and nonciliated (Fig. 21.12). Their relative numbers, and activity, are influenced by the level of circulating estrogens. Early in the **follicular phase** of the cycle, the cells become taller and begin to form cilia. In the **preovulatory phase**, the mean percentage of ciliated cells on the fimbriae is 48%, but it declines to about 4% in the late **luteal phase**. Cyclic changes are also evident in the non-ciliated cells, which show evidence of increased synthetic activity, reaching a peak at mid-cycle and declining thereafter.

The beating of cilia on the fimbriae creates currents in the overlying film of fluid that move the fertilized ovum into the infundibulum of the oviduct, and the cilia of the ampulla and isthmus contribute to its transport to the uterus. The function of the non-ciliated cells is less well understood. Although the nature of their secretion is not known, it probably creates an intralumenal environment that sustains the motility of the spermatozoa and enables them to undergo **capacitation**, a series of biochemical changes that enables them to fertilize the ovum. The environment must also enable the fertilized ovum to develop to the multicellular blastocyst stage during its passage down the oviduct.

The muscularis of the oviducts was traditionally described as consisting of concentric layers of longitudinal and circular smooth muscle. Scanning micrographs of oviducts subjected to maceration and ultrasonic bombardment, have now shown this interpretation to be erroneous. There are no distinct layers. In the ampulla and infundibulum, the smooth muscle cells form a loose network of bundles oriented in many directions. Towards the isthmus, longitudinally oriented smooth muscle bundles predominate. *In vivo* observations have shown that, in midcycle, contraction of smooth muscle in the infundibulum brings the ostium of the oviduct into contact with the ovary and the fimbriae sweep over its surface, facilitating entry of the ovum into the oviduct. It has previously been assumed that rhythmic waves of contraction (peristalsis) moving along the oviduct towards the isthmus contribute to transport of the ovum to the uterus. In view of the absence of concentric layers of consistently oriented smooth muscle, this interpretation now seems less likely.

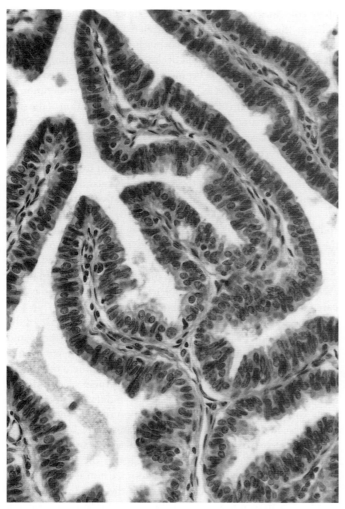

Figure 21.12 Photomicrograph of one of the folds of the mucosa in the oviduct showing its ciliated columnar epithelium.

UTERUS

The human **uterus** is a pear-shaped organ with a thick muscular wall. It is about 7 cm long, 4 cm wide at its upper end, and 2.5 cm in depth (Fig. 21.1). It is slightly flattened anteroposteriorly and is normally tipped forward. Its rounded upper portion is referred to as the **fundus**, and its wide upper two-thirds is its body, or **corpus**. A narrower portion below this is the **isthmus**, and a cylindrical lower segment is the **cervix** (Fig. 21.1). The lower end of the cervix that projects into the vagina is its **portio vaginalis**. The flattened uterine cavity is triangular in outline and is continuous with the lumen of the initial segment of the oviducts on either side of the fundus. At its narrow lower end, the lumen is continuous with the **cervical canal**, which opens into the vagina.

Myometrium

The muscle of the uterine wall, called the **myometrium**, is 1.25 cm thick and is made up of interlacing bundles of smooth muscle

separated by connective tissue. Four indistinctly defined layers can be distinguished. In the two innermost layers, the orientation of the smooth muscle is mainly longitudinal. The next layer is less compact and contains numerous blood vessels. Peripheral to this is a layer in which circularly oriented fibers predominate, and in the thin outermost layer, they are again longitudinal. The two outermost layers are continuous with the muscularis of the oviducts. Smooth muscle decreases and connective tissue increases in the isthmus of the uterus, and the cervix consists almost exclusively of dense connective tissue containing many elastic fibers. During pregnancy, considerable enlargement of the uterus is required to accommodate the growing fetus. This is accomplished by hypertrophy of the existing smooth muscle cells and addition of new cells. There is also an increase in the collagen content of the uterine wall. After pregnancy, these changes are reversed by a decrease in the size and number of smooth muscle cells.

The cervix surrounds a **cervical canal** about 3 cm in length that is continuous above with the uterine lumen, through a constriction called the **internal os**. It is continuous below with the vagina, through a narrow opening called the **external os**. The canal is lined by tall columnar epithelial cells with nuclei displaced to the base by mucous droplets that occupy much of the cytoplasm. Highly branched **cervical glands**, extending into the submucosa, are lined by a similar epithelium. The mucus secreted by these glands contains the enzyme lysozyme. It cleaves the proteoglycans of bacterial cell walls and is believed to be important in the defense against the bacterial flora of the lower reproductive tract. Near the external os, there is an abrupt transition from simple columnar epithelium to stratified squamous epithelium, which covers the portion of the cervix that projects into the vagina. The wall of the cervix contains few smooth muscle cells and is composed mainly of dense connective tissue. Late in pregnancy, changes in its fibrous and amorphous components make the cervix softer and more pliable, facilitating its dilatation by the advancing head of the fetus.

Leiomyoma uteri (or fibroid tumor) is the most common tumor of women. It is a benign tumor derived from smooth muscle of the myometrium. There is often more than one in the wall of the uterus and, when small, they may be without symptoms and may go undetected for years. Larger tumors may cause pain and disturbances of the menstrual cycle, with bleeding between periods. Treatment is by hysterectomy (surgical removal of the uterus).

Endometrium

Endometrium is the term applied to the mucosa lining the uterine cavity. It consists of a simple columnar epithelium containing ciliated cells and cells with microvilli only (Fig. 23–13). Tubular glands extend downwards into a very thick lamina propria, commonly referred to as the **endometrial stroma**. From puberty until menopause, the endometrium undergoes monthly cyclic changes in its thickness and histological appearance, in response to fluctuating levels of ovarian hormones. At the end of a cycle in which no ovum is fertilized, the greater part of its thickness sloughs off,

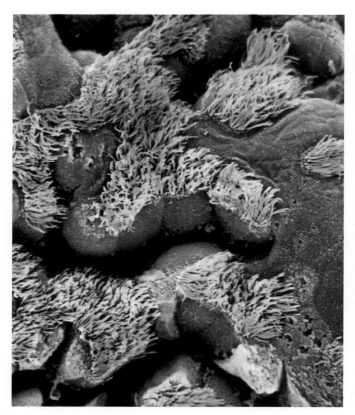

Figure 21.13 Scanning electron micrograph of the surface epithelium of the endometrium. (Color added: blue, cilia; yellow, microvilli.) The dark areas between groups of ciliated cells are the openings of endometrial glands. (Micrograph courtesy of Professor P. Motta, University of Rome La Sapienza.)

accompanied by extravasation of blood from the vessels of its stroma. The products of these degenerative changes appear as a bloody vaginal discharge, the **menstrual flow**, that continues for 3–5 days.

Two zones of the endometrium are distinguished. The upper half to two-thirds portion, which will be sloughed off at the next menstrual flow, is called the **functionalis**, whereas the deeper portion, which persists and regenerates the functionalis in the next cycle, is called the **basalis**. To understand the changes occurring in menstruation, some knowledge of the blood supply is needed. The uterine arteries course longitudinally in the broad ligament along the sides of the uterus. Branches penetrate to the vascular layer of the myometrium. Their branches, called **arcuate arteries**, take a circumferential course to the midline, where they anastomose with arcuate arteries from the other side. Penetrating branches of the arcuate arteries, called the **straight arteries**, give off lateral branches that supply the basalis of the endometrium and continue as **coiled** or **spiral arteries** that supply the functionalis. Late in the menstrual cycle, there is a vasoconstriction of the coiled arteries that leads to the necrotic changes in the endometrium culminating in menstruation.

Cyclic changes of the endometrium

For descriptive purposes, the menstrual cycle is divided into **proliferative**, **secretory**, and **menstrual phases**. The proliferative

phase coincides with the secretion of estrogens by the developing follicles; the secretory phase is correlated with the secretion of progesterone by the functional corpus luteum; and the menstrual phase is associated with a rapid decline in hormonal stimulation.

The **proliferative phase** begins at the end of the menstrual flow, on about day 5 of the cycle, and extends to day 14. Proliferation of cells in the epithelium of the basalis results in restoration of the surface epithelium and a progressive lengthening of the endometrial glands. This is accompanied by active proliferation of the stromal cells. These regenerative changes in the first 2 weeks of an ideal 28-day cycle, result in growth of the endometrium from a postmenstrual thickness of 0.5 mm to 2–3 mm. The glands are lined by columnar epithelium and are, initially, relatively straight. Later, they become more sinuous (Fig. 21.14A,B) and their columnar epithelial cells accumulate glycogen, displacing the nucleus towards the apex. Concurrent with these changes, the coiled portions of the branches of the arcuate arteries that were lost during menses, regenerate and take on a spiral course as they lengthen. By day 14 of the cycle, the endometrium has completed its regeneration and is prepared for receipt of an implanting blastocyst.

In the **secretory phase**, extending from day 15 to day 28 of the cycle, the glands of the functionalis become more tortuous and acquire lateral sacculations that result in a larger lumen, which is irregular in outline (Fig. 21.14C). The glycogen content of the cells diminishes and the lumen contains a glycoprotein secretion. The glands in the basalis remain more slender and their walls are relatively straight. Elongation and convolution of the coiled arteries continues and the stroma becomes edematous.

In the **menstrual phase** of a cycle in which an ovum is not fertilized, marked vascular changes begin in the endometrium about 2 weeks after ovulation. The endometrium is blanched for hours at a time, owing to constriction of the coiled arteries. The glands cease to secrete and the stroma is invaded by large numbers of leukocytes. After about 2 days of intermittent interruption of blood flow, the vasoconstriction of the coiled arteries becomes continuous, depriving the functionalis of oxygenated blood, while blood flow to the basalis is uninterrupted. The ischemic (blood-deficient) functionalis begins to degenerate. Several hours later, the constricted arteries reopen, but the walls of their distal portions, now damaged by ischemia, rupture and blood escapes into the stroma and breaks out into the uterine lumen. This is followed by shedding of clumps of necrotic endometrium, and by day 3 or day 4 of menses, the entire functionalis of the endometrium has sloughed off. Blood loss is normally about 35 ml, but larger amounts are common. The basalis remains intact and soon begins to regenerate a new functionalis.

Endometriosis is a condition in which endometrial tissue occurs in sites outside of the uterus. Small plaques of endometrium may be present on an ovary, in the broad ligament of the uterus, or on the floor of the pelvis. Opinion is divided as to its cause. Some attribute it to reflux of bits of viable endometrium through the oviducts during menstruation and their implantation on various surfaces in the pelvis. Others believe the ectopic endometrium arises by local metaplasia of the mesothelium and its underlying stroma. The patients have abdominal pain and dysmenorrhea (painful menstruation). It is treated with some success with steroid hormones to suppress the cycling of the endometrium.

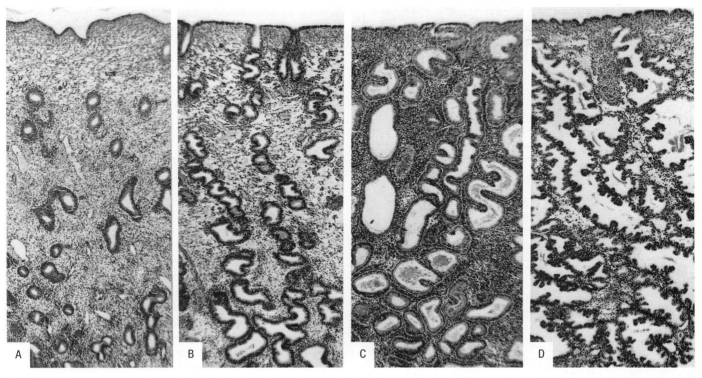

Figure 21.14 Photomicrographs of the endometrium in different stages of the menstrual cycle. (A) Proliferative phase (day 9). (B) Early secretory phase (day 15). (C) Late secretory phase (day 19). (D) Gestational endometrium. (Photomicrographs courtesy of A. Hertig.)

Histophysiology of the uterus

The interactions between the hypophysis, ovary, and endometrium are depicted in Fig. 21.15. The growth and maturation of ovarian follicles is controlled by secretion of FSH and LH by the hypophysis. A surge of secretion of these hormones in mid-cycle triggers ovulation (Fig. 21.15). The changes in the uterine endometrium are regulated by the ovarian hormones, estrogen and progesterone. After menstruation, increasing production of estrogen by granulosa cells of a developing follicle stimulates regeneration of the functionalis of the endometrium. A peaking of circulating estrogen shortly before mid-cycle acts upon the hypophysis to induce the mid-cycle surge of LH and FSH secretion. After the resulting ovulation, an increase in secretion of progesterone by the corpus luteum stimulates further changes in the endometrium, which prepare it for reception of a fertilized ovum. If the ovum is not fertilized, degeneration of the corpus luteum results in a precipitous drop in progesterone that triggers the vascular changes in the endometrium that culminate in menstruation (Fig. 21.15). On the other hand, if fertilization and implantation of an ovum do occur, chorionic gonadotrophins, hormones produced by cells of the developing placenta, result in maintenance of a functional corpus luteum, the so-called corpus luteum of pregnancy.

FERTILIZATION

While ovulation is in progress, the fimbria of the oviduct are motile and are sweeping over the surface of the ovary. Beating of cilia on their epithelium creates currents in the film of fluid on that surface, drawing the ovum into the oviduct, where spermatozoa await its arrival. The granulosa cells adhering to the ovum's **zona pellucida** are quickly dispersed, exposing its surface. The zona is composed of three glycoproteins that have been designated **ZP1**, **ZP2**, and **ZP3**. In its formation in the developing ovarian follicle, molecules of ZP2 and ZP3 copolymerize to form microfilaments that are cross-linked by molecules of ZP1 to form a firm meshwork within the zona. Certain oligosaccharides of ZP3 serve as sperm receptors. A specific protein in the plasmalemma of the sperm head binds to the receptors on the zona. This binding triggers the **acrosome reaction** of the spermatozoon (Fig. 21.16). This involves fusion of the acrosomal membrane with the overlying sperm plasmalemma at multiple sites, creating openings through which enzymes of the acrosome are released. These digest a channel through the zona pellucida, through which the vigorously motile spermatozoon enters the space between the zona and the plasmalemma of the ovum (the oolemma). The membrane on the postacrosomal region of the sperm head then fuses with the oolemma and the sperm nucleus enters the cytoplasm of the ovum, where its chromatin begins to decondense. Fusion of the membranes triggers the **cortical reaction** of the ovum. Thousands of **cortical granules** in its peripheral cytoplasm undergo exocytosis, releasing enzymes into the space beneath the zona pellucida (perivitelline space). These destroy the sperm-receptors of the zona pellucida, thus preventing the binding and entry of other spermatozoa.

Entry of the spermatozoon into the ovum initiates completion of its second meiotic division, with production of a second polar body. The spermatozoon contains an unusually high

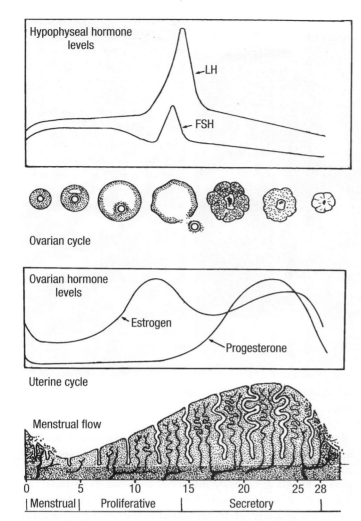

Figure 21.15 Diagram of the hormone levels and correlated morphological changes in the developing follicle in the ovary (above) and ovarian hormone levels, correlated with changes in the uterine endometrium (below). FSH, follicle-stimulating hormone; LH, luteinizing hormone.

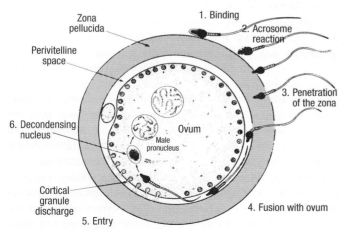

Figure 21.16 Diagram of the successive events in the fertilization of an ovum. (1) Binding of the sperm head to the zona pellucida. (2) Acrosome reaction of the spermatozoon. (3) Penetration of the zona. (4) Fusion with the oolemma, followed by decondensation of the nucleus in preparation for fusion with the oocyte nucleus.

amount of nitric oxide synthase. Upon contact and entry into the ovum, the sperm releases nitric oxide, which causes calcium release, thereby stimulating the ovum's nitric oxide synthase. More calcium is then released, triggering a cascade of chemical reactions that initiate division in the ovum. Completion of fertilization occurs by fusion of the decondensed sperm nucleus with the nucleus of the ovum, restoring the diploid chromosome number.

IMPLANTATION

As the fertilized ovum passes down the oviduct, it divides repeatedly, forming a small spherical mass of cells, called the **morula.** Upon reaching the lumen of the uterus on about day 4, it consists of many more cells, which have become arranged in a hollow sphere called the **blastocyst.** After a day or two in the lumen of the uterus, the blastocyst attaches to the surface of the secretory endometrium (Fig. 21.17A). At this stage, there is a cluster of cells at one pole of the blastocyst, called the **inner cell mass,** that is destined to form the embryo proper. The remainder of the sphere consists of **trophoblast cells** that actively invade the endometrium (Fig. 21.17A). Rapid proliferation of the trophoblast gives rise to an inner layer of **cytotrophoblast,** made up of separate cells, and an outer layer of **syncytiotrophoblast,** which is a multinucleate layer of protoplasm in which no cell boundaries are discernible. The cytotrophoblast is mitotically active and the newly formed cells fuse with, and are incorporated into, the surrounding syncytiotrophoblast.

Erosion of the endometrium by the trophoblast enables the embryo and its investments to sink deeper into it. By day 9 to day 11, it is entirely within the endometrium, surrounded by a thin layer of cytotrophoblast and a thicker layer of syncytiotrophoblast (Fig. 21.17B). As this outer layer continues to invade the endometrium, it becomes permeated by a labyrinthine system of intercommunicating spaces (lacunae), filled with blood liberated from endometrial blood vessels eroded by the syncytiotrophoblast. At day 11 after ovulation, the embryo proper is a bilaminar disk, consisting of a plate of columnar epithelial cells, the **ectoderm,** and a thinner layer of cuboidal cells, the **endoderm.** At its margins, the ectodermal plate is continuous with a thin layer of squamous cells that enclose a small **amniotic cavity** (Fig. 21.17B). The endoderm is continuous at its margins with a sheet of squamous cells that enclose the **yolk sac.** Between these structures and the trophoblast is a space, called the **exocelom,** which is traversed by thin strands of **extraembryonic mesenchyme.** The broad peripheral zone of trophoblast is henceforth referred to as the **chorion.**

From day 15 onwards, cords of trophoblast grow deeper into the endometrium, forming the **primary chorionic villi.** These are soon invaded at their base by mesenchyme that advances in their interior to their tips, converting the primary villi into **secondary chorionic villi** (Fig. 21.18). These consist of an outer layer of syncytiotrophoblast and an inner layer of cytotrophoblast around a core of mesenchyme (Fig. 21.19). The villi are bathed by blood flowing sluggishly through a system of lacunae that collectively

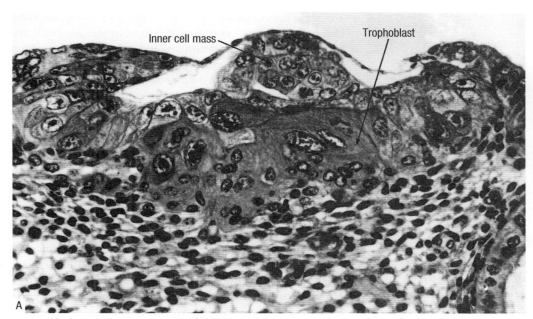

Inner cell mass

Trophoblast

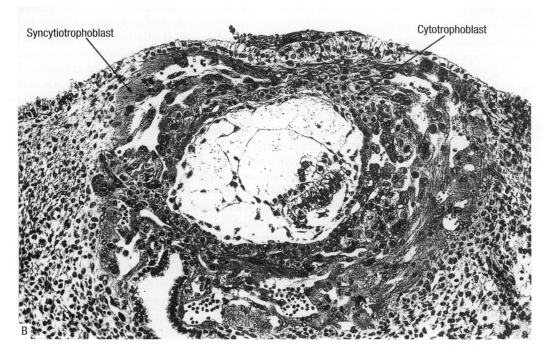

Syncytiotrophoblast

Cytotrophoblast

Figure 21.17 Photomicrographs of early human implantation sites. (A) At day 7 the embryo is a small sphere of cells, called the inner cell mass. Beneath it the trophoblast is penetrating the endometrium. (B) At day 9, the embryo is a bilaminar disk, and the trophoblast has differentiated into cytotrophoblast and syncytiotrophoblast. (Reproduced from A. Hertig and J. Rock *Carnegie Contributions to Embryology*, No 125, 1941. Courtesy of the Carnegie Institution of Washington.)

form the **intervillous space**. From the ends of the secondary chorionic villi, columns of syncytiotrophoblast grow across this intervillous space, and upon reaching the other side, they spread along it, coalescing with similar outgrowths of neighboring villi to form a continuous **trophoblastic shell**, interrupted only at sites of communication of maternal blood vessels with the intervillous space. Throughout the remainder of the pregnancy, the intervillous space is lined by trophoblast and traversed by villi that are fixed to the maternal tissue by their continuity with the trophoblastic shell or **basal plate**. The villi absorb nutrients from the surrounding maternal blood and excrete waste products into it.

Meanwhile, endothelial-lined spaces have developed in the mesenchyme within the cores of the villi and these coalesce to form blood vessels that communicate with vessels that are developing in the **body stalk** (later to become the umbilical cord). By day 22, the embryo has developed a heart, and fetal blood then begins to circulate through the vessels of the placental villi. Later in pregnancy, the villi begin to branch and their branching continues in the weeks that follow, increasing their total surface area.

The endometrium responds to invasion by the trophoblast with changes in its stroma. The fusiform stromal cells enlarge and take on a polygonal epithelioid form and are henceforth called **decidual cells**. They are pale-staining and their cytoplasm is rich in glycogen. The endometrium, so modified, is referred to as the

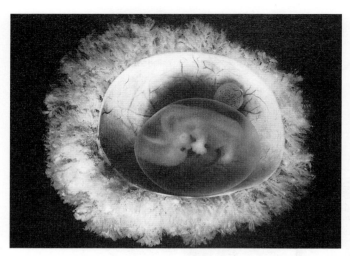

Figure 21.18 Photograph of a human embryo at 40 days of gestation, showing the numerous placental villi projecting from the entire periphery of the chorion frondosum. (Reproduced from D.G. McKay and M.V. Richardson *Am J Obst Gynec* 1935; 69:735.)

decidua. The portion of the decidua beneath the developing embryo is termed the **decidua basalis**; the portion extending over its adlumenal surface is called the **decidua capsularis**; that lining

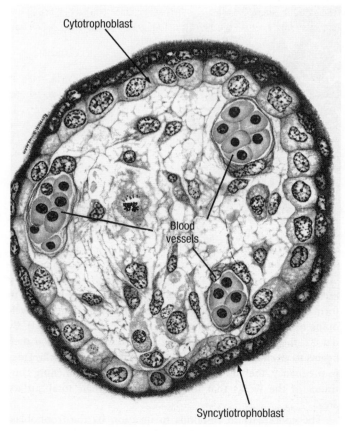

Figure 21.19 Drawing of a cross-section of a placental villus. Notice the cytotrophoblast on the inside, and the darker syncytiotrophoblast on the outside. The fetal blood vessels in the interior of the villus contain nucleated primitive erythroblasts.

the rest of the uterus, away from the products of conception, is the **decidua vera**. The contact of the fetal trophoblast with the maternal decidua is a confrontation between cells of different genotypes. Why fetal cells bearing antigens inherited from the father are not subject to immunological rejection is still not understood.

During the first 8 weeks of pregnancy, villi are equally numerous around the entire circumference of the chorion (Fig. 21.18), but thereafter the villi penetrating the decidua basalis rapidly increase in number and length, whereas those penetrating the decidua capsularis degenerate. By the third month, the adlumenal portion of the chorion, now devoid of villi, is smooth and relatively avascular and is called the **chorion laeve**. The portion invading the decidua basalis is now called the **chorion frondosum**. This discoid basal area of long trophoblastic villi will progress to form the fetal portion of the definitive **placenta**. By that time, the branching of the villi has continued until their total surface area is about 10 m². The additional surface area achieved by the microvilli of the syncytiotrophoblast would probably bring the total surface area to nearly 90 m².

By four and a half months of gestation, the uterine lumen is largely obliterated by the growing fetus and its membranes. The decidua capsularis has degenerated and the chorion laeve has fused with the decidua vera on the opposite side of the uterine lumen. The subsequent development of the placenta involves a great increase in the number and length of the villi of the chorion frondosum and expansion of the blood-filled intervillous spaces (Fig. 21.20).

In the fetal portion of the developing placenta, the cytotrophoblast cells cease to divide and progressively decrease in number; by the fifth month, those remaining no longer form a continuous layer. These remnants ultimately fuse with and are incorporated into the syncytiotrophoblast. The syncytiotrophoblast is not of uniform thickness. Thick areas containing clusters of nuclei alternate with thin areas devoid of nuclei. Dilated fetal capillaries, in the core of the villi, are closely applied to the thin areas, so the barrier between the fetal and maternal blood is little more than 2 μm in thickness, facilitating gas exchange between them. During the first trimester, nucleated red blood cells can be observed in the capillaries of the villi. Mature non-nucleated erythrocytes appear during mid-pregnancy.

Histophysiology of the placenta

Blood, poor in oxygen, is carried from the fetus to the placenta in the **umbilical arteries** and circulates in the capillaries of the placental villi. Venous blood returning from the villi is carried via the **umbilical veins** to their junction with the inferior vena cava near the heart. On the maternal side of the circulation, blood from the arcuate arteries of the uterus passes through coiled arteries of the decidua into the intervillous space, where it flows over the surface of the placental villi and through communications between the intervillous space and veins of the decidua basalis. Oxygen, carbon dioxide, fatty acids, and electrolytes can pass through the syncytiotrophoblast by diffusion. Amino acids cross the barrier by active transport. Immunoglobulins and other macromolecules are

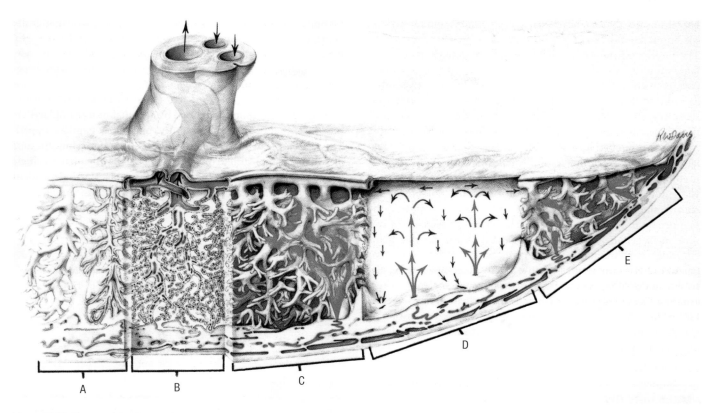

Figure 21.20 Diagram of the placenta showing its structure and the maternal and fetal circulation. (A) The tree of branching villi. (B) Fetal circulation of the villi in section. (C) Maternal circulation. (D) Pathway of maternal blood through the intervillous spaces. (E) Placental marginal zone. (Reproduced from E.M. Ramsey and J.W. Harris *Carnegie Contributions to Embryology*, No 261 1966; Vol. 38:61.)

taken up by receptor-mediated endocytosis and moved across the barrier in transport vehicles.

The placenta is a major endocrine organ producing hormones essential for maintenance of pregnancy. **Chorionic gonado-trophin**, one of the hormones secreted by the trophoblast, is detectable very early in pregnancy and increases rapidly up to the fifth month. It is similar to LH of the hypophysis and serves to maintain the corpus luteum in the maternal ovary and to stimulate its secretion of progesterone. The placenta also secretes **progesterone** which acts locally on the endometrium, stimulating proliferation of cells of the decidua. It also acts on the myometrium, inhibiting uterine contraction during pregnancy. In many mammals, the placenta also secretes **placental lactogen**, a hormone that stimulates development of the mammary gland of the mother, in anticipation of lactation. No such secretion has been verified for the human.

FEMALE EXTERNAL GENITALIA

The genitalia of the female include the **vagina, clitoris, labia majora**, and the **labia minora**. The vagina is a fibromuscular tube 8–9 cm in length extending from the uterine cervix to the vestibule of the external genitalia. In the virgin, its opening is partially closed by a crescentic fold, or fenestrated membrane, called the **hymen**. The vaginal mucosa consists of stratified squamous

epithelium, 150–200 μm thick, with a lamina propria rich in elastic fibers. As in the epidermis, antigen-presenting Langerhans cells are present in the lower layers of the epithelium. The superficial cells of the epithelium undergo very little keratinization. Their cytoplasm is filled with glycogen in the middle of the menstrual cycle, but this diminishes later in the cycle. Cells are constantly exfoliating from the epithelium of the cervix and vagina, and leukocytes, which abound in the lamina propria, migrate through the epithelium into the lumen. The vaginal epithelium has no associated glands and the film of fluid that lubricates its surface is evidently contributed, in large measure, by the glands in the cervix. The relatively thin muscularis of the vagina is composed of interlacing bundles of smooth muscle oriented both longitudinally and circumferentially, with longitudinal bundles greatly predominating in the outer half of the muscular coat.

Cancer of the cervix is one of the most common forms of cancer in women. Its early detection by examination of the cells continually exfoliated from the cervical and vaginal epithelium has greatly reduced the mortality from this form of cancer. This simple technique involves swabbing the surface of the vagina and smearing the cells onto a glass microscope slide. It is commonly called the Papanicolaou test, or PAP test after its originator. Cancer cells can be detected by their distinctive morphology and staining properties.

The female genital region is called the **vulva**. It is bounded by the **labia majora**, two rounded, longitudinal folds that extend from the mons pubis anteriorly to the perineum posteriorly. On their lateral surface, the skin bears coarse hairs. On their inner surface, the skin is smooth, hairless, and contains many sebaceous glands. The interior of the folds consists mainly of adipose tissue. The **labia minora**, medial to the labia majora, are thin, flexible folds covered with stratified squamous epithelium that has a very thin keratinized layer. It is devoid of hairs, but contains numerous sebaceous glands. The labia minora have a core of spongy connective tissue containing networks of elastic fibers. Unlike the labia majora, they contain no adipose tissue. The space between the two labia minora is called the **vestibule**. It contains the orifices of the urethra, anteriorly, and of the vagina, posteriorly. The labia converge anteriorly and form a thin fold over the dorsum of the **clitoris**, the homolog of the penis. This fold is comparable to the prepuce on the penis, in the male. The clitoris is made up of two very small cylinders of erectile tissue that end in a small **glans clitoridis**, corresponding to the glans penis of the male. Two **glands of Bartholin**, about 1 cm in diameter, open onto the medial surface of the labia minora. They are tubuloalveolar glands corresponding to the bulbourethral glands of the male. They secrete a lubricating mucus. Several smaller mucus-secreting **vestibular glands** around the opening of the urethra correspond to the glands of Littré in the male.

MAMMARY GLANDS

Although not strictly a part of the reproductive tract, the mammary glands are important accessory glands that have evolved in mammals to nourish their offspring. In the human female, they reach their greatest development at about the age of 20 years.

Atrophic changes begin at 40 years and become marked after the menopause. In addition to these long-term changes related to age, the breasts undergo slight changes in size in each menstrual cycle, and striking changes in size and functional activity during pregnancy and lactation.

The mammary gland is a compound tubuloalveolar gland consisting of 15–20 lobes drained by an equal number of **lactiferous ducts** that open at the tip of the **mammary papilla** (nipple). The lobes are separated by connective tissue and varying amounts of adipose tissue. Unlike other major glands, which have a single large duct, the mammary gland is an assemblage of independent units, each having its own excurrent duct. Within the nipple, each lactiferous duct is slightly dilated to form a **lactiferous sinus**.

Mammary adenocarcinoma (cancer of the breast) is one of the most common malignancies of women, having an incidence of 10%. As in other cancers, the cause is unknown, but there is a genetic component. A woman whose mother or sister has had breast cancer is at significantly greater risk. With early detection by annual mammogram, the probability of survival is far greater than for most cancers. Surgical removal of the entire breast may be preferable to partial mastectomy, in some cases.

Inactive gland

At birth, the gland is devoid of acini, consisting only of short branching ducts. As puberty approaches, the rising level of ovarian hormones stimulates growth and branching of the lactiferous ducts of the mammary gland and small masses of epithelial cells are formed at the ends of the smallest branches. These do not have

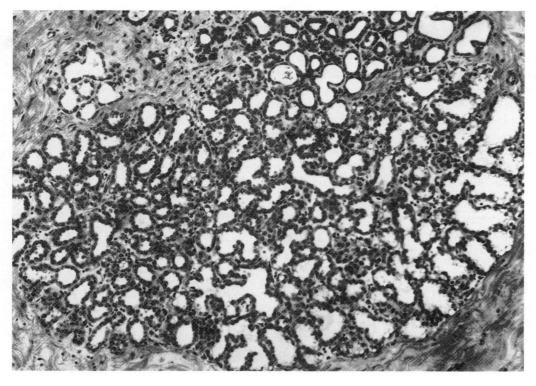

Figure 21.21 Photomicrograph of a section of mammary gland late in pregnancy. The gland has hypertrophied in preparation for lactation but is not yet secreting.

a lumen but are capable of developing into functional acini later in response to appropriate hormonal stimulation. In the adult, cyclic changes in the glandular tissue are minimal and the slight increase in breast size and sense of fullness experienced by some women at mid-cycle are probably caused by an increase in blood flow and some edema of the connective tissue of the breast.

Active gland

The elevated levels of estrogens and progesterone during pregnancy bring about major changes in the mammary glands. There is a rapid increase in length and branching of the duct system, an expansion of the pre-existing spherical masses of cells at the ends of the smallest ducts and their differentiation into acini that are somewhat atypical in having a larger lumen than those of other glands (Fig. 21.21). Between their lining epithelium and the basal lamina are stellate **myoepithelial cells** that have several long radiating cell processes. These adhere to the processes of other myoepithelial cells to form a wide-meshed network around the acinus (Fig. 21.22A). Stimulation of the nipple by a suckling baby leads to contraction of the myoepithelial cells constricting the acini and expressing milk from their lumen into the duct system. As in other contractile cells their cytoplasm is very rich in actin filaments and the myoepithelial cells can be selectively stained with fluorescent antibody to actin (Fig. 21.22B).

In histological sections of a lactating mammary gland, the appearance of different regions varies considerably, suggesting that not all areas are in the same functional state at the same time. In some areas, the walls of the acini are thin and their lumen contains many droplets of the lipid component of milk (Fig. 21.23). In other areas the epithelium of the acini is taller, and their lumen is smaller and contains few or no lipid droplets. The taller cells are generally eosinophilic with some basophilia in the basal cytoplasm.

In electron micrographs, there are arrays of parallel cisternae of rough endoplasmic reticulum in the basal cytoplasm and there is a large supernuclear Golgi complex. Two distinct types of secretory

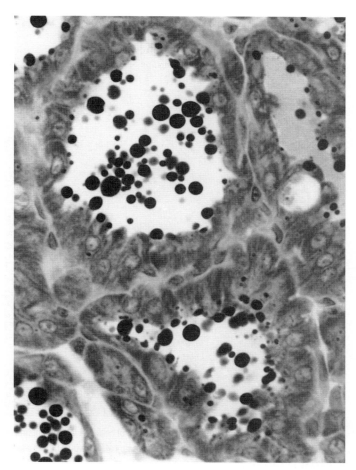

Figure 21.23 Photomicrograph of a lactating rodent mammary gland, fixed in osmium to preserve lipid of the milk. There are many secreted lipid droplets in the lumen. (Courtesy of N. Feder.)

product are identifiable: (1) vacuoles containing multiple small dense granules; and (2) large droplets of lipid. The mode of secretion of these two products differs. The sizable vacuoles containing the dense protein granules fuse with the plasmalemma as in other glandular cells (Fig. 21.24A). The large lipid droplets project into the lumen of the acinus covered only by the plasmalemma, and these are then pinched off, with the lipid now enclosed in a portion of the cell membrane (Fig. 21.24B).

Histophysiology of the mammary gland

The growth and differentiation of the ducts and acini of the gland, initiated by increased estrogens and progesterone in the early weeks of pregnancy, continue after the placenta becomes the dominant source of these hormones. Actual secretion of milk is suppressed until birth of the baby. After delivery of the placenta, there is a precipitous drop in the hormones that had inhibited secretion by the prepared gland. In the absence of this inhibition, **prolactin**, secreted by the pars distalis of the hypophysis, is a powerful lactogenic stimulus, and full lactation is established within a few days.

Once lactation is initiated, the cells secrete continuously, but

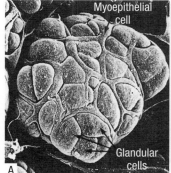
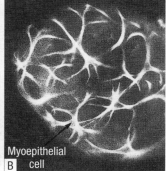

Figure 21.22 (A) Scanning electron micrograph of an acinus of the mammary gland, showing the network of myoepithelial cells occupying grooves in the base of the epithelium. (B) Acinus of a mammary gland stained with a fluorescent probe for actin. (A. Reproduced from T. Nagano *Cell Tis Res* 1980; 209:1. B. Reproduced from J. Emerman and W. Vogl *Anat Rec* 1986; 216:405.)

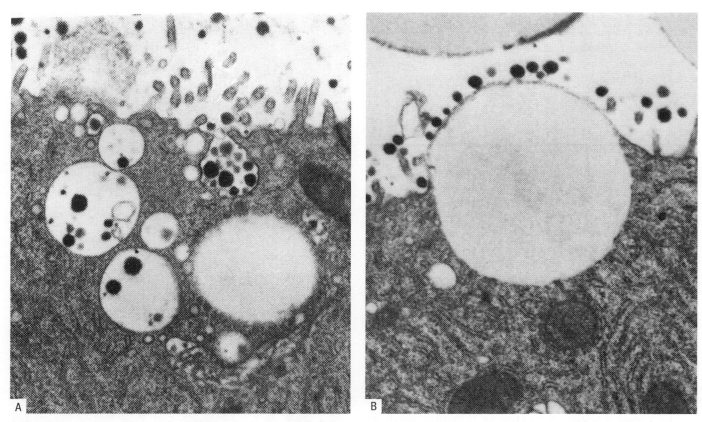

Figure 21.24 Electron micrograph of the apical portion of cells of a lactating mammary gland. (A) Exocytosis of vesicles containing granules of milk protein. (B) Lipid droplet protruding into the lumen covered by plasma membrane. Later, it would be extruded, enveloped in a detached portion of the plasmalemma. (Micrograph courtesy of A. Ichikawa.)

release of milk is episodic. Between breast feedings, milk is stored in the acini and small ducts. At feeding time, psychic and sensory stimuli associated with handling the baby are relayed to the hypophysis, resulting in the release of a surge of **prolactin** from its anterior lobe and **oxytocin** from its posterior lobe. Prolactin causes increased secretion into the acini, and oxytocin causes contraction of the myoepithelial cells around the alveoli, resulting in expulsion of the accumulated milk. When these complex mechanisms proceed smoothly, the average milk production of a mother feeding one baby is in excess of 1100 ml/day, and a mother of twins may produce over 2100 ml/day. Milk contains water and electrolytes (88%), protein (1.3%), and carbohydrate (3.3%), plus immunoglobulins (IgE and IgA) produced by plasma cells in the connective tissue of the gland. The principal protein component is **casein** and the principal carbohydrate is **lactose**.

The initial product of the mammary gland following birth is **colostrum**. Colostrum differs from milk in its higher immunoglobulin component, mainly IgA, which provides the baby with some initial immunologic protection. Colostrum is also high in protein content, but lower in fat content than milk.

After weaning of the baby, interruption of the neurohormonal stimuli and distension of the gland result in cessation of secretion, collapse of the acini, sloughing and autolysis of cells, and elimination of their residues by macrophages. Despite the widespread autolytic activity, some viable epithelial cells remain, forming acini without a lumen, and the myoepithelial cells persist. In a subsequent pregnancy, growth and differentiation of a functioning gland is repeated. In old age, the gland undergoes gradual atrophy of the acini and terminal portions of the duct system, with the gland returning to the prepubertal condition.

Questions

1 Which part of the oviduct has the most complex folding of its mucosa?
  a ampulla
  b medulla
  c fundus
  d fimbria
  e isthmus

2 Which one of the following lacks glands?
  a vagina
  b cervix of the uterus
  c endometrium, secretory phase
  d oviduct
  e endometrium, proliferative phase

3 Which statement best describes the corpus luteum?
  a it is composed primarily of dense regular connective tissue
  b it produces and secretes progesterone
  c it exhibits the stigma on one side
  d it produces and secretes HCG
  e it contains the zona pellucida

4 Which statement is true of the ovary?
  a it contains about one million ova at birth
  b it produces ova from its well developed medullary layer
  c it contains five million ova by age ten
  d it produces ova until puberty
  e it is essentially an avascular organ

5 Large numbers of nucleated erythrocytes in vessels of the chorionic villi indicate which one of the following?
  a early pregnancy
  b late pregnancy
  c damage to maternal blood vessels
  d loss of the cytotrophoblast
  e loss of the syncytiotrophoblast

6 Milk ejection is caused by which one of the following hormones?
  a prolactin
  b estradiol
  c oxytocin
  d dopamine
  e FSH

7 The oviduct is lined by which of the following types of epithelia?
  a simple columnar, often ciliated
  b stratified squamous non-keratinized
  c pseudostratified columnar with microvilli
  d simple columnar, never ciliated
  e simple cuboidal

8 Which of the following statements is correct?
  a the primary follicle exhibits a well defined antrum
  b the oocyte completes the second meiotic division at the time of ovulation
  c the cumulus oophorus is well developed in the secondary oocyte
  d the glassy membrane is a basement membrane between the theca interna and the stratum granulosum
  e the primary follicle has at least four layers of follicular cells surrounding it

9 Which of the following is not part of the placental barrier?
  a syncytial trophoblast
  b cytotrophoblast
  c endometrium
  d connective tissue
  e capillary endothelium

10 Which diagnostic feature of the uterus denotes pregnancy?
  a nucleated red blood cells
  b presence of glycogen-rich secretions in the glands
  c decidual reaction
  d engorgement of the spiral arteries
  e thickening of the stratum basale

11 From what structure does the corpus albicans arise?

12 In what structure does fertilization normally occur?

13 Nucleated red blood cells can be observed in what structure?

14 What region of the oviduct is closest to the ovary?

15 What hormone is required for the maintenance of the corpus luteum?

16 The chorionic frondosum will become what structure?

17 IgA is found in large amounts in what secretion?

18 The zona pellucida surrounds what structure?

19 What is the name of the structure analogous to Cowper's gland in the male?

20 When would the ovary display corpora lutea and albicantia, but no Graafian follicles?

Chapter twenty-two

Eye

The eyes are complex photoreceptor organs that enable us to sense the form, color and movement of objects in our field of vision. Each eye occupies an **orbit**, a hemispherical cavity in the front of the skull that protects it and permits a range of eye movements. The wall of the eyeball is made up of three layers: (1) a thick, fibrous, outer layer, the **corneoscleral coat**; (2) a vascular middle layer, the **uvea**; and (3) a photosensitive inner layer, the **retina** (Fig. 22.1). The corneoscleral layer has a transparent anterior portion, the **cornea**, and an opaque posterior region, the **sclera**. Together these encapsulate the greater part of the eyeball, and protect the delicate structures within the organ. The transparency of the cornea permits light to enter the eye and reach the retina at the back of the eye. The sclera and the intraocular fluid pressure maintain the spherical shape of the eye. Its blood supply is carried by blood vessels within the uvea. The anterior margin of the uvea includes the **ciliary body**, a belt-like specialization, encircling the cornea near to its junction with the sclera (Fig. 22.2). It contains smooth muscle that can change the shape of the lens to bring light from different distances to focus on the retina. Thus, the ciliary body is the agent of **visual accommodation**, corresponding to the focusing device on a camera. The **iris**, a thin continuation of the ciliary body anterior to the lens, is able to constrict or dilate to vary the diameter of the pupil and thus control the amount of light entering the eye. It is, therefore, an adjustable optical diaphragm, corresponding to the aperture-setting device on a camera. The multilayered retina lining the posterior two-thirds of the eye contains the **rods** and **cones**, which are the receptors for light. It also contains complex neural networks that encode visual information and send it through the optic nerve to the **visual cortex** of the brain.

The interior of the eye has three chambers: (1) the **anterior chamber** between the cornea and the iris; (2) the **posterior chamber** between the iris and the lens, anteriorly, and the vitreous body, posteriorly; and (3) the **vitreous cavity**, the large spherical space between the lens and the retina (Fig. 22.3). The transparent media in the path of light are, in sequence, the **cornea**, the **aqueous humor** (the fluid content of the anterior chamber), the **lens**, and the **vitreous body**, a gelatinous translucent substance that fills the posterior chamber.

SCLERA

The sclera is a thick, fibrous layer, ranging in thickness from 0.6 mm near the corneoscleral junction to 1.0 mm at the posterior pole of the eye. It consists of flat bundles of collagen fibers, networks of elastic fibers, and occasional flattened fibroblasts between the fiber bundles. It is connected by loose strands of thin collagen fibers to **Tenon's capsule**, a thin sheet of connective tissue separating the eyeball from the adipose tissue that fills the bony orbit behind the eyeball. A narrow **episcleral space** between the sclera and Tenon's capsule permits the eyeball to rotate. Movements of the eyeball depend on extraocular muscles with origins on the wall of the orbit, and insertions onto the sclera.

CORNEA

The cornea is slightly thicker than the sclera, measuring 1.1 mm in the center and 0.6 mm at its periphery. Within it, five layers are

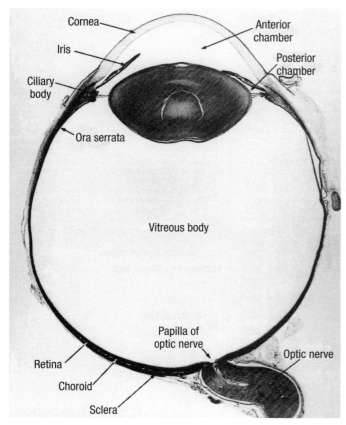

Cornea
Anterior chamber
Iris
Posterior chamber
Ciliary body
Ora serrata
Vitreous body
Papilla of optic nerve
Retina
Optic nerve
Choroid
Sclera

Figure 22.1 Photomicrograph of a meridional section of a monkey eye. (Micrograph courtesy of H. Mizoguchi.)

The cornea is avascular and depends upon diffusion of oxygen from the atmosphere or from the aqueous humor in the anterior chamber. Its transparency is attributable, at least in part, to the uniform diameter and changing orientation of the collagen fibers in its successive layers. With this arrangement, scattered rays of light cancel each other by destructive interference. When corneal edema occurs, the increase in the amount of fluid between the collagen fibers results in cloudiness of the cornea.

SCLEROCORNEAL JUNCTION

The transition from the highly ordered, transparent cornea to the opaque connective tissue of the sclera is called the **sclerocorneal junction**, or the **limbus**. On its inner surface, there is a shallow depression occupied by a **trabecular meshwork** made up of strands of connective tissue covered by an endothelium that is continuous with that on the posterior surface of the cornea (Figs 22.2, 22.4). Aqueous humor, percolating through the maze of endothelium-lined spaces of the limbus, finds its way into **Schlemm's canal**, a slender, tubular space that encircles the periphery of the cornea. Twenty-five to fifty slender channels, radiating from the outer wall of the canal, communicate with deep veins of the limbus, which drain into the episcleral veins. Thus, aqueous humor, following this path, drains into the circulatory system.

In individuals over 60 years of age, impaired flow of fluid through the trabecular meshwork and Schlemm's canal may lead to **glaucoma**. The resulting increase in intraocular pressure results in nerve damage and progressive loss of peripheral vision. Glaucoma is a major cause of blindness. Medications may slow the progress of the disorder. If this fails, laser surgery on the trabecular meshwork may improve fluid drainage and lower intraocular pressure.

The corneal epithelium is continuous at the limbus with the epithelium of the **conjunctiva**, the mucous membrane that covers the anterior surface of the eyeball peripheral to the cornea. At its margins, the conjunctiva is reflected from the eyeball onto the inner surface of the eyelids. At the edge of the cornea, Bowman's membrane terminates and is replaced by connective tissue underlying the epithelium of the conjunctiva. Radially arranged loops of blood capillaries in the conjunctiva extend a few millimeters into the cornea. Metabolites diffusing from these vessels contribute to the nutrition of the avascular central portion of the cornea.

UVEA

The uvea is the middle layer of the wall of the eyeball. It has three regions: the **choroid**, the **ciliary body**, and the **iris**. The **choroid** is a highly vascular portion of the uvea that underlies the retina and provides it with oxygen and other metabolites. The **ciliary body** is a specialized anterior region of the uvea that extends from the anterior margin of the retina, the **ora serrata**, to the sclerocorneal

identifiable in histological sections: (1) the **corneal epithelium**; (2) **Bowman's membrane**; (3) the **substantia propria** (corneal stroma); (4) **Descemet's membrane**; and (5) the **endothelium** (Fig. 22.2).

The epithelium consists of about five layers of unkeratinized cells. It has a very rich supply of sensory nerve endings, and has a remarkable capacity for regeneration. Minor injuries are repaired by a gliding movement of neighboring cells to fill the defect, followed by an increased rate of mitosis in the basal layer. **Bowman's membrane**, beneath the epithelium, is not a membrane in the usual sense of the word, but is a lamina 10–12 μm thick, consisting of a dense meshwork of randomly oriented thin fibrils of collagen. It ends abruptly at the margin of the cornea. The **substantia propria** (stroma), making up 90% of the thickness of the cornea, is an unusual connective tissue, having a highly ordered arrangement of its bundles of collagen fibers (Fig. 22.3). They form thin lamellae arranged in many layers. Within each lamella, the fibers are parallel, but those of successive lamellae change direction so that they are nearly at a right angle to those of the adjacent lamellae. The cells are thin, flattened fibroblasts lodged in narrow clefts between successive lamellae. Cells and fibers are embedded in a ground substance, rich in chondroitin sulfate and keratan sulfate. **Descemet's membrane** is simply a very thick basal lamina (7–10 μm) consisting of a hexagonal array of very thin, atypical collagen fibrils. It is a product of the simple squamous **endothelium** on the inner surface of the cornea (Fig. 22.3).

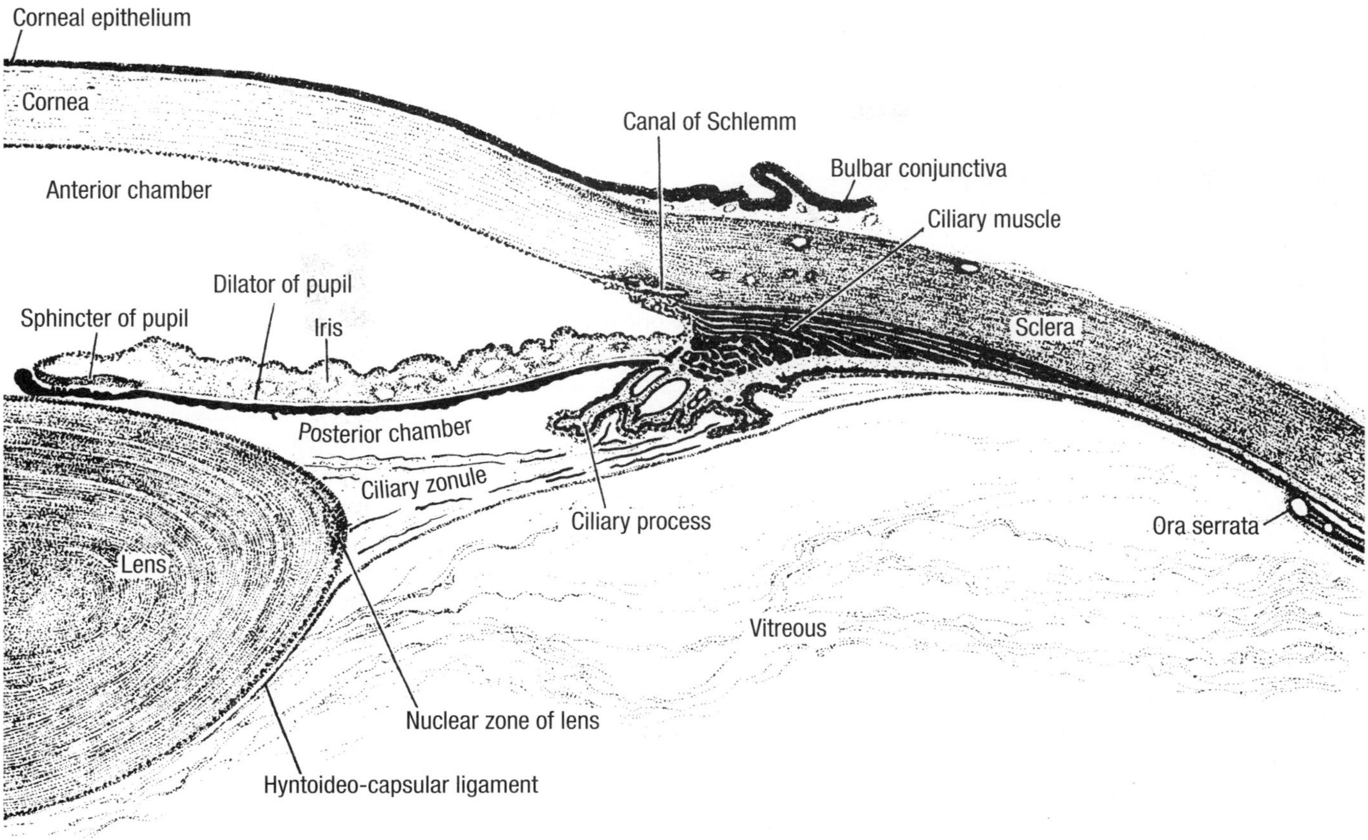

Figure 22.2 Drawing of the sclerocorneal junction, iris, lens and ciliary body as seen in a meridional section. (Modified after Schaffer.)

junction (Figs 22.3, 22.4). The **iris** is a thin diaphragm that continues from the ciliary body over the anterior surface of the lens. Its inner edge outlines the **pupil** of the eye.

Choroid

The choroid is a thin, highly vascular layer immediately beneath the sclera. It contains many blood vessels within loose connective tissue rich in fibroblasts, macrophages, lymphocytes, and plasma cells. Melanocytes, are also present in limited numbers, giving this layer a brown color. The inner portion of this layer, the **choriocapillaris**, contains a dense network of capillaries that is essential for the nutrition of the overlying retina. These vessels are lined by endothelium that is fenestrated on the side towards the retina. Between the choroid and the retina is **Bruch's membrane**, a structureless refractile layer 1–4 μm in thickness, resembling a thick basal lamina. The choroid ends anteriorly at the irregularly scalloped posterior margin of the ciliary body, called the **ora serrata**.

Ciliary body

The **ciliary body** is a circumferential thickening of the uvea between the ora serrata and the cornea. It is involved in suspension of the lens, and in changes of its shape necessary to bring the

rays of light into focus upon the retina (accommodation). In a meridional section of the eyeball, the shape of the ciliary body is that of a slender, inverted triangle with its base towards the anterior chamber (Fig. 22.2). About 70 radially oriented ridges, the **ciliary processes**, project from its base towards the lens (Fig. 22.4). These are covered by a bilaminar epithelium and have a core of loose connective tissue. Slender **zonula fibers**, originating in the basal lamina of the ciliary epithelium, pass between its cells and insert into the capsule of the lens, holding it in place (Fig. 22.2).

The bilaminar **ciliary epithelium** is an anterior continuation of the retinal layer. Because of its origin from the two layers of the invaginated embryonic optic cup, the ciliary epithelium is exceptional in that the apices of the cuboidal cells of its outer layer are apposed to the apices of the cells in the lower layer, and there is a basal lamina on both surfaces of the epithelium. The cell apices in the two layers are joined by desmosomes, but there are small intercellular spaces between them. The cells of the layer adjacent to the core of the ciliary processes are filled with melanin pigment granules (Fig. 22.4). Those of the unpigmented outer layer contain many mitochondria and cisternae of rough endoplasmic reticulum (rER). The plasmalemma adjacent to the basal lamina is elaborately infolded, as in other epithelia transporting water and ions. The ciliary epithelium produces the **aqueous humor**, a clear fluid containing most of the soluble constituents of the blood, but very little protein. This fluid moves from the posterior chamber through the pupil into the anterior chamber. It is drained from

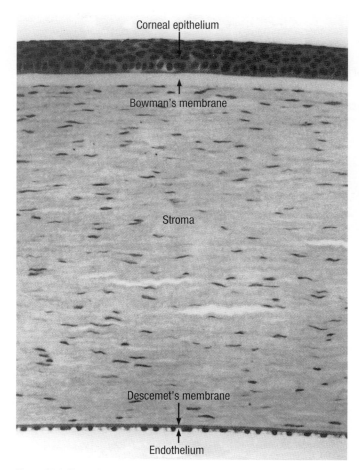

Figure 22.3 Photomicrograph of a section of the human cornea. (Reproduced courtesy of T. Kuwabara from R.O. Greep (ed.) *Histology*, 2nd edn, McGraw-Hill Book Co., New York, 1966.)

there through the trabecular meshwork and canal of Schlemm into the blood. Maintenance of the optimal intraocular pressure depends on an accurate balance between the rate of its production by the ciliary epithelium and the rate of its outflow to the episcleral veins. When this balance is disturbed, intraocular pressure is increased, resulting in serious damage to the optic nerve and retina.

The bulk of the ciliary body consists of the **ciliary muscle**, the muscle of accommodation. It is made up of bundles of smooth muscle of differing orientation. One group close to the sclera is oriented anteroposteriorly and stretches the sclera. Other groups of muscle fibers radiate medially, towards the vitreous, and still others, at the base of the ciliary processes, are oriented circularly. Contraction of the circular fibers eases tension on the zonula fibers, permitting the lens to become more convex, thus changing its refractive power. Connective tissue of the ciliary body and blood vessels from the highly vascular choroid form the core of the ciliary processes.

Iris

The iris arises from the ciliary body and projects towards the anteroposterior axis of the eye, anterior to the lens, separating the anterior chamber of the eye from the posterior chamber. It consists of highly vascular, loose connective tissue, covered on its posterior surface by a continuation of the ciliary epithelium. The layer that was not pigmented on the ciliary body, becomes heavily pigmented on the iris. The other pigmented layer becomes less pigmented on the iris and its cells are transformed into myoepithelial cells with long radiating processes filled with actinfilaments. Collectively, the myoepithelial cells of the iris constitute the **dilator pupillae**, which increases the diameter of the

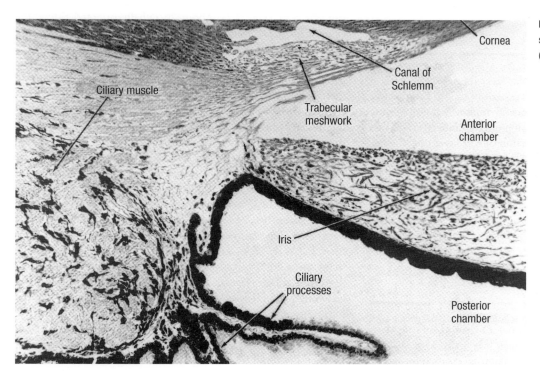

Figure 22.4 Photomicrograph of the sclerocorneal angle of the human eye. (Micrograph courtesy of T. Kuwabara.)

pupil. In the stroma of the iris near the pupil, there is a thin ring of circumferentially oriented smooth muscle cells, which form the **sphincter pupillae** (Fig. 22.5). Its contraction reduces the diameter of the pupil. The ability to change the diameter of the pupil permits vision over a wide range of light intensities. Moreover, when the pupil constricts in bright light, the depth of focus is increased and aberrations (imperfections in the refraction of a lens) are minimized. The anterior surface of the iris is not covered by epithelium but is made up of a discontinuous layer of fibroblasts and melanocytes. The stroma of the iris consists of loose connective tissue containing many small blood vessels, which are atypical in that they lack smooth muscle in their wall, regardless of their size. The color of the iris depends on the number of melanocytes in its stroma. If they are few, the light reflected from the pigmented epithelium on its posterior surface will appear blue. If they are abundant, the iris will appear brown. The pattern of pigmentation and of the vessels is unique for each person. Photographs of the iris are now being used for individual identification in place of fingerprints.

REFRACTIVE MEDIA

The refractive media of the eye are the **cornea**, the **lens**, and the **vitreous body**. The structure of the cornea has been described above. Its refractive power, which is a function of its index of refraction (1.376) and its radius of curvature (7.8 mm), is twice as high as that of the lens.

Lens

The lens is biconvex and is sufficiently elastic to permit slight changes in its shape. It is about 10 mm in diameter and 3.7–4.0 mm in thickness, but its thickness increases to 4.5 mm in accommodation (the bringing of near objects into focus). The lens is covered by a homogenous, highly retractile lens capsule rich in type IV collagen and proteoglycans (Fig. 22.6). On the anterior surface of the lens, beneath its capsule, is a layer of cuboidal epithelial cells, called the **subcapsular epithelium**. Towards the equator of the lens these cells become columnar. During lens development, elongation and differentiation of cells in this equatorial region results in their transformation into long **lens fibers**. The term lens 'fiber' is unfortunate, for each of these is actually a

modified epithelial cell, shaped like a six-sided prism 7–10 mm long, 8–12 μm wide, and only 2 μm thick (Fig. 22.7). They number about 2000 in the human lens, and have a curved course parallel to the convex anterior and posterior surfaces of the lens. The outer fibers are nucleated, but the deeper fibers have lost their nuclei. They are arranged in precise rows in multiple layers that converge towards the equator of the lens, where their surfaces are elaborately interdigitated (Fig. 22.7). Elsewhere, their sides are straight but have occasional short, rounded processes that fit into depressions of conforming shape in the adjacent fiber (Fig. 22.6B). The cytoplasm of the lens fibers contains very few organelles, but is filled with longitudinally oriented intermediate filaments, and a large amount of a special protein called **crystallin**.

Aging, drugs, or metabolic disorders may lead to the development of **cataracts**, a progressive opacification of the lens of the eye that results in blurred vision. It is very common and early in onset in persons with diabetes. The condition is very successfully treated by extraction of the lens from its capsule and its replacement with a plastic lens.

Vitreous body

The vitreous body that fills the eye globe between the lens and the retina, is a colorless, transparent, gelatinous substance. It is 99% water, with a liquid phase and a solid phase. The liquid phase contains highly hydrated long molecules of hyaluronic acid, and the solid phase consists of a network of very thin collagen fibers, 6–15 nm in diameter. Near its periphery, there are a few cells called **hyalocytes**. These are believed to synthesize the collagen and much of the hyaluronic acid of the vitreous body.

RETINA

The retina contains the **rods** and **cones**, the photoreceptors that are essential for vision. The photosensitive portion of the retina extends from the papilla of the optic nerve at the back of the eye, to the posterior margin of the ciliary body. Its outermost layer, the **pigment epithelium**, is separated from the choroid by Bruch's membrane, the thin, structureless layer on the inner surface of the choroid. The supranuclear cytoplasm of the pigment epithelial cells contains many melanin granules. These also

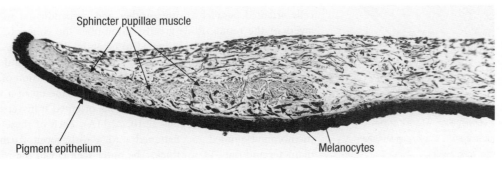

Figure 22.5 Photomicrograph of a section through the portion of the iris nearest to the pupil, showing the pigment epithelium and the sphincter pupillae muscle. (Micrograph courtesy of T. Kuwabara.)

Sphincter pupillae muscle

Pigment epithelium

Melanocytes

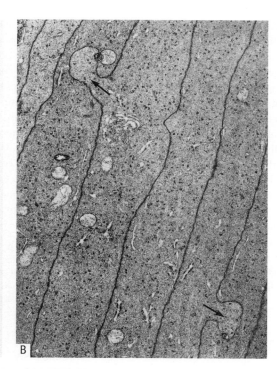

Figure 22.6 (A) Photomicrograph of the bow area of the human lens, where the epithelial cells become greatly elongated to form lens fibers. (B) Electron micrograph of fibers of the human lens. Note the short lateral processes occupying a concavity in the surface of the adjacent fiber (at arrows). (Micrographs courtesy of T. Kuwabara.)

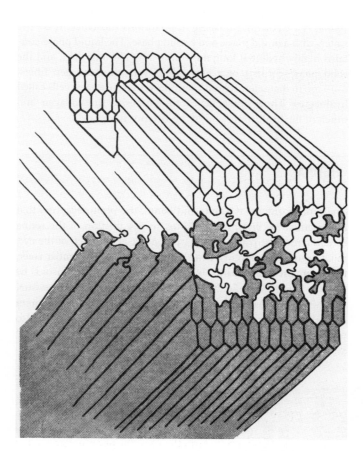

Figure 22.7 Drawing of the arrangement of the lens fibers. Their cross-sectional profile is hexagonal except in the area of their convergence, where there is considerable interdigitation of fibers. (Reproduced from T. Wanko and M. Green (eds) *Structure of the Eye*, Academic Press, New York, 1969.)

extend into long apical cell processes that occupy narrow spaces between the outer segments of the rods and cones of the retina. The melanin granules absorb light that has passed through the photoreceptor layer of the retina, preventing its reflection from the outer tunics of the eyeball. The basal cytoplasm of the pigment epithelial cells contains abundant smooth endoplasmic reticulum (sER) that is thought to be the site of storage of vitamin A, which is needed by the rods and cones. The plasmalemma at the cell base is infolded and interdigitated with basal processes of neighboring cells.

With aging, there may be accumulation of extracellular material in the pigment epithelium, breaks in Bruch's membrane, and an associated proliferation of subretinal blood vessels. These changes lead to **macular degeneration** with slowly progressing loss of vision.

Photoreceptor cells

The photoreceptor cells, the rods and cones, are long, slender cells oriented parallel to one another and perpendicular to the layers of the retina. Rods greatly outnumber the cones. In the human, their number is estimated to be about 120 million. The cones are very regularly distributed among the rods, a uniform distance apart (Figs 22.8, 22.9). The photosensitive portion of the rod is its cylindrical **outer segment**, which is made up of a very large number of closely spaced, flat disks oriented transverse to the long axis of the cell (Figs 22.10, 22.11A). Each of these is a membrane-bounded sac flattened into a disk about 2 μm in diameter and only 14 nm thick. The outer segment of the rod is

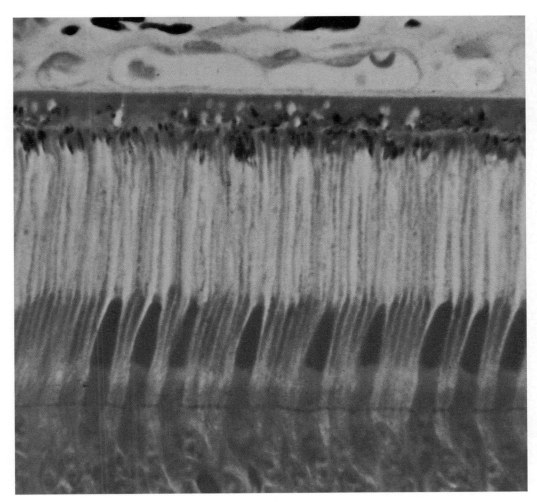

Figure 22.8 Photomicrograph of the outermost layers of the monkey retina. The cones are distinguishable from the rods by the greater size and deeper staining of their inner segment. The back of the eye is at the top of the figure. (Courtesy of J. Rostgaard.)

continuously renewed. Disks at its tip are exfoliated and ingested by the cells of the underlying pigment epithelium. New disks are formed, at the same rate, at the base of the outer segment. The outer segment is totally renewed in 10–14 days. The outer segment is connected to the **inner segment** by a slender stalk, containing a short cilium that emerges from a basal body in the distal end of the inner segment (Fig. 22.11A). The outer portion of the rod inner segment is filled with long mitochondria (Fig. 22.12). Below, it is continuous with an ovoid cell body containing the nucleus, a small Golgi complex, occasional tubules of endoplasmic reticulum, and longitudinally oriented microtubules. Towards the vitreous cavity, the cell body tapers down to a thin cell process called the **inner fiber**. This ends in a terminal expansion, the **spherule**, which synapses with the second of a series of neurons that conduct the visual stimulus to the brain (Fig. 22.10, 22.13). The spherule envelopes postsynaptic elements that are dendrites of the **bipolar cells** of the retina. The cytoplasm of the spherule contains a dense **synaptic rod**, or ribbon, that is surrounded by a halo of synaptic vesicles (Fig. 22.13).

The membrane of the disks in the outer segment of the rod contains **rhodopsin (visual purple)**, which consists of a pigment, **retinene**, bound to a large protein molecule. When exposed to light, retinene dissociates from this protein (a process called

'**bleaching**'). In the dark, the retinene–protein complex is reconstituted. Bleaching of rhodopsin by light initiates the visual stimulus. Rhodopsin is synthesized in the inner segment of the rod, transported through the stalk to the outer segment, and incorporated in the new disks being formed there.

The cones number 6–7 million. Like the rods, they consist of an outer segment connected to an inner segment by a slender stalk. However, the shape of the outer segment is conical instead of cylindrical (Figs 22.8, 22.10). Near its base, the two membranes of the disks are occasionally continuous with the plasmalemma along one side, suggesting that they may form by invagination of this membrane. Tracer studies provide no evidence of movement of the cone disks from base to tip, and there appears to be no exfoliation of disks. Cones are responsible for color vision and they contain no rhodopsin. There are at least three functional types of cones that cannot be distinguished morphologically. Each type contains a photopigment, **iodopsin**, which absorbs photons in one of three regions of the light spectrum; 419 nm (blue), 531 nm (green), and 558 nm (red). As in the rods, the outer portion of the inner segment is rich in mitochondria (Fig. 22.12). The cell body, containing the nucleus, is relatively short. The inner fiber of the cone is thicker than that of the rod and, as it approaches the next layer of the retina, it expands into a broader ending, called the

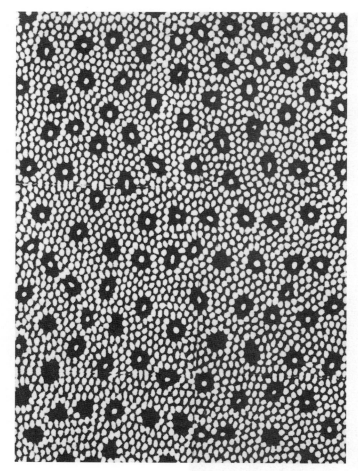

Figure 22.9 Photomicrograph of a horizontal section through the outer segments of the photoreceptors of monkey retina, showing their relative numbers and uniform distribution. The micrograph was printed as a negative, so the white dots outlined by a dark space are the cones. (Courtesy of E. Raviola.)

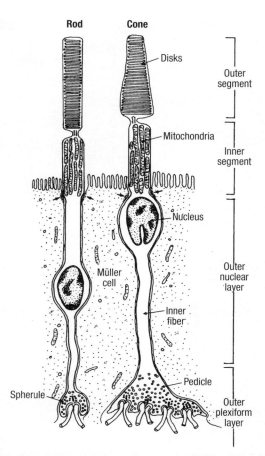

Figure 22.10 Diagram of a rod (left) and a cone (right) and their supporting Müller cells. Note the different shape of their outer segment and the greater size of the cone inner fiber and its pedicle.

pedicle, which contains multiple invaginated synapses with the bipolar and horizontal cells (Fig. 22.10).

Layers of the retina

In histological sections, seven layers are recognizable above the pigment epithelium: **photoreceptor layer, outer nuclear layer, outer plexiform layer, inner nuclear layer, inner plexiform layer, ganglion cell layer,** and the **nerve fiber layer** (Figs 22.14, 22.15). The photoreceptor layer consists of the outer segments of the rods and cones. The densely staining, outer nuclear layer includes the myriad nuclei of the rods and cones and the base of their inner fibers. The lightly staining, outer plexiform layer is largely devoid of nuclei and contains the spherules of the rods, the pedicles of the cones, and their synapses. The inner nuclear layer contains the cells bodies and nuclei of three cell types: the **bipolar cells**, the **horizontal cells**, and the **amacrine cells**. One type of bipolar cell, oriented perpendicular to the layers of the retina, connects the photoreceptor cells with large neurons in the ganglion cell layer. Its dendrites are in synaptic contact with the

spherules of two or three rods, and its axon contacts up to four ganglion cells. A second type of bipolar cell (monosynaptic bipolar cell) connects a single rod cell to a small type of **ganglion cell**. A third type connects several cone pedicles to both large and small ganglion cells. The horizontal cells, oriented parallel to the layers of the retina, have very long processes that branch into groups of shorter processes in the inner plexiform layer (Fig. 22.15). Some horizontal cells contact 10 or more rod spherules. Others make contact with six or seven cone pedicles. The function of the horizontal cells is poorly understood. They do not appear to have an axon and may simply serve to integrate the stimuli of groups of photoreceptors. The function of the several kinds of amacrine cells is equally obscure. They are situated in the inner portion of the inner nuclear layer and have numerous dendrites, but no recognizable axon. Their processes contact the axonal endings of bipolar cells, and dendrites of multiple ganglion cells (Fig. 22.15).

Owing to the way in which the eye develops in the embryo, light must pass through all of the above layers before reaching the photoreceptors. This orientation of the retina would seem opposite to that which would maximize light reception by the rods and cones, but it functions very well.

The ganglion cell layer contains the cell bodies of large neurons that have been called ganglion cells only because of their

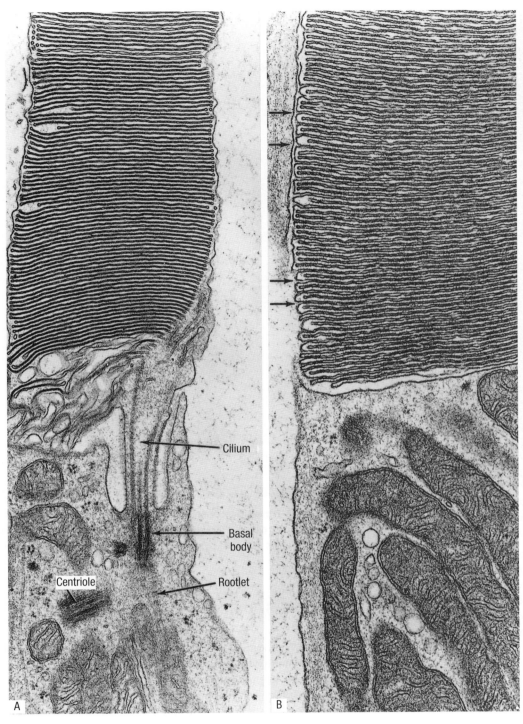

Figure 22.11 (A) Electron micrograph of the proximal portion of a rod outer segment, and a portion of the inner segment. Note the cilium and basal body in the stalk connecting them. (B) Corresponding region of a cone. Observe that some of the bilaminar discs are open to the extracellular space (at arrows). (Courtesy of T. Kuwabara.)

resemblance to cells in the peripheral ganglia of the nervous system. They are the terminal link in the chain of neurons between the photoreceptor cells and the brain. They receive input from the bipolar cells, and their long axons become one of the many fibers of the optic nerve running from the retina to the visual cortex of the brain. There are at least two categories of ganglion cells in the primate retina, differing greatly in size. Their axons, in the nerve fiber layer at the inner surface of the retina, converge upon the optic nerve (**optic papilla**). This small, round area, of the retina, devoid of photoreceptors, is the so-called 'blind spot' of the retina.

As a specialized portion of the central nervous system, the retina contains supporting elements comparable to the neuroglia of the brain. Among these are the radially oriented **Müller cells**, which are supporting cells unique to the retina. The cell body is a long slender pillar of varying width, crossing the layers of the retina and extending throughout the greater part of its thickness. At the inner and outer plexiform layers, it gives off many lateral

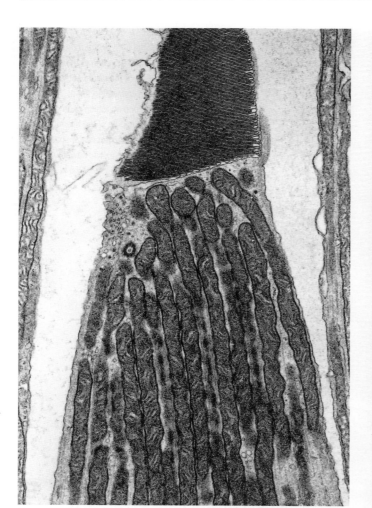

Figure 22.12 Electron micrograph of the outer part of the cell body of a cone, illustrating the high concentration of mitochondria near the outer segment.

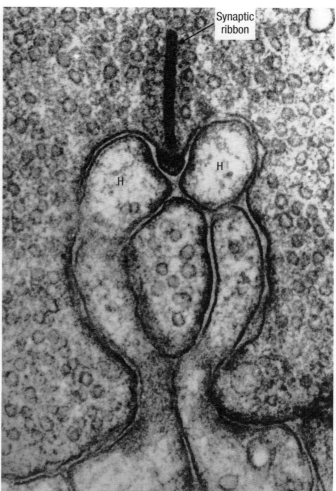

Figure 22.13 Electron micrograph of the invaginated synapse of a rod spherule in rabbit retina. Two processes (H) inserted between the principal elements of the synapse may arise from a horizontal cell. (Courtesy of E. Raviola.)

branches that occupy the spaces between the neuronal processes in those layers. In electron micrographs, there is a conspicuous row of zonulae adherentes between the outer ends of the Müller cells and the cell bodies of the photoreceptor cells. Early histologists, using the light microscope, erroneously described this dark line as an 'outer limiting membrane'. The term is no longer used.

Fovea

Immediately lateral to the optic nerve, there is a yellowish oval area called the **macula lutea**. In its center is a shallow depression about 1.5 mm in diameter called the **fovea** (Fig. 22.16). This small area contains no rods, but up to 30 000 closely packed cones, and the cell bodies of the overlying bipolar and ganglion cells are displaced laterally, making this the thinnest part of the retina. Light focused upon it passes to the outer segments of the cones unimpeded by passing through thick nuclear and ganglion cell layers. Therefore the fovea, no larger than the head of a pin, is the area of greatest visual acuity, and for detailed color vision, the light must be focused upon it.

HISTOPHYSIOLOGY OF VISION

Rays of light from an illuminated object are refracted by the cornea onto the lens, which bends them further to come to focus on the photosensitive retina. There, a greatly reduced inverted image of the object is formed, and the quanta of incident light are transduced by the rods and cones into neural signals. These are processed by the overlying network of retinal neurons and translated into nerve impulses that are conducted to the brain over the axons of the optic nerve.

The rods and cones differ in their sensitivity to light. Rods are active in dim illumination (**scotopic vision**) and cones are active in daylight conditions (**photopic vision**). The retinal rod is extremely sensitive to light, being able to respond to a single photon (the smallest unit of light energy). Many more photons are required to activate a cone. As ambient light decreases, so does color vision. Thus, night vision is in shades of gray to black.

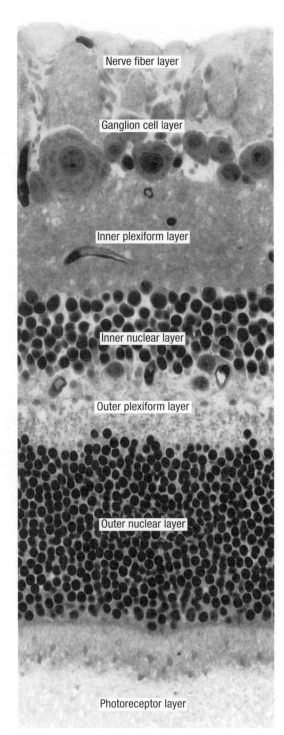

Figure 22.14 Photomicrograph of the retina of a cat, showing its principal layers. The innermost layer is at the top of the figure. (Courtesy of A.J. Ladman.)

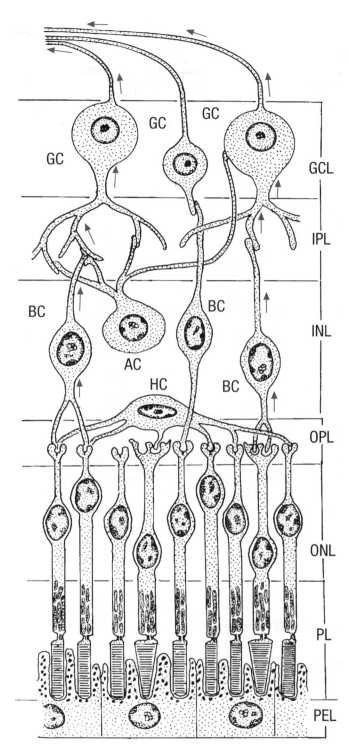

Figure 22.15 Simplified diagram of the principal cell types of the retina: AC, amacrine cell; BC, bipolar cell; GC, ganglion cell; HC, horizontal cell. Layers of the retina: GCL, ganglion cell layer; INL, inner nuclear layer; IPL, inner plexiform layer; ONL, outer nuclear layer; OPL, outer plexiform layer; PEL, pigment epithelial layer; PL, photoreceptor layer.

In the dark, the visual pigment **rhodopsin** accumulates in the membrane of the disks in the outer segment of the rod. It is broken down by exposure to light. The biochemical mechanism of activation of the rods is complex. It depends mainly upon thousands of ion channels in their membranes. In darkness, these are held open by their binding of cyclic guanosine monophosphate. The open channels permit inflow of Na^+ ions into the outer segment that results in a depolarization that keeps the Ca^{2+} channels open, permitting more-or-less continuous release of neurotransmitter to the bipolar cells. When light

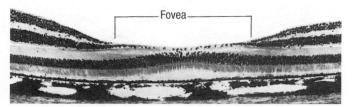

Figure 22.16 Photomicrograph of the fovea of a monkey retina, showing the marked reduction in thickness of the retina in this area of maximal visual acuity. (Courtesy of H. Mizoguchi.)

triggers breakdown of rhodopsin in the outer segment, cyclic guanosine monophosphate is enzymatically degraded and ion channels are closed, interrupting inflow of Na^+ and Ca^{2+} ions and causing a hyperpolarization of the cell that inhibits its release of neurotransmitter. In the rods, turning off signaling (hyperpolarization) conveys information to the bipolar cells as effectively as depolarization does in other neural cells that generate action potentials. The signal spreads from the bipolar cells to the ganglion cells and these generate action potentials that are conducted to the visual cortex of the brain. In the recovery phase of the process, visual pigment is regenerated in the disks of the outer segment and calcium is pumped out of the presynaptic portion of the synapse. These events require energy generated by the numerous mitochondria of the rod inner segment.

All cones are morphologically similar, but there are actually three kinds that have three different visual pigments, called **photopsins**, that are sensitive to different wavelengths of the visual spectrum, blue, green, or red. The perception of intermediate hues depends upon the relative numbers of the three kinds of cones that are simultaneously activated. To the extent that they have been analyzed, the breakdown and regeneration of the visual pigments of cones seem to be similar to that of rods.

ACCESSORY STRUCTURES

Eyelids

The eyelids form during embryonic life as folds of skin that advance over the front of the eyeball. The skin on their outer side is thinner than that elsewhere on the face, and its stratified squamous epithelium has few papillae. There are a few sebaceous glands, and fine hairs are visible only with magnification. Deep to the subcutaneous loose connective tissue, there are transversely oriented bundles of striated muscle that constitute the palpebral portion of the **orbicularis oculi muscle**, which closes the eyelids. The upper lid is raised by the **levator palpebrae superioris muscle**. Its origin is in the roof of the orbit and it terminates in a thin fascia that inserts onto the **superior tarsus**, a convex, hemispherical plate of dense connective tissue that stiffens the lid and makes it conform to the curvature of the underlying eyeball (Fig. 22.17).

Embedded within the tarsus are 20 or more parallel **Meibomian glands** that have individual ducts opening in a single row along the free edge of the lid. A much smaller **inferior tarsus**, containing about 20 Meibomian glands, is found in the lower lid. The secretion of these modified sebaceous glands forms a thin lipid layer over the tear film, thereby retarding evaporation.

The eyelashes are coarse hairs set obliquely in three or four rows along the edge of the lids. They are replaced at intervals of 100–150 days. Associated with their follicles are modified sweat glands, called the **glands of Moll**, and modified sebaceous glands, the **glands of Zeis** (Fig. 22.17). The secretion of both is delivered into the follicles of the eyelashes.

Conjunctiva

At the lid margins, the skin on their outer surface is continuous with the **palpebral conjunctiva** on their inner surface. This thin, transparent mucous membrane lines the inner surface of the lids, and at their base, continues onto the front of the eyeball as the **bulbar conjunctiva**, which terminates at the margin of the cornea. The conjunctival epithelium is stratified with two or three layers of cells. The basal layer is columnar and those at the surface are low cuboidal or squamous. There are a few goblet cells in this epithelium and their secretion contributes to the tear film. The potential space between the eyelids and the eyeball is called the **conjunctival sac**.

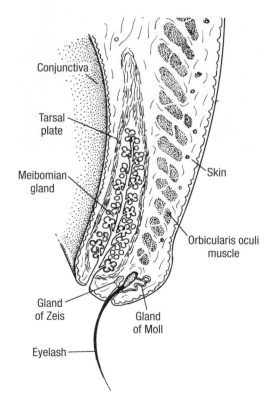

Figure 22.17 Diagram of a section of an eyelid, showing the location of its principal components.

Lacrimal glands

An almond-shaped lacrimal gland is situated above the temporal quadrant of each eyeball. It consists of several lobules drained by 6–12 ducts that open into the conjunctival sac. It is a tubuloalveolar gland in which the alveoli are somewhat distended and lined by serous columnar cells containing pale secretory granules. Intercellular secretory canaliculi can be found between the cells. Between the epithelium and its basal lamina are branching myoepithelial cells that contribute to expulsion of the secretion from the acini. The secretion of the lacrimal gland forms the tear film over the bulbar conjunctiva and the cornea. This fluid is drained into two tiny orifices, the **lacrimal puncta**, one on the rim of each lid at its medial end. These are the openings of two short **lacrimal ducts** about 1 mm in diameter and 8 mm long and lined by stratified squamous epithelium. These join to form a single very short duct opening into the **lacrimal sac**, which is the expanded upper end of a **nasolacrimal duct** that courses downwards to open into the inferior meatus of the nasal cavity. The lacrimal sac and nasolacrimal duct are lined by ciliated pseudostratified columnar epithelium containing some goblet cells.

The secretion of the lacrimal gland contains antibodies and the antibacterial enzyme lysozyme, and the secretion both lubricates and protects the conjunctiva and cornea. The secretion of tears in excess (weeping), in response to pain or strong emotions, is confined to humans and its physiological significance, if any, is not understood. The volume of lacrimal secretion diminishes in old age, resulting in dryness and irritation of the front of the eye. This can be relieved by plugging the nasolacrimal duct to retain the tears in the conjunctival sac.

Questions

1 Aqueous humor is drained from the eye via the
   a canal of Schlemm
   b ciliary channels
   c central retinal vein
   d optic papilla
   e lacrimal duct

2 Which of the following is the most highly vascular tissue of the eye?
   a choroid
   b sclera
   c cornea
   d lens capsule
   e tunica fibrosa

3 Among the five recognized histological layers of the cornea, which of the following makes up the bulk of its structure?
   a substantia propria
   b Bowman's membrane
   c Descemet's membrane
   d epithelium
   e endothelium

4 The limbus of the eye marks the junction of the
   a neural retina and pigmented epithelium
   b ciliary body and iris
   c pars iridica and pars caeca
   d cornea and sclera
   e anterior and posterior chambers

5 The portion of the retina specialized for highest acuity vision is the
   a optic papilla
   b area enriched for rods
   c lamina vitrea
   d ellipsoid
   e fovea

6 The primary refractive structure of the eye is the
   a lens
   b cornea
   c vitreous humor
   d aqueous humor
   e retina

7 Glaucoma can result from an obstruction of the
   a uveal tract
   b Tenon's space
   c lacrimal duct
   d canal of Schlemm
   e choriocapillaris

8 The cell type that carries neural transmission from the retina to the brain is the
   a ganglion cell
   b amacrine cell
   c bipolar cell
   d horizontal cell
   e lateral geniculate cell

9 In the eye, the zonule is composed of suspensory ligaments which connect the
   a iris and ciliary body
   b ciliary body and ciliary muscles
   c cornea and sclera
   d anterior and posterior chambers
   e lens and ciliary body

10 Aqueous humor is produced by the
   a zonule of Zinn
   b iris
   c ciliary processes
   d retina
   e cornea

11 The ciliary body is continuous with what pigmented structure?

12 What fluid drains from the eye through the canal of Schlemm?

13 What is the name of the structure that lies just below the corneal epithelium?

14 The layer of the retina closest to the choroid contains large amounts of what substance?

15 What is the first tissue layer of the eye that light rays encounter?

16 What area is defined by the space bordered by the iris, lens, ciliary processes, and zonular attachments?

17 Tissues associated with the anterior chamber of the eye are avascular, so they are dependent on what to supply nutrients?

18 The fovea contains a large number of what type of cell?

19 What structure marks the anterior limit of both the retina and choroid and the start of the ciliary body?

20 The lens is held in place by what structure?

Ear

The ear is a sensory organ that has two important functions: (1) the detection of sound (hearing), and (2) the maintenance of balance. These functions are subserved by three distinct regions of the organ: the **external ear**, the **middle ear**, and the **inner ear**. In hearing, sound impinging upon the **external ear** is directed into a short tube that is closed at its end by a taut membrane, the eardrum. Sounds of frequencies ranging from 16 to 20 000 cycles per second induce vibration of the same frequency in the eardrum. These oscillations are amplified by three minute articulated bones in the **middle ear** that transmit them to a second membrane across the opening of a spiral duct of the inner ear. There, they are translated into nerve impulses that are interpreted in the auditory center of the brain. The balancing function of the ear resides in three semi-circular ducts of the inner ear. These sense sudden linear or rotational acceleration of the head and generate nerve impulses that trigger the corrective body movements necessary to restore the state of equilibrium.

EXTERNAL EAR

The **auricle (pinna)** is an irregularly shaped plate of elastic cartilage with a perichondrium rich in elastic fibers. It is covered by skin that is closely adherent to the perichondrium, except on the posterior surface of the ear where there is a small amount of subcutaneous connective tissue. The skin bears a few fine hairs and their associated sebaceous glands. Sweat glands are few or absent.

The **external auditory meatus (acoustic meatus)** is a canal about 2.5 cm in length, extending inwards from the auricle (Fig. 23.1). Coarse hairs project into its outer third and the sebaceous glands associated with their follicles are exceptionally large. The skin lining the canal also contains **ceruminous glands**. These

coiled, tubular glands are modified sweat glands. They secrete **cerumen**, a brownish waxy material. The ducts of the glands open either onto the surface of the skin or into the necks of the hair follicles. The **auditory canal** is closed, at its inner end, by the ovoid, translucent **tympanic membrane** or eardrum (Fig. 23.1). This is covered on its outer surface by a thin layer of epidermis, and on its inner surface by a squamous epithelium that lines the **tympanic cavity**. Between the two epithelia of the eardrum, there is a tough layer of connective tissue containing both collagenous and elastic fibers. In its anterior upper quadrant, the tympanic membrane is thinner, and this region is referred to as **Shrapnell's membrane**. Vibration of the tense tympanic membrane by sound waves initiates the hearing process.

MIDDLE EAR

The middle ear, or **tympanic cavity**, is an irregular space within the **temporal bone**, bounded laterally by the tympanic membrane. It communicates posteriorly with air-filled spaces within the mastoid process of the temporal bone, and anteriorly with the **eustachian tube** that courses downwards from the middle ear to the nasopharynx (Fig. 23.1). The cavity is lined by squamous epithelium. A thin lamina propria intervenes between the epithelium and the periosteum of the surrounding bone. Near the inner end of the eustachian tube, there is a transition from squamous epithelium to the ciliated pseudostratified epithelium that lines the tube. The act of swallowing, or yawning, briefly opens the eustachian tube, allowing the pressure in the tympanic cavity to equalize with that of the atmosphere. The contents of the tympanic cavity include the **auditory ossicles** and the **tensor tympani** and **stapedius muscles**.

The auditory ossicles are a chain of three very small bones, the

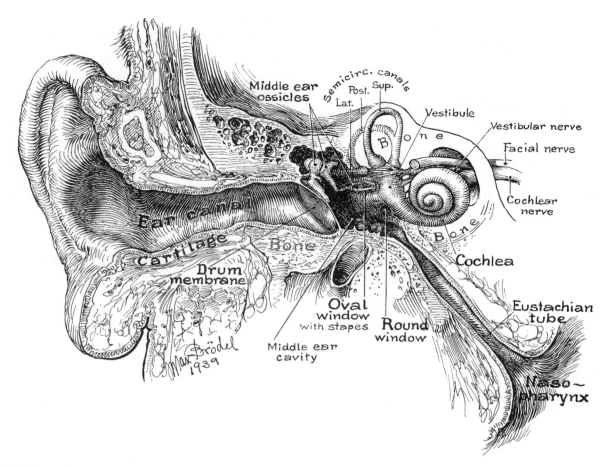

Figure 23.1 Drawing of the structure of the external, middle and inner ear (Reproduced from W. Brodel, in J. Malone, M. Guild, and B. Crowe (eds) *Three Unpublished Drawings of the Human Ear*, W.B. Saunders Co. Philadelphia, 1946.)

incus, malleus, and **stapes,** that articulate with one another to extend across the tympanic cavity from the tympanic membrane to the **oval window,** an opening in the bony wall between the middle ear and the inner ear (Fig. 23.1). The three bones articulate at diarthrodial joints and are covered by the squamous epithelium lining the cavity. Their piston-like action transforms the energy of the vibrating tympanic membrane into forceful oscillations of pressure in the fluid of the inner ear.

A common complication of an upper respiratory infection is **otitis media,** a bacterial infection of the middle ear. There is fever and pain as the lining of the tympanic cavity thickens and an inflammatory exudate (pus) accumulates within it. This may lead to perforation of the tympanic membrane and drainage into the auditory canal. If not successfully treated with antibiotics, the infection may spread into the air-spaces of the mastoid process, causing **mastoiditis.** If infection there persists, surgical removal of the mastoid process (mastoidectomy) may be necessary.

INNER EAR

The several components of the inner ear occupy a series of communicating cavities in the petrous portion of the temporal bone

that collectively comprise the **osseous labyrinth.** This contains the **membranous labyrinth,** consisting of: two small sacs, the **utricle** and **saccule;** three **semicircular ducts** (anterior, posterior and lateral), emanating from the utricle; and the **cochlear duct** in the spiral bony canal of the osseous labyrinth (Fig. 23.2). All portions of the membranous labyrinth contain a fluid, called the **endolymph.**

The wall of the membranous labyrinth is separated from the

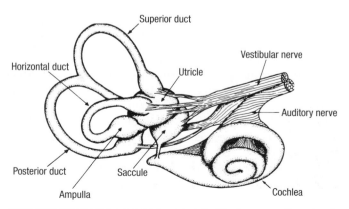

Figure 23.2 Drawing of the membranous labyrinth of the human ear. (Reproduced from D.E. Parker *Sci Am* 1980; 243:120.)

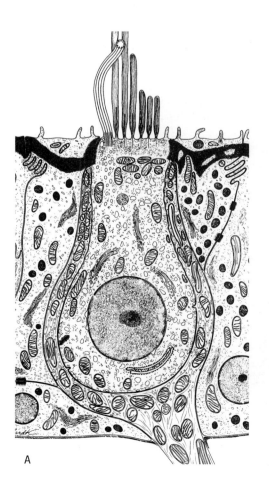

Figure 23.3 Drawing of the macula utriculi showing the relation of the otolithic membrane to the hair cells. The drawing is cut away at the left to show the stereocilia on the rows of hair cells. (Reproduced from D.E. Parker *Sci Am* 1980; 243:120.)

wall of the osseous labyrinth by a **perilymphatic space**, which contains a fluid of different composition, called the **perilymph**. The central portion of the osseous labyrinth, called the **vestibule**, contains the utricle and saccule and these are often referred to as the **vestibular organs**. Their function is to maintain the normal position of the body. They respond to acceleration of the head by generating nerve impulses to the brain, which initiate reflexes that restore normal body position.

Utricle and saccule

The **utricle** and the **saccule** are two small sac-like structures that occupy concavities in the wall of the central portion of the vestibule. Their wall consists of an outer fibrous layer, a more delicate intermediate layer of highly vascular connective tissue, and an inner layer of low-cuboidal epithelium. In certain specialized receptor regions, however, the epithelium is more complex. There is an area, 2–3 mm in diameter, in the floor of the utricle called the **macula utriculi**, which consists of columnar **hair cells** and **supporting cells** (Fig. 23.3). On the free surface of each hair cell, there is a bundle of 40–80 unusually long and thick stereocilia (the 'hairs') and a single cilium (Figs 23.4, 23.5). The interior of each stereocilium is filled with closely packed microfilaments of actin that extend downwards into a thick terminal web. The stereocilia within the bundle are aligned in rows, with those in the successive rows increasing in length from 1 μm, on one side, to 100 μm on the side adjacent to the cilium. The cilium has the usual '9 + 2' arrangement of doublet microtubules, but the pair of single microtubules in the center may be absent in its distal portion. Because its internal structure is typical of cilia elsewhere in the body, it has been regarded as a kinocilium (a motile cilium), but its motility is in question.

Two kinds of hair cells are distinguishable in histological sections. **Type I** is flask-shaped, with a rounded base and a narrower neck. For the greater part of its length, it is surrounded

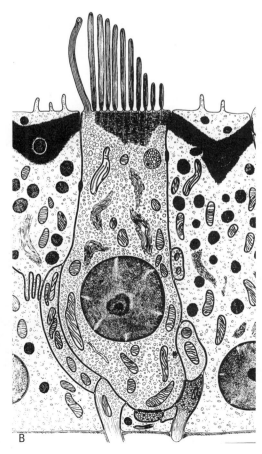

Figure 23.4 (A) Drawing of a type I vestibular hair cell showing the neural calyx enveloping much of its length. (B) A comparable depiction of the type II hair cell, which lacks a surrounding calyx.

A

B

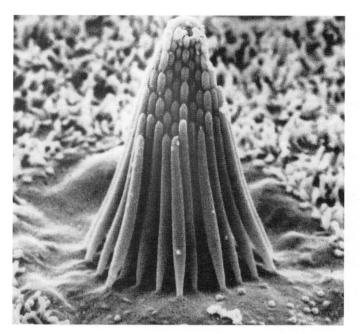

Figure 23.5 Scanning electron micrograph of the bundle of stereocilia on a hair cell of a bullfrog. The bundle on vestibular hair cells of the human is very similar. (Micrograph courtesy of D. Corey.)

by a deep, chalice-shaped afferent nerve ending, called the **calyx** (Fig. 23.5A). **Type II** is more columnar in shape, and it is not enclosed in a calyceal nerve ending. Instead, there are multiple, small afferent nerve endings in contact with its base. Dense structures called synaptic ribbons are found in the peripheral cytoplasm adjacent to each afferent nerve ending. Between the hair cells are columnar **supporting cells** that bear numerous short microvilli on their free surface, but they are otherwise unspecialized.

The stereocilia and kinocilium of the hair cells project into the underside of a moderately thick layer of a gelatinous glycoprotein that is probably secreted by the supporting cells. Traditionally, this layer has been called the **otolithic membrane**, but 'membrane' is clearly an inappropriate term. Embedded in the upper surface of this gel-like layer of glycoprotein are a multitude of crystalline bodies 3–5 μm in diameter, called **otoliths** or **otoconia** (Fig. 23.3). These consist of calcium carbonate in a protein matrix, and are thought to give the layer of glycoprotein additional inertia, resisting displacement. Thus, when linear acceleration is applied to the head, this gelatinous layer and its otoliths tend to remain stationary, while the hair cells beneath are moved slightly, bending the stereocilia (hairs). This triggers membrane depolarization in the calyceal nerve endings and the resulting nerve impulses are transmitted to the brain.

The smaller **saccule** is lined by an epithelium similar to that lining the utricle. On its anterior wall, there is an area called the **macula sacculi**, which has a structure similar to that of the macula utriculi. However, this macula is on the vertical anterior wall of the saccule, whereas that of the utricle is on its horizontal floor. The hair cells of the two maculae therefore respond to head movements in different directions (see below).

SEMICIRCULAR DUCTS

The three **semicircular ducts** occupy the bony semicircular canals. One end of each duct emerges from the utricle and returns to it at the other end of the semicircle. The ducts are lined by cuboidal epithelium and contain the fluid called **endolymph**. Each has a small dilatation near the utricle, called the **ampulla**. In the floor of each ampulla is a transverse ridge, called the **crista ampullaris** (Fig. 23.6). As in other sensory areas of the inner ear, the epithelium over the top of the crista consists of hair cells and supporting cells. Here, the hair cells do not extend down to the basal lamina but occupy rounded recesses between neighboring supporting cells. On their free surface, they have a tuft of stereocilia and a single kinocilium. The ends of these extend upwards into the base of a conical, gelatinous structure, called the **cupula**, which projects into the lumen of the ampulla (Fig. 23.6).

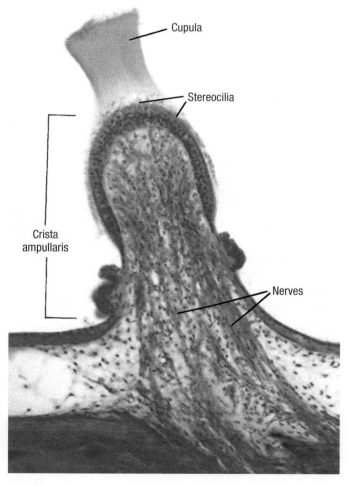

Figure 23.6 Photomicrograph of a transverse section of a crista ampullaris on the floor of the ampulla of a semicircular duct. The stereocilia on the epithelium project into an overlying cupula consisting of a gelatinous material. (Reproduced from D.E. Parker *Sci Am* 1980; 243:120.)

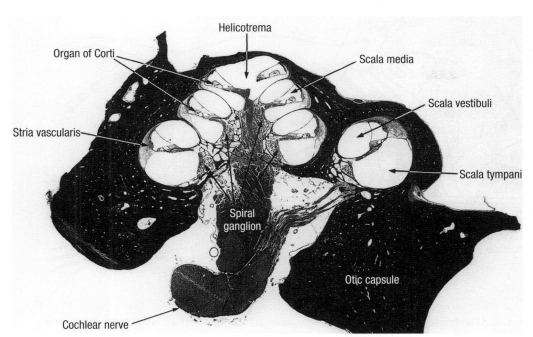

Figure 23.7 Photomicrograph of a section through the axis of the cochlea, showing the scala vestibuli, scala tympani, and the organ of Corti on the basilar membrane of the scala media. (Micrograph courtesy of H. Mizoguti.)

COCHLEA

The **cochlea** is located anteromedial to the vestibule and is conical in form, 5 mm in height and 9 mm in breadth across its base. It consists of a spiral bony canal about 35 mm in length that makes two and three-quarters turns around a central pillar of spongy bone, called the **modiolus** (Figs 23.1, 23.7). At its base, the **cochlear canal** communicates with the tympanic cavity through two openings in its lateral wall: the **oval window** (fenestra vestibuli) and the **round window**. The oval window is closed by the foot-plate of the stapes, the third of the three articulated auditory ossicles in the tympanic cavity. The round window is closed by a membrane.

A narrow ridge projects from the modiolus of the cochlea into the spiral cochlear canal. From its edge, the **basilar membrane** extends across the canal to join a thickening of the endosteum on the opposite side. A second membrane, the **vestibular membrane** (Reissner's membrane), extends obliquely across the canal at an angle to the basilar membrane (Figs 23.7, 23.8). The lumen of the canal is thus divided into three spiral chambers: the **scala vestibuli**, above the vestibular membrane; the **scala media**, between the vestibular membrane and the basilar membrane; and the **scala tympani**, below the basilar membrane (Fig. 23.8). The scala media, also called the **cochlear duct**, contains **endolymph** and ends blindly at the tip of the spiral. The scala vestibuli and scala tympani contain **perilymph** and the two communicate at the apex of the cochlea through a small opening, called the **helicotrema**.

Histologists traditionally called anything that appeared in section as a thin line, a 'membrane'. Much of their terminology has persisted, but students should be aware that the so-called membranes of the cochlea are not membranes in the contemporary meaning of the word (namely a bimolecular layer of phospholipids).

The **vestibular membrane** consists of two layers of squamous epithelium and their shared intervening basal lamina. The epithelium on the side towards the scala vestibuli is extremely thin. That on the side towards the scala media is slightly thicker and its cells have short clavate microvilli on their free surface. In both epithelia, the cells are joined by tight junctions, their lateral surfaces are interdigitated, and the cell base is elaborately infolded. These features suggest that they are involved in water and electrolyte transport. The epithelium on the side towards the scala media is continuous at the lateral wall of the canal, with a thicker stratified epithelium, the **stria vascularis**, which contains an intraepithelial plexus of capillaries. The superficial cells of the stria have many microvilli, and their base is infolded to form a labyrinthine system of narrow cell processes filled with mitochondria. The cells of the basal layer, surrounding the intraepithelial capillaries, contain fewer mitochondria and have processes that interdigitate with

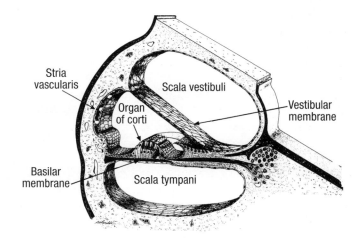

Figure 23.8 Schematic depiction of a section through one of the turns of the spiral cochlea, showing the organ of Corti on the basilar membrane.

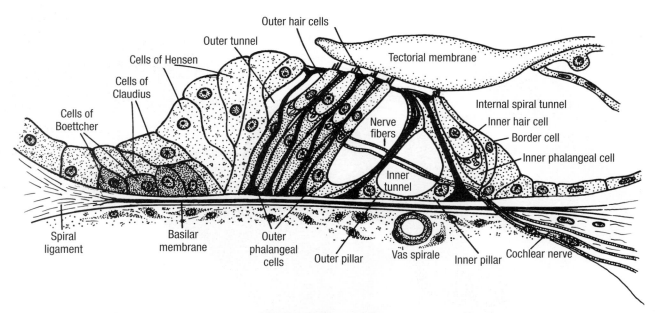

Figure 23.9 Drawing of a sectiion through the organ of Corti from the upper part of the first coil of the human cochlea. (Reproduced and slightly modified after J. Held *Untersuchungen über der feineren Bau des Ohrlabyrinthes*, Vol 1, Teubner, Leipzig, 1908.)

cells of the upper layer. The specialized epithelium of the stria vascularis is involved in water transport and maintenance of the electrolyte composition of the endolymph in the scala media.

On the **basilar membrane**, the epithelium is columnar and is highly specialized to form the **organ of Corti**, the receptor for auditory stimuli (Figs 23.9,23.10). It consists of hair cells and several types of supporting cells. One of the latter, the **phalangeal cells**, have a columnar basal portion with a cup-shaped upper end that is occupied by the rounded base of a hair cell. A slender lateral process of the same cell extends upwards to the surface of the epithelium and there expands into a platelike structure joined to the terminal web region of the hair cell, and to surrounding supporting cells by junctional complexes (Fig.23.11). The cell body contains conspicuous bundles of filaments and microtubules that converge upon the lateral process and continue in it to the surface of the epithelium. This well-developed cytoskeleton of these phalangeal cells gives them the stiffness necessary to maintain the position of the hair cells. Two rows of a second type of supporting cell, the **outer** and **inner pillar cells**, are separated at their base by a wide intercellular space, called the **inner tunnel** (Figs 23.9,23.10.) Their apices, however, are in contact with each other and with the hair cells in the rather stiff **reticular lamina**, which is a mosaic made up of the apical ends of the hair cells and the plate-like heads of their supporting phalangeal cells. The pillar cells, on either side

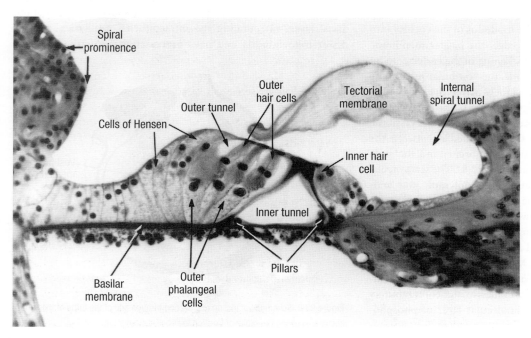

Figure 23.10 Photomicrograph of the organ of Corti of a cat. The tectorial membrane has been lifted off the hair cells during specimen preparation. (Photomicrograph courtesy of H. Engstrom.)

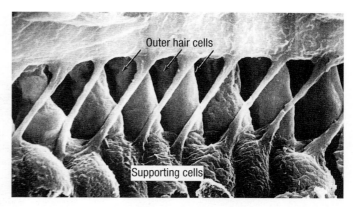

Figure 23.12 Scanning electron micrograph of a row of outer hair cells and the lateral processes of their supporting phalangeal cells. (Micrograph courtesy of H. Engstrom.)

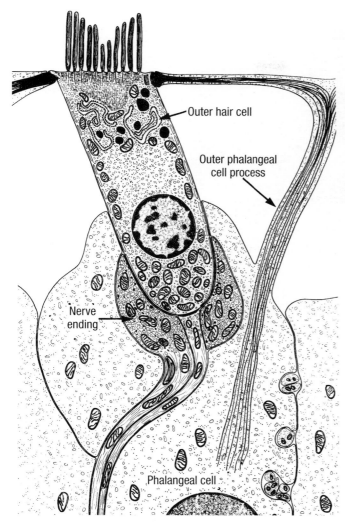

Figure 23.11 Drawing of the relationship between an outer hair cell and the flat head of the lateral process of its supporting phalangeal cell.

of the tunnel, are tall cells with an unusual shape. They have a broad base containing the nucleus, but they narrow to a slender cylindrical portion that is not in contact with neighboring cells. This then widens, at the apex, into a thin plate, which is attached by junctional complexes to other cells of the reticular lamina (Figs 23.9,23.11,23.12). Microtubules arising in the basal cytoplasm converge into a dense bundle that completely fills the slender pillar of the cell. Interspersed among the microtubules are 6nm microfilaments. In the apical plate, the microtubules diverge and many of them end in the junctional complexes with adjacent cells. These bundles of microtubules give the pillars the stiffness to buttress the reticular plate containing the upper ends of the hair cells.

The hair cells of the organ of Corti are arranged in parallel ranks. The **inner hair cells** form a single row along the entire length of the organ (Fig.23.13). On the apical surface of each is a U-shaped bundle of 50–60 hairs. A kinocilium is lacking. Some distance lateral to the inner hair cells are three rows of taller **outer hair cells**, with their stereocilia distributed in a V- or W-shaped pattern (Fig.23.14). The stereocilia are stiffened by a dense bundle of actin filaments in their interior. They vary in length in a step-

wise manner, so that the bundle has a short side and a long side. A thin fiber called a **tip-link** runs diagonally from the tip of each stereocilium to the tip of the next stereocilium in the row (Fig.23.15). The tips of the stereocilia are embedded in the **tectorial membrane**. Again, this is not a true membrane but a gelatinous sheet of glycoprotein stiffened by integral 4nm filaments of a protein related to keratin (Figs 23.9,23.10). The rounded base of each hair cell is set up in a cup-shaped depression in the body of the supporting phalangeal cell, with afferent and efferent nerves interposed between the supporting cell and the hair cell.

HISTOPHYSIOLOGY OF THE INNER EAR

Vestibular function

During any disturbance of equilibrium, the vestibular apparatus, consisting of the utricle, saccule, and semicircular ducts, responds to acceleration of the head by sending nerve impulses to the brain that initiate reflexes to restore the body to its normal position. The receptor for linear acceleration of the head is the horizontally oriented **macula utriculi**. When the head undergoes linear acceleration, the otolith membrane remains relatively stationary, while the hair cells beneath it move slightly with the wall of the utricle, causing a deflection of the stereocilia in the direction opposite to that of the head movement. The information relayed to the brain initiates the corrective movements. The orientation of the **macula sacculi**, on the other hand, is nearly vertical and it responds to sudden movements of the head at a right angle to those that activate the macula of the utricle.

The receptors that detect angular acceleration of the head are situated in the ampullae of the three semicircular canals. The anterior (or superior) semicircular duct and the posterior semicircular duct are oriented approximately vertically, at an angle to one another, and the lateral duct is nearly horizontal. Angular acceleration of the head causes motion of the wall of one of the canals relative to the endolymph in the lumen. As the cupula is displaced, the stereocilia of the underlying hair cells are flexed in the opposite direction, resulting in depolarizing of the cells and

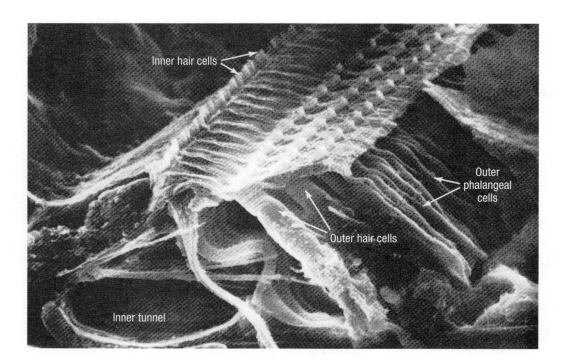

Figure 23.13 Scanning electron micrograph of a guinea pig organ of Corti cut transversely and viewed obliquely. Note the rows of hair cells (top), and the outer phalangeal cells at the right. (Micrograph courtesy of H. Engstrom.)

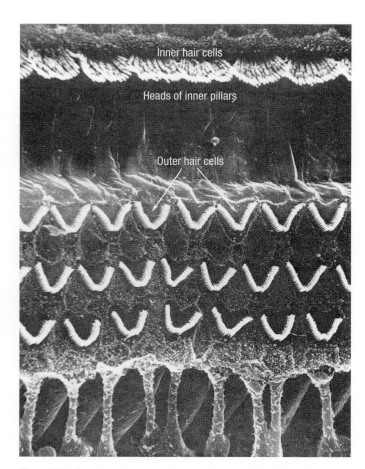

Figure 23.14 Scanning micrograph of a guinea pig organ of Corti viewed from above. The bundles of stereocilia appear V-shaped. In the human they have a W-shape, but otherwise, the structure of the organ is the same. (Micrograph courtesy of H. Engstrom.)

an increase in frequency of their impulses to the brain. Thus, the hair cells act as minute strain-gauges, responding to movement of their stereocilia towards the kinocilium. The brain responds by activating muscles influencing the position of the eyes and other muscle groups that tend to correct the disturbance of equilibrium. The three canals in each ear are slightly displaced

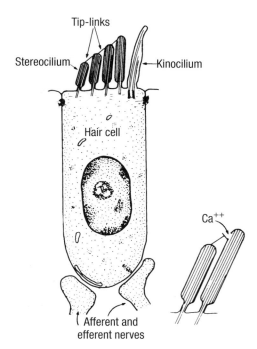

Figure 23.15 Drawing of a vestibular hair cell showing the tip-links between them. Deflection of the stereocilia opens ion channels, permitting influx of Ca^{2+} ions. (Reproduced from J.T. Corwin and M.E. Warhol *Am Rev Neurosci* 1991; 13:301.)

off the center axis so that the brain receives information from six different sources (angles), rather than from each of three canals whose orientation is identical.

Auditory function

Sound waves produce vibrations of the tympanic membrane that are transmitted, via the malleus, incus, and the stapes, to the fluid in the cochlear canal. The auditory ossicles have an amplifying effect, transforming a very low pressure on the eardrum to a 20-fold greater pressure on the fluid in the cochlea. The foot-plate of the stapes acts like a piston, alternately compressing and easing the pressure on the endolymph. The induced pressure wave-front progresses through the endolymph of the scala media, resulting in a vibration of the basilar membrane that causes a rocking motion of the organ of Corti. The resulting shearing forces move the stereocilia with respect to the overlying tectorial membrane. When the bundle is deflected towards its tall side, the tip-links between successive rows of stereocilia are stretched, resulting in opening of **transduction channels** near the tips of the stereocilia. These permit entry of Ca^{2+} ions, creating an inward current that depolarizes the hair cell membrane. This triggers an increase in the release of neurotransmitters at the basolateral surface of the hair cells, activating the sensory nerve endings. The tip-links thus serve as gating springs, opening the ion channels. Deflection of the bundle towards its short side tends to close the channels.

Thus, unlike other types of sensory cells, hair cells do not depend upon a cascade of chemical reactions to generate a signal. Such a process would be too slow for detection of sound. To process sound in the high frequencies of human hearing, it is estimated that the hair cells would have to turn current on and off more than 10 000 times a second. Instead, the mechanism that makes hearing possible depends on the tip-links and the fact that the inner resting potential of the hair cells is negative, whereas that of the surrounding endolymph is positive, making the transmembrane potential across the apices of the hair cells higher than that of any other cell type. This increases their sensitivity to slight movement of their hairs. A deflection of only 3 nm is the threshold of hearing. This is comparable to deflection of the top of the Eiffel Tower by a thumb's breadth. A deflection of 50–120 nm results in a near maximal response.

The perception of sound intensity (loudness) is called **amplitude discrimination**. This sense is dependent on the degree of displacement of the basilar membrane at any given frequency. The ability of the ear to distinguish the **frequency** (pitch) of a sound has long been attributed to differences in width of the basilar membrane along its length and to differences in length of the stereocilia on the hair cells. Each tone was believed to produce maximal amplitude of vibration in a particular region of the membrane, with sound of high frequency having the greatest effect on the membrane near the base of the cochlea, and sound of low frequency producing maximal vibration near the helicotrema. Nerve fibers from each level along the membrane are thought to conduct impulses to an area of the brain where there are neurons that are activated by specific frequencies. Interpretation of this passive mechanism, based on the differing width of the basilar membrane along its length, still holds true, but there is recent experimental evidence for an active fine-tuning of frequency, namely, selectivity by motor activity of the hair cells. The outer hair cells normally vary in length, from 20–50 μm near the base of the cochlea to 75–90 μm near its apex. Isolated hair cells, in the absence of a basilar membrane, have been found to respond to mechanical or electrical stimulation by a slight change in their length. Long cells respond best to low frequencies, and short cells to high frequencies. The best frequency for inducing a motor response, in a given cell, is correlated with the length of the cell and its original position in the cochlea.

There are only about 16 000 hair cells in the human cochlea and they have little or no capacity for regeneration. Millions of people suffer from impaired hearing as a result of loss of, or damage to, their hair cells. We live in an environment in which loud sounds are common, and about 40% of our hair cells are lost by the age of 65. In experimental animals, a 2 h exposure to a loud noise, such as a loud rock band, is enough to damage seriously the bundles of stereocilia in the inner ear.

Questions

1 What is the source of the endolymph in the membranous labyrinth of the inner ear?

  a Reissner's membrane

  b stria vascularis

  c tympanic membrane

  d helicotrema

  e endolymphatic sac

2 Which structure connects the middle ear with the oral cavity or nasopharynx?

  a oval window

  b malleus

  c cochlea

  d auditory (eustachian) tube

  e round window

3 Which of the following space(s) is/are filled with air?

  a tympanic cavity

  b vestibule

  c auditory tube

  d a and c

  e b and c

4 Which cells serve a supportive function in the organ of Corti?

  a Hensen's cells

  b inner pillar cells

  c outer pillar cells

  d both phalangeal cell types

  e all of the above

5 In the ear, the tectorial membrane

  a separates air from endolymph

  b separates air from perilymph

  c is surrounded by air

  d separates endolymph from perilymph

  e is surrounded by endolymph

6 Within the cochlea, hair cells of the inner ear project their stereocilia into which structure?

  a Reissner's membrane

  b basilar membrane

  c tympanic membrane

  d vestibular membrane

  e tectorial membrane

7 Within the inner ear, where are the maculae located?

  a one in the saccule and one in the utricle

  b two in the saccule

  c two in the utricle

  d one in each semicircular canal

  e in the cochlea

8 In the auditory apparatus, which of the following structures serves a function similar to that of the cupula and otolithic membrane in the vestibular apparatus?

  a Reissner's membrane

  b basilar membrane

  c tympanic membrane

  d vestibular membrane

  e tectorial membrane

9 The ability of the cochlea to distinguish different frequencies of sound is principally because of differences in properties of

  a regions of the tectorial membrane

  b kinocilia on hair cells

  c regions of the tympanic membrane

  d synapses made by sensory neurons of the spiral ganglion

  e regions of the basilar membrane

10 The oval window separates

  a air from endolymph

  b air from perilymph

  c air from air

  d endolymph from perilymph

  e air from ectolymph

11 What structure produces endolymph?

12 What ossicle is connected to the tympanic membrane?

13 What structure of the ear is associated with hairs and sebaceous and ceruminous glands?

14 What surrounds the tectorial membrane?

15 What is the name of the structures in the inner ear that are composed primarily of calcium carbonate?

16 What is the name of the structure in the organ of Corti that supports the inner and outer hair cells, cells of Henson, and the inner and outer phalangeal cells?

17 The varying width of what membrane allows the perception of different frequencies of sound?

18 What structure connects the middle ear with the nasopharynx?

19 Changes in angular acceleration are detected by what structures?

20 Transmission of sound from air to fluid occurs at what structure in the ear?

Glossary

A-band
The dark band of the sarcomere in skeletal and cardiac muscle containing the myosin filaments and a short segment of the actin filaments of the adjacent I-bands.

A-cell (α-cell)
A cell type in the Islets of Langerhans of the pancreas that secretes the hormone glucagon.

Acidophils
Cells of the hypophysis that have a high affinity for acid dyes. They include the somatotrophs, secreting growth hormone, and lactotrophs, secreting prolactin.

Acetylcholine
A neurotransmitter released at neuromuscular junctions and at some synapses of the autonomic nervous system.

Acinus
A spherical functional subunit of an exocrine gland, consisting of pyramidal epithelial cells around a small lumen.

ACTH
(See *adrenocorticotrophic hormone*)

Actin
A protein that polymerizes to form the microfilaments of the cytoskeleton. Actin filaments interact with myosin filaments in muscle contraction and in cell locomotion.

Active transport
An energy-dependent carrier-mediated transport of molecules across a membrane against an electrochemical gradient.

Adenosine triphosphate (ATP)
A molecule that releases energy upon transfer of phosphate to various substrates. It serves as a store of free energy needed for many of the biochemical reactions of cell metabolism.

Aldosterone
A hormone of the adrenal cortex acting upon the kidney to control body fluid balance.

Adrenocorticotrophic hormone
A hormone of the anterior hypophysis that stimulates the adrenal cortex to release its hormones (cortisol, aldosterone, and androgens).

Alveolus
A thin-walled subunit of the lung where exchange of O_2 and CO_2 takes place between the blood and the inspired air

Ameloblast
The cell type of a developing tooth that produces the enamel.

Amnion
The innermost of the fetal membranes that forms the wall of a fluid-filled sac surrounding the embryo.

Anabolism
Synthetic processes of metabolism, as opposed to catabolism, the degradation of substances to smaller units.

Anaphase
The stage of mitosis in which chromatids separate and move to opposite poles of the spindle.

Androgens
A generic term for the male sex hormones.

Anemia
A deficiency of red blood cells, or of hemoglobin.

Aneuploidy
Any departure from the normal number of chromosomes for a given species.

Angiogenesis
The formation of new blood vessels by sprouting from pre-existing blood vessels.

Ankyrin
A protein that links the actin-binding protein spectrin to an integral membrane protein of the erythrocyte.

Antibody
A protein produced by B-lymphocytes that binds to a specific antigen (foreign protein) in the humoral immune response.

Antigen
Any substance inducing an immune response, usually a protein foreign to the body.

Antigen-presenting cell
A phagocytic cell that digests foreign protein and presents antigenic peptides to B or T-lymphocytes to elicit an immune response.

Apical domain
The portion of the plasma membrane on the free surface of an epithelial cell.

Apocrine secretion
A mode of secretion in which the apical portion of the cell, containing accumulated secretory product is shed into the lumen.

Apoptosis
Programmed cell death. An active process distinct from **necrosis**, cell death resulting from toxins or cell injury.

Argentaffin cells — Cells of the gastrointestinal tract in which cytoplasmic deposits of metallic silver are formed when stained with silver salts. This is due to their content of the neurotransmitter, serotonin.

Astrocyte — A type of glial cell in the brain and spinal cord that provides mechanical and metabolic support for the neurons.

ATP (adenosine triphosphate) — A molecule that yields free energy upon hydrolysis of the terminal phosphate. It serves as a store of energy for many of the biochemical reactions of cell metabolism.

Autoantibody — An antibody that binds to a normal constituent of the body, instead of to a foreign protein.

Autoimmunity — An abnormal condition in which the body mounts an immune response against one of its own tissues.

Autonomic ganglia — Bodies containing the cell bodies of post-ganglionic neurons of the autonomic nervous system.

Autonomic nervous system — The division of the peripheral nervous system that innervates cardiac and smooth muscle and glands. Also called the **involuntary nervous system**.

Autophagy — Destruction of cytoplasmic organelles by enclosing them in a membrane to which lysosomes fuse releasing hydrolytic-enzymes that digest the organelle.

Axon — The long cell process of a neuron that carries impulses from the cell body to a synapse on an effector cell.

Axoneme — The cytoskeleton of cilia and flagella consisting of 2 single microtubules surrounded by 9 triplet microtubules.

Axoplasm — The cytoplasm of an axon, the long cell process of a neuron that is capable of exhibiting action potentials.

Azurophilic granules — Cytoplasmic granules of neutrophils containing hydrolytic enzymes. They are functionally equivalent to lysosomes.

B-cells (β-cells) — Cells of the islets of Langerhans in the pancreas that synthesize and release the hormone, insulin.

B-lymphocytes — A class of lymphocytes that synthesize immunoglobulins (antibodies) that mediate the humoral immune response.

Band cells — Immature neutrophils that do not yet have a polymorphous nucleus. They are released into the blood from the bone marrow, usually in response to an infection.

Basal body — A structure at the base of a cilium. It resembles a centriole and nucleates tubulin polymerization to form the microtubules of the axoneme of the cilium.

Basal lamina — The compact layer of extracellular matrix immediately beneath the cells of an epithelium. Formerly called the **basement membrane**.

Basolateral domain — That portion of the plasma membrane of a polarized epithelial cell which is in contact with adjacent cells, and with the basal lamina.

Basophilia — The preferential binding of basic dyes to certain components of cells.

Basophil — A type of leukocyte that has in its cytoplasm large basophilic granules containing histamine.

Basophilic erythroblast — An early stage in development of an erythrocyte. It is a large cell with a heterochromatic nucleus and a cytoplasm rich in ribosomes.

Bile — The fluid secreted by cells of the liver (hepatocytes) and stored in the gall bladder. It facilitates lipid absorption in the intestine.

Bile canaliculi — Minute channels between hepatocytes that conduct bile to a system of larger hepatic ducts.

Blast cells — A general term for cells at the earliest stage in the differentiation of any of the hemopoietic cell lineages in the bone marrow.

Bowman's capsule — A double-walled cup at the proximal end of a nephron that contains the glomerulus. Also called the **glomerular capsule**.

Brown fat — A form of adipose tissue specialized for lipid storage and heat production. Also called **multilocular adipose tissue**.

Brunner's glands — Glands in the submucosa of the duodenum secreting an alkaline mucin that neutralizes the acidic gastric secretions.

Brush border — A specialization of the apical surface of certain epithelial cells, consisting of closely spaced microvilli.

Bundle of His — A bundle of specialized myocytes that conduct impulses from the atrioventricular node to the cardiac muscle of the ventricles. Also called the **atrioventricular bundle**.

Cadherins — A class of membrane proteins involved in calcium-dependent adhesion of neighboring epithelial cells.

Calcitonin — A hormone secreted by the parafollicular cells of the thyroid gland. It decreases the activity of osteoclasts to lower blood calcium.

Calcium channel — A protein complex in the cell membrane forming a channel through which calcium ions can enter the cell.

Canaliculi — Narrow channels in the calcified matrix of bone connecting the lacunae containing osteocytes.

Capacitation — Changes occurring in the plasma membrane of the sperm head in preparation for fertilization.

Capillary — A very small, thin-walled blood vessel that conducts blood from an arteriole to a venule.

Carotid body — A small body at the bifurcation of the carotid artery containing cells that sense the oxygen concentration of the blood and influence respiratory rate.

Carotid sinus — A specialized region of the common carotid artery serving as a baroreceptor sensitive to changes in blood pressure.

Carrier protein — A protein that selectively binds to small molecules and transports them across a membrane.

Catabolism — The breakdown of substances to smaller units, as opposed to **anabolism**, the synthetic activities of metabolism.

Catecholamines — The hormones of the adrenal medulla (epinephrine, and norepinephrine).

Cell body — The portion of a cell between the nucleus and the plasmalemma. The term is most often used to specify the perinuclear portion of a neuron, while excluding its axon and dendrites. Also called the **perikaryon**.

Cell cortex — A firm layer of cytoplasm underlying the plasma membrane, consisting of a meshwork of cross-linked actin filaments.

Cell cycle — The sequence of events between two cell divisions. It is divided into four stages designated G_1, S, G_2, and M (mitosis). Cells that are not cycling are said to be in a fifth stage, G_0.

Cell-mediated immune response — An immune response in which cytotoxic T-lymphocytes are the active agents, releasing substances that lyse foreign or virus-infected cells.

Centriole — A short cylindrical organelle consisting of 9 triplet microtubules around a central cavity. Centrioles occur in pairs with their long axes oriented perpendicular to one another.

Centromere — The primary constriction of a chromosome where sister chromatids are adherent to one another at metaphase of mitosis.

Centrosome — An organelle, containing two centrioles embedded in an amorphous matrix that is the site of nucleation of tubulin to form microtubules. The centrosome divides prior to cell division and daughter centrosomes form the poles of the mitotic spindle.

Channel proteins — Integral proteins of the plasma membrane which form pores that permit passage of ions and small molecules through the membrane down a concentration gradient.

Chemotaxis — A process in which motile cells migrate up the concentration gradient of a diffusible substance. It is important for the mobilization of neutrophils and macrophages at a site of bacterial invasion.

Chiasma — A crossing over of the free arms of chromatids in the tetrads formed in prophase of meiosis I. It results in exchange of segments of the genome of homologous chromosomes.

Cholecystokinin — A peptide released by the I-cells of the duodenal mucosa that stimulates gall bladder contraction and release of bile to facilitate digestion of fats in the jejunum.

Cholesterol — An important molecule that is synthesized in the liver. It is a major component of cell membranes and is a precursor in the synthesis of steroid hormones.

Chondrocyte — The principal cell type of hyaline cartilage.

Choroid — The vascular layer of the eye located between the sclera and the retina.

Choroid plexus — Highly vascular folds of the ependyma and pia mater projecting into the ventricles of the brain. It is involved in formation of the cerebrospinal fluid.

Chorion — The outermost layer of the early embryo that gives rise to the trophoblast of the placenta.

Chromaffin tissue — Tissue in the medulla of the adrenal gland that produces the hormones epinephrine and norepinephrine.

Chromatid — One of the two subunits of a mitotic chromosome.

Chromatin — Clumps of basophilic material in the interphase nucleus consisting of coiled molecules of DNA and associated histone proteins.

Chromosomes — Rod-like structures formed in the nucleus at prophase of cell division. Each contains two molecules of DNA and associated histone proteins and has a characteristic length and banding pattern.

Cilia — Slender, motile, cell processes on some epithelial cells, that beat to-and-fro in synchrony to move a film of mucus across the surface of the epithelium.

Cisternae — Membrane-bounded flat saccules that are often arranged parallel to one another. They are found in the rough endoplasmic reticulum and in the Golgi complex.

Clara cell — A non-ciliated cell type of the bronchiolar epithelium.

Clathrin — A protein that polymerizes to form a basket-like lattice around a vesicle during the process of receptor-mediated endocytosis.

Clonal deletion — Destruction of self-reactive T-lymphocytes in the thymus.

Clone The cells resulting from successive divisions of a single cell.

Coated pit A clathrin coated invagination of the plasmalemma involved in endocytosis.

Codon The basic unit of the genetic code consisting of a group of three nucleotides of DNA (or RNA) that code for a single amino acid.

Collagen A structural protein that polymerizes to form collagen fibers which are found in abundance in the extracellular connective tissues.

Colon The segment of the intestinal tract that extends from the caecum to the end of the sigmoid flexure. Also called the **large intestine.**

Complement A group of proteins of the blood plasma which are activated to increase inflammatory or immune responses.

Connexon The functional unit of the gap-junction consisting of six membrane proteins around a central pore.

Cornea The transparent tissue at the front of the eye made up of orthogonal arrays of collagen fibers covered by outer and inner layers of squamous epithelium

Cortical meshwork The dense meshwork of cross-linked actin filaments responsible for the gel-like consistency of the cell cortex.

Crenation A distortion of the plasma membrane of erythrocytes exposed to a hypertonic solution which results in a spiny appearance of the cell.

Cristae ampullaris Ridges on the floor of the ampullae of the semicircular ducts in the middle ear that bear hair-cells detecting head movement.

Crossing-over Breakage and exchange of segments between the free arms of chromatids in the tetrads, during prophase of meiosis I.

Crypts Shallow invaginations of the epithelium between intestinal villi.

Cytokines Molecules secreted to stimulate, or otherwise alter the behavior of near-by cells, in contrast to hormones which are blood-borne molecules affecting distant target cells.

Cytokinesis Cleavage of the cell body after movement of the chromosomes to the poles of the spindle in mitosis and meiosis II.

Cytoplasm The substance of the cell between the nucleus and the plasma membrane.

Cytoskeleton Cytoplasmic protein filaments of several kinds that form an internal structural framework stabilizing the shape of static cells, and contributing to the shape changes of motile cells.

Cytosol The matrix of the cytoplasm in which the membrane-bounded organelles and other formed elements are suspended.

Cytotoxic T-cells A type of T-lymphocyte that kills foreign, or virus infected cells, by lysis, in the cell-mediated immune response.

Defensins Cationic peptides that have an antimicrobial function. They are found in the azurophilic granules of neutrophils and in certain cell types of the skin and intestinal mucosa.

Dendrites Branching processes of neurons that receive electrical or chemical signals, from other neurons and carry them to the cell body.

Dendritic cells Antigen-presenting phagocytic cells in the skin, spleen and lymph nodes that process antigen and stimulate proliferation of neighboring lymphocytes. Also called Langerhans cells.

Depolarization A shift in the electrical potential of a cell, towards zero, relative to its environment.

Dermis A layer of dense connective tissue underlying the epidermis of the skin.

Desmin A protein forming the intermediate filaments characteristic of muscle cells.

Desmosome A type of junction that binds adjacent cells together and anchors the actin filaments of their cytoskeletons.

Diaphysis The shaft of a developing long bone between the distal and proximal epiphyses.

Differentiation The developmental process by which cells become biochemically and structurally specialized for a specific function.

Diploid cell A cell containing two copies of each chromosome.

DNA (deoxyribonucleic acid) The genetic material of all cells. A polymer of four nucleotides: adenine, cytosine, guanine and thymine. The sequence of nucleotides encodes the information necessary for synthesis of all the different RNAs and proteins of the body.

DNA replication The process in which copies of the DNA molecules are made prior to cell division, insuring that both of the daughter cells will contain the informational content of the entire genome.

Duodenum The first 8–10 inches of the small intestine.

Dynein A large cytoskeletal motor protein that moves vesicles or organelles along microtubules toward their minus end. It is also involved in generating the bending movements of cilia.

E-face In freeze-fracture preparations of cells, membranes are cleaved between the two layers of phospholipid molecules. In electron mcrographs, the E-face is the inner face of the outer lipid monolayer of the membrane. The **P-face** is the opposing surface of the inner leaflet of the bilayer.

Echinocyte   An erythrocyte that has shrunken in hypertonic medium and has spiny radiating surface projections.

Ectoderm   The outermost of the three primary germ layers (ectoderm, mesoderm, endoderm) of the early embryo. It gives rise to the epidermis of the skin and the nervous system.

Elastin   A glycoprotein that forms the elastic fibers of connective tissue.

Endocrine gland   A ductless gland secreting one or more hormones that are transported in the blood to a distant target organ.

Endocytosis   Uptake of material into cells by the formation of invaginations of the plasma membrane that pinch off and move into the cytoplasm as membrane-bounded vesicles.

Endoderm   The innermost germ layer of the early embryo which gives rise to the GI-tract and much of the respiratory tract.

Endomitosis   Multiple nuclear divisions without cytokinesis, resulting in a multinucleate giant cell.

Endoplasmic reticulum   An organelle consisting of a system of membrane-bounded tubules and cisternae that ramify throughout the cytoplasm. 'Rough' and 'smooth' endoplasmic reticulum are distinguished by the presence or absence of adherent ribosomes.

Endothelium   The simple squamous epithelium that lines blood and lymphatic vessels.

Enteroendocrine cells   Widely scattered solitary endocrine cells in the epithelium of the gastrointestinal tract.

Eosinophil   A granular leukocyte that contains eosinophilic granules. Eosinophils are increased in number in allergic reactions and parasitic infections.

Eosinophil cationic protein   A protein in the granules of eosinophils that is toxic for certain parasites of humans.

Ependyma   A cuboidal epithelium lining the ventricles of the brain.

Epidermis   The stratified squamous epithelium forming the outermost layer of the skin.

Epididymis   A highly convoluted epithelial tubule on the posterior surface of the testis in which spermatozoa are stored and complete their maturation.

Epiphysis   An end segment of a developing long bone separated from the diaphysis by an intervening layer of hyaline cartilage, called the epiphyseal plate.

Epithelium   A sheet of cells covering an outside surface, or lining the lumen of a body cavity or hollow internal organ.

Equatorial plate   The plane midway between the poles of the mitotic spindle, on which the chromosomes become aligned in metaphase of mitotic and meiotic cell divisions.

Erythroblast   A nucleated cell of the bone marrow that undergoes further differentiation to give rise to an erythrocyte.

Erythrocyte   An anucleate cell of the blood containing hemoglobin for transport of O_2 to the tissues. Also called a **red blood cell**.

Erythropoiesis   The production of erythrocytes in the bone marrow.

Erythropoietin   A glycoprotein produced in the kidneys, that regulates production of erythrocytes by the bone marrow.

Estrogens   Female sex hormones produced by the ovaries (viz. estradiol and estrone).

Euchromatin   The unstained portion of the chromatin of the interphase nucleus that is in a decondensed state to make its nucleotide sequences accessible for transcription.

Exocrine glands   Glands that release their product into a system of ducts opening onto an internal or external surface.

Exocytosis   Release of a substance from a cell by fusion of the limiting membrane of a vesicle (or secretory granule) with the plasma membrane.

Extracellular matrix   The ground substance and fibrous components the connective tissues of the body.

Fallopian tube   (See *Oviduct*)

Fibrillar center   A pale-staining region of a nucleolus, containing a segment of the chromosome that is being transcribed to generate RNA molecules that bind to protein to form ribonucleoproteins that condense to form the pars granulosa of the nucleolus.

Fibrin   A fibrous protein formed by interaction of thrombin and fibrinogen during blood clotting.

Fibrinogen   A large soluble protein present in blood plasma that gives rise to fibrin during blood clotting.

Fibroblast   A major cell type of connective tissue that synthesizes collagen, which polymerizes extracellularly to form the collagen fibers of the extracellular matrix. Also called a **fibrocyte**.

Filamin   One of the actin-binding proteins that cross-link actin filaments into a dense meshwork that gives the cytosol its gel-like consistency.

Filopodium   A long slender cell process of motile cells that binds, at its tip to extracellular components.

Fimbrin   An actin-binding protein that cross-links the actin filaments in the core of each microvillus of the brush-border of epithelial cells.

Flagellum   A long motile cell process containing an axoneme like that of a cilium. The spermatozoon is propelled by bending movements of its long flagellum.

Follicle   A structure in the cortex of the ovary, consisting of an ovum enveloped by one or more layers of epithelial cells.

Follicle-stimulating hormone   A glycoprotein hormone of the hypophysis that stimulates development of ovarian follicles and their production of estrogens.

Freeze-fracture   A method of specimen preparation in which tissue is rapidly frozen and then fractured. A heavy metal is then evaporated onto the fracture surface, followed by deposition of a carbon film over it. The tissue is then digested away and the resulting replica of the fracture face is examined with an electron microscope.

FSH   (See *follicle-stimulating hormone*)

Gamete   A sex cell: either a spermatozoon or an ovum.

Ganglion   A cluster of neuronal cell-bodies outside of the central nervous system.

Gap junction   A junctional specialization in which hexagonal arrays of transmembrane proteins (connexons) in the membranes of adjacent cells, surround a pore that permits movement of small molecules between cells.

Gastrin   A peptide secreted by the G-cells in the gastric mucosa that stimulates secretion by the gastric glands.

Gene   A segment of a DNA molecule that encodes a particular protein or ribonucleic acid molecule.

Gene expression   Transcription and translation of the information encoded in a gene for the synthesis of a particular protein.

Gland   An organ consisting of epithelial cells specialized for synthesis and release of a product. In exocrine glands the product is released into a system of ducts. In endocrine glands it is released into the blood.

Glial cells   Non-neuronal cells of the nervous system that provide mechanical and metabolic support and insulation for the neurons.

Glomerulus   A cluster of contorted capillaries at the upper end of each nephron that filter the blood to form urine.

Glucagon   A polypeptide hormone secreted by the A-cells of the islets of Langerhans of the pancreas. It increases the blood glucose level, as opposed to insulin, which lowers blood glucose.

Glycocalyx   A poorly staining fuzzy layer on the free surface of certain epithelia, consisting of the long carbohydrate chains of integral membrane glycoproteins at the tips of the microvilli.

Glycogen   A polymer of glucose formed for short term storage of carbohydrate in the cell cytoplasm.

Goblet cell   A cell type in the epithelia of the intestinal and respiratory tracts that secretes mucus. The name is descriptive of their shape, in which the cell base is narrow while the apical region is expanded with accumulated secretory product.

Gonads   The reproductive organs: testes in the male, ovaries in the female.

Gonadotropins   A general term for hormones of the anterior pituitary that stimulate the growth and functioning of the gonads.

Graafian follicle   The mature ovarian follicle.

Granulocyte   Any of the white blood cells that have conspicuous granules in their cytoplasm (neutrophil, eosinophil and basophil).

Growth hormone   A hormone of the anterior pituitary that stimulates growth. Also called somatotropin.

Hair cells   Receptor cells in the labyrinth and cochlea of the inner ear that possess stereocilia which detect gravity, acceleration or sound.

Hair follicles   Epithelial extensions of the epidermis into the dermis that generate hairs.

Haploid   Having a single set of unpaired chromosomes.

Hassall's corpuscles   Aggregations of concentrically arranged flat epithelial cells found in the medulla of the thymus.

Haversian system   A subunit of compact bone consisting of concentric layers of calcified bone matrix around a central canal (Haversian canal) occupied by a capillary.

Helicotrema   A small opening between the scala vestibuli and the scala tympani at the apex of the cochlear duct.

Helper T-cell   T-lymphocytes that respond to an antigen by secreting cytokines that stimulate B-lymphocytes specific for the same antigen.

Hemopoiesis   The process of blood cell formation in the bone marrow.

Hemoglobin   The oxygen-transporting protein of erythrocytes.

Hemopoietic stem cell   A pluripotential cell of the bone marrow which divides repeatedly, giving rise to blast cells of different lineages that differentiate into the several types of blood cells.

Hepatocytes	Epithelial cells of the parenchyma of the liver.
Heterochromatin	The clumps of basophilic material of the interphase nucleus that consist of condensed chromatin thought to be transcriptionally inactive.
Histamine	A small molecule stored in the granules of mast cells, and released upon contact of these cells with an antigen. It initiates inflammation.
Histogenesis	The process of formation of a tissue by proliferation, aggregation and differentiation of its cells.
Holocrine secretion	A mode of secretion in which entire cells containing a secretory product are shed into the lumen of the gland.
Homologous chromosomes	Pairs of chromosomes (maternal and paternal) that are of the same length and have comparable genetic loci.
Hormone	A secretory product that is carried in the blood to affect distant target cells that have specific receptors for that molecule.
Humoral immune response	An immune response involving B-lymphocyte production of antibodies against a foreign protein (antigen).
Hyperplasia	Growth of a tissue beyond its normal size due to increase in cell number through cell division.
Hyperthyroidism	Excess production of thyroid hormone. Also called **Grave's disease**.
Hypertrophy	Enlargement of an organ due to increase in size of its cells.
I-band	A pale-staining segment of the sarcomere of striated muscle consisting of actin filaments.
IL-l	An interleukin produced by macrophages that activates antibody production by B-lymphocytes.
IL-2	An interleukin produced by helper-lymphocytes that promotes B-lymphocyte proliferation.
Ileum	The distal portion of the small intestine, extending from the end of the jejunum to the caecum.
Immune response	An activation of the immune system. It may involve production of antibodies by B-lymphocytes, or lysis of foreign, or virus infected cells by cytotoxic T-lymphocytes.
Inflammation	A response of tissues to injury or bacterial invasion involving vasodilatation, and mobilization of large numbers of neutrophils, and macrophages to phagocytize the bacteria or damaged cells.
Insulin	A polypeptide hormone secreted by the B-cells of the islets of Langerhans that lowers blood glucose by enhancing its trans-membrane transport into muscle, liver and adipose tissue.

Integrins	A class of integral membrane proteins that bind to components of the extracellular matrix.
Intercalated disc	An interdigitated junctional complex between cardiac muscle cells.
Interleukins	Cytokines produced by cells of the immune system to activate, or induce proliferation of, other cells of the system. Eighteen or more different interleukins have been identified.
Intermediate filaments	A class of cytoskeletal filaments about 10 nm in diameter. They consist of different proteins in different cell types (viz. keratin, vimentin, desmin).
Interphase	The period when a cell is not in division. It includes the G_1, S, and G_2 stages of the cell cycle.
Interstitial cells	Cells in the interstices between the seminiferous tubules of the testis that secrete testosterone. Also called Leydig cells.
Ion channels	Pores formed by integral proteins of the plasma membrane through which ions can diffuse into or out of the cell down their concentration gradient.
Ion pump	A membrane protein that uses the energy released by ATP hydrolysis for active transport of ions across a membrane against their concentration gradient.
Jejunum	The segment of the small intestine between the duodenum and the ileum.
Juxtaglomerular apparatus	Specialized cells in the distal tubule and the adjacent afferent arteriole of a renal glomerulus. Those in the wall of the arteriole secrete renin, a molecule that increases blood pressure.
Karyotype	A complete set of the paired homologous chromosomes of a given species.
Keratin	An intermediate filament protein found in cells of the skin and certain other epithelia, and in hair and nails.
Keratinocytes	Cells in the upper layers of the epidermis that contain large amounts of keratin.
Kinesin	A cytoskeletal motor protein that uses the energy released by ATP hydrolysis to move vesicles and other cargo along a microtubule towards its plus end.
Kinetochore	A proteinaceous layer on the outer surface of the centromere of chromosomes, to which microtubules of the spindle attach.
Kupffer cells	A type of macrophage (fixed macrophage) associated with the endothelium lining the sinusoids in the liver.

Lacunae Cavities in the calcified matrix of bone, occupied by osteocytes. Also, similar cavities in cartilage matrix that are occupied by chondrocytes.

Lamella One layer of a multilayered structure such as an Haversian system of bone.

Lamellipodium A broad flat cell process involved in the actin-based motility of fibroblasts and other cell types.

Lamins A class of intermediate filament-like proteins (lamins A, B and C) that make up the nuclear lamina.

Laminin A glycoprotein that is a major component of the basal lamina of epithelia.

Langerhans cells Phagocytic cells in the epidermis specialized for presentation of antigen to lymphocytes. They are comparable to the **dendritic cells** of lymph nodes and spleen.

Leukocyte A general term for any of the white blood cell types.

Leydig cells Testosterone-secreting cells located between the seminiferous tubules of the testis. Also called **interstitial cells** of the testis.

LH (See *luteinizing hormone*).

Ligand A molecule that binds specifically to another molecule, viz. a hormone bound to its receptor is its ligand.

Lipids A heterogeneous group of compounds that are insoluble, or only slightly soluble, in water (viz. fats, oils, waxes).

Low density lipoprotein (LDL) An important component of the blood plasma with the primary function of transporting cholesterol to and from the tissues.

Luteinizing hormone (LH) A pituitary hormone that stimulates maturation of ovarian follicles and triggers ovulation. In the male, it stimulates secretion of testosterone by the Leydig cells of the testis.

Lumen The cavity within a hollow organ such as the intestine, or a blood vessel.

Lymph The fluid in the lymphatic vessels that returns excess extracellular fluid to the blood.

Lymphocyte A type of leukocyte that occurs in two morphologically similar, but functionally distinct forms: the B-lymphocyte, that produces antibodies in the humoral immune response, and the T-lymphocyte which is the agent of the cell-mediated immune response.

Lymph node A small organ that filters lymph and mounts an immune response to bacteria, and other foreign proteins.

Lymphoid tissue A tissue rich in lymphocytes, macrophages and reticular cells (viz. lymph nodes, thymus, spleen and Peyer's patches).

Lymphokines Signaling molecules produced by lymphocytes, and macrophages, that act upon neighboring cells to enhance their function or stimulate their proliferation.

Lysis Disintegration of a cell by breakdown of its plasma membrane and loss of its cytoplasm.

Lysosome A cell organelle rich in hydrolytic enzymes involved in the degradation of substances taken up by endocytosis, and in the elimination of aged or damaged cell organelles.

M-cells Solitary cells in the intestinal epithelium overlying lymphoid nodules, that take up antigens from the lumen and pass them on to macrophages for presentation to lymphocytes that occupy a recess in the base of the cell. These then enter the underlying lymphoid tissue and initiate an immune response to those antigens.

Macrophage A cell type specialized for phagocytosis and presentation of antigens to T-lymphocytes. The macrophage develops by further differentiation of a monocyte.

Macula A receptor organ in the vestibule of the inner ear involved in maintaining the body's equilibrium by detecting gravity and linear acceleration.

Mammary gland The milk-secreting gland within a female breast.

Marginal band An equatorial ring-like bundle of microtubules that maintains the flattened shape of blood platelets.

Mast cell A cell type of connective tissue that has many meta-chromatic granules in its cytoplasm containing histamine, a mediator of inflammation and the symptoms of allergy.

Megakaryocyte A large multinucleated cell of the bone marrow that gives rise to the blood platelets.

Meiosis A process of producing haploid gametes. An initial division (meiosis-I), after DNA replication, is immediately followed by a second division (meiosis-II), without prior replication of the DNA, resulting in four haploid daughter cells.

Melanin A brown to black pigment produced by specialized cells (melanocytes) of the epidermis. It is also present in hair and contributes to eye-color.

Melanocyte A cell of the epidermis, dermis or iris producing melanin granules (melanosomes).

Melanosomes Membrane-bounded cytoplasmic granules containing melanin, which are produced by melanocytes. They may be transferred to other cell types such as the keratinocytes of the epidermis.

Melatonin A hormone secreted by the pineal gland that inhibits release of gonadotropins from the hypophysis. It is also involved in maintenance of the circadian rhythm of metabolism.

Merocrine secretion A mode of secretion in which, the limiting membrane of secretory granules fuses with the plasma membrane to release the cell product.

Mesenchyme The embryonic tissue that gives rise to the connective tissue of the adult.

Mesoderm The middle of the three primary germ layers of the early embryo that gives rise to the musculoskeletal, blood-vascular, and urogenital systems.

Mesothelium The simple squamous epithelium that lines the peritoneal, pericardial and pleural cavities.

Messenger ribonucleic acid (mRNA) A long RNA molecule that serves as a template for protein synthesis.

Metaplasia The transformation of one type of adult tissue into another.

Metastasis The establishment of a secondary malignant tumor by transport of cells of the primary tumor through blood or lymphatic vessels to a new site in the body.

Microtubule A long cytoplasmic tubule, with a diameter of about 25 nm and a wall 5 nm thick, that is a heteropolymer of the proteins α-tubulin and β-tubulin. Microtubules serve as tracks along which vesicles or organelles can be moved from place to place by motor proteins.

Microvilli Slender processes of uniform length and diameter on the apical surface of certain epithelial cells. Hundreds of closely spaced microvilli constitute the brush border of absorptive epithelia.

Mitochondrion A bacilliform cytoplasmic organelle that synthesizes ATP which provides the energy needed for many of the biochemical reactions of cell metabolism.

Mitosis The process of somatic cell division which insures that the two daughter cells will each have the same number of pairs of homologous chromosomes as the parent cell.

Monocyte A type of blood leukocyte that will later migrate through the wall of a capillary and differentiate into a macrophage of the connective tissue.

Motor end plate The specialized junction between the end of a nerve axon and a skeletal muscle fiber, where release of acetylcholine from the axon stimulates the muscle to contract. Also called a **neuromuscular junction**.

Myelin sheath An insulating layer consisting of many layers of membrane wrapped around a nerve axon. It is formed by Schwann cells in the peripheral nerves, or by oligodendrocytes, in the central nervous system.

Myelocyte A cell of the bone marrow that is an intermediate stage in the development of a granular leukocyte of the blood.

Myocardium The thick layer of cardiac muscle making up most of the wall of the heart.

Myoepithelial cells Stellate contractile cells found between the epithelium and the basal lamina of the acini in certain glands (viz. mammary gland). Their contraction is believed to constrict the acini of the gland contributing to movement of the secretion into the duct system.

Myometrium The smooth muscle layer in the wall of the uterus.

Myosin A motor protein found in nearly all cells. In muscle cells, myosin polymerizes into thick filaments that interact with actin-containing thin filaments to generate muscle contraction.

Necrosis Death and disintegration of cells due to injury, disease or oxygen deprivation. Necrosis is distinct from apoptosis, which is a programmed cell death for elimination of excess or senescent cells.

Nephron A structural and functional unit of the kidney consisting of a renal corpuscle, and a renal tubule.

Nerve impulse A wave of self-propagating membrane depolarization that moves along the membrane of an axon.

Neuroglia Non-neuronal cells of the nervous system. They include the astrocytes, oligodendroglia, and ependymal cells.

Neuromuscular junction (See *motor end plate*).

Neuron A cell of the nervous system specialized for generation and transmission of electrical impulses along its long axon.

Neurosecretory cells Neurons that have a secretory function, releasing a hormone into the bloodstream.

Neurotransmitter A chemical that is released at the end of a nerve axon in response to depolarization of its membrane. It then diffuses across the narrow intercellular space, binds to a receptor and activates, or inhibits, a second cell. Examples of neurotransmitters are acetylcholine and serotonin.

Neutrophil A type of polymorphonuclear leukocyte specialized for taking up bacteria by phagocytosis and destroying them.

Nissl bodies   Coarse basophilic bodies in the cytoplasm of neurons. Electron microscopy has revealed that these are arrays of parallel cisternae of the rough endoplasmic reticulum. The term is seldom used now.

Norepinephrine   A neurotransmitter released at the synapses of neurons of the sympathetic nervous system.

Nucleoplasm   The content of the cell nucleus. Also called karyoplasm.

Nuclear envelope   The structure that encloses the nucleoplasm, consisting of two membranes separated by a narrow cisternal space.

Nuclear lamina   A layer of fine filaments associated with the inner surface of the nuclear envelope. Filaments of the protein lamin-A predominate in the inner half of the lamina, while the outer half consists mainly of filaments of lamin-B.

Nuclear pore   A discontinuity in the nuclear envelope, where its inner membrane is continuous with its outer membrane around a 10nm opening which permits passage of proteins and RNAs between the nucleoplasm and cytoplasm.

Nucleation   The first step initiating polymerization of monomers to form a larger structure made up of repeating subunits such as a microtubule or an actin filament.

Nucleolus   A structure within the nucleus made up of branching and rejoining strands consisting of closely packed ribonucleic acid particles. The nucleolus is the site of synthesis of the subunits of the ribosomes.

Nucleosomes   Repeating units of chromatin structure consisting of DNA wrapped around a core of eight histone molecules.

Odontoblast   A cell type of the developing tooth that secretes dentin.

Olefactory epithelium   The sensory epithelium located in the upper portion of the nasal cavity which contains the receptors for the sense of smell.

Oligodendrocyte   A type of glial cell that forms the myelin sheaths of axons in the central nervous system.

Oocyte   The developing female gamete that will ultimately be released from the ovary as an ovum.

Opsonin   A substance that binds to the surface of particles and enhances their uptake by phagocytic cells.

Organelles   Structures within the cytoplasm that carry out specific cellular functions. They are usually membrane bounded.

Osmosis   The movement of water through a membrane to balance the concentration of a solute on the two sides of the membrane.

Osteoblast   The cell type that gives rise to bone matrix.

Osteoclast   A large multinucleated cell that breaks down bone matrix and releases calcium ions into the blood.

Osteocytes   The relatively inactive bone cells that occupy lacunae in the calcified matrix of bone.

Osteoid   The initial uncalcified bone matrix secreted by osteoblasts.

Osteon   A structural subunit of bone, also called a **Haversian system**.

Ovarian follicle   A spherical structure in the cortex of the ovary made up of epithelial cells surrounding an oocyte. Later in its development it has a cavity containing follicular fluid.

Oviduct   A tubular organ into which ova are released from the ovary for transport to the uterus. Also called the **Fallopian tube**.

Oxyntic cell   An eosinophilic cell type of the gastric mucosa that secretes hydrochloric acid. Also called **parietal cell** or **chloridogenic cell**.

Oxytocin   A peptide hormone synthesized in the hypothalamus and released from the posterior lobe of the pituitary. It induces contraction of smooth muscle of the uterus, and of the myoepithelial cells of the mammary gland.

Pancreas   A major gland of the gastrointestinal tract that secretes a number of digestive enzymes into the duodenum.

Paneth cell   An eosinophilic cell type in the glands of the intestinal mucosa that secretes antimicrobial peptides, called cryptidins or defensins.

Parafollicular cells   Pale-staining solitary cells found at the base of the epithelium of thyroid follicles. Their secretory granules contain calcitonin, a polypeptide hormone involved in the regulation of blood calcium. Also called **calcitonin cells**.

Parathyroid hormone (PTH)   A peptide hormone secreted by the parathyroid glands. It stimulates osteoclasts to degrade calcified bone matrix to increase blood calcium.

Parenchyma   The specialized functional portion of an organ, excluding its connective tissue stroma.

Parietal cell   (See *oxyntic cell*).

Pepsin   A proteolytic enzyme secreted by the chief cells of gastric glands. It is activated at the low pH of the stomach contents.

Perforin A chemical produced by cytotoxic T-lymphocytes that forms holes in the plasma membrane of a target cell resulting in its lysis.

Perichondrium The layer of dense connective tissue surrounding hyaline or elastic cartilage.

Periosteum The layer of connective tissue enveloping bones. It is a source of osteogenic cells.

Pepsin An enzyme that digests proteins in the acidic environment of the gastric contents. It is secreted by the chief cells (zymogenic cells) of the gastric glands.

Pepsinogen The inactive precursor of pepsin in the secretory granules of the chief cells of the gastric glands.

Peroxisome A cytoplasmic organelle containing peroxidase and catalase.

Peyer's patches Aggregations of lymphoid tissue in the submucosa of the small intestine. Their abundant B-lymphocytes, T-lymphocytes and dendritic cells are involved in immune responses to the bacterial antigens in the gut lumen.

Phagocyte Any cell capable of phagocytosis (neutrophils, macrophages and dendritic cells).

Phagocytosis The uptake of particulate material, such as bacteria, by extending pseudopodia around it and drawing it into the cytoplasm in a large vacuole derived from the cell membrane.

Photoreceptor A sensory receptor cell that responds to photons of light viz. the rods and cones of the retina.

Plasma The fluid component of the blood.

Plasma cell A cell of the immune system arising by terminal differentiation of an antigen-stimulated B-lymphocyte. It secretes a large amount of specific antibody.

Platelet A flat, anucleate cell type of the blood that is involved in blood clotting. Also called a **thrombocyte** or **thromboplastid.**

Plicae circulares Transversely oriented folds of the intestinal mucosa and submucosa projecting into the lumen.

Podocyte A cell type with multiple cell processes that surrounds the capillaries in the glomeruli of the kidney. Narrow spaces between the cell processes, called filtration slits, permit passage of the plasma filtrate to form urine.

Polyribosome A number of ribosomes associated with a single molecule of messenger RNA.

Primary immune response The immune response to a first exposure to an antigen.

Progesterone A steroid hormone, secreted by the corpora lutea of the ovary, that promotes proliferation of the endometrium of the uterus in preparation for implantation of a fertilized ovum.

Prophase An early stage of cell division in which the chromosomes condense and the nuclear envelope breaks down.

Pseudopod A broad cell process involved in phagocytosis or amoeboid cell motility.

Purkinje fibers Specialized muscle fibers of the cardiac conduction system.

Pyknosis A terminal inactivation of the nucleus in which all of the chromatin is heterochromatin, and the nucleus appears as a small dense body of irregular shape.

Receptor A molecule that binds another molecule (its ligand) with high specificity.

Releasing hormones A generic term for hormones of the hypothalamus that cause the release of specific hormones from cells of the anterior pituitary (viz. gonadotropin-releasing hormone (GnRH) causing release of follicle-stimulating hormone (FSH) and luteinizing hormone (LH)).

Renal Referring to the kidney.

Renin An enzyme released by specialized cells in the wall of the afferent arterioles of the renal glomeruli, when blood flow is reduced. It generates a vasoactive molecule that increases the blood pressure.

Resting potential The electrical potential that exists across the plasma membrane of an excitable cell in the resting state. The potential results from unequal distribution of positively and negatively charged ions on the two sides of the plasma membrane.

Reticular fibers Fine fibers of a protein, reticulin, found in the extracellular matrix of lymphoid organs, liver and smooth muscle.

Reticulocytes Immature erythrocytes found in the bone marrow, and in limited numbers in the circulation. An increase in their number in the peripheral blood is indicative of an increase in rate of erythrocyte production.

Reticuloendothelial system A term applied to the total population of phagocytic cells in the body, including fixed macrophages of the spleen and Kuppfer cells of the liver. This term has now been replaced by **mononuclear phagocyte system.**

Retina The light sensitive layer of nervous tissue at the back of the eye, containing the photoreceptors: rods and cones.

Ribosomes Small particles in the cytoplasm that are involved in translation of the information encoded in messenger RNAs to synthesize proteins.

Rough endoplasmic reticulum (rER) A cytoplasmic organelle consisting of a network of tubules and cisternae limited by a membrane bearing adherent polyribosomes.

Sarcolemma
The plasma membrane of a muscle fiber.

Sarcomere
The repeating unit of the myofibrils of striated muscle extending between successive Z-lines. In the resting muscle, it includes the A-band and half of its two flanking I-bands.

Sarcoplasm
The cytoplasm of striated muscle fibers.

Sarcoplasmic reticulum
The specialized endoplasmic reticulum of striated muscle which sequesters and releases calcium.

Schwann cell
A type of glial cell that forms the insulating myelin sheath around the axon of neurons in the peripheral nervous system.

Sclera
The thick, fibrous, outer layer of the eyeball which is continuous with the cornea anteriorly and with the sheath of the optic nerve posteriorly.

Sebum
The oily substance secreted by the sebaceous glands of the skin.

Secondary immune response
The robust immune response to a second, and subsequent exposures, to the same antigen.

Secretin
A peptide hormone secreted by S-cells of the duodenal mucosa that stimulates secretion of bile and pancreatic enzymes.

Sertoli cells
Cells of the seminiferous epithelium that support the developing germ cells. Occluding junctional complexes between neighboring Sertoli cells create a blood–testis permeability barrier.

Serum
The amber-colored fluid left behind when blood clots, trapping the erythrocytes, leukocytes and platelets in a meshwork of fibrin filaments.

Sinoatrial node
A network of specialized cardiac myocytes that constitute the pacemaker controlling the rhythmic contractions of the heart.

Smooth endoplasmic reticulum (sER)
A cytoplasmic organelle consisting of a network of membrane-bounded tubules throughout the cytoplasm. It is described as 'smooth' because, unlike rER, it does not have ribosomes associated with it limiting membrane.

Smooth muscle
A type of muscle made up of fusiform cells containing long actin filaments, and relatively short myosin filaments. Its contraction is by a sliding filament mechanism that is not subject to voluntary control.

Somatotropin
A pituitary hormone that stimulates growth. Also called **growth hormone**.

Spectrin
A protein associated with the membrane of erythrocytes that forms, with actin, a unique cytoskeleton that allows reversible deformation of erythrocytes in their passage through capillaries.

Spinal ganglion
An expansion of the dorsal root of the spinal cord that contains the cell bodies of sensory neurons.

Spindle fibers
The bundles of microtubules in the mitotic spindle.

Stem cell
A primitive cell that divides to produce one daughter cell that replaces the original stem cell, and another daughter cell that differentiates into a specialized cell type.

Stereocilia
Stiff non-motile cell processes, filled with actin filaments, found only on sensory epithelial cells of the inner ear.

Stratified epithelium
An epithelium composed of multiple layers of cells.

Stress fibers
Bundles of actin filaments extending across the cytoplasm and terminating at sites of cell to substrate adhesion.

Striated muscle
Muscle in which the sarcomeres of the myofibrils are in register across the cell, resulting in a cross-banded appearance. Both skeletal and cardiac muscle are examples of striated muscle.

Stroma
The connective tissue framework of an organ.

Substrate
(1) The substance upon which an enzyme acts, or (2) the solid surface upon which cells adhere and move.

Surfactant
A surface-active lipid material secreted by Type II cells of the pulmonary alveoli that reduces the surface tension of water, preventing collapse of the alveoli upon exhalation.

Synapse
A specialized communicating junction between two neurons (an axo-dendritic synapse) or between a nerve axon and a muscle cell (a neuromuscular junction).

Synapsis
The pairing of chromatids of homologous chromosomes during prophase of meiosis-I.

Synaptic cleft
The narrow intercellular space at a synapse across which a neurotransmitter diffuses to bind to receptors on the post-synaptic effector cell.

T-tubules
Tubular invaginations of the sarcolemma of skeletal muscle that conduct a wave of depolarization inwards to cause release of calcium ions from the sarcoplasmic reticulum, triggering contraction.

Telomere
Repeats of a non-coding sequence of DNA at the ends of chromosomes.

Telophase
The final phase of mitosis when chromosome separation is completed, the nuclear envelope is reforming, and cytokinesis is in progress.

Template
A structure that determines the way in which the subunits of a developing structure will be assembled.

Terminal web A thick layer of cross-linked actin filaments that crosses an epithelial cell immediately beneath its brush border.

Testosterone The steroid hormone secreted by the interstitial cells (Leydig cells) of the testis.

Thick filaments Polymers of myosin 12-14nm in diameter located in the A-band of striated muscle.

Thin filaments Polymers of actin with associated proteins (troponin and tropomyosin) making up the I-bands of striated muscle and extending into the A-band between its myosin filaments.

Thrombin A plasma enzyme that cleaves fibrinogen to fibrin during the clotting of blood.

Thrombosis The formation of a blood clot that occludes the lumen of a blood vessel.

Thymus A substernal lymphoid organ in which T-lymphocytes of the immune system multiply in an antigen independent manner and acquire immunocompetence. Its epithelial cells produce hormones (thrombopoietin and thymosin) that are believed to be essential for development of immunocompetence.

Thyroxin A hormone secreted by the thyroid gland that increases metabolic rate, heat production, and blood pressure. Also called **T4**.

Tight junction Synonym for the zonula occludens, a sealing junction closing the paracellular pathway across an epithelium.

Totipotent Capable of giving rise to all cell types of an organism.

Transcription The synthesis of RNA, by the enzyme RNA polymerase, using a sequence of nucleotides in DNA as a template.

Translation The synthesis of a polypeptide using information encoded in a molecule of messenger RNA that specifies the sequence of amino acids.

Trophoblast A layer of epithelium that develops around the blastocyst, attaches it to the endometrium of the uterus, and forms the outer layer of the placenta.

Ubiquitin A cytoplasmic protein that binds to other proteins selected for proteolytic degradation by large protein complexes called proteasomes.

Utricle A small saccule in the vestibule of the inner ear from which the semicircular ducts originate.

Uvea The pigmented layer of the eye, that includes the iris, ciliary body, and choroid.

Vacuole Any large membrane-bounded vesicle found in the cytoplasm.

Vasa vasorum Blood vessels on the surface of large elastic arteries, extending branches inward to supply the thick tunica media.

Vascular An adjective referring to the blood vessels. Also used to mean richly supplied with blood vessels.

Villin An actin-binding protein in the microvilli of the brush border.

Vimentin A protein forming the intermediate filaments of fibroblasts, smooth muscle, and endothelial cells.

Volkmann's canals Transverse or oblique channels which connect the Haversian canals of bone to each other, and to the marrow cavity.

von Willebrandt factor A component of plasma which is produced and stored in endothelial cells of large arteries. It is involved in platelet adhesion during blood clotting.

Weibel-Palade bodies Cytoplasmic granules in the endothelial cells of arteries. They are sites of storage of von Willebrandt factor.

Z-lines (Z-disks) Dense transverse lines across the myofibrils of striated muscle located at either end of each sarcomere. The actin filaments of the myofibrils are anchored to the Z-lines by α-actinin.

Zona pellucida A translucent layer around the mammalian ovum that contains receptors for spermatozoa.

Zonula adherens A belt-like junctional complex around columnar epithelial cells to which actin filaments of the terminal web attach. It is one of several devices for maintaining cell cohesion.

Zonula occludens A belt-like junctional complex of epithelial cells that closes the intercellular space preventing movement of molecules across the epithelium via a paracellular route.

Zymogen granules Secretory granules of the pancreatic acinar cells containing inactive precursors of proteolytic enzymes.

Answers

Chapter one

1	B	11	microtubule
2	D	12	lipofuchsin granules
3	C	13	glycogen
4	D	14	axoneme
5	B	15	pinocytosis
6	B	16	nucleolus
7	D	17	polyribosome
8	C	18	glycocalyx
9	D	19	dynein
10	C	20	codons

Chapter two

1	D	11	stratified squamous non-keratinized epithelium
2	C	12	simple squamous
3	A	13	mesothelium
4	D	14	zonula occludens
5	E	15	ciliated pseudostratified columnar
6	C	16	desmosome
7	C	17	ciliated pseudostratified columnar
8	A	18	transitional
9	B	19	axoneme
10	E	20	gap junction

Chapter three

1	D	11	eosinophil
2	B	12	neutrophil
3	A	13	megakaryocyte
4	D	14	platelets
5	A	15	lymphocyte
6	C	16	proerythroblast
7	A	17	myeloblast
8	D	18	normoblast
9	E	19	megakaryocyte
10	A	20	promyelocyte

Chapter four

1	D	11	type II collagen
2	D	12	reticular fibers
3	C	13	type III collagen
4	D	14	adipocyte
5	C	15	macrophage
6	E	16	fibroblast
7	A	17	tropocollagen
8	B	18	macrophage
9	D	19	mast cell
10	E	20	elastic fiber

Chapter five

1	C	11	type I collagen
2	D	12	keratan sulfate
3	C	13	type II
4	A	14	chondrocyte
5	A	15	diffusion
6	B	16	perichondrium
7	D	17	elastic cartilage
8	E	18	somatomedin-C
9	C	19	hyaline cartilage
10	D	20	isogenous group

Chapter six

1	A	11	Haversian system
2	D	12	endosteum
3	E	13	hydroxyapatite
4	D	14	osteoclast
5	B	15	osteoclast
6	C	16	inner circumferential lamellae
7	D	17	Haversian canal
8	C	18	canaliculi
9	E	19	Volkmann's canals
10	C	20	spongy bone

Chapter seven

1	B	11	cardiac muscle
2	B	12	myofibrils
3	E	13	Z-line
4	E	14	cardiac muscle
5	D	15	calmodulin
6	B	16	skeletal muscle
7	C	17	endomysium
8	A	18	sarcomere
9	B	19	pacemaker
10	A	20	skeletal muscle

Chapter eight

1	A	11	axon
2	A	12	gray matter
3	D	13	pseudounipolar
4	E	14	microglia
5	B	15	sensory
6	A	16	presynaptic vesicle
7	D	17	neuromuscular spindle
8	C	18	salutatory
9	C	19	acetylcholine
10	C	20	glia

Chapter nine

1	B	11	endothelial
2	D	12	epicardium
3	C	13	pericyte
4	D	14	external elastic lamina
5	B	15	Purkinje fibers
6	C	16	sinoatrial node
7	B	17	tunica intima
8	B	18	vasa vasorum
9	A	19	tunica adventitia
10	A	20	tunica media

Chapter ten

1	C	11	spleen
2	D	12	plasma cell
3	C	13	thymus
4	A	14	spleen (white pulp)
5	A	15	B-lymphocyte
6	A	16	T-lymphocyte (cytotoxic)
7	D	17	antibodies
8	A	18	T-lymphocyte (cytotoxic)
9	B	19	spleen
10	A	20	plasma cell

Chapter eleven

1	C	11	stratum corneum
2	B	12	dermis
3	D	13	epidermis
4	E	14	arrector pili
5	B	15	stratum basale
6	A	16	melanosome
7	E	17	keratinocyte
8	D	18	rete pegs
9	A	19	Langerhans cell
10	C	20	stratum granulosum

Chapter twelve

1	B	11	tongue
2	D	12	serous gland
3	A	13	circumvallate papillae
4	E	14	ameloblast
5	C	15	saliva
6	D	16	sublingual gland
7	A	17	dentin
8	C	18	soft palate
9	C	19	filiform papilla
10	E	20	IgA

Chapter thirteen

1	B	11	pyloric and cardiac regions
2	B	12	simple columnar mucigenous bordered
3	A	13	parietal (oxyntic) cell
4	A	14	parietal cell
5	D	15	parietal (oxyntic) cell
6	B	16	ph 2.0
7	A	17	gastrin
8	D	18	lamina propria
9	A	19	fundus/corpus
10	E	20	pepsinogen

Chapter fourteen

1	D	11	taeniae coli
2	E	12	simple columnar striated bordered epithelium
3	D	13	Brunner's gland
4	D	14	Auerbach's plexus
5	C	15	goblet cell
6	B	16	peristalsis
7	D	17	plicae circulares
8	D	18	serotonin
9	C	19	ileum
10	D	20	lacteal

Chapter fifteen

1 D

2 C

3 E

4 E

5 C

6 B

7 A

8 E

9 A

10 B

11 Kupffer's cell

12 bile

13 gallbladder

14 hepatocyte

15 hepatic acinus

16 space of Disse

17 portal vein

18 space of Disse

19 bile canaliculus

20 Kupffer's cell

Chapter sixteen

1 B

2 C

3 E

4 C

5 B

6 E

7 C

8 A

9 A

10 A

11 D-cell

12 pancreas

13 striated

14 somatostatin

15 glucagon

16 somatostatin

17 glucagon

Chapter seventeen

1 D

2 D

3 D

4 C

5 B

6 C

7 B

8 B

9 E

10 C

11 larynx

12 type II pneumocyte

13 olfactory epithelium

14 vocalis muscle

15 conducting subdivision

16 elastic fiber

17 parasympathetic

18 alveolus

19 type II pneumocyte

20 bronchioles

Chapter eighteen

1 D
2 A
3 A
4 B
5 B
6 D
7 E
8 B
9 D
10 C

11 renal corpuscle
12 glomerulus
13 proximal convoluted tubule
14 transitional epithelium
15 erythropoietin and renin
16 arcuate
17 renin
18 filtration slit
19 renin
20 loop of Henle

Chapter nineteen

1 C
2 D
3 E
4 B
5 E
6 C
7 B
8 A
9 A
10 E

11 pancreas
12 pars nervosa
13 calcitonin
14 thyrotrope
15 supraoptic and paraventricular nuclei of the hypothalamus
16 somatotropin
17 pregnant uterus and breast
18 pineal gland
19 thyrocalcitonin
20 zona reticularis

Chapter twenty

1 A
2 A
3 C
4 E
5 B
6 B
7 C
8 D
9 C
10 E

11 ejaculatory duct
12 spermiation
13 corpus spongiosum
14 prostate gland
15 Sertoli cell
16 ductus deferens
17 pseudostratified columnar epithelium
18 testosterone
19 prostate gland
20 mitochrondria

Chapter twenty-one

1 D
2 A
3 B
4 A
5 A
6 C
7 A
8 D
9 C
10 C

11 corpus luteum
12 oviduct
13 placenta
14 fimbria
15 HCG
16 fetal placenta
17 colostrum
18 oocyte
19 Bartolin's gland
20 post-menopause

Chapter twenty-two

1 A
2 A
3 A
4 D
5 E
6 B
7 D
8 A
9 E
10 C

11 iris
12 aqueous humor
13 Bowman's membrane
14 pigment
15 corneal epithelium
16 posterior chamber
17 aqueous humor
18 cone photoreceptors
19 ora serrata
20 suspensory ligaments

Chapter twenty-three

1 B
2 D
3 D
4 E
5 E
6 E
7 A
8 E
9 E
10 B

11 stria vascularis
12 malleus
13 external auditory meatus
14 endolymph
15 otoliths
16 basilar membrane
17 basilar membrane
18 eustachian tube
19 cristae ampullares
20 oval window

Index

Note: page numbers in *italics* refer to tables, page numbers in **bold** refer to figures.

islets of Langerhans 266
parathyroid 259–61, **260**
pineal 264–6, **265, 266**
thyroid 257–9, **257–9**
endocytosis 11, 19–21
phagocytosis 19, 20–1, **20**
pinocytosis 19, **19, 20**
receptor-mediated 19–20, **20**
endoderm 292
endolymph 316, 318, 319, 320, 323
endometrial stroma 289–90, 293
endometriosis 290
endometrium 289–91, **290–2**, 292, 293–4
endomysium 101
endoneurium 125
endoplasmic reticulum (ER) 6, 7–9, **7, 9**, 67
see also sarcoplasmic reticulum
rough (rER) **2**, 8, **8**, 39, **39**, 118, 210, **211**
smooth (sER) **2**, 8, **8**, 9, 118, 210, 211, **211, 212**
endosomes 20
early 11, **12**
late 11, **12**
endosteum 87, 88, 94
endothelial adhesion molecule-1 (selectin) 69
endothelium 30
corneal 302
enteroendocrine cells
gastric mucosa 191, 192–3, 194, **194**
intestinal 200, 204, 220
eosinophil-derived neurotoxin 48
eosinophilic cationic protein (ECP) 48
eosinophilic metamyelocytes 57, **58**
eosinophils **47**, 48, **49, 54**, 55, **56**, 66, 69–70
ependymal cells 130
epicardium 135
epidermal-melanin unit 166
epidermis 163–7
Langerhans cells 166–7, **167**
Merkel cells 167, **167**
pigmentation 165–6
thick skin 163–5, **164, 165**
thin skin 165, **166**
epidermolysis bullosa 16
epididymus 269, **269**, 270, 278–9, **278, 279**
epidural space 132
epiglottis 227–8
epimysium 101
epinephrine 263, 264
epineurium 125
epiphyseal plate 81, **83**, 84, 87–8, **88**, 93, 94, **95, 97**
epiphysis 87–8, **88**, 93, 94
closure 94
episcleral space 301
epithelium 29–41
see also ciliated epithelium; *specific types*
absorptive 37, 38
basal lamina 36
cell cohesion 32–5
cell communication 35
cell transport 33, 38
classification 29–32, **30, 31**
ciliated 29, **31**, 32, 37, **38**
columnar 29, 30, **30, 31, 32**, 33, 36, 225, 228–9, 230
cuboidal 29, 30, **30, 32**, 225, 228–9, 230
keratinized stratified squamous 30, **31**

pseudostratified 30–2, **30, 31**, 225–6, 228, 230
simple 29–30, **30, 31**
squamous 29, 30, **30, 31**, 32, **32**, 163, 177, 225
stratified 29, 30, **30, 31, 32**, 163, 177, 225
transitional 32
defining 29
polarity 32, **34**
renewal 37–8
secretory 38–40
surface specializations 36–7, **37**
eponychium 171
equatorial plate 23, **23**, 24
erectile dysfunction 281
erection 281
erythroblasts 55, 57
erythrocytes 43–4, **44, 46**, 60
biconcave shape 16
hemopoiesis 51, 53, **53–4**, 55, **55–7**
mature 55
in the spleen 159, 160–1
erythrocytopoiesis 51, 53, **53–4**, 55, **55–7**
erythropoietin 60, 237, 246
esophagus 188–90, **188**, 195
estradiol 285, 286, 287
estrogen 291
estrone 286
euchromatin 5
Eustachian tube 315, **316**
excurrent ducts 277–9, **278, 279**
exocelom 292
exocrine glands 39–40, **39**
expiration 228, 234
external auditory meatus 315, **316**
external lamina
elastic, of the arteries 136, **137**, 138, 139, **139**
of skeletal muscle 101
of smooth muscle 114
external os 289
extracellular fibers 64–6, **64**
collagen 64–6, **64, 65**
elastic **64**, 66
reticular 66, **66**
extraembryonic mesenchyme 292, 293
extrusion zones 204
eye 301–14, **302**
accessory structures 312–3
anterior chamber 301
cornea 301–2, **302, 304**
histophysiology of vision 310–2
posterior chamber 301
refractive media 305
retina 301, 302, 303, 305–12, **307–12**
sclera 301, **302**
sclerocorneal junction 302, **303, 304**
uvea 301, 302–5
vitreous cavity 301
eyelids 312, **312**

F-cells (PP-cells), of the islets of Langerhans 220, 221
facial nerve 179
factor 3 213
familial hypercholesterolemia 20
fat cells *see* adipose cells
female reproductive system 283–99, **287**

external genitalia 283, **283**, 295–6
fertilization 291–2, **292**
implantation 292–5, **293**
mammary glands 296–8, **296–8**
ovaries 283–7, **284–8**, 291, **292**
oviducts 283, **283**, 287–8, **288, 289**, 291
uterus 283, **283**, 289–91, **290, 291**
ferritin 161
fertilization 291–2, **292**
fibrillar centers 5
fibrin 46
fibrinogen 46, 213
fibrinolysin 280
fibroblasts 65–6, 66, 67, **67, 68**, 72–3
intermediate filaments 16
fibrocartilaginous callus 84, 97
fibroid tumor 289
fibronectin 64
fibrous sheath 274, **274**
filaggrin 165
filamin 15
filopodia 21
filtration slits 239, 245
fingerprints 163
first polar body 285, **286**
flagella 19
focal adhesions 16
follicle-stimulating hormone (FSH) 252, 255, 277, 286–7, 291, **292**
follicular atresia 285
foot processes (pedicels) 129, 239, **240**
fossa navicularis 248
fovea 310, **312**
foveolae *see* gastric pits
fracture repair 97
frequency (pitch) 323
functionalis 290

G_0 phase, of cell division 22
G_1 phase, of cell division 22
G_2 phase, of cell division 22, 23
G-cells
of the gastric mucosa 193, 194
intestinal 200
gallbladder 207, 212, 213–5
gallstones 214
gametes 25–6
ganglia 117, 131
celiac 131
ciliary 131
dorsal root 128
mesenteric 131
otic 131
paravertebral 131
pterygopalatine 131
submandibular 131
thoracic sympathetic 234
ganglion cells (retinal) 308–9, 312
gap junction 32, 35, **35**
gaseous exchange 230
gastric glands 190–1, **190, 191**, 192, **193**, 194
gastric intrinsic factor 192
gastric mucosa 189, **189–92**, 190–3, 194
gastric pits (foveolae) 190–1, **190**, 193
gastric ulcer 192
gastrin 191, 194
gastro-esophageal reflux disorder 190

Bloom & Fawcett's
Concise Histology

Second Edition